Topics in Bone Biology Volume 6

Series Editors

Felix Bronner, PhD
Department of Reconstructive Sciences
University of Connecticut Health Center
Farmington, CT
USA

Mary C. Farach-Carson, PhD
Department of Biochemistry and Cell Biology
Rice University
Houston, TX
USA

Felix Bronner, Mary C. Farach-Carson
and Helmtrud I. Roach (Eds.)

Bone and Development

Springer

Felix Bronner, PhD
Department of Reconstructive
Sciences
University of Connecticut
Health Center
Farmington, CT
USA

Mary C. Farach-Carson, PhD
Department of Biochemistry
and Cell Biology
Rice University
Houston, TX
USA

Helmtrud I. Roach, PhD
Bone & Joint Research Group
Southhampton General Hospital
Southampton
UK

ISBN 978-1-84882-821-6 e-ISBN 978-1-84882-822-3
DOI: 10.1007/978-1-84882-822-3

Library of Congress Control Number: 2009938953

Printed on acid-free paper

springer.com

Preface

This book, Vol. 6 in the series *Topics in Bone Biology*, deals with bone development from growth to mineralization. Understanding tissue development involves combining embryological and histological information with the increasing knowledge from molecular and genetic studies. In each developmental stage, some genes are expressed and others silenced. Disease, especially disease progression, also is characterized by changes in gene expression that then are transmitted to daughter cells. In both situations, the choreography of gene expression and partial or complete silencing often are the result of the interaction between the genome and the epigenome, i.e., between a very stable set of structures and rapidly changing environmental factors.

Chapter 1, by O'Connor, Farach-Carson, and Schanen, is an overview of the field and of topics discussed in greater detail in subsequent chapters. After discussing bone development in terms of intramembranous and endochondral ossification, the chapter describes gene expression in osteoblasts and osteoclasts, bone cell coupling, and the regulatory effects of steroid hormones. Primary genetic defects that lead to various bone diseases – Marfan's syndrome, Paget's disease, and juvenile osteoporosis, among others – are analyzed. The chapter ends with a section on the epigenetic regulation of bone development, including methylation, histone modifications, and imprinting. This chapter, like all others, has an extensive bibliography and figures to illustrate principal points.

Colnot and Alliston, in Chap. 2, describe the complex cellular and molecular interactions that control patterning and morphogenesis during embryonic development of the skeleton. The chapter describes chondrocyte and osteoblast differentiation, their interaction, and the regulatory role of the perichondrium. The chapter then proceeds to the signal pathways that stimulate maturation of the perichondrium and the recruitment of perichondrial cells to become matrix-synthesizing osteoblasts. The authors discuss the role of angiogenesis and of matrix resorbing cells and raise the question about continuing tissue interactions in postnatal life. They conclude by calling attention to animal models and genetic approaches.

The complicated structure that constitutes the epiphyseal growth plate is discussed in Chap. 3, by Anderson and Shapiro. They describe the architecture, detailed anatomy, and cellular dynamics of the growth plate, the role of the many regulators, such as parathyroid hormone-related protein, thyroxin, glucocorticoids, and leptins, and analyze in detail the mineralization process. Chondrocytes play an important metabolic role in the growth plate, but must ultimately be removed from the organ. This occurs either by apoptosis via the intrinsic pathway, regulated, in part, by the Bcl-2 gene family, or by the extrinsic pathway via cell death ligand receptors. Alternatively, autophagy may result in degradation of cellular components. The last section of the chapter discusses diseases such as rickets, achondroplasia, and enchondromas.

Discovered in *Drosophila* and largely conserved up to humans, the signaling pathway called Hedgehog affects cellular behavior, including proliferation, differentiation, and survival. Regard, Mak, Gordon, and Yang, in Chap. 4, describe the effect of two of the three genes that make up the hedgehog family in vertebrates, Sonic Hedgehog, Indian Hedgehog, and Desert Hedgehog, with the expression by the latter confined to the gonads. The chapter describes in detail the Hedgehog signaling pathway and its role in human genetics and skeletal patterning, including craniofacial development. The authors then describe the role of the Sonic Hedgehog, particularly in digit formation and limb outgrowth and point out that Sonic Hedgehog has emerged as a master regulator of early embryonic pattern formation and craniofacial morphogenesis, but that Indian Hedgehog is the key regulator of endochondral bone growth and ossification. The chapter concludes with discussions of the role of Hedgehog in joint formation and skeletal homeostasis.

MicroRNAs constitute the most abundant mode of posttranscriptional regulation in the genome. They play an important role in development and differentiation. Chap. 5, by Gradus and Hornstein, reviews the biology of these molecules and the evidence that microRNAs are an integral component of the genetic hierarchies that govern skeletal and limb development. MicroRNAs are involved in Hedgehog signaling, and as discussed by the authors, the specific microRNA-214 is regulated by Twist, a transcription factor, haploinsufficiency of which causes the Saethre-Chotzen syndrome. MicroRNAs are linked to bone morphogenetic protein and fibroblast growth factor signaling, with the cartilage-specific microRNA-140 modulating the platelet-derived growth factor. The authors conclude by pointing out that growing understanding of the regulatory role played by these molecules should lead to better knowledge of development and of diseases due to mutations that affect microRNA expression.

Pierre Marie, in Chap. 6, discusses in detail the fibroblast growth factor/fibroblast growth factor receptor signaling pathway, first in the growth plate, then in chondrodysplasias and the mutations that lead to these diseases. In cranial bone, fibroblast growth factor signaling upregulates osteogenesis and missense mutations in the receptor lead to premature fusions of the cranial sutures and to many skeletal disorders, including Apert and Crouzon syndromes. Marie concludes that the genes induced by fibroblast growth factor receptor signaling and implicated in the pathogenesis of dysplasias need to be identified.

Embryogenesis proceeds under conditions of hypoxia before the circulatory system is established. Chap. 7, by Schipani and Khatri, discusses hypoxia-inducible factor-1, a transcription factor that is a major regulator of cellular adaptation to hypoxia. Hypoxia-inducible factor-1α acts on two other factors that are involved in sensing variations in oxygen pressure. The authors discuss these interactions and other target genes of factor-1α, relationships to energy metabolism, angiogenesis, and autophagy. Further discussion is on relationship to chondrocytes, their survival, proliferation, and differentiation. Hypoxia-inducible factor-1α also plays a role in joint development, in articular cartilage, and, as analyzed by the authors, in osteoblasts, osteoclasts, and in bone modeling and remodeling.

Bone morphogenetic proteins, discovered over 40 years ago, but identified and purified much later, play major roles in patterning, tooth development, and regulation of apoptosis, among others. Estrada and Lyons, in Chap. 8, describe the signaling pathway of these proteins, their role in mesenchymal condensation that leads to chondrogenesis, the effect of bone morphogenetic protein expression on Sox9, a transcription factor, expressed in all cartilage primordia, and crosstalk with other signaling pathways such as Indian Hedgehog, parathyroid hormone-related protein, and fibroblast growth factor. These proteins also play a signaling role in osteogenesis, modulating the RANKL-osteoprotegerin pathway. The authors point out that the canonical bone morphogenetic protein signaling pathway has been implicated in the regulation of the transcription factor Runx2, as well as in adipogenesis and energy metabolism.

Chapter 9, by Bodine, describes another important signaling pathway, that of the Wnts, a large family of polypeptides that play a key signaling function in embryogenesis, organogenesis, and morphogenesis. The chapter describes loss of function and gain of function mutations in LRP5, the human Wnt coreceptor, and then proceeds to a description of dickkopf expression in osteoblast function and bone formation. Bodine analyzes the effects of SOST/sclerostin, which blocks signaling by the bone morphogenetic protein and Wnt. Evidently, sclerostin inhibits bone formation by blunting the canonical Wnt pathway. The chapter describes the effects of several Wnts, of the dickkopf factors, and of the secreted frizzled-related proteins on bone formation and development. Additional discussion deals with β-catenin, the adenomatous polyposis coli gene product, and the T-cell specific transcription factor in skeletogenesis.

The craniofacial complex, head, face, and mouth, provides individual identity and therefore is the most distinguishing feature of the human body. D'Souza, Ruest, Hinton, and Svoboda, in Chap. 10, detail the structure and development of the components of this complex. They describe mandible development, its molecular regulation, and patterning of the mandibular neural crest cells in terms of the genes and signal pathways involved. The chapter then deals with the temporomandibular joint, its morphogenesis, postnatal growth, and maturation. Morphogenesis and molecular mechanisms in palatal development are discussed, again with much emphasis on the various signaling pathways, followed by analysis of palate ossification and palate deformities. The final section deals with tooth development, signaling interactions, and the role of the extracellular matrix in tooth morphogenesis and cytodifferentiation.

Chapter 11, by MacDougall and Javed, complements the previous chapter and compares mineralization in dentin and bone. After discussion of odontogenesis and of primary and secondary dentinogenesis, the cytodifferentiation of osteoblasts and odontoblasts is described and compared, and transcriptional control of differentiation and regulation by growth factors and hormones is analyzed, as are the effects of mechanical factors. The discussion of remodeling, repair, and genetic syndromes and diseases is concluded by a comparison of bone and dentin.

In Chap. 12, Wang and Lee discuss how bone proteins evolved. Emphasis is on the genes of extracellular matrix proteins, many of which are specific to mineralized tissues with no counterparts in tissues of nonmineralizing organisms. After reviewing the process of gene duplication, of importance for the development of higher organisms, the authors discuss collagens, osteocalcin, matrix Gla proteins, and their evolutionary links. The chapter then discusses the secretory calcium-binding proteins. These have only limited sequence homology, but gene structure and biochemical characteristics determine their evolutionary relationships. Other topics discussed include small leucine-rich proteoglycans and the evolution of apatite-binding peptides. The chapter concludes with an evaluation of the evolutionary approach to understanding bone formation and ossification.

Osteogenesis imperfecta is a heritable disorder encountered in perhaps 0.02% children at birth, leading to early mortality in many and bone fragility in the survivors. Arundel and Bishop, in Chap. 13, discuss the biology of the disease, animal models, and the brittle bones due to the disease, and then detail the clinical approach. The authors discuss history and examination of the patient, including dental manifestations, differential diagnosis, and tests for the disease. These include biochemical analyses, radiography, and histomorphometry. Evaluation of treatment by calcitonin, growth hormone, and bisphosphonates is followed by an analysis of the problems encountered in adults, specifically, hearing impairment, cardiovascular, and respiratory problems.

Kaplan, Groppe, Seemann, Pignolo, and Shore, in Chap. 14, discuss fibrodysplasia ossificans progressiva, the result of a recurrent heterozygous missense mutation of one of the receptors for bone morphogenetic protein, namely, Activin receptor A, type I. The mutation leads to abnormal skeletal morphogenesis and tissue repair, skeletal metamorphosis of connective tissue, degenerative joint disease, and benign skeletal neoplasms. The chapter describes the clinical and molecular features of the disease, diagnosis and misdiagnosis, the signaling pathways, and the gene, followed by discussion of the dysregulation of morphogenesis, metamorphosis, oncogenesis, and joint function brought about by this morphogene. Neither definitive treatment nor cure is available for fibrodyplasia ossificans progressiva, but the authors discuss possible approaches such as intervention in the signaling pathway or blocking the trigger to inflammation.

Bone mineral homeostasis results from the interactions of the vitamin D and parathyroid hormone regulatory systems. Peterlik, in Chap. 15, describes in molecular detail how 1,25-dihydroxyvitamin D_3 and extracellular calcium ions act as co-regulators of cellular proliferation, differentiation, and function in many organs and cell systems. The chapter describes how, during development, bone mineral homeostasis is maintained by the joint actions of parathyroid hormone and the parathyroid hormone-related protein. Postnatally, however, there is the additional strong input by the vitamin D endocrine system, through the CYP24A1-encoded enzyme, 25-hydroxy-D3–24-hydroxylase. Peterlik discusses the dysfunction of short-term and long-term regulation of mineral metabolism, with emphasis on vitamin D status and calcium intake. He then analyzes rickets and osteomalacia, osteoporosis, cancer, diabetes mellitus type I, hypertension, chronic vascular disease, and chronic kidney disease in terms of the roles played by the two endocrine regulatory systems and their effect on the calcium receptor of cell membranes.

Takeda, in Chap. 16, calls attention to the now recognized important relationship between the skeleton and energy and glucose metabolism. He discusses the role of leptin in regulating bone mass and bone remodeling, pointing out that animal experiments indicate a clear separation of the actions of leptin on appetite and bone metabolism, with the latter mediated by leptin receptors in the ventromedial hypothalamus. This indicates a role by the sympathetic nervous system. Neuropeptides that affect appetite, melacortins, neuromedin, and neuropeptide Y, and their relationship to bone mass are discussed, with the final sections of the chapter devoted to bone cell regulation of glucose metabolism and the role of osteocalcin.

With sufficient information, it becomes possible to model a system and to predict relationships that can then be experimentally verified. Chen, Schuetz, and Pearcy, in Chap. 17, describe and simulate mechanobiological regulation of bone growth, remodeling, and fracture healing. They describe bone function and form and provide an equation relating stress to the fraction of bending moment/bending resistance, multiplied by the external radius of the bone. This is not yet a model, but predicts that stress will decrease if the internal radius increases, provided the area remains constant. Based on available evidence, the authors then present the concept of an osteogenic index and formulas that define distortional stress and hydrostatic stress. If the apparent density of bone is considered characteristic of internal structure, then this can describe remodeling both for cancellous and cortical bone. The final section of the chapter deals with fracture healing and the publications that have proposed simulations of fracture healing.

This book, as previous volumes in this series, reflects the conceptual interaction between medical science and practice, and how effective practice benefits from advances in knowledge, yet makes clear how far we remain from fully understanding the skeleton and its function as an organ system. We thank all authors for their dedication to their subjects and the opportunity to integrate a large and often exciting body of knowledge. We are grateful to Springer, our publisher, for their help in assuring intellectual and aesthetic quality.

Felix Bronner
Farmington, CT

Mary C. Farach-Carson
Houston, TX

Helmtrud I. Roach
Southampton, UK

Contents

Contributors

Tamara Alliston, PhD
Department of Orthopaedic Surgery
University of California
San Francisco, CA, USA

H. Clarke Anderson, MD
Department of Pathology and Laboratory Medicine
University of Kansas Medical Center
Kansas City, KS, USA

Paul Arundel, MBBS, DCH
Academic Unity of Child Health, Sheffield Children's Trust
University of Sheffield
Sheffield, UK

Nicholas J. Bishop, MRCP, MD
Academic Unity of Child Health, Sheffield Children's Trust
University of Sheffield
Sheffield, UK

Peter V.N. Bodine, PhD
Department of Women's Health and Musculoskeletal Biology
Wyeth Research
Collegeville, PA, USA

Felix Bronner, PhD
Department of Reconstructive Sciences
University of Connecticut Health Center
Farmington, CT, USA

Gongfa Chen, BSc Meng, PhD
Institute of Health and Biomedical Innovation
Queensland University of Technology
Brisbane, Queensland, AUS

Céline Colnot, PhD
Department of Orthopaedic Surgery
University of California at San Francisco
San Francisco General Hospital
San Francisco, CA, USA

Rena N. D'Souza, DDS, PhD
Department of Biomedical Sciences
Baylor College of Dentistry
Texas A&M University Health Science Center
Dallas, TX, USA

Kristine D. Estrada, BS
Department of Orthopaedic Surgery
Department of Molecular, Cell and Developmental Biology
University of California at Los Angeles
Los Angeles, CA, USA

Mary C. Farach-Carson, PhD
Department of Biochemistry and Cell Biology
Rice University
Houston, TX, USA

Joshua A. Gordon, BA
Genetic Disease Research Branch
National Human Genome Research Institute
National Institutes of Health
Bethesda, MD, USA

Ben Gradus, BSc, MSc
Department of Molecular Genetics
Weizmann Institute of Science
Rehovot, ISR

Jay C. Groppe, PhD
Department of Biomedical Sciences
Baylor College of Dentistry
Texas A&M University Health Science Center
Dallas, TX, USA

Robert J. Hinton, PhD
Department of Biomedical Sciences
Baylor College of Dentistry
Texas A&M University Health Science Center
Dallas, TX, USA

Eran Hornstein, MD, PhD
Department of Molecular Genetics
Weizmann Institute of Science
Rehovot, ISR

Amjad Javed, MS, PhD
Department of Oral and Maxillofacial Surgery
University of Alabama at Birmingham
School of Dentistry
Birmingham, AL, USA

Frederick S. Kaplan, MD
Division of Molecular Orthopaedic Medicine
Department of Orthopaedic Surgery
The University of Pennsylvania
School of Medicine
Philadelphia, PA, USA

Richa Khatri, BS
Endocrine Unit
Medicine MGH-Harvard Medical School
Boston, MA, USA

Mary J. MacDougall, PhD
Department of Oral and Maxillofacial Surgery
University of Alabama at Birmingham
School of Dentistry
Birmingham, AL, USA

Kingston K. Mak, PhD
Genetic Disease Research Branch
National Human Genome Research Institute
National Institutes of Health
Bethesda, MD, USA

Seung-Wuk Lee, PhD
Department of Bioengineering
University of California at Berkeley
Berkeley, CA, USA

Karen M. Lyons, PhD
Department of Orthopaedic Surgery
Department of Molecular, Cell and Developmental Biology
University of California at Los Angeles
Los Angeles, CA, USA

Pierre J. Marie, PhD
Laboratory of Osteoblast Biology and Pathology
University Paris 7, Hôpital Lariboisière
Paris, FRA

Rose D. O'Connor, PhD
Department of Biological Sciences
University of Delaware
Newark, DE, USA

Mark Pearcy, PhD, FIEAust, CPEng (Biomed)
Institute of Health and Biomedical Innovation
School of Engineering Systems
Queensland University of Technology
Brisbane, Queensland, AUS

Meinrad Peterlik, MD, PhD
Department of Pathophysiology
Medical University of Vienna
Vienna, AUT

Robert J. Pignolo, MD, PhD
Department of Medicine
University of Pennsylvania
School of Medicine
Philadelphia, PA, USA

Jean B. Regard, PhD
Genetic Disease Research Branch
National Human Genome Research Institute
National Institutes of Health
Bethesda, MD, USA

Helmtrud I. Roach, PhD
Bone & Joint Research Group
Southampton General Hospital
Southampton, UK

L-Bruno Ruest, PhD
Department of Biomedical Sciences
Baylor College of Dentistry
Texas A&M University Health Science Center
Dallas, TX, USA

N. Carolyn Schanen, MD, PhD
Nemours Biomedical Research
A. I. duPont Hospital for Children
Wilmington, DE, USA

Ernestina Schipani, MD, PhD
Endocrine Unit
Medicine MGH-Harvard Medical School
Boston, MA, USA

Michael Schuetz, MD, PhD
School of Engineering Systems / IHBI
Queensland University of Technology
Brisbane, Queensland, AUS

Petra Seemann, PhD
Berlin-Brandenburg Center for Regenerative Therapies
Institution Charité Universitätsmedizin Berlin
Berlin, GER

Irving M. Shapiro, BDS, PhD
Department of Orthopaedic Surgery
Jefferson Medical College
Thomas Jefferson University
Philadelphia, PA, USA

Eileen M. Shore, PhD
Department of Orthopaedic Surgery
University of Pennsylvania School of Medicine
Philadelphia, PA, USA

Kathy K.H. Svoboda, PhD
Department of Biomedical Sciences
Baylor College of Dentistry
Texas A&M University Health Science Center
Dallas, TX, USA

Shu Takeda, MD, PhD
Section of Nephrology, Endocrinology and Metabolism
Department of Internal Medicine
Keio University
Tokyo, JPN

Eddie Wang, BS
Department of Bioengineering
University of California at Berkeley
Berkeley, CA, USA

Yingzi Yang, PhD
Genetic Disease Research Branch
National Human Genome Research Institute
National Institute of Health
Bethesda, MD, USA

Abbreviations

1,25-$(OH)_2D_3$	1,25-Dihydroxyvitamin D_3
24,25-$(OH)_2D_3$	24,25-Dihydroxyvitamin D_3
25-(OH)D	25-Hydroxyvitamin D
aBMD	Areal bone mineral density
ACVR1/ALK2	Activin receptor A type 1/activin-like kinase 2, a bone morphogenetic protein type I receptor
AD	Autosomal dominant
ADAM	A disintegrin and metalloprotease domain
adrb	Beta-adrenergic receptor
AER	Apical ectodermal ridge
AHO	Albright's hereditary osteodystrophy
ALP	Alkaline phosphatase
AMBN	Ameloblastin
AMEL	Amelogenin
AMP	Adenosine monophosphate
AMPK	Adenosine monophosphate kinase
AMTN	Amelotin
AP1 (or AP-1)	Activator protein 1
APAF-1	Apoptotic peptidase activating factor 1
APC	Adenomatous polyposis coli or anaphase-promoting complex
APO2L	Tumor necrosis factor-related apoptosis-inducing ligand
AR	Androgen receptor; autosomal recessive
ARC	Arcuate
ARF	Activation, resorption, and formation
ARNT	Aryl hydrocarbon nuclear translocator
ATF4	Activating transcription factor 4
ATG (or Atg)	Autophagy related genes
ATPase	Adenosine triphosphoesterase
AVβ5	Annexin V beta 5
BAD	Bcl-2-associated death promoter (BAD) protein
BAFF	B-cell activating factor of the TNF family
Bapx1	Bagpipe homeobox homolog 1 (also called Nkx3.2)
BAT	Brown adipose tissue
Bcl-2, Bcl XL	B-cell lymphoma-2, B cell lymphoma-2 long form

BDA2	Brachydactyly type A2
BDC	Brachydactyly type C
bFGF	Basic fibroblast growth factor
BGP	Bone γ-carboxyglutamate protein (osteocalcin)
BH3	Bcl2 homology domain 3
bHLH	Basic helix-loop-helix
Bid	BH3 interacting domain death agonist
Bim	Bcl2-interacting mediator of cell death
BLYS	B lymphocyte stimulator
BMC	Bone mineral content
BMD	Bone mineral density
BMF	Bcl2 modifying factor
BMP	Bone morphogenetic protein
BMPR	Bone morphogenetic protein receptor
BMPR1A	Bone morphogenetic protein 1A, a BMP type I receptor
BMPR1B	Bone morphogenetic protein receptor 1B, a BMP type I receptor
BMSC	Bone marrow mesenchymal stem cell
BMU	Basic multicellular unit
Bnip3	Bcl-2-binding protein Nip3
BrdU	Bromodeoxyuridine
BSP	Bone sialoprotein
CamKII	Calmodulin-dependent protein kinase II
cAMP	Cyclic-adenosine monophosphate
CaP	Calcium phosphate
CaR	Calcium-sensing receptor
Cart	Cocaine- and amphetamine-regulated transcript
CCD	Cleidocranial dysplasia
cDNA	Complementary DNA
C/EBPs	CCAAT-enhancer-binding proteins
Ci	Cubitus interuptus
CK	Casein kinase
CL/P	Cleft lip with or without cleft palate
CNC	Cranial neural crest
CNTF	Ciliary neurotrophic factor
Col1a1	Collagen type I alpha 1
Col1a2	Collagen type I alpha 2
COMP	Cartilage oligomeric matrix protein
Cos2	Costal2
COX4	Cytochrome C oxidase 4
CP	Cerebral palsy; chondroprogenitor; cleft palate
CREB	Cyclic AMP response element binding protein
CRTAP	Cartilage associated protein
CT	Computed tomography
C-TAD	Carboxy-terminal transcriptional activation domain
CTGF	Connective tissue growth factor
CTP cell	Connective tissue progenitor cell
CVJ	Costovertebral joint

CYP24A1	25-Hydroxyvitamin D-24-hydroxylase
CYP27B1	25-Hydroxyvitamin D-1α-hydroxylase
CZ	Calcifying zone
DD	Dentin dysplasia
DECM	Dentin extracellular matrix
DEXA	Dual-energy X-ray absorptiometry
DGI	Dentinogenesis imperfecta
DHCR7	7-Dehydrocholesterol reductase
Dhh	Desert hedgehog
DI	Dentinogenesis imperfecta
Disp	Dispatched
Dkk	Dickkopf
Dlx5	Distal-less homeobox 5
DMP1 (or Dmp1)	Dentin matrix protein 1
DMPI	Dentin matrix acidic phosphoprotein I
DNA	Deoxyribonucleic acid
Dnm3	Dynamin3
DNMTs	DNA methyl-transferase enzymes
DPP	Dentin phosphoprotein
Dsh	Disheveled
DSP	Dentin sialoprotein
DSPP	Dentin sialophosphoprotein
DSP-PG	Proteoglycan form of DSP
DXA	Dual energy X-ray absorptiometry
E11.5 m	Embryonic, as in "embryonic day 11.5 in the mouse"
ECF	Extracellular fluid
ECM	Extracellular matrix
Edn1	Endothelin-1
Ednra	Endothelin-A receptor
EF-2	Activity elongation factor
EMP	Enamel matrix protein
EMT	Epithelial-mesenchymal transition
ENAM	Enamelin
ER	Endoplasmic reticulum
ERα	Estrogen receptor α
ERK	Extracellular signal-regulated kinase
EXT	Exostoses
EXT1	Multiple hereditary exostoses gene 1
EXT2	Multiple hereditary exostoses gene 2
FASL	FAS ligand
FBN1	Fibrillin 1
FEM	Finite element method
FGF	Fibroblast growth factor
FGFR	Fibroblast growth factor receptor
FIH	Factor inhibiting Hif
FKBP12	An inhibitory protein that binds to all the GS-domains of all TGF-β and BMP type I receptors and prevents promiscuous activation in the absence of ligand

FOP	Fibrodysplasia ossificans progressiva
FZD	Frizzled
GAS-1	Growth arrest specific-1
GCPS	Greig cephalopolysyndactyly syndrome
GDF5	Growth differentiation factor 5
GFP-Rac-1	Green fluorescent protein binding to Rac-1
GH	Growth hormone
Gla	γ-Carboxyglutamate
Gli	Glioblastoma
GM-CSF	Granulocyte-macrophage colony-stimulating factor
Groucho/TLE	Groucho/transducin like enhancer
GS activation domain	Glycine-serine activation domain; important intracellular activation domain of all type I TGF-β and BMP receptors
GSK	Glycogen synthase kinase
HA (or HAP)	Hydroxyapatite
HBM	High bone mass
HC	Hypertrophic chondrocyte
HDAC4	Histone deacetylase 4
HDACi	Histone deacetylase inhibitor
HERS	Hertwig's epithelial root sheath
Hh	Hedgehog
HIF	Hypoxia-inducible factor
HIP	Hedgehog interacting protein
HME	Hereditary multiple exostoses syndrome
HMG	High mobility group
HPE	Holoprosencephaly
HRE	Hypoxia responsive element
HSC	Hematopoietic stem cell
HSPG	Heparin sulfate proteoglycan
Hyp mice	Hypophosphatemic mice
HZ	Hypertrophic zone
ICAM-1	Inter-cellular adhesion molecule 1
ICR	Imprinting control region
ICV	Intracerebroventricular
IGF(-1)	Insulin-like growth factor(-1)
Ihh	Indian hedgehog
IJO	Idiopathic juvenile osteoporosis
IL-1	Interleukin 1
IL-6	Interleukin-6
iNOS	Inducible nitric oxide synthase
IP3	Inositol 1,4,5-trisphosphate
JNK	c-Jun NH2-terminal kinase
Krm	kremen
LC3	Microtubule-associated protein light chain 3
LDH	Lactic dehydrogenase
LDL	Low-density lipoprotein (LDL)
LEF (or Lef)	Lymphoid-enhancer binding factor
LepR	Leptin receptor

LFA-1	Lymphocyte function-associated antigen 1
LIF	Leukemia inhibitory factor
Lrp 5, Lrp6	Low-density lipoprotein receptor-related protein 5/6
LRP	LDL receptor-related protein
LRR	Leucine rich repeats
MAPK	Mitogen-activated protein kinase
MAR	Mineral apposition rate
MBD	Methyl binding domain; methylation binding domain
Mcar	Melanocortin 4 receptor
MCC	Mandibular condylar cartilage
MCP-1	Monocyte chemotactic protein-1
M-CSF	Macrophage colony stimulating factor
MCT	Monocarboxylate transporter
Mechanobiology	The study of how mechanical or physical conditions regulate biologic processes
Mechanotransduction	The mechanism by which cells convert mechanical stimulus into chemical activity
Mecp2	Methylation CpG binding protein
MEE	Medial edge epithelia
MEF	Mouse embryo factor
MEPE	Matrix extracellular phosphoglycoprotein
MES	Midline epithelial seam
MGP	Matrix γ-carboxyglutamate protein
MHE	Multiple hereditary exostoses
miRNA	MicroRNA
MMP (or Mmp)	Matrix metalloproteinase
MP	Mid-palatal
MRI	Magnetic resonance imaging
mRNA	Messenger ribonucleic acid
MSC	Mesenchymal stem cell
Msx1	Msh homeobox 1
Msx2	Hsh (Drosophila) homeo box homolog 2 (mus musculus)
mTOR	Mammalian target of rapamycin
MTP	Mineralized tissue proteins
MVs	Matrix vesicles
Mya	Million years ago
NAD	Nicotinamide adenine dinucleotide
NAI	Nonaccidental injury
NC	Nasal capsular cartilages
NCC	Neural crest cells
NCPs	Noncollagenous proteins
NFAT	Nuclear factor of activated T cells
NF-Y	Nuclear transcription factor Y
NHE	Na^+/H^+ exchanger
NLS	Nuclear localization signal
NMU	NeuromedinU
NMUR	NeuromedinU receptor

NO	Nitrous oxide
NOXA	Phorbol-12-myristate-13-acetate-induced protein 1,
NPY	Neuropeptide Y
ns	Nasal septum
NS	Nonsyndromic
OB	Osteoblast
OC (or Ocn)	Osteocalcin
OCY	Osteocyte
ODAM	Odontogenic ameloblast associated protein
ODDD	Oxygen-dependent degradation domain
OG2	Osteocalcin gene 2
OI	Osteogenesis imperfecta
ONJ	Osteonecrosis of the jaw
OO	Orbicularis oris
OP	Osteoprogenitor
OPG	Osteoprotegerin
OPN	Osteopontin; secreted phosphoprotein 1
OPPG	Osteoporosis pseudoglioma
OSC	Osteocalcin
OSM	Oncostatin M
OSN	Osteonectin
OST-PTP	Osteotesticular protein tyrosine phosphatase
Osx	Osterix
p.c.6 wk-h	Post conception, as in "post conception 6 weeks in humans"
P3H	Prolyl 3-hydroxylase
P4Ha	Prolyl-4-hydroxylase
PAP-A	Postaxial polydactyly type A
PAS	PER/ARNT/SIM
PDG	Platelet derived growth factor
PDGrα	Platelet derived growth factor receptor alpha
PFC	Phosphokinase C
PGK-1	Phosphoglycero kinase-1
PHD	Prolyl-hydroxylase domain
PHEX	Phosphate regulating gene with homologies to endopeptidases
PHP	Pseudohypoparathyroidism
PHS	Pallister-Hall syndrome
Pi	Inorganic phosphate
PI3K	Phosphatidyl-inositol 3-kinase
PIM2	Provirus integration site for Moloney murine leukemia virus 2
PKA	Protein kinase A
PKC	Protein kinase C
PLC	Phospholipase C
PLOD2	Procollagen-lysine, 2-oxoglutarate 5-dioxygenase 2
PO_4	Orthophosphate
POH	Progressive osseous heteroplasia
PP1	Protein phosphatase 1
PPAR	Peroxisome proliferator activated receptor

Ppiase	Inorganic pyrophosphatase
pre-HC	Pre-hypertrophic
pre-OB	Pre-osteoblast
pri-miRNA	Primary miRNA precursor
PSM	Presomitic mesoderm
Ptc (or Ptch)-1	Patched-1
PTH	Parathyroid hormone
PTHr1	Parathyroid hormone receptor 1
PTHrP	Parathyroid hormone-related protein
PTHrpR	Parathyroid hormone related peptide receptor
PUMA	p53-Up-regulated modulator of apoptosis
pVHL	von Hippel Lindau tumor suppressor protein
PYY	Peptide YY
PZ	Proliferative zone
QCT	Quantitative computed tomography
RAGE	Receptor for advanced glycation end products
RANK	Receptor activator of nuclear factor κ B
RANKL	RANK ligand
RANTES	Chemokine (C-C motif) ligand 5
Rb	Retinoblastoma
RCT	Randomized controlled trial
rGH	Recombinant growth hormone
rho GTPase	Rho family of GTPases
RISC	RNA induced silencing complex
ROS	Reactive oxygen species
RTS	Rubinstein-Taybi syndrome
RTT	Rett syndrome
Runx2	Runt-related transcription factor 2
RZ	Reserve (resting) zone
Satb2	Special AT-rich sequence binding protein 2
SCPP	Secretory calcium binding phosphoprotein
SCS	Saethre-Chotzen syndrome
sFRP	Secreted frizzled-related protein
SHED cells	Stem cells from human exfoliated deciduous teeth
Shh	Sonic hedgehog
Shn3	Schnurri-3
SIBLINGs	Small integrin-binding ligand N-linked glycoproteins
siRNA	Small inhibitory RNA
SLOS	Smith-Lemli-Opitz syndrome
SLRP	Small leucine rich proteoglycans
SMAD	Class of transcription factors in the TGF-β and BMP signaling pathway
SM-FKBP12	Smad/Smurf - FKBP12 complex
Smo	Smoothened
Smurf	Smad ubiquitin regulatory factor
SNS	Sympathetic nervous system
Sox9	SRY (sex determining region Y)-box 9
SPARC	Secreted protein, acidic, cysteine-rich or osteonectin

SPARCL1	Secreted protein, acidic, cysteine-rich like 1 protein
SPC	Skeletal progenitor cell
STAT (or Stat)	Signal transducer and activator of transcription
Stat1	Signal transducers and activators of transcription protein 1
Stat2	Signal transducers and activators of transcription protein b2
STI	Signal transduction inhibitor
Sufu	Suppressor of fused
SUMO	Small ubiquitin-like modifier
SV40	Simian virus 40
Syk	Spleen tyrosine kinase
T3	Thyroid hormone (triodothyroxine)
TBI	Traumatic brain injury
TBV	Trabecular bone volume
TCA	Tricarboxylic acid
TCF (or TCT)	T cell-specific transcription factor
TCF/LEF family	T-cell factor-lymphoid enhancer-binding factor/ lymphoid enhancement factor
	Terminal deoxynucleotide triphosphate transferase-mediated deoxyuridine
TGFβ	Transforming growth factor beta
TIMP	Tissue inhibitor of metalloproteinase
TMJ	Temporomandibular joint
TNAP	Tissue nonspecific alkaline phosphatase
TNF	Tumor necrosis factor
TP	Trans-palatal
TRACP	Tartrate-resistant acid phosphatase
TRAIL	Tumor necrosis factor-related apoptosis-inducing ligand
TRAP	Tartrate-resistant acid phosphatase
TRD	Transcriptional repression domain
TSP	Thrombospondin
TUNEL	Triphosphate nick end-labeled
Twist	Basis helix-loop-helix family of transcription factors
UCP	Uncoupling protein
UPR	Unfolded protein response
UTR	Untranslated region
VAGF	Vascular angiogenic growth factor
vBMD	Volumetric BMD
VDR	Vitamin D receptor
VDRE	Vitamin D response element
VEGF	Vascular endothelial growth factor
VKD	Vitamin K dependent
VMH	Ventromedial hypothalamic
VPA	Valproate
VPI	Velopharyngeal incompetence

WAT	White adipose tissue
WGD	Whole genome duplication
WIF	Wnt inhibitory factor
Wnt	Group of Wingless/int-1 genes
Wnt	Wingless int
ZPA	Zone of polarizing acitivity
β-Cat	β-catenin

1. Genetic and Epigenetic Aspects of Bone Development

Rose D. O'Connor, Mary C. Farach-Carson, and N. Carolyn Schanen

1.1 Introduction

It now is widely accepted that genes provide the template for the cell and ultimately for the organism, but that was not always the case. Gregor Mendel first developed the hypothesis that a hereditary force was at work when he crossed green and yellow pea plants in the mid 1800s [40]. Although Mendel was unable to identify what we now know to be genes, several years later, Oswald Avery led us to that discovery [40]. Genes carry the information needed to develop in utero, grow postnatally, and mature into adult beings. As development proceeds into adulthood, various genes are expressed at different times. Most humans carry 23 pairs of chromosomes with 22 pairs made up by somatic chromosomes and 1 pair determining whether an individual will be a male (XY) or a female (XX). Major advances in the DNA technology and high throughput sequencing have shown that there are fewer than 30,000 genes that encode proteins in the human body, and even fewer than that number are expressed and still a smaller subset is expressed at any one time in an individual differentiated cell. Nonetheless, the transcriptome of a cell is complex and may include more than tens of thousands of gene products than the active genes owing to the alternative exon utilization, allelic preferences, and transcript processing. The osteoblast transcriptome has been analyzed and compared with those in similar cells, such as chondrocytes and fibroblasts [50]. As expected, while there are many common gene products expressed, the osteoblast transcriptome is unique and endows this specialized bone cell with its characteristic properties. The combined forces of inherited genetic sequence and epigenetic control of gene expression further refine the transcriptome of each individual human being, such that no two individuals possess exactly identical bone cells. These differences account for the fundamental variation in bone shape, length, subarchitecture, mineral density, and responses to stimuli that occur in the human population.

1.2 Overview of Human Genetic Disorders of Bone Development

Given the complexity of the temporal and spatial interplay of the diverse cell types required for proper bone morphogenesis and homeostasis, it is perhaps not surprising that disruption of expression of numerous genes by mutation has contributed a host of human skeletal disorders.

F. Bronner et al. (eds.), *Bone and Development*, Topics in Bone Biology 6,
DOI 10.1007/978-1-84882-822-3_1, © Springer-Verlag London Limited 2010

These include genes that encode proteins that are critical mediators of cell-cell communication, such as growth factors and their receptors, matrix proteins, and key transcription factors that define the program of gene activity of the cells within the bone. In addition, from examining the numerous human skeletal dysplasias for which the causative genes have been identified, it is clear that different mutations in the same gene (allelic heterogeneity) can have disparate clinical outcomes, indicating that some pathways are involved in multiple stages of skeletal formation and growth. As might be predicted, disruption of pathways that are critical for early stages of bone formation often lead to abnormalities in both patterning and bone morphogenesis, and may affect other organ systems, while those that interfere with specific aspects of bone growth or mineralization are associated with disorders that show more normal overall skeletal patterning, but lead to abnormalities in limb length, improper maintenance of normal mineralization, focal bony overgrowth, or ectopic mineralization. Numerous, complex skeletal malformation syndromes have been identified in humans. Only in the past two decades, has it been possible to separate the ones that are genetically related, because many syndromes share common phenotypic features such as shortening of long bones, vertebral flattening, thinning of ribs, and involvement of skull or facial bones. DNA diagnostics have made a major impact on the classification and diagnosis of human skeletal dysplasias, which in turn, has provided a wealth of information on the role of a given gene product in skeletal formation, growth, and function (for review, see [28] and references therein).

1.3 Bone Development

Ossification, or the development of the hard component of bone, is generally described as taking place through two separate processes, intramembranous vs. endochrondral ossification, although evidence from human skeletal dysplasias suggests that the demarcation between the two processes is not always clearly defined. Intramembranous ossification refers to the process by which flat bones, including those of the cranial vault, some facial bones, and the lateral aspect of the clavicle, develop directly from the mesenchymal precursor cells [108]. These mesenchymal cells form condensations, which are then invaded by a network of vasculature and induce differentiation into mature osteoblasts [109]. The osteoblasts mature and secrete osteoid, directly laying down the foundation that will become that particular bone [18]. A more complex process termed as endochondral ossification utilizes an intermediary step of cartilage formation for the development of long bones as well as other bones of the skeleton [41]. In endochondral ossification, embryonic mesenchymal cells condense to form a cartilaginous template in the approximate size and shape of the developing bone (reviewed in [35]). The cartilage cells or chondrocytes differentiate and undergo a period of hypertrophic growth before becoming vascularized and invaded by osteoclasts, osteoblasts, and other precursor cells [47]. The mesenchymal to chondrocyte and then to osteoblast transitions are processes that are tightly regulated by differential expression of many genes, several of which are transcription factors that play central roles in coordinating the timing of the expression of genes involved in growth and differentiation of the numerous cell types found in the developing bone. Osteoclasts, derived from hematopoietic precursors, are multinucleated cells that resorb bone [168], whereas bone-forming osteoblasts arise from pluripotent mesenchymal stem cells [7]. Both these cell types were the subjects of earlier volumes in this series, and will not be described in detail here. Briefly, osteoblasts secrete new osteoid, which then becomes mineralized, while osteoclasts resorb the old bone in a defined pattern. This balance of new bone formation by osteoblasts and subsequent resorption by osteoclasts allows the bones to grow to the correct size and shape (reviewed in [119]). The proper development of bony structures requires not only the activity of the cells involved in bone formation, but also the carefully controlled balance with the activity of nearby osteoclasts.

1.4 Gene Expression in Osteoblast Development

1.4.1 Sox9

One of the earliest transcription factors expressed by mesenchymal cells as they transition toward bone development is Sox9. Although Sox9 expression has been identified in the mesenchymal cells that are destined to become either osteoblasts or chondrocytes, it is likely that the transcriptional regulatory activity of Sox9 induces chondrocyte maturation while inhibiting osteoblast differentiation [187]. Sox9 has been repeatedly shown to have an essential role in cartilage development, whereby it induces chondrogenesis under the control of bone morphogenetic proteins (BMPs) [60]. In humans, the *SOX9* gene lies on chromosome 17q24.3-q25.1 and heterozygosity for the loss of function mutations in the gene are responsible for campomelic dysplasia (OMIM #114290) [43]. Clinically, the disorder is characterized by prenatal curvature of the long bones with dimpling of the overlying, modestly flattened vertebral bodies, 11 pairs of ribs, and "wingless" scapulae [72]. Most notably, it is also associated with sex reversal or ambiguity of external genitalia in the affected XY individuals, because Sox9 is a critical regulator in testes development. The bones of the face are also affected, leading to a low nasal bridge and micrognathia, and frequently with cleft palate (Pierre Robin sequence) [169]. Sox9 directly regulates the expression of type II collagen [11], and disruption in cartilage formation leads to abnormalities in the upper airway. Respiratory insufficiency is a common cause of death in many newborns with mutations in this gene [72]. Development in patients with this disorder ranges from normal to moderately delayed, and there is progressive scoliosis and hearing loss over time, although the vast majority succumb to respiratory insufficiency in the newborn period (for review, see [169]). Genotype-phenotype correlations are not straightforward and variability within the families argues for genetic background effects [102, 140]. Curiously, although Sox9 is expressed in the cells that will become both chondrocytes and osteoblasts, the skeletal phenotype in campomelic dysplasia appears to reflect deficiencies primarily in endochondral ossification.

1.4.2 Runx2

Runx2 (Cbfa1/Osf2/AML3/PEBP2αA), is a runt domain containing transcription factor that is essential for both chondrocyte and osteoblast maturation. Expression of Runx2 in mesenchymal stem cells inhibits differentiation of these cells into adipocytes or chondrocytes, while allowing these fated cells to differentiate into preosteoblasts and osteoblasts (reviewed in [86]). Although Runx2 has other functions beyond its role in regulation of gene expression, it is the transcription factor function of Runx2 that is critical for bone development, as Runx2 preferentially binds to and regulates many genes that are essential for osteoblast differentiation in both endochondral and intramembraneous ossification [86, 171]. Knockout studies of Runx2 in a mouse model system caused a complete lack of skeletal mineralization, which resulted in embryonic lethality [87].

In humans, the autosomal dominant disorder, cleidocranial dysplasia (Fig. 1.1) (OMIM #119600), is caused by mutation of the *RUNX2* gene on chromosome 6p21. Mutations generally result in the loss of function alleles leading to haploinsufficiency for the protein product, with functional analyses of mutant alleles indicating that some may have dominant negative effects [99, 121, 129]. Because of the central importance of RUNX2 in osteoblast differentiation, the bones that are most obviously abnormal in cleidocranial dysplasia are those that arise from intramembranous ossification – the skull and clavicle, although virtually all bones are affected [72]. The phenotype is characterized by abnormalities in the formation of the frontal, parietal, and occipital bones with delayed closure of the cranial sutures. Decreased growth of facial bones gives the appearance of facial flattening [108]. The clavicle is rarely completely absent, but is hypoplastic. Preservation of the medial aspect of this bone, which expresses type II collagen and Sox9, which are markers of cartilage lineage, has been used to argue that this bone is

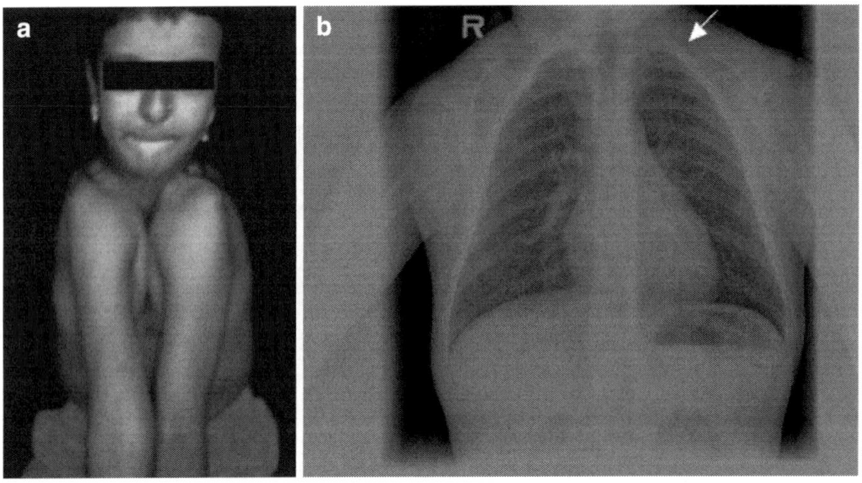

Figure 1.1. (**a**) Patient with cleidocranial dysostosis showing the absence of clavicles and curvature of the humeri. (**b**) Radiograph of the patient in *panel A* showing hypoplasia of the clavicles (*arrow*), resulting in downsloping shoulders. (Adapted with permission from Kumar [88]).

of mixed origin in terms of formation via endochondral vs. intremembranous mechanisms [68]. In addition, patients with cleidocranial dysplasia have delayed secondary tooth eruption. Overall growth is affected with short stature that is relatively proportionate, with decreased bone mineral density (BMD) and growth plate abnormalities, evident radiographically [72].

1.4.3 Dlx5

Dlx5, a homeobox gene, which is the mammalian homolog of Drosophila Distal-less (Dll) genes, encodes a transcription factor expressed primarily in the developing brain and bone. Dlx5 protein expression is essential for both axial and appendicular skeletal development. *Dlx6*, another homeobox gene, shares functional redundancy with Dlx5. Knockout models in which both Dlx5/Dlx6 are deleted, show abnormal chondrocyte/osteoblast differentiation as well as disruption of the proximal–distal patterning in the limb bud [136]. The condensed cartilage that ultimately forms the bones of the limbs undergoes both longitudinal and appositional growth. Dlx5 has a particularly important role in the conversion of immature chondrocytes to hypertrophic chondrocytes, highlighted by a chick limb model in which misexpression of Dlx5 resulted in increased chondrocyte maturation and severe shortening of long bones [160]. In addition to its role in limb development, Dlx5 is involved in normal bone remodeling by regulating transcription of osteocalcin [137, 138]. Dlx5 can also interact with Msx2, another protein in a set of expressed homeobox genes, which serves an essential role in skeletal formation and development of the nervous system. Dlx5 and Msx2 regulate the expression of alkaline phosphatase, as Msx2 transcriptionally represses alkaline phosphatase until Dlx5 expression increases to a threshold that allows it to counteract Msx2 and induce alkaline phosphatase levels [78]. Additionally, Msx2 inhibits osteocalcin gene expression in osteoblasts until the later stage of maturation, when Dlx5 inhabits the osteocalcin promoter region and upregulates expression of the gene [58, 78]. Msx2 and Dlx5 are likely to have reciprocal roles in osteoblast proliferation and maturation by the stimulation of osteocalcin and alkaline phosphatase expression at the appropriate times during development and differentiation [116]. To date, no human disorder has been identified that is caused by mutation in either the *DLX5* or *DLX6* loci on chromosome 7q21.3–22.1, although they are considered as positional candidates for the autosomal dominant split-hand split-foot malformation (OMIM%183600), because they lie in the critical region for this disorder [141, 142]. Loss of function mutations in *MSX2*, which lies on chromosome 5q34-q35 lead to craniosynostosis, type 2, (OMIM #604747), a relatively rare dominant disorder arising from premature closure of the cranial sutures [71]. Notably, patients with trisomy of this region may also have craniosynostosis, suggesting that expression levels need to be tightly balanced for normal sutural closure [149, 175].

1.4.4 Twist1

A basic helix-loop-helix transcription factor, Twist1, has emerged as an important regulator of bone development. TWIST1 has been shown to particularly induce Runx2 expression in human calvarial osteoblasts [51, 185], and loss of Twist1 has led to decreased expression of osteoblast-specific genes, such as FGFR2 [51]. Additionally, Twist1 plays an important role in mouse limb development by regulating the expression of Fgf, Shh, and Bmp-2, whereby growth and differentiation of the limb bud are regulated [118]. In a heterozygous Twist1 mouse model, the forelimbs are unaffected while the hindlimbs show preaxial polydactyly [15]. Twist1 knockout mice exhibited severely retarded limb bud formation, as forelimb and hindlimb bud growth was prematurely arrested [118]. Conversely, in the mouse preosteoblastic cell line, MC3T3-E1 cells were used to reveal that the Twist1 suppression of osteoblastic differentiation is accomplished through the inhibition of BMP signaling [59]. Specifically, activation of HDAC1 interaction with Smad4 accounted for this decrease in osteogenesis [59]. Recently, Twist1 has also been implicated in murine chondrocyte regulation through inhibition of Runx2 and ultimately Fgf-18, even though Twist1 expression is limited to chondrocytes in the perichondrium [66]. Although the data on Twist1 regulation of bone development is often contradictory and not yet fully understood, we can be sure that Twist1 does have a role in bone development. This is evident through studies on Saethre–Chotzen syndrome, which is also known as acrocephalysyndactyly III (ACS III. OMIM#101400), where mutations in TWIST1 that result in loss of TWIST1 activity cause premature fusion of the cranial sutures, facial dysmorphisms, and digit defects. The coronal sutures are most frequently involved, although others may also undergo premature closure. Segmentation defects involving the bones of the thumb and cervical vertebrae as well as radioulnar synostosis, occur in this syndrome, suggesting a role for TWIST1 in pattern formation and segmentation (see [130] for review).

1.5 Gene Expression in Osteoclast Development

1.5.1 Initiation and Coupling

Cytokines, including RANKL and M-CSF, produced by osteoclast-supporting marrow stromal cells, induce intracellular cascades (Fig. 1.2) in hematopoietic precursors and immature osteoclasts that express receptors for these cytokines (reviewed in [184]). The interaction of the cytokine receptor-activator nuclear factor κ B (RANK) with its receptor RANKL on the surface of preosteoclasts and mature osteoclasts plays a key role in the initiation of this process. In receiving cells, signal cascades activate downstream transcription factors such as c-Fos/AP-1 and NF-κB (reviewed in [184]). These transcription factors cue hematopoietic precursors and immature osteoclasts to express osteoclast-specific proteins that ultimately support osteoclast differentiation [74, 156, 164].

Coupling of osteoblasts and osteoclasts is essential in both bone development as well as remodeling that occurs throughout life. In development, this coupling process results in bone patterning which produces and maintains the bones of the skeleton in correct size and shape. Developmental bone patterning is regulated by specific patterning genes such as those in the Hox, Pax, and Sox families, as well as growth factors such as FGF and TGFβ, in addition to matrix proteins and integrins, including fibronectin and laminin. This process of bone patterning has been explored in detail in an earlier book in this series which focused on bone formation.

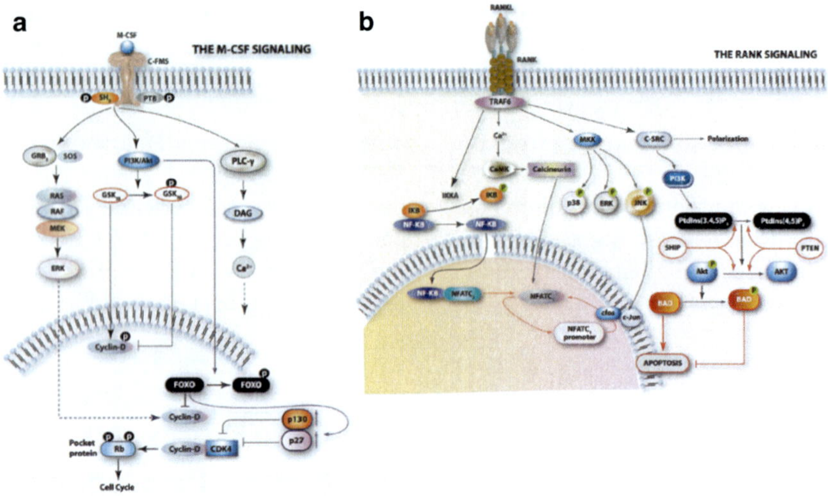

Figure 1.2. (**a**) M-CSF signaling cascade in osteoclasts. M-CSF interacts with the c-FMS receptor to induce the Ras/Rak/ERK/MEK pathway as well as the PI3K/Akt and PLC-γ pathways, which converge on regulation of the cell cycle through cyclin D1. (**b**) The essential RANKl/RANK signaling pathway works through TRAF6 to induce translocation of NF-κB to the nucleus along with the transcription factors NFATc1, c-Fos, and c-Jun. Activation of this pathway is critical for osteoclastogenesis from osteoclast progenitor cells. (Adapted with permission from Yavropoulou [184]).

1.5.2 Transcription Factors

Other essential transcription factors in the process of osteoclast maturation are PU.1, MITF, and c-FOS [184]. Specifically, PU.1 knockout mice not only lack osteoclasts, but also do not have any macrophages [165]. Ultimately, PU.1 goes on to stimulate the production of RANK. The cytokine M-CSF actually mediates the transcription of its sole receptor, c-FMS, by stimulating PU.1. In the absence of M-CSF, there is a decrease in tissue macrophages, which ultimately leads to osteopetrosis, an increased BMD, owing to the reduction in the number of osteoclasts [31]. MITF is another transcription factor which plays a role in osteoclast differentiation and survival. Probably, it is the interaction of MITF with PU.1 that specifically regulates the target genes during osteoclastic differentiation [69, 153]. The transcription factor, AP-1, a heterodimer of FOS proteins such as c-FOS, also aids in the regulation of osteoclast differentiation. Mice lacking c-FOS also have an osteopetrosis phenotype, even though the number of macrophages increases [49]. Several years ago, a transcription factor NFATc1, nuclear factor of activated T cells, was shown to be a necessary transcription factor in osteoclastogenesis [70, 162]. Even though NFATc1 is not an osteoclast-specific transcription factor, several studies have shown that deletion of NFATc1 from an osteoclast model system resulted in reduced osteoclastogenesis [3, 24] and even reversal of osteoclastic differentiation [24]. NFATc1 has another interesting characteristic in that it can autoregulate; thus, upregulation of NFATc1 by RANK signaling causes a constitutive increase in NFATc1 expression driving osteoclast maturation and longevity through the regulation of several osteoclast-specific genes (reviewed in [161]).

1.5.3 Differentiation and Activation

After the onset of osteoclastogenesis, an entirely new set of genes play a large role in osteoclast differentiation, including those that guide the fusion and multinucleation of preosteoclasts, as they form mature osteoclastic cells. One such protein is the receptor for advanced glycation end (RAGE) products, which augments differentiation, maturation, and function of osteoclast precursors. In a RAGE-deficient mouse model, an increase in bone mass and BMD with decreased bone resorptive activity was reported [37, 189]. Osteoclasts lacking RAGE had a disrupted actin ring and impaired sealing zone structures, which hindered osteoclast maturation and reduced bone resorption [189]. A subsequent study [188] reported that HMGB1, a high-mobility group protein, could act as an autocrine ligand for RAGE. The authors further showed that RANKL stimulation of HMGB1 led to the extracellular release of HMGB1, an essential component of RANKL-induced osteoclast differentiation.

In addition to the differentiation induced by the RANKL:RANK pathway, ICAM-1 and LFA-1 have been implicated in promoting cell–cell contact between osteoclast precursors during the stage when immature mononuclear osteoclasts fuse to form multinucleated cells (reviewed in [184]). The production of chemokines MCP-1 and RANTES generate chemotactic signals, which also lead to mononuclear osteoclast fusion [77]. Several cytokines and colony-stimulating factors including IL-1, 3, 6, and 11, as well as LIF, OSM, CNTF, TNF, and GM-CSF play vital roles in initiating this cell-to-cell contact (reviewed in [95]). After the final stage of osteoclast multinucleation, activation of these cells is mediated by the principal osteoclastic integrin $\alpha_v\beta_3$, c-SRC kinase, and SYK, ultimately leading to Rac activation, which is essential for cytoskeletal reorganization in the osteoclast (reviewed in [184]).

1.6 Steroid Hormone Receptors in Skeletal Development

The sex steroids estrogen and testosterone play major roles in skeletal development and maintenance (reviewed in [159]). Traditionally, estrogen and testosterone were defined by their gender-specific skeletal effects, with estrogen being the main sex steroid in women and testosterone in men. However, the evolving view of estrogen and testosterone effects on bone now includes a role for both the sex steroids in the maintenance of the male and female skeleton [120, 135, 173].

1.6.1 Estrogens

Sims et al. [152] performed an elegant knockout experiment of the estrogen receptors ERα and ERβ, both of which are critical mediators for the downstream effects of estrogen. Several conclusions were made from this study. First, deletion of only ERα reduced bone turnover that ultimately increased trabecular bone volume in both male and female mice. Second, in the ERβ knockouts, the male mice were largely unaffected, while the female mice had decreased bone resorption with increased trabecular bone volume. Third, the double ERα/β knockouts demonstrated a suppression of bone turnover in females, and consequently, a decrease in trabecular bone volume, suggesting a compensatory mechanism of ERα and ERβ in the regulation of bone mass in female mice. In contrast to the female mice, the male double ERα/β knockouts showed reduced bone resorption, ultimately leading to an increase in trabecular bone volume. Careful interpretation of the results of these knockout studies are required, however, because the skeletal phenotype of the ER knockouts can be attributed to both direct and indirect effects of circulating estrogen and testosterone levels, as there may be a compensatory mechanism in place in the event of a total knockout. Additionally, several ER allelic variants have been implicated in low BMD susceptibility. ERα polymorphisms may contribute to multigenic disorders such as osteoporosis [45], predict responsiveness to raloxifene treatment [64], or otherwise, be linked to BMD [133]. Allelic variants of ERβ have also been associated with changes in BMD [172].

1.6.2 Androgens

In contrast to the osteoprotective effect of estrogen in the female skeleton, the role of androgens has not been as well established, although one female androgen receptor (AR) knockout model showed no skeletal abnormalities (reviewed in [159]). The role of androgens in maintaining the male skeleton has been better characterized, and data show that androgens can affect the skeleton through either direct activation of the AR or indirectly after aromatization into estrogens, which thereby activate the ERs [76]. Loss of estrogens or androgens increases the rate of bone remodeling by two methods: suppression of osteoblastogenesis and osteoclastogenesis as well as altering the lifespan of osteoclasts and osteoblasts [98]. These actions can then disrupt the balance of bone resorption and formation [98]. It has been hypothesized that testosterone chiefly affects mature osteoblasts and osteocytes, while estrogen has a major role in the regulation of osteoblastic activity through the many stages of differentiation (reviewed in [159]). Interestingly, polymorphisms in aromatase, the product of the CYP19 gene and the key enzyme in the conversion of testosterone to estradiol, have been correlated with the differences in cortical bone size, but not with trabecular vBMD [97].

1.6.3 Vitamin D

The sometimes controversial roles of vitamin D hormones on bone development and homeostasis were recently reviewed [154]. Clearly, it is increasingly certain that vitamin D hormones exert their effects on bone, both directly and indirectly. In addition to influencing bone growth by modulating bioavailability of calcium and phosphate, the secosteroid interacts with the gene products that are the 25-hydroxyvitamin D-1alpha-hydroxylase and the vitamin D receptor (VDR). Polymorphisms in these genes thus can affect both osteoblasts and growth-plate chondrocytes, and ultimately bone shape, length, and BMD [96, 104, 154]. Molecular genetic studies have shown clear roles for the hormonally active metabolite of vitamin D, 1,25-$(OH)_2D_3$, in growth-plate chondrocytes [5, 16, 154]. Functional ablation of the VDR in collagen type II-expressing chondrocytes reduces RANKL expression and delays osteoclastogenesis. The net effect of this is an increase in bone volume at the primary spongiosa [154]. Mice in which the VDR is ablated in chondrocytes have reduced circulating levels of FGF23 and elevated serum phosphate concentrations [154]. It has been suggested that this occurs because 1,25-$(OH)_2D_3$, acting through specific receptors, causes a factor to be secreted from chondrocytes, which in paracrine fashion, alters FGF23 production by osteoblasts.

1.7 Primary Genetic Defects Affecting Bone Development

The following genetic disorders of bone development were chosen among many candidate genes to illustrate the basic principles linking genetics and bone development. The list is meant to be illustrative rather than comprehensive. Genetic disorders of bone development and their clinical manifestations can be grouped into three basic categories: (a) primary skeletal dysplasias presenting with abnormal bone and cartilage development; (b) systemic or localized homeostatic imbalances resulting in uncoupled processes of bone formation and resorption; and (c) mineralization defects resulting in bone fragility. The occurrence of these syndromes as a consequence of genetic mutation has provided much information about the function of these genes in normal bone and during bone growth.

1.7.1 Achondroplasia (OMIM#100800)

Occurring in 1 in 15,000 to 1 in 40,000 live births, achondroplasia is the most common primary skeletal dysplasia associated with disproportionate growth of long bones. The patients have rhizomelic shortening of the limbs (relative shortening of the proximal segments), large heads with frontal bossing and flattening of the midface, and thoracolumbar lordosis (Fig. 1.3). Achondroplasia is an autosomal dominant condition caused by mutations in the *FGFR3* gene on chromosome 4p16.3, with 99% of patients carrying a mutation that alters the same residue in the transmembrane domain of the protein leading to a constitutively active receptor [44, 67, 72]. FGFR3 is a receptor tyrosine kinase with a split intracellular kinase domain. It acts as a negative regulator of bone growth by repression of BMP4 expression and Hedgehog signaling [115], as well as activation of Stat1 pathways [57]. The achondroplasia mutations lead to ligand-independent activation of the receptor resulting in shortening of the long bone growth at the level of the growth plate, as discussed in Chap. 3 of this volume, by inhibiting chondrocyte proliferation, and decreasing the rate of chondrocyte differentiation [115]. Moreover, in

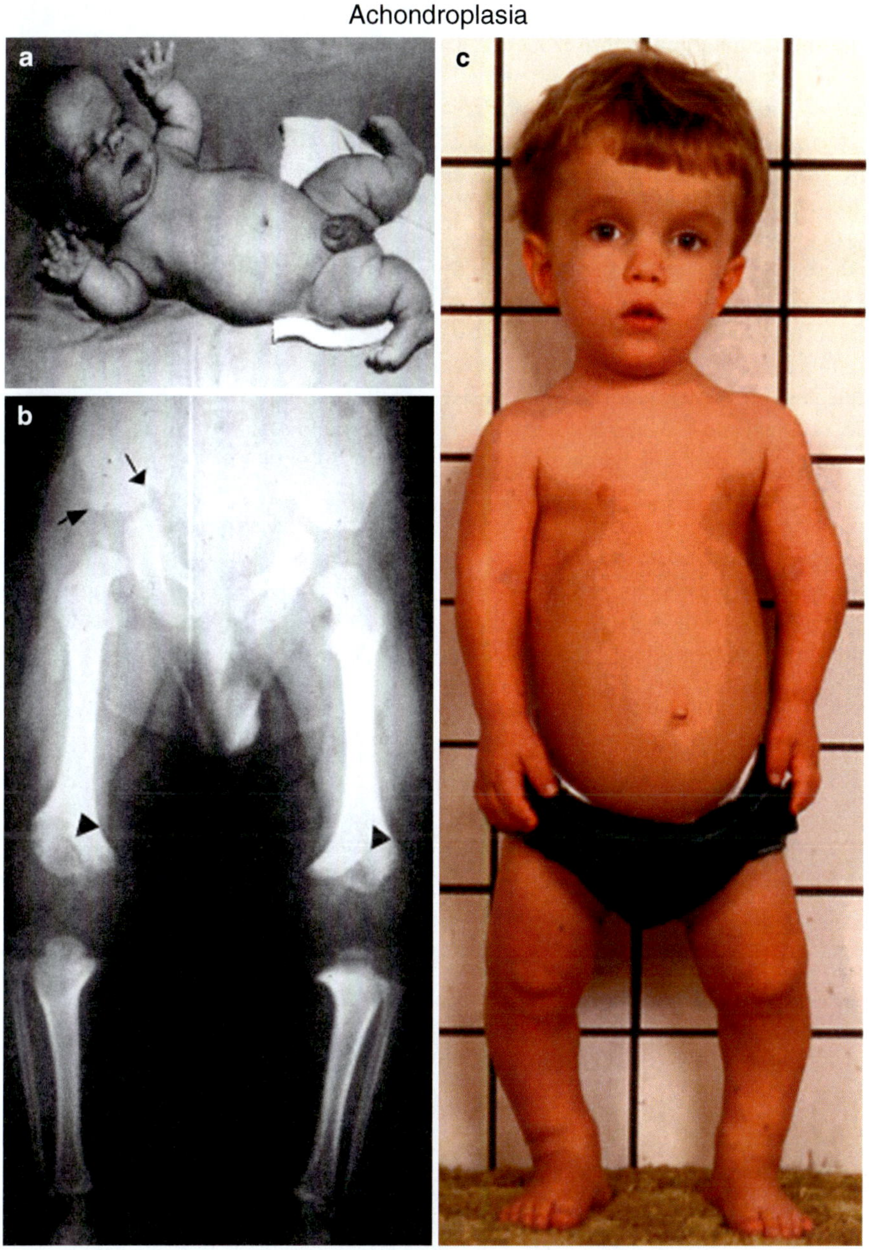

Figure 1.3. (**a**) Infant with achondroplasia who has macrocephaly with frontal bossing and flattening of the bones in the midface. The thorax is narrow and extremities are short, with bowing of the long bones in the legs. Note the joint laxity and redundant skin folds. (**b**) Radiograph from a child with achondroplasia showing squared off of the roof of the acetabulum and small sacrosciatic notches (*arrows*). The femur, tibia, and fibula are short with "chevron deformities" in the distal femur (*arrow heads*) caused by protrusion of the epiphysis into the metaphyseal space. In the distal portion of the leg, note the extension of the fibula beyond the end of the tibia. (**c**) Depicts a 3-year-old boy with achondroplasia, who has rhizomelic (proximal) shortening of the extremities, small thoracic cage, frontal bossing, and a flattened midface. Curvature of the tibia is evident. (Reprinted from Horton et al. [85]. Copyright 2007, with permission from Elsevier).

a murine model of the disorder, endochondral ossification is disrupted with abnormalities in vascularization of the growth plate [146]. Notably, mutations in the tyrosine kinase domains of the FGFR3 receptor lead to thanataphoric dysplasia (type II), a severe skeletal dysplasia that is almost uniformly lethal in the neonatal period. Type I thanatophoric dysplasia, which is distinguished clinically by curved femurs, is often caused by mutations at the termination codon of the gene, although other mutations have been identified [163]. The thanatophoric dysplasia mutations are also caused by the gain of function alleles, which are more active than the achondroplasia alleles, but have also been shown to cause apoptosis of the cells in response to growth stimuli [90, 158]. More information on these syndromes can be found in Chap. 6 of this volume. On the other end of the spectrum, a milder phenotype, hypochondroplasia, is also caused by mutations in *FGFR3* [128], which have been identified in Muenke coronal craniosynostosis (OMIM# 602849) [38] and Crouzon syndrome with acanthosis nigricans (dark pigmentation of the skin) (OMIM#612247) [103], demonstrating the wide variable expressivity of mutations in the gene.

Pseudoachondroplasia (OMIM #177170). Babies with pseudoachondroplasia (Fig. 1.4) have normal lengths at birth, but typically, are diagnosed at the time they begin to walk, because of a waddling gait. Growth of the long bones is disparately affected, and these individuals develop a short-limbed form of short stature by the age of 2 years. Facial features are normal. Joint pain begins in childhood and often is progressive [29]. The disorder is caused by heterozygous mutations in the *COMP* gene encoding a large extracellular matrix glycoprotein, cartilage oligomeric matrix protein [63]. It is transmitted in an autosomal dominant manner, but new mutations account for a substantial portion of the cases. Approximately one-third of the individuals with pseudoachondroplasia have the same mutation, involving deletion of an aspartic acid in a calmodulin-like calcium-binding domain of the protein [17]. The remaining mutations are typically missense alleles that interfere with domain-folding and processing of the protein [25, 34, 84]. The retention of COMP in the endoplasmic reticulum (ER) of the chondrocytes leads to ER stress and unfolded protein response, which contribute to

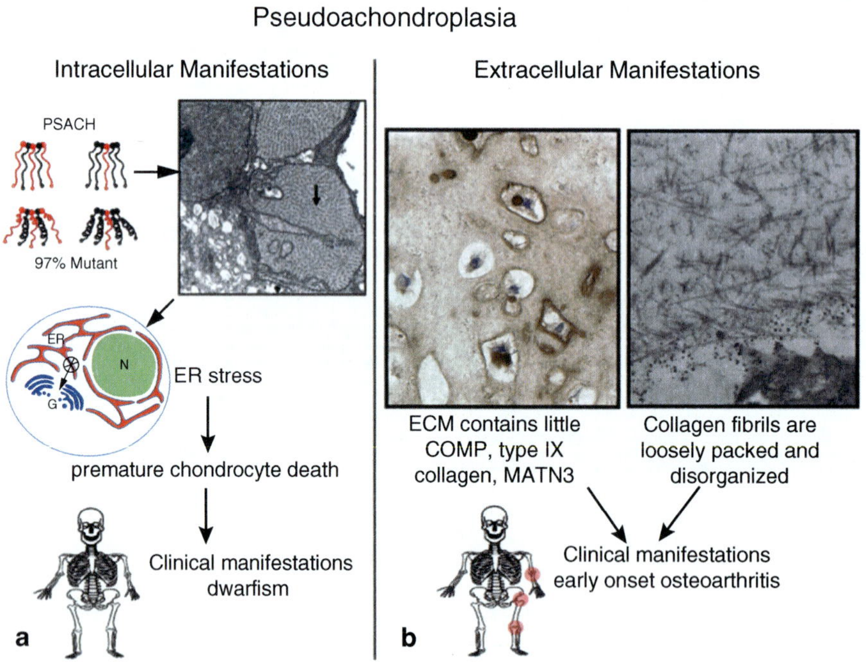

Figure 1.4. Effects of COMP mutations on skeletal development. (**a**) Intracellular manifestations of *COMP* mutations in pseudoachondroplasia. The mutant COMP protein is improperly folded and retained within the rough endoplasmic reticulum (ER). The resulting ER stress causes apoptotic death of the chondrocytes at the growth plate leading to short stature. (**b**) Extracellular outcomes of *COMP* mutations. Decreases in abundance of COMP as well as type IX cartilage, and Matrilin 3 in the extracellular matrix. In addition, disorganization and reduction in collagen fibrils in the matrix make it prone to erosion and account for early-onset osteoarthritis in the affected individuals. (Reprinted with permission from Posey et al. [127]).

the pathogenesis of the disorder by causing apoptosis of the chondrocytes [62].

1.7.2 Marfan Syndrome (OMIM# 154700)

This is an autosomal dominant connective tissue disorder caused by the mutation of the gene encoding the extracellular matrix protein, fibrillin 1 (FBN1). Clinically, the hallmark features of Marfan syndrome are disproportionate growth of the long bones leading to tall stature and arachnodactyly, with aortic dilation and dislocation of the lens in the eye. The gene lies on chromosome 15q21.1 and numerous types of mutations have been identified with a relatively high frequency of cysteine substitution mutations in the EGF-like repeat domains of the protein. The pathogenesis of the skeletal overgrowth is not known, however, FBN1 is expressed in bone and osteoblast-like cells [80].

1.7.3 Osteogenesis Imperfecta

Osteogenesis imperfecta (OI) includes a group of disorders associated with variable bone fragility, hearing loss, and in some cases, dentinogenesis imperfecta [155]. The disorder is divided into seven types, which differ dramatically in severity that can range from a relatively mild form with few fractures, mild short stature (or normal stature) and normal teeth (type I), to a perinatal lethal form associated with poor ossification of the skeleton, multiple fractures, and deformity of type II. The majority of the cases of OI types I–IV are caused by mutation in the genes encoding the alpha chains of procollagen, *COL1A1* and *COL1A2*. Inheritance is autosomal dominant, with new mutations underlying the severe forms. Although genotype–phenotype correlations are not always completely predictable, mutations that lead to decreases in the production of protein are associated with milder phenotypes (type 1) [180]. In contrast, missense mutations that lead to the production of a stable, but misfolded procollagen fibril can be incorporated into the triple helix of a collagen strand and have dominant negative effects [155]. Studies in an animal model of a moderate form of OI suggest that disruption of normal collagen synthesis results in an early reduction in bone formation and an increase in osteoclast production, leading to poorly mineralized bone [170].

1.7.4 Hereditary Multiple Exostosis

Mutations in the *EXT1* (chromosome 8q24.11; OMIM#133700) or *EXT2* (chromosome 11p12-p11; OMIM#133702) genes cause hereditary multiple exostoses, a syndrome which is inherited in an autosomal dominant manner. The *EXT1* [122] and the *EXT2* genes encode the proteins exostosin-1 and exostosin-2, respectively, which associate to form a functional complex in the Golgi of the cells actively secreting heparan sulfate [186]. Both the proteins are ER-resident type II transmembrane glycosyltransferases responsible for the chain elongation step of heparan sulfate biosynthesis. Mutations in the *EXT1* gene cause the type I form of multiple exostoses, which is typically more severe than mutations in EXT2, which lead to the type II form of the syndrome. A minority of patients with hereditary multiple exostoses do not have mutations in either the EXT1 or the EXT2 gene, and it is not known why multiple exostoses occur in these patients [122, 186]. Interestingly, it has been reported that the periochondrium may be the source of the stem cells that initiate the formation of new exostoses [61]. The formation of what are essentially new auxiliary growth plates in patients with hereditary multiple exostosis indicates that heparan sulfate-dependent processes play a primary role in the initiation and control of the processes that regulate bone growth and growth-plate development.

1.7.5 Paget's Disease of Bone

Paget's disease of bone (PDB, OMIM#602080) is a late-onset disorder characterized by focal areas of increased bone turnover containing enlarged hyperactive bone resorbing osteoclasts [65]. Mutations in sequestosome 1 (SQSTM1; chromosome 5q35) are associated with familial and sporadic disease in up to 40% of cases [65], supporting the notion that this condition has a strong genetic component. Additional genetic loci almost certainly exist, but are yet to be definitively identified. Sequestosome 1 is a multifunctional protein that, among other activities, binds ubiquitin and modulates the nuclear factor kappa-B (NF-κB) signaling pathway. As an intracellular scaffolding or adaptor protein, sequestosome 1 plays a central role in coordinating signaling pathways that modulate osteoclast activation. The focal disturbances in bone turnover and homeostasis lead to a variety of clinical complications, such as bone pain, deformity, pathological fractures, and deafness [32]. Given the common theme of skeletal dysplasia in persons suffering from mutations affecting TNF family member receptors, NFκB signaling pathways, transcriptional targets downstream of NFκB, and scaffolding proteins modulating these pathways, there is no doubt that this is a fundamental pathway in bone growth and development as has been described [177].

1.7.6 Familial Expansile Osteolysis (OMIM#174810)

Mutations in RANK/TNFRSF11A (chromosome 18q22.1) lead to the development of a relatively rare primary skeletal dysplasia with many manifestations that include osteolytic lesions mainly located in the long bones. This is classified as a disabling deformity associated with a high risk of pathological fracture, with deafness and loss of dentition [177]. The dysplasia is inherited as an autosomal dominant disorder with some phenotypic overlap with Paget's disease of bone [65]. The syndrome is a direct result of mutations that lead to constitutive activation of RANK and a chronic state of rapid skeletal remodeling.

1.7.7 Hyperphosphatasia (OMIM#239000)

Inactivating mutations in the TNFRSF11B gene (chromosome 8q24), which encodes osteoprotegerin (OPG), are responsible for idiopathic hyperphosphatasia, a severe bone homeostatic disorder that shares phenotypic similarity with PDB and which is inherited in an autosomal recessive fashion. In essence, loss of both alleles encoding OPG leads to unregulated RANKL signaling, excessive osteoclast activation, and chronic osteolysis. The symptoms of hyperphosphatasia mimic many of those of familial expansile osteolysis including high bone turnover, deafness during early childhood, "idiopathic external lysis" of adult teeth, and may involve focal lesions in appendicular bones that mimic active PDB [177]. Interestingly, till date, no mutations in RANKL itself have been associated with human disease. However, mutations that result in enhanced RANK signaling through inactivation of OPG or activation of RANK are associated with hyperphosphatasia and familial expansile osteolysis, respectively [12].

1.7.8 Juvenile Osteoporosis (OMIM 259750)

The subject of osteoporosis affecting the adult population was thoroughly discussed in Vol. 2 in this book series. The juvenile version of this disease, however, appears to have a complex genetic etiology. No single gene is the culprit, and disruption of no single pathway appears to be the root cause. As is discussed in the subsequent section, for children with Rett syndrome, certain genetic syndromes are predictably associated with low bone mass. In addition to these occurrences, many more subtle but nonetheless important factors can influence the accumulation of bone mass during bone growth. Such factors include genetics, gender, ethnicity, nutrition (e.g., calcium, vitamin D, and protein), hormonal factors (e.g., sex steroids and insulin-like growth factor I), physical activity, and exposure to various risk factors (e.g., alcohol, smoking, and certain medications) [14]. Family and twin studies have estimated that 60–80% of peak bone mass variability in the general population is attributable to genetic factors [14]. It is clear that bone growth in individuals responds differently to external factors including diet and exercise. As more is learned about the interactions among gene products expressed by bone cells, it is hoped that molecular signatures will be developed to assist in predicting personalized responses to external factors, especially among growing children.

1.7.9 X-linked Hypophosphatemia (OMIM#307800)

Familial hypophosphatemia is a rare genetic disease that is transmitted as an X-linked dominant trait. Mutations on the phosphate-regulating gene with homologies to endopeptidases on the X-chromosome (PHEX) gene (chromosome Xp22.2-p22.1) are responsible for the familial form of the disease. The PHEX protein is a transmembrane endopeptidase that belongs to the type II integral membrane zinc-dependent endopeptidase family. Numerous reports demonstrate that PHEX is involved in mineralization of bone and dentin, as well as in renal phosphate reabsorption. Interestingly, the metallopeptidase PHEX is a heparin-binding protein that binds to heparan sulfate in the extracellular matrix and may modulate its enzymatic activity, protein stability, and cellular trafficking [8]. The exact substrates for PHEX, whose cleavage is dysregulated by mutations in PHEX, are the subject of much active research. This research has focused on FGF23 (reviewed in [110]) and more recently, on the matrix extracellular phosphoglycoprotein (MEPE). Hyp mice having an inactivating mutation of the PHEX gene have bones with increased levels of MEPE [1, 6]. An acidic, serine- and aspartic acid-rich motif (ASARM) is located in the C-terminus of MEPE and some other matrix proteins in the mineralized tissues. It was recently proposed that pASARM inhibits mineralization by binding to hydroxyapatite and that this inhibitor can be cleaved by PHEX, which provides a mechanism explaining how loss of PHEX activity can lead to extracellular matrix accumulation of ASARM resulting in the osteomalacia of X-linked hypophosphatemia [1]. This hypothesis is intriguing, but remains to be unequivocally proven.

1.8 Epigenetic Regulation in Development

1.8.1 Methylation

In addition to genetic regulation in bone development, epigenetic gene regulation can also lead to differences in bone formation and maintenance. Epigenetics refers to the heritable changes in the genome that are not caused by differences in the DNA sequence. These epigenetic modifications include methylation of the 5′ carbon of cytosines within a cytosine–guanine dinucleotides, and acetylation or methylation of lysine residues on histones. Methylation of CpG dinucleotides within a stretch of DNA traditionally has been thought to lead to transcriptional silencing, whereas methylation and acetylation at the different lysine residues on histones can either have transcriptional activation or repression activities depending on whether it allows the chromatin to open up or forces it to condense. In a normal developmental state, reprogramming of major epigenetic marks such as methylation of the 5′ carbon of cytosines are erased from the gametes during fertilization and replaced with embryonic marks that are important for early embryonic development and beyond (Fig. 1.5) [131, 134, 157]. These specific "marks" on the DNA are referred to as epigenetic modifications, and although it is largely unknown, there is a mechanism within the cell that can specifically read these modifications. For example, methylated cytosines can be bound and regulated by methyl-binding domain (MBD) containing proteins, such as a protein in a family of MBDs, Mecp2, which contains an MBD domain [100, 101, 114].

1.8.2 Imprinting

Another epigenetic phenomenon is called imprinting, indicating that certain genes are expressed from only one chromosome in a parent-of-origin dependent manner [9, 132]. These allele-specific differences are often maintained by differential methylation patterns [132], although there may be other imprints on DNA as well. The properties of DNA methyl-transferase enzymes (DNMTs) make them uniquely suited to play a role in imprinting, as they are needed to maintain DNA methylation, which is an important imprinting mark (reviewed in [126]). Fewer than 1% of all mammalian genes are imprinted, totaling just over 30 genes discovered to date. Imprinted genes are not found sporadically throughout the genome, but rather they tend to

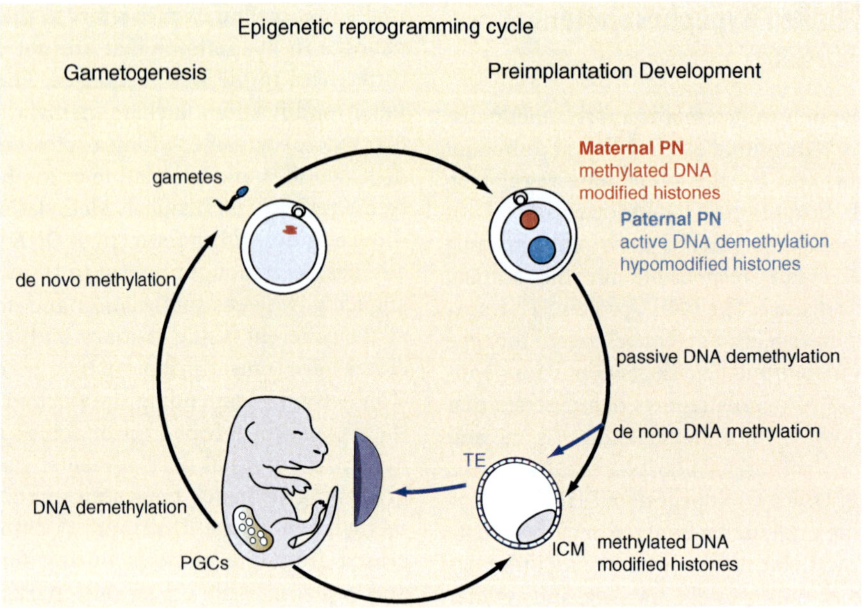

Figure 1.5. The cycle of epigenetic reprogramming in mammalian cells. Epigenetic modifications are reprogrammed twice during development. Early in the preimplantation development cycle, the parental imprint is erased by DNA demethylation in the pronucleus (PN), followed by reprogramming via de novo DNA methylation to reestablish the parental imprints. After fertilization, DNA demethylation and removal of histone modifications occurs, although imprinted genes maintain their methylation marks. De novo methylation in the primordial germ cells (PGCs) restores the epigenetic modifications in the first two lineages of the blastocyte stage, while the inner cell mass (ICM) remains hypermethylated when compared with the trophoectoderm (TE). (Adapted with permission from Morgan et al. [105]).

cluster together [126]. Often these clusters of two or more imprinted genes are regulated by a region called the imprinting control region (ICR), which determines the allele-specific expression of those particular genes [79]. For this small subset of genes, it is very important that only the correct allele is expressed for each particular gene that can be either maternal or paternal. Disease often results in the case where the incorrect allele is expressed or mutations are found on the expressed allele.

In this section, we will explore a few representative disorders that illustrate the consequence of impaired imprinting and epigenetic gene regulation. The Gnas gene that encodes the G-coupled protein receptor α subunit is located within a cluster of imprinted genes, with transcript-specific transcription in both the sense and antisense directions [125, 182]. Methylation of the proximal Gnas exon 1 promoter has not been associated with the imprinting status of Gnas exon 1, and rather within this cluster of genes around the Gnas exon 1 locus, there have been several ICRs that have been shown to directly regulate Gnas exon 1 tissue-specific expression [93, 94, 178, 179]. Gnas exon 1 is biallelically expressed in most tissues, but shows an inclination toward maternal expression in several tissues, including renal proximal tubes and brown and white adipose tissue (reviewed in [124]).

Phenotypic abnormalities have been associated with the loss of imprinting or allele-specific mutations in many of the genes encoded within the Gnas locus (reviewed in [124]). Interestingly, parental-specific inheritance of mutations in the Gnas exon 1 transcript leads to a particular set of problems. Pseudohypoparathyroidism (PHP) results from mutations in Gnas exon 1 transcript, but several distinct PHP disorders have been identified, including PPHP and PHP type1a. In addition to hormonal resistance to parathyroid hormone (PTH), PHP type1a cases have features of Albright's hereditary osteodystrophy (AHO). While PPHP also shows features of AHO, these cases do not exhibit hormone resistance to PTH [36, 181]. AHO refers to a collection of features including short stature, obesity, brachydactyly, ectopic ossifications, and mental retardation (reviewed in [10]). While PPHP and PHP type1a share several common features, they actually arise from mutations on different parental alleles. Production of PHP type1a is a direct effect of mutations on the maternally derived allele, while PPHP results from mutations on the paternal allele [176]. Several other disorders have also resulted from mutations on the Gnas exon 1 gene. Progressive osseous heteroplasia (POH), a devastating disease resulting from widespread ossification in childhood and progressive ossification of the skeletal muscle and deep tissue, has also been shown to be a consequence of paternally inherited mutations in Gnas exon 1 gene [2, 23, 150]. From the abovementioned examples, it is clear that epigenetic dysregulation can play a large role in disease state, specifically with regard to bone.

1.8.3 Epigenetic Regulation of Mediators of Bone Formation and Remodeling

Several instances of epigenetic regulation affecting bone formation, remodeling, and ultimately, BMD have been documented. Epigenetic modulation of *RANKL* expression was initially described in late passage mouse stromal ST2 cells [83]. In these cells, methylation of two CpG dinucleotide clusters, one near a putative vitamin D response element (VDRE) and other near the start site of transcription in the mouse *RANKL* gene was coincident with a decrease in the ability of osteoblastic cells to support *in vitro* osteoclastogenesis [82]. Sequences near the VDRE were methylated in both early and late passage cells; however, cytosine methylation status increased dramatically from early to late passage cells in the region flanking the transcription initiation site coincident with the downregulation of RANKL expression [83]. Additionally, data from the Rubin laboratory demonstrated complex modulation of histone modifications associated with *RANKL* promoter activity and gene expression, with the SWI/SNF chromatin remodeling complex being implicated in the control of osteoblast differentiation [42]. Further studies by Kitazawa even suggest a direct connection between Mecp2 and *RANKL* in late passage ST2 cells [81], a time when RANKL expression is downregulated.

1.8.4 Histone Modifications

Epigenetic regulation of bone has been reported to correlate histone deacetylation with the regulation of osteoblast differentiation. Clinically, it has been observed that children with epilepsy [52] as well as adult epilepsy patients [13, 139] treated with valproate (VPA), a histone deacetylase inhibitor (HDACi), had a reduction in skeletal growth and bone mass and decreased BMD, respectively. Even though gene profile studies have linked VPA to the up or downregulation of several sets of genes, the exact mechanism by which VPA accelerates bone differentiation, ultimately leading to reduced BMD has not yet been elucidated [27, 144]. Additionally, there is evidence linking HDACi with accelerated osteoblast differentiation through inhibition of the interaction of HDAC3 and Runx2 [143, 145]. Other studies have highlighted the importance of epigenetic regulation in bone, as increased histone 3 acetylation was observed in the bone sialoprotein promoter [89], and both reduced CpG methylation and increased acetylation levels have been implicated in osteocalcin transcriptional activation [147, 148, 151, 174]. Acceleration of osteoblast differentiation as a result of HDAC inhibition has been reported using both osteoblastic cell lines as well as clinical observations [27, 143, 145]. While gene profiling studies have been performed to uncover key genes that are disrupted with HDACi treatment, a mechanism that would lead to reduced BMD is not yet clear.

1.8.5 DNA Methylation and Rett Syndrome

Over 95% of all patients with the neurodevelopmental disorder, Rett syndrome (RTT), are females who present with neurological dysfunction that becomes apparent after the first few months of life [55, 56]. In addition to the prominent neurological symptoms, children with RTT frequently have reductions in skeletal growth and low BMD, which lead to pathological fractures in childhood and early adolescence [54, 91, 93]. One of the first studies to document the risk of osteopenia in RTT compared bone mineralization in RTT girls with normal controls and individuals diagnosed with cerebral palsy (CP), who have impaired mobility and risks for disuse atrophy similar to patients with RTT [54]. Despite adequate calcium and vitamin D intake, RTT patients, when compared with both the control populations had decreases in whole body and spinal BMD as well as bone mineral content (BMC) even when corrected for age. Longitudinal and cross-sectional studies of RTT patients revealed that bone mass increases over time in RTT girls at a much lower rate than in normal controls [19, 20, 106, 190]. The reduction in cortical bone thickness and BMD is further exacerbated by anticonvulsant use, immobility, and scoliosis, which compound the morbidity imparted by bone fragility in RTT patients [21, 48, 75, 107].

Most cases of RTT are caused by mutations in *MECP2* (murine ortholog *Mecp2***) [4], the most notable in a family of MBD proteins that all share sequence homology with the MBD of Mecp2 [100, 101, 112]. In addition to the MBD, a transcriptional repression domain (TRD) [111] and nuclear localization signal (NLS) have been identified. As mentioned previously, DNA methylation of cytosines in CpG dinucleotides is an epigenetic modification that is important for transcriptional regulation [26, 33, 39], and imprinting [123]. Mecp2 was identified as a protein that would preferentially bind to methylated CpG dinucleotides [112, 114] in the genome and repress transcription by recruiting corepressors such as mSin3A, c-Ski, N-CoR [85], as well as histone deacetylases [73, 113], although there is evidence that Mecp2 can repress transcription independent of methylation state [46].

Until recently, it was believed that Mecp2 acted solely as a global transcriptional repressor, even though microarray analyses using Mecp2 deficient systems did not yield much information regarding specific targets of Mecp2 [30, 166, 167]. Recent studies have demonstrated that Mecp2 binding is neither limited to the promoter regions of the genes [183], nor is Mecp2 now confined to its role as a long-term transcriptional silencer. Further work has shown that Mecp2 has the ability to bind and transcriptionally regulate genes through both transcriptional repression and activation [22].

Several Mecp2-deficient mouse models have been developed, which harbor various inactivating mutations in the Mecp2 locus. The strain developed by the Bird laboratory, B6.129P2(C)-Mecp2tm1.1Bird/J, carries a deletion of exons 3 and 4 generated by a constitutive Cre-mediated recombination event [53]. While extensive work has established many neurological similarities between this mouse model and RTT patients, our laboratory is investigating whether this mouse model can recapitulate the bone phenotype and provide insight into the mechanism by which Mecp2 regulates BMD. The results of our work reveal that the $Mecp2^{-/yBIRD}$ mice have an abnormal skeletal phenotype that may be similar to the aberrant phenotype in RTT patients, which often results in decreased BMD [117]. Further analysis is needed to determine the exact mechanism by which Mecp2 regulates BMD; however, this is another example of epigenetic dysregulation leading to irregular BMD.

1.9 Summary and Conclusions

Here, we describe the importance of genes and genetics in the regulation of skeletal development, expressively emphasizing several genetic mutations that can lead to disorders of the bone. Specifically, Sox9, Runx2, Dlx5, and Twist1 have essential roles in bone development, whereby a mutation in each of these genes can lead to differential, yet destructive effects on the skeleton. In addition to these genes that are expressed in the osteoblast, it is also crucial to think about the role of the osteoclast in proper bone formation, patterning, and development. Our brief discussion regarding genes that are necessary for osteoclast initiation, coupling, and differentiation, as well as the critical transcription factors, only highlights some of the genes that regulate osteoclastogenesis. Steroid hormones such as estrogens, androgens, and vitamin D also have an effect on bone development and each one has a significant impact on proper skeletogenesis and maintenance of bone mineral density. Several primary genetic defects that result in bone abnormalities have been examined as examples of disorders that fit into one of the three criteria: primary skeletal dysplasias, systemic or localized homeostatic imbalances, and mineralization defects.

In addition to the effect of DNA sequence-specific genetic mutations on bone development, it is necessary to explore the role of epigenetics on skeletal development and disorders of the bone. Epigenetic modifications including DNA methylation and histone methylation and acetylation have been implicated in the regulation of proper bone mineral density. Mutations in genes that participate in epigenetic gene regulation (*Mecp2*) or are acted upon by epigenetic modifications (*Gnas*) have been shown to result in reduced bone volume and cause skeletal defects. Additionally, bone development can be affected by improper control of genes with a role in epigenetic regulation, such as histone deacetylases. Coupled together, this illustrates the importance of epigenetic modifications and regulation of epigenetically controlled genes in the development and maintenance of the skeleton. The information presented in this chapter leads to a good overview of the mechanisms whereby bone development is controlled, but there is undoubtedly much more to learn. The understanding of skeletal development and bone biology as a whole will continue to improve as we identify more genes that are critical in bone development and maintenance, uncover genes that are involved in epigenetic regulation, and learn more about the mechanism by which cells place an imprint on particular genes.

References

1. Addison WN, Nakano Y, Loisel T, Crine P, McKee MD (2008) MEPE-ASARM peptides control extracellular matrix mineralization by binding to hydroxyapatite: an inhibition regulated by PHEX cleavage of ASARM. J Bone Miner Res 23: 1638–1649
2. Adegbite NS, Xu M, Kaplan FS, Shore EM, Pignolo RJ (2008) Diagnostic and mutational spectrum of progressive osseous heteroplasia (POH) and other forms of GNAS-based heterotopic ossification. Am J Med Genet A 146A:1788–1796
3. Aliprantis AO, Ueki Y, Sulyanto R, Park A, Sigrist KS, Sharma SM, Ostrowski MC, Olsen BR, Glimcher LH (2008) NFATc1 in mice represses osteoprotegerin during osteoclastogenesis and dissociates systemic osteopenia from inflammation in cherubism. J Clin Invest 118:3775–3789
4. Amir RE, Van den Veyver IB, Wan M, Tran CQ, Francke U, Zoghbi HY (1999) Rett syndrome is caused by mutations in X-linked MECP2, encoding methyl-CpG-binding protein 2. Nat Genet 23: 185–188
5. Anderson PH, Atkins GJ (2008) The skeleton as an intracrine organ for vitamin D metabolism. Mol Aspects Med 29:397–406
6. Argiro L, Desbarats M, Glorieux FH, Ecarot B (2001) Mepe, the gene encoding a tumor-secreted protein in oncogenic hypophosphatemic osteomalacia, is expressed in bone. Genomics 74:342–351
7. Aubin JE (1998) Bone stem cells. J Cell Biochem Suppl 30–31:73–82
8. Barros NM, Nascimento FD, Oliveira V, Juliano MA, Juliano L, Loisel T, Nader HB, Boileau G, Tersariol IL, Carmona AK (2008) The critical interaction of the metallopeptidase PHEX with heparan sulfate proteoglycans. Int J Biochem Cell Biol 40:2781–2792
9. Bartolomei MS, Tilghman SM (1997) Genomic imprinting in mammals. Annu Rev Genet 31: 493–525
10. Bastepe M, Juppner H (2005) GNAS locus and pseudohypoparathyroidism. Horm Res 63:65–74
11. Bell DM, Leung KK, Wheatley SC, Ng LJ, Zhou S, Ling KW, Sham MH, Koopman P, Tam PP, Cheah KS (1997) SOX9 directly regulates the type-II collagen gene. Nat Genet 16:174–178
12. Blair JM, Zheng Y, Dunstan CR (2007) RANK ligand. Int J Biochem Cell Biol 39:1077–1081
13. Boluk A, Guzelipek M, Savli H, Temel I, Ozisik HI, Kaygusuz A (2004) The effect of valproate on bone mineral density in adult epileptic patients. Pharmacol Res 50:93–97
14. Bonjour JP, Chevalley T, Rizzoli R, Ferrari S (2007) Gene-environment interactions in the skeletal response to nutrition and exercise during growth. Med Sport Sci 51:64–80
15. Bourgeois P, Bolcato-Bellemin AL, Danse JM, Bloch-Zupan A, Yoshiba K, Stoetzel C, Perrin-Schmitt F (1998) The variable expressivity and incomplete penetrance of the twist-null heterozygous mouse phenotype resemble those of human Saethre-Chotzen syndrome. Hum Mol Genet 7:945–957
16. Boyan BD, Jennings EG, Wang L, Schwartz Z (2004) Mechanisms regulating differential activation of membrane-mediated signaling by 1alpha,25(OH)2D3 and 24R,25(OH)2D3. J Steroid Biochem Mol Biol 89–90:309–315
17. Briggs MD, Mortier GR, Cole WG, King LM, Golik SS, Bonaventure J, Nuytinck L, De Paepe A, Leroy JG, Biesecker L, Lipson M, Wilcox WR, Lachman RS, Rimoin DL, Knowlton RG, Cohn DH (1998) Diverse mutations in the gene for cartilage oligomeric matrix protein in the pseudoachondroplasia-multiple epiphyseal dysplasia disease spectrum. Am J Hum Genet 62:311–319

18. Bruder SP, Caplan AI (1989) Cellular and molecular events during embryonic bone development. Connect Tissue Res 20:65–71
19. Budden SS, Gunness ME (2001) Bone histomorphometry in three females with Rett syndrome. Brain Dev 23(suppl 1):S133–S137
20. Budden SS, Gunness ME (2003) Possible mechanisms of osteopenia in Rett syndrome: bone histomorphometric studies. J Child Neurol 18:698–702
21. Cepollaro C, Gonnelli S, Bruni D, Pacini S, Martini S, Franci MB, Gennari L, Rossi S, Hayek G, Zappella M, Gennari C (2001) Dual X-ray absorptiometry and bone ultrasonography in patients with Rett syndrome. Calcif Tissue Int 69:259–262
22. Chahrour M, Jung SY, Shaw C, Zhou X, Wong ST, Qin J, Zoghbi HY (2008) MeCP2, a key contributor to neurological disease, activates and represses transcription. Science 320:1224–1229
23. Chan I, Hamada T, Hardman C, McGrath JA, Child FJ (2004) Progressive osseous heteroplasia resulting from a new mutation in the GNAS1 gene. Clin Exp Dermatol 29:77–80
24. Chang EJ, Ha J, Huang H, Kim HJ, Woo JH, Lee Y, Lee ZH, Kim JH, Kim HH (2008) The JNK-dependent CaMK pathway restrains the reversion of committed cells during osteoclast differentiation. J Cell Sci 121: 2555–2564
25. Chen TL, Posey KL, Hecht JT, Vertel BM (2008) COMP mutations: domain-dependent relationship between abnormal chondrocyte trafficking and clinical PSACH and MED phenotypes. J Cell Biochem 103:778–787
26. Chen WG, Chang Q, Lin Y, Meissner A, West AE, Griffith EC, Jaenisch R, Greenberg ME (2003) Derepression of BDNF transcription involves calcium-dependent phosphorylation of MeCP2. Science 302:885–889
27. Cho HH, Park HT, Kim YJ, Bae YC, Suh KT, Jung JS (2005) Induction of osteogenic differentiation of human mesenchymal stem cells by histone deacetylase inhibitors. J Cell Biochem 96:533–542
28. Cohen MM Jr (2006) The new bone biology: pathologic, molecular, and clinical correlates. Am J Med Genet A 140:2646–2706
29. Cohn DH (1995) Pseudoachondroplasia. GeneReviews at GeneTests: Medical Information Resource (database online). University of Washington, Seattle
30. Colantuoni C, Jeon OH, Hyder K, Chenchik A, Khimani AH, Narayanan V, Hoffman EP, Kaufmann WE, Naidu S, Pevsner J (2001) Gene expression profiling in postmortem Rett syndrome brain: differential gene expression and patient classification. Neurobiol Dis 8:847–865
31. Dai XM, Ryan GR, Hapel AJ, Dominguez MG, Russell RG, Kapp S, Sylvestre V, Stanley ER (2002) Targeted disruption of the mouse colony-stimulating factor 1 receptor gene results in osteopetrosis, mononuclear phagocyte deficiency, increased primitive progenitor cell frequencies, and reproductive defects. Blood 99:111–120
32. Daroszewska A, Ralston SH (2006) Mechanisms of disease: genetics of Paget's disease of bone and related disorders. Nat Clin Pract Rheumatol 2:270–277
33. Darwanto A, Kitazawa R, Maeda S, Kitazawa S (2003) MeCP2 and promoter methylation cooperatively regulate E-cadherin gene expression in colorectal carcinoma. Cancer Sci 94:442–447
34. Deere M, Sanford T, Ferguson HL, Daniels K, Hecht JT (1998) Identification of twelve mutations in cartilage oligomeric matrix protein (COMP) in patients with pseudoachondroplasia. Am J Med Genet 80: 510–513
35. DeLise AM, Fischer L, Tuan RS (2000) Cellular interactions and signaling in cartilage development. Osteoarthr Cartil 8:309–334
36. de Nanclares GP, Fernandez-Rebollo E, Santin I, Garcia-Cuartero B, Gaztambide S, Menendez E, Morales MJ, Pombo M, Bilbao JR, Barros F, Zazo N, Ahrens W, Juppner H, Hiort O, Castano L, Bastepe M (2007) Epigenetic defects of GNAS in patients with pseudohypoparathyroidism and mild features of Albright's hereditary osteodystrophy. J Clin Endocrinol Metab 92:2370–2373
37. Ding KH, Wang ZZ, Hamrick MW, Deng ZB, Zhou L, Kang B, Yan SL, She JX, Stern DM, Isales CM, Mi QS (2006) Disordered osteoclast formation in RAGE-deficient mouse establishes an essential role for RAGE in diabetes related bone loss. Biochem Biophys Res Commun 340:1091–1097
38. Doherty ES, Lacbawan F, Hadley DW, Brewer C, Zalewski C, Kim HJ, Solomon B, Rosenbaum K, Domingo DL, Hart TC, Brooks BP, Immken L, Lowry RB, Kimonis V, Shanske AL, Jehee FS, Bueno MR, Knightly C, McDonald-McGinn D, Zackai EH, Muenke M (2007) Muenke syndrome (FGFR3-related craniosynostosis): expansion of the phenotype and review of the literature. Am J Med Genet A 143A:3204–3215
39. Drewell RA, Goddard CJ, Thomas JO, Surani MA (2002) Methylation-dependent silencing at the H19 imprinting control region by MeCP2. Nucleic Acids Res 30:1139–1144
40. Dunn PM (2003) Gregor Mendel, OSA (1822–1884), founder of scientific genetics. Arch Dis Child Fetal Neonatal Ed 88:F537–F539
41. Erlebacher A, Filvaroff EH, Gitelman SE, Derynck R (1995) Toward a molecular understanding of skeletal development. Cell 80:371–378
42. Fan X, Roy EM, Murphy TC, Nanes MS, Kim S, Pike JW, Rubin J (2004) Regulation of RANKL promoter activity is associated with histone remodeling in murine bone stromal cells. J Cell Biochem 93:807–818
43. Foster JW, Dominguez-Steglich MA, Guioli S, Kwok C, Weller PA, Stevanovic M, Weissenbach J, Mansour S, Young ID, Goodfellow PN et al (1994) Campomelic dysplasia and autosomal sex reversal caused by mutations in an SRY-related gene. Nature 372:525–530
44. Francomano CA (2008) Achondroplasia. GeneReviews at GeneTests: Medical Information Resource (database online). University of Washington, Seattle
45. Gennari L, Becherini L, Masi L, Mansani R, Gonnelli S, Cepollaro C, Martini S, Montagnani A, Lentini G, Becorpi AM, Brandi ML (1998) Vitamin D and estrogen receptor allelic variants in Italian postmenopausal women: evidence of multiple gene contribution to

bone mineral density. J Clin Endocrinol Metab 83: 939–944
46. Georgel PT, Horowitz-Scherer RA, Adkins N, Woodcock CL, Wade PA, Hansen JC (2003) Chromatin compaction by human MeCP2. Assembly of novel secondary chromatin structures in the absence of DNA methylation. J Biol Chem. 278: 32181–32188
47. Gerber HP, Vu TH, Ryan AM, Kowalski J, Werb Z, Ferrara N (1999) VEGF couples hypertrophic cartilage remodeling, ossification and angiogenesis during endochondral bone formation. Nat Med 5:623–628
48. Gonnelli S, Caffarelli C, Hayek J, Montagnani A, Cadirni A, Franci B, Lucani B, Rossi S, Nuti R (2008) Bone ultrasonography at phalanxes in patients with Rett syndrome: a 3-year longitudinal study. Bone 42:737–742
49. Grigoriadis AE, Wang ZQ, Cecchini MG, Hofstetter W, Felix R, Fleisch HA, Wagner EF (1994) c-Fos: a key regulator of osteoclast-macrophage lineage determination and bone remodeling. Science 266:443–448
50. Grundberg E, Brandstrom H, Lam KC, Gurd S, Ge B, Harmsen E, Kindmark A, Ljunggren O, Mallmin H, Nilsson O, Pastinen T (2008) Systematic assessment of the human osteoblast transcriptome in resting and induced primary cells. Physiol Genomics 33: 301–311
51. Guenou H, Kaabeche K, Mee SL, Marie PJ (2005) A role for fibroblast growth factor receptor-2 in the altered osteoblast phenotype induced by Twist haploinsufficiency in the Saethre-Chotzen syndrome. Hum Mol Genet 14:1429–1439
52. Guo CY, Ronen GM, Atkinson SA (2001) Long-term valproate and lamotrigine treatment may be a marker for reduced growth and bone mass in children with epilepsy. Epilepsia 42:1141–1147
53. Guy J, Hendrich B, Holmes M, Martin JE, Bird A (2001) A mouse Mecp2-null mutation causes neurological symptoms that mimic Rett syndrome. Nat Genet 27:322–326
54. Haas RH, Dixon SD, Sartoris DJ, Hennessy MJ (1997) Osteopenia in Rett syndrome. J Pediatr 131: 771–774
55. Hagberg B (1985) Rett's syndrome: prevalence and impact on progressive severe mental retardation in girls. Acta Paediatr Scand 74:405–408
56. Hagberg B, J. Aicardi, K. Dias, O. Ramos (1983) A progressive syndrome of autism, dementia, ataxia, and loss of purposeful hand use in girls: Rett's syndrome: report of 35 cases. Ann Neurol 14:471–479
57. Hart KC, Robertson SC, Donoghue DJ (2001) Identification of tyrosine residues in constitutively activated fibroblast growth factor receptor 3 involved in mitogenesis, Stat activation, and phosphatidylinositol 3-kinase activation. Mol Biol Cell. 12:931–942
58. Hassan MQ, Javed A, Morasso MI, Karlin J, Montecino M, van Wijnen AJ, Stein GS, Stein JL, Lian JB (2004) Dlx3 transcriptional regulation of osteoblast differentiation: temporal recruitment of Msx2, Dlx3, and Dlx5 homeodomain proteins to chromatin of the osteocalcin gene. Mol Cell Biol. 24:9248–9261
59. Hayashi M, Nimura K, Kashiwagi K, Harada T, Takaoka K, Kato H, Tamai K, Kaneda Y (2007) Comparative roles of Twist-1 and Id1 in transcriptional regulation by BMP signaling. J Cell Sci 120:1350–1357
60. Healy C, Uwanogho D, Sharpe PT (1999) Regulation and role of Sox9 in cartilage formation. Dev Dyn 215:69–78
61. Hecht JT, Hayes E, Haynes R, Cole WG, Long RJ, Farach-Carson MC, Carson DD (2005) Differentiation-induced loss of heparan sulfate in human exostosis derived chondrocytes. Differentiation 73:212–221
62. Hecht JT, Makitie O, Hayes E, Haynes R, Susic M, Montufar-Solis D, Duke PJ, Cole WG (2004) Chondrocyte cell death and intracellular distribution of COMP and type IX collagen in the pseudoachondroplasia growth plate. J Orthop Res 22:759–767
63. Hecht JT, Nelson LD, Crowder E, Wang Y, Elder FF, Harrison WR, Francomano CA, Prange CK, Lennon GG, Deere M et al (1995) Mutations in exon 17B of cartilage oligomeric matrix protein (COMP) cause pseudoachondroplasia. Nat Genet 10:325–329
64. Heilberg IP, Hernandez E, Alonzo E, Valera R, Ferreira LG, Gomes SA, Bellorin-Font E, Weisinger JR (2005) Estrogen receptor (ER) gene polymorphism may predict the bone mineral density response to raloxifene in postmenopausal women on chronic hemodialysis. Ren Fail 27:155–161
65. Helfrich MH, Hocking LJ (2008) Genetics and aetiology of Pagetic disorders of bone. Arch Biochem Biophys 473:172–182
66. Hinoi E, Bialek P, Chen YT, Rached MT, Groner Y, Behringer RR, Ornitz DM, Karsenty G (2006) Runx2 inhibits chondrocyte proliferation and hypertrophy through its expression in the perichondrium. Genes Dev 20:2937–2942
67. Horton WA, Hall JG, Hecht JT (2007) Achondroplasia. Lancet 370:162–172
68. Huang LF, Fukai N, Selby PB, Olsen BR, Mundlos S (1997) Mouse clavicular development: analysis of wild-type and cleidocranial dysplasia mutant mice. Dev Dyn 210:33–40
69. Hu R, Sharma SM, Bronisz A, Srinivasan R, Sankar U, Ostrowski MC (2007) Eos, MITF, and PU.1 recruit corepressors to osteoclast-specific genes in committed myeloid progenitors. Mol Cell Biol. 27:4018–4027
70. Ishida N, Hayashi K, Hoshijima M, Ogawa T, Koga S, Miyatake Y, Kumegawa M, Kimura T, Takeya T (2002) Large scale gene expression analysis of osteoclastogenesis in vitro and elucidation of NFAT2 as a key regulator. J Biol Chem 277:41147–41156
71. Jabs EW, Muller U, Li X, Ma L, Luo W, Haworth IS, Klisak I, Sparkes R, Warman ML, Mulliken JB et al (1993) A mutation in the homeodomain of the human MSX2 gene in a family affected with autosomal dominant craniosynostosis. Cell 75:443–450
72. Jones KL (ed) (2006) Smith's recognizable patterns of human malformation, 6th edn. Elsevier Saunders, Philadelphia, pp 390–391; 462–465
73. Jones PL, Veenstra GJ, Wade PA, Vermaak D, Kass SU, Landsberger N, Strouboulis J, Wolffe AP (1998) Methylated DNA and MeCP2 recruit histone deacetylase to repress transcription. Nat Genet 19: 187–191
74. Karsenty G, Wagner EF (2002) Reaching a genetic and molecular understanding of skeletal development. Dev Cell 2:389–406

75. Keret D, Bassett GS, Bunnell WP, Marks HG (1988) Scoliosis in Rett syndrome. J Pediatr Orthop 8: 138–142
76. Khosla S, Melton LJ III, Riggs BL (2002) Clinical review 144: estrogen and the male skeleton. J Clin Endocrinol Metab 87:1443–1450
77. Kim MS, Day CJ, Morrison NA (2005) MCP-1 is induced by receptor activator of nuclear factor-{kappa}B ligand, promotes human osteoclast fusion, and rescues granulocyte macrophage colony-stimulating factor suppression of osteoclast formation. J Biol Chem 280:16163–16169
78. Kim YJ, Lee MH, Wozney JM, Cho JY, Ryoo HM (2004) Bone morphogenetic protein-2-induced alkaline phosphatase expression is stimulated by Dlx5 and repressed by Msx2. J Biol Chem 279:50773–50780
79. Kinoshita T, Ikeda Y, Ishikawa R (2008) Genomic imprinting: a balance between antagonistic roles of parental chromosomes. Semin Cell Dev Biol 19:574–579
80. Kitahama S, Gibson MA, Hatzinikolas G, Hay S, Kuliwaba JL, Evdokiou A, Atkins GJ, Findlay DM (2000) Expression of fibrillins and other microfibril-associated proteins in human bone and osteoblast-like cells. Bone 27:61–67
81. Kitazawa R, Kitazawa S (2007) Methylation status of a single CpG locus 3 bases upstream of TATA-box of receptor activator of nuclear factor-kappaB ligand (RANKL) gene promoter modulates cell- and tissue-specific RANKL expression and osteoclastogenesis. Mol Endocrinol 21:148–158
82. Kitazawa R, Kitazawa S, Maeda S (1999) Promoter structure of mouse RANKL/TRANCE/OPGL/ODF gene. Biochim Biophys Acta 1445:134–141
83. Kitazawa S, Kitazawa R (2002) Epigenetic control of mouse receptor activator of NF-kappa B ligand gene expression. Biochem Biophys Res Commun 293: 126–131
84. Kleerekoper Q, Hecht JT, Putkey JA (2002) Disease-causing mutations in cartilage oligomeric matrix protein cause an unstructured Ca2+ binding domain. J Biol Chem 277:10581–10589
85. Kokura K, Kaul SC, Wadhwa R, Nomura T, Khan MM, Shinagawa T, Yasukawa T, Colmenares C, Ishii S (2001) The Ski protein family is required for MeCP2-mediated transcriptional repression. J Biol Chem 276:34115–34121
86. Komori T (2006) Regulation of osteoblast differentiation by transcription factors. J Cell Biochem 99: 233–1239
87. Komori T, Yagi H, Nomura S, Yamaguchi A, Sasaki K, Deguchi K, Shimizu Y, Bronson RT, Gao YH, Inada M, Sato M, Okamoto R, Kitamura Y, Yoshiki S, Kishimoto T (1997) Targeted disruption of Cbfa1 results in a complete lack of bone formation owing to maturational arrest of osteoblasts. Cell 89:755–764
88. Kumar S, Scott JX, Kanagalakshmi (2006) Cleido-Cranial Dysplasia: A Case Report. Internet J Ped Neonatol, Vol 6
89. Lamour V, Detry C, Sanchez C, Henrotin Y, Castronovo V, Bellahcene A (2007) Runx2- and histone deacetylase 3-mediated repression is relieved in differentiating human osteoblast cells to allow high bone sialoprotein expression. J Biol Chem 282:36240–36249
90. Legeai-Mallet L, Benoist-Lasselin C, Delezoide AL, Munnich A, Bonaventure J (1998) Fibroblast growth factor receptor 3 mutations promote apoptosis but do not alter chondrocyte proliferation in thanatophoric dysplasia. J Biol Chem 273:13007–13014
91. Leonard H, Thomson M, Bower C, Fyfe S, Constantinou J (1995) Skeletal abnormalities in Rett syndrome: increasing evidence for dysmorphogenetic defects. Am J Med Genet 58:282–285
92. Leonard H, Thomson MR, Glasson EJ, Fyfe S, Leonard S, Bower C, Christodoulou J, Ellaway C (1999) A population-based approach to the investigation of osteopenia in Rett syndrome. Dev Med Child Neurol 41:323–328
93. Liu J, Chen M, Deng C, Bourc'his D, Nealon JG, Erlichman B, Bestor TH, Weinstein LS (2005) Identification of the control region for tissue-specific imprinting of the stimulatory G protein alpha-subunit. Proc Natl Acad Sci U S A 102:5513–5518
94. Liu J, Yu S, Litman D, Chen W, Weinstein LS (2000) Identification of a methylation imprint mark within the mouse Gnas locus. Mol Cell Biol 20: 5808–5817
95. Li Z, Kong K, Qi W (2006) Osteoclast and its roles in calcium metabolism and bone development and remodeling. Biochem Biophys Res Commun 343: 345–350
96. Lorentzon M, Lorentzon R, Nordstrom P (2000) Vitamin D receptor gene polymorphism is associated with birth height, growth to adolescence, and adult stature in healthy caucasian men: a cross-sectional and longitudinal study. J Clin Endocrinol Metab 85: 1666–1670
97. Lorentzon M, Swanson C, Eriksson AL, Mellstrom D, Ohlsson C (2006) Polymorphisms in the aromatase gene predict areal BMD as a result of affected cortical bone size: the GOOD study. J Bone Miner Res 21: 332–339
98. Manolagas SC (2000) Birth and death of bone cells: basic regulatory mechanisms and implications for the pathogenesis and treatment of osteoporosis. Endocr Rev 21:115–137
99. Matheny CJ, Speck ME, Cushing PR, Zhou Y, Corpora T, Regan M, Newman M, Roudaia L, Speck CL, Gu TL, Griffey SM, Bushweller JH, Speck NA (2007) Disease mutations in RUNX1 and RUNX2 create nonfunctional, dominant-negative, or hypomorphic alleles. EMBO J 26:1163–1175
100. Meehan RR, Lewis JD, Bird AP (1992) Characterization of MeCP2, a vertebrate DNA binding protein with affinity for methylated DNA. Nucleic Acids Res 20:5085–5092
101. Meehan RR, Lewis JD, McKay S, Kleiner EL, Bird AP (1989) Identification of a mammalian protein that binds specifically to DNA containing methylated CpGs. Cell 58:499–507
102. Meyer J, Sudbeck P, Held M, Wagner T, Schmitz ML, Bricarelli FD, Eggermont E, Friedrich U, Haas OA, Kobelt A, Leroy JG, Van Maldergem L, Michel E, Mitulla B, Pfeiffer RA, Schinzel A, Schmidt H, Scherer G (1997) Mutational analysis of the SOX9 gene in campomelic dysplasia and autosomal sex reversal: lack of genotype/phenotype correlations. Hum Mol Genet 6: 91–98

103. Meyers GA, Orlow SJ, Munro IR, Przylepa KA, Jabs EW (1995) Fibroblast growth factor receptor 3 (FGFR3) transmembrane mutation in Crouzon syndrome with acanthosis nigricans. Nat Genet 11:462–464
104. Minamitani K, Takahashi Y, Minagawa M, Yasuda T, Niimi H (1998) Difference in height associated with a translation start site polymorphism in the vitamin D receptor gene. Pediatr Res 44:628–632
105. Morgan HD, Santos F, Green K, Dean W, Reik W (2005) Epigenetic reprogramming in mammals. Hum Mol Genet. 14: R47-58
106. Motil KJ, Ellis KJ, Barrish JO, Caeg E, Glaze DG (2008) Bone mineral content and bone mineral density are lower in older than in younger females with Rett syndrome. Pediatr Res 64:435–439
107. Motil KJ, Schultz RJ, Abrams S, Ellis KJ, Glaze DG (2006) Fractional calcium absorption is increased in girls with Rett syndrome. J Pediatr Gastroenterol Nutr 42:419–426
108. Mundlos S (1999) Cleidocranial dysplasia: clinical and molecular genetics. J Med Genet 36:177–182
109. Mundlos S, Olsen BR (1997) Heritable diseases of the skeleton. Part II: molecular insights into skeletal development-matrix components and their homeostasis. FASEB J 11:227–233
110. Murthy AS (2009) X-linked hypophosphatemic rickets and craniosynostosis. J Craniofac Surg 20: 439–442
111. Nan X, Campoy FJ, Bird A (1997) MeCP2 is a transcriptional repressor with abundant binding sites in genomic chromatin. Cell 88:471–481
112. Nan X, Meehan RR, Bird A (1993) Dissection of the methyl-CpG binding domain from the chromosomal protein MeCP2. Nucleic Acids Res 21: 4886–4892
113. Nan X, Ng HH, Johnson CA, Laherty CD, Turner BM, Eisenman RN, Bird A (1998) Transcriptional repression by the methyl-CpG-binding protein MeCP2 involves a histone deacetylase complex [see comments]. Nature 393:386–389
114. Nan X, Tate P, Li E, Bird A (1996) DNA methylation specifies chromosomal localization of MeCP2. Mol Cell Biol 16:414–421
115. Naski MC, Ornitz DM (1998) FGF signaling in skeletal development. Front Biosci 3:d781–94
116. Newberry EP, Latifi T, Towler DA (1998) Reciprocal regulation of osteocalcin transcription by the homeodomain proteins Msx2 and Dlx5. Biochemistry 37: 16360–16368
117. O'Connor RD, Zayzafoon M, Farach-Carson MC, Schanen NC (2009) Mecp2 deficiency decreases bone formation and reduces bone volume in a rodent model of Rett syndrome. Bone 45(2):346–356
118. O'Rourke MP, Soo K, Behringer RR, Hui CC, Tam PP (2002) Twist plays an essential role in FGF and SHH signal transduction during mouse limb development. Dev Biol 248:143–156
119. Olsen BR, Reginato AM, Wang W (2000) Bone development. Annu Rev Cell Dev Biol 16:191–220
120. Orwoll ES (2003) Men, bone and estrogen: unresolved issues. Osteoporos Int 14:93–98
121. Otto F, Kanegane H, Mundlos S (2002) Mutations in the RUNX2 gene in patients with cleidocranial dysplasia. Hum Mutat 19:209–216
122. Pannier S, Legeai-Mallet L (2008) Hereditary multiple exostoses and enchondromatosis. Best Pract Res Clin Rheumatol 22:45–54
123. Pedone PV, Pikaart MJ, Cerrato F, Vernucci M, Ungaro P, Bruni CB, Riccio A (1999) Role of histone acetylation and DNA methylation in the maintenance of the imprinted expression of the H19 and Igf2 genes. FEBS Lett 458:45–50
124. Peters J, Holmes R, Monk D, Beechey CV, Moore GE, Williamson CM (2006) Imprinting control within the compact Gnas locus. Cytogenet Genome Res 113: 194–201
125. Peters J, Wroe SF, Wells CA, Miller HJ, Bodle D, Beechey CV, Williamson CM, Kelsey G (1999) A cluster of oppositely imprinted transcripts at the Gnas locus in the distal imprinting region of mouse chromosome 2. Proc Natl Acad Sci U S A 96: 3830–3835
126. Pfeifer K (2000) Mechanisms of genomic imprinting. Am J Hum Genet 67:777–787
127. Posey KL et al. (2008) Thrombospondins: from structure to therapeutics. Cell Mol Life Sci 65:687–699
128. Prinos P, Costa T, Sommer A, Kilpatrick MW, Tsipouras P (1995) A common FGFR3 gene mutation in hypochondroplasia. Hum Mol Genet 4:2097–2101
129. Puppin C, Pellizzari L, Fabbro D, Fogolari F, Tell G, Tessa A, Santorelli FM, Damante G (2005) Functional analysis of a novel RUNX2 missense mutation found in a family with cleidocranial dysplasia. J Hum Genet 50:679–683
130. Ratisoontorn C, Cunningham ML (2005) Saethre-Chotzen syndrome. GeneReviews at GeneTests: Medical Information Resource (database online). University of Washington, Seattle
131. Reik W, Dean W, Walter J (2001) Epigenetic reprogramming in mammalian development. Science 293: 1089–1093
132. Reik W, Walter J (2001) Genomic imprinting: parental influence on the genome. Nat Rev Genet 2: 21–32
133. Riancho JA, Zarrabeitia MT, Valero C, Sanudo C, Mijares V, Gonzalez-Macias J (2006) A gene-to-gene interaction between aromatase and estrogen receptors influences bone mineral density. Eur J Endocrinol 155:53–59
134. Rideout WM III, Eggan K, Jaenisch R (2001) Nuclear cloning and epigenetic reprogramming of the genome. Science 293:1093–1098
135. Riggs BL, Khosla S, Melton LJ III (1998) A unitary model for involutional osteoporosis: estrogen deficiency causes both type I and type II osteoporosis in postmenopausal women and contributes to bone loss in aging men. J Bone Miner Res 13:763–773
136. Robledo RF, Rajan L, Li X, Lufkin T (2002) The Dlx5 and Dlx6 homeobox genes are essential for craniofacial, axial, and appendicular skeletal development. Genes Dev 16:1089–1101
137. Ryoo HM, Hoffmann HM, Beumer T, Frenkel B, Towler DA, Stein GS, Stein JL, van Wijnen AJ, Lian JB (1997) Stage-specific expression of Dlx-5 during osteoblast differentiation: involvement in regulation of osteocalcin gene expression. Mol Endocrinol 11:1681–1694

138. Samee N, Geoffroy V, Marty C, Schiltz C, Vieux-Rochas M, Levi G, de Vernejoul MC (2008) Dlx5, a positive regulator of osteoblastogenesis, is essential for osteoblast-osteoclast coupling. Am J Pathol 173:773–780
139. Sato Y, Kondo I, Ishida S, Motooka H, Takayama K, Tomita Y, Maeda H, Satoh K (2001) Decreased bone mass and increased bone turnover with valproate therapy in adults with epilepsy. Neurology 57: 445–449
140. Savarirayan R, Robertson SP, Bankier A, Rogers JG (2003) Variable expression of campomelic dysplasia in a father and his 46, XY daughter. Pediatr Pathol Mol Med. 22:37–46
141. Scherer SW, Poorkaj P, Allen T, Kim J, Geshuri D, Nunes M, Soder S, Stephens K, Pagon RA, Patton MA et al (1994) Fine mapping of the autosomal dominant split hand/split foot locus on chromosome 7, band q21.3-q22.1. Am J Hum Genet 55:12–20
142. Scherer SW, Poorkaj P, Massa H, Soder S, Allen T, Nunes M, Geshuri D, Wong E, Belloni E, Little S et al (1994) Physical mapping of the split hand/split foot locus on chromosome 7 and implication in syndromic ectrodactyly. Hum Mol Genet 3:1345–1354
143. Schroeder TM, Kahler RA, Li X, Westendorf JJ (2004) Histone deacetylase 3 interacts with runx2 to repress the osteocalcin promoter and regulate osteoblast differentiation. J Biol Chem 279: 41998–42007
144. Schroeder TM, Nair AK, Staggs R, Lamblin AF, Westendorf JJ (2007) Gene profile analysis of osteoblast genes differentially regulated by histone deacetylase inhibitors. BMC Genomics 8:362
145. Schroeder TM, Westendorf JJ (2005) Histone deacetylase inhibitors promote osteoblast maturation. J Bone Miner Res 20:2254–2263
146. Segev O, Chumakov I, Nevo Z, Givol D, Madar-Shapiro L, Sheinin Y, Weinreb M, Yayon A (2000) Restrained chondrocyte proliferation and maturation with abnormal growth plate vascularization and ossification in human FGFR-3(G380R) transgenic mice. Hum Mol Genet 9:249–258
147. Shen J, Hovhannisyan H, Lian JB, Montecino MA, Stein GS, Stein JL, Van Wijnen AJ (2003) Transcriptional induction of the osteocalcin gene during osteoblast differentiation involves acetylation of histones h3 and h4. Mol Endocrinol 17: 743–756
148. Shen J, Montecino M, Lian JB, Stein GS, Van Wijnen AJ, Stein JL (2002) Histone acetylation in vivo at the osteocalcin locus is functionally linked to vitamin D-dependent, bone tissue-specific transcription. J Biol Chem 277:20284–20292
149. Shiihara T, Kato M, Kimura T, Hayasaka K, Yamamori S, Ogata T (2004) Craniosynostosis with extra copy of MSX2 in a patient with partial 5q-trisomy. Am J Med Genet A 128A:214–216
150. Shore EM, Ahn J, Jan de Beur S, Li M, Xu M, Gardner RJ, Zasloff MA, Whyte MP, Levine MA, Kaplan FS (2002) Paternally inherited inactivating mutations of the GNAS1 gene in progressive osseous heteroplasia. N Engl J Med 346:99–106
151. Sierra J, Villagra A, Paredes R, Cruzat F, Gutierrez S, Javed A, Arriagada G, Olate J, Imschenetzky M, Van Wijnen AJ, Lian JB, Stein GS, Stein JL, Montecino M (2003) Regulation of the bone-specific osteocalcin gene by p300 requires Runx2/Cbfa1 and the vitamin D3 receptor but not p300 intrinsic histone acetyltransferase activity. Mol Cell Biol 23:3339–3351
152. Sims NA, Dupont S, Krust A, Clement-Lacroix P, Minet D, Resche-Rigon M, Gaillard-Kelly M, Baron R (2002) Deletion of estrogen receptors reveals a regulatory role for estrogen receptors-beta in bone remodeling in females but not in males. Bone 30:18–25
153. So H, Rho J, Jeong D, Park R, Fisher DE, Ostrowski MC, Choi Y, Kim N (2003) Microphthalmia transcription factor and PU.1 synergistically induce the leukocyte receptor osteoclast-associated receptor gene expression. J Biol Chem 278:24209–24216
154. St-Arnaud R (2008) The direct role of vitamin D on bone homeostasis. Arch Biochem Biophys 473:225–230
155. Steiner RD, Pepin MG, Byers PH (2005). Osteogenesis imperfecta. GeneReviews at GeneTests: Medical Information Resource (database online). University of Washington, Seattle
156. Suda T, Takahashi N, Udagawa N, Jimi E, Gillespie MT, Martin TJ (1999) Modulation of osteoclast differentiation and function by the new members of the tumor necrosis factor receptor and ligand families. Endocr Rev 20:345–357
157. Surani MA (2001) Reprogramming of genome function through epigenetic inheritance. Nature 414:122–128
158. Su WC, Kitagawa M, Xue N, Xie B, Garofalo S, Cho J, Deng C, Horton WA, Fu XY (1997) Activation of Stat1 by mutant fibroblast growth-factor receptor in thanatophoric dysplasia type II dwarfism. Nature 386:288–292
159. Syed F, Khosla S (2005) Mechanisms of sex steroid effects on bone. Biochem Biophys Res Commun 328: 688–696
160. Tadic T, Dodig M, Erceg I, Marijanovic I, Mina M, Kalajzic Z, Velonis D, Kronenberg MS, Kosher RA, Ferrari D, Lichtler AC (2002) Overexpression of Dlx5 in chicken calvarial cells accelerates osteoblastic differentiation. J Bone Miner Res 17:1008–1014
161. Takayanagi H (2007) The role of NFAT in osteoclast formation. Ann N Y Acad Sci 1116:227–237
162. Takayanagi H, Kim S, Koga T, Nishina H, Isshiki M, Yoshida H, Saiura A, Isobe M, Yokochi T, Inoue J, Wagner EF, Mak TW, Kodama T, Taniguchi T (2002) Induction and activation of the transcription factor NFATc1 (NFAT2) integrate RANKL signaling in terminal differentiation of osteoclasts. Dev Cell 3:889–901
163. Tavormina PL, Shiang R, Thompson LM, Zhu YZ, Wilkin DJ, Lachman RS, Wilcox WR, Rimoin DL, Cohn DH, Wasmuth JJ (1995) Thanatophoric dysplasia (types I and II) caused by distinct mutations in fibroblast growth factor receptor 3. Nat Genet 9:321–328
164. Teitelbaum SL (2000) Bone resorption by osteoclasts. Science 289:1504–1508
165. Tondravi MM, McKercher SR, Anderson K, Erdmann JM, Quiroz M, Maki R, Teitelbaum SL (1997)

Osteopetrosis in mice lacking haematopoietic transcription factor PU.1. Nature 386:81–84
166. Traynor J, Agarwal P, Lazzeroni L, Francke U (2002) Gene expression patterns vary in clonal cell cultures from Rett syndrome females with eight different MECP2 mutations. BMC Med Genet 3:12
167. Tudor M, Akbarian S, Chen RZ, Jaenisch R (2002) Transcriptional profiling of a mouse model for Rett syndrome reveals subtle transcriptional changes in the brain. Proc Natl Acad Sci U S A 99: 15536–15541
168. Udagawa N, Takahashi N, Akatsu T, Tanaka H, Sasaki T, Nishihara T, Koga T, Martin TJ, Suda T (1990) Origin of osteoclasts: mature monocytes and macrophages are capable of differentiating into osteoclasts under a suitable microenvironment prepared by bone marrow-derived stromal cells. Proc Natl Acad Sci U S A 87: 7260–7264
169. Unger S, Scherer G, Superti-Furga A (2008). Campomelic dysplasia. GeneReviews at GeneTests: Medical Information Resource (database online). University of Washington, Seattle
170. Uveges TE, Collin-Osdoby P, Cabral WA, Ledgard F, Goldberg L, Bergwitz C, Forlino A, Osdoby P, Gronowicz GA, Marini JC (2008) Cellular mechanism of decreased bone in Brtl mouse model of OI: imbalance of decreased osteoblast function and increased osteoclasts and their precursors. J Bone Miner Res 23:1983–1994
171. Vaes BL, Ducy P, Sijbers AM, Hendriks JM, van Someren EP, de Jong NG, van den Heuvel ER, Olijve W, van Zoelen EJ, Dechering KJ (2006) Microarray analysis on Runx2-deficient mouse embryos reveals novel Runx2 functions and target genes during intramembranous and endochondral bone formation. Bone 39: 724–738
172. Valero C, Zarrabeitia MT, Hernandez JL, Zarrabeitia A, Gonzalez-Macias J, Riancho JA (2005) Bone mass in young adults: relationship with gender, weight and genetic factors. J Intern Med 258:554–562
173. Vanderschueren D, Vandenput L, Boonen S, Lindberg MK, Bouillon R, Ohlsson C (2004) Androgens and bone. Endocr Rev 25:389–425
174. Villagra A, Gutierrez J, Paredes R, Sierra J, Puchi M, Imschenetzky M, Wijnen Av A, Lian J, Stein G, Stein J, Montecino M (2002) Reduced CpG methylation is associated with transcriptional activation of the bone-specific rat osteocalcin gene in osteoblasts. J Cell Biochem 85:112–122
175. Wang JC, Steinraths M, Dang L, Lomax B, Eydoux P, Stockley T, Yong SL, Van Allen MI (2007) Craniosynostosis associated with distal 5q-trisomy: further evidence that extra copy of MSX2 gene leads to craniosynostosis. Am J Med Genet A 143A:2931–2936
176. Weinstein LS, Yu S, Warner DR, Liu J (2001) Endocrine manifestations of stimulatory G protein alpha-subunit mutations and the role of genomic imprinting. Endocr Rev 22:675–705
177. Whyte MP (2006) Paget's disease of bone and genetic disorders of RANKL/OPG/RANK/NF-kappaB signaling. Ann N Y Acad Sci 1068: 143–164
178. Williamson CM, Ball ST, Nottingham WT, Skinner JA, Plagge A, Turner MD, Powles N, Hough T, Papworth D, Fraser WD, Maconochie M, Peters J (2004) A cis-acting control region is required exclusively for the tissue-specific imprinting of Gnas. Nat Genet 36:894–899
179. Williamson CM, Turner MD, Ball ST, Nottingham WT, Glenister P, Fray M, Tymowska-Lalanne Z, Plagge A, Powles-Glover N, Kelsey G, Maconochie M, Peters J (2006) Identification of an imprinting control region affecting the expression of all transcripts in the Gnas cluster. Nat Genet 38:350–355
180. Willing MC, Deschenes SP, Slayton RL, Roberts EJ (1996) Premature chain termination is a unifying mechanism for COL1A1 null alleles in osteogenesis imperfecta type I cell strains. Am J Hum Genet 59:799–809
181. Wilson LC, Hall CM (2002) Albright's hereditary osteodystrophy and pseudohypoparathyroidism. Semin Musculoskelet Radiol 6:273–283
182. Wroe SF, Kelsey G, Skinner JA, Bodle D, Ball ST, Beechey CV, Peters J, Williamson CM (2000) An imprinted transcript, antisense to Nesp, adds complexity to the cluster of imprinted genes at the mouse Gnas locus. Proc Natl Acad Sci U S A 97: 3342–3346
183. Yasui DH, Peddada S, Bieda MC, Vallero RO, Hogart A, Nagarajan RP, Thatcher KN, Farnham PJ, Lasalle JM (2007) Integrated epigenomic analyses of neuronal MeCP2 reveal a role for long-range interaction with active genes. Proc Natl Acad Sci U S A 104:19416–19421
184. Yavropoulou MP, Yovos JG (2008) Osteoclastogenesis – current knowledge and future perspectives. J Musculoskelet Neuronal Interact 8:204–216
185. Yousfi M, Lasmoles F, Marie PJ (2002) TWIST inactivation reduces CBFA1/RUNX2 expression and DNA binding to the osteocalcin promoter in osteoblasts. Biochem Biophys Res Commun 297:641–644
186. Zak BM, Crawford BE, Esko JD (2002) Hereditary multiple exostoses and heparan sulfate polymerization. Biochim Biophys Acta 1573:346–355
187. Zhou G, Zheng Q, Engin F, Munivez E, Chen Y, Sebald E, Krakow D, Lee B (2006) Dominance of SOX9 function over RUNX2 during skeletogenesis. Proc Natl Acad Sci U S A 103:19004–19009
188. Zhou Z, Han JY, Xi CX, Xie JX, Feng X, Wang CY, Mei L, Xiong WC (2008) HMGB1 regulates RANKL-induced osteoclastogenesis in a manner dependent on RAGE. J Bone Miner Res 23:1084–1096
189. Zhou Z, Immel D, Xi CX, Bierhaus A, Feng X, Mei L, Nawroth P, Stern DM, Xiong WC (2006) Regulation of osteoclast function and bone mass by RAGE. J Exp Med 203:1067–1080
190. Zysman L, Lotan M, Ben-Zeev B (2006) Osteoporosis in Rett syndrome: a study on normal values. Scientific World J 6:1619–1630

2. Tissue Interactions in Long Bone Development

Céline Colnot and Tamara Alliston

2.1 Introduction

Most skeletal elements of the adult vertebrate are composed of several tissues: cartilage, bone, bone marrow, and blood vessels. Tissue organization within the skeletal elements is established during embryonic development through various stages of patterning, cellular condensation, differentiation, and morphogenesis. The tissues at the sites of skeletogenesis constitute a unique microenvironment that coordinates the development of each bone [14, 44, 45, 51, 72]. Coordination among bone, cartilage, vasculature, and hematopoietic cells is mediated by conserved signaling pathways, including those initiated by the hedgehog, Wnt, fibroblast growth factor (FGF), transforming growth factor-β (TGF-β), and bone morphogenetic protein (BMP) family ligands. The fact that the function of all resident cell types is controlled by a common set of regulatory pathways is integral to the inter-tissue interactions that are required for skeletal development. Growth factor cues from the microenvironment intersect with cell-intrinsic factors, such as growth factor receptors or the lineage-specific transcription factors, Sox9 and Runx2. Each cell type expresses a unique complement of cell-intrinsic factors that dictate its response to the same growth factor signal. In addition, the specific localization or compartmentalization of the receptors and ligands establishes feedback loops that finely tune skeletal growth and development.

Discrimination of the effects of these cascades on the differentiation of each cell type is complicated. Recently, the use of tissue-specific genetic mouse models has added a powerful new tool that complements classical embryological approaches and allows dissection of the role of each pathway in the tissue interactions that lead to skeletal development. This chapter will review the tissue interactions required for long bone development, where the interdependent development of bone and cartilage is particularly evident. In addition, it will review the current understanding of the cell's intrinsic and extrinsic factors that coordinate the development of multiple tissue types during skeletogenesis.

2.2 Cell Fate Decisions in Early Bone Development

While most bones of the cranial skeleton form via intramembranous ossification, bones of the axial and appendicular skeletons form via endochondral ossification. Both processes are initiated by the condensation of mesenchymal cells.

F. Bronner et al. (eds.), *Bone and Development*, Topics in Bone Biology 6,
DOI 10.1007/978-1-84882-822-3_2,

The signals that induce these condensations are still poorly understood, but close physical contact between the mesenchymal cells is critical in promoting skeletal cell fate decisions and subsequent differentiation [34]. Mesenchymal cells differentiate directly into osteoblasts during intramembranous ossification, but give rise to chondrocytes and osteoblasts during endochondral ossification. Cell fate selection and cell differentiation are directed by the expression of essential lineage-specific transcription factors, Sox9 and Runx2. Secreted factors, such as Wnts, shift the balance of activity between the chondrogenic Sox9 and the osteogenic Runx2 to drive the differentiation pathway selected by the common osteochondroprogenitors. During intramembranous ossification, cells are first exposed to high levels of Wnt signaling, which leads to increased *Runx2* and decreased *Sox9* expression, and guides the cells toward osteogenesis. However, the opposite occurs in endochondral ossification [21]. Shortly after the initial condensation of limb mesenchyme, cells in the center of the condensation begin to differentiate into chondrocytes, while those at the periphery elongate and form the perichondrium (Fig. 2.1). Later, during endochondral ossification, cells in the perichondrium are exposed to higher levels of Wnt signaling, and thus, are driven to osteogenesis.

The early emergence of two cell lineages from a common mesenchymal progenitor establishes interactions that govern endochondral ossification. Thus, cartilage–perichondrium interactions are central to early long bone development. Following initial tissue interactions, more complex interactions occur because of the arrival of blood vessels (Fig. 2.1). This triggers the replacement of the cartilage template by bone and bone marrow, and regulates osteoblast differentiation. Blood vessels also bring in cells that will form the hematopoietic compartment of the bone marrow, as well as matrix-resorbing cells that remove the cartilage matrix and cooperate with osteoblasts to build, maintain, and remodel the bone matrix throughout life [28, 54, 60].

2.3 Intrinsic Re gulation of Chondrogenesis and Osteogenesis

2.3.1 Chondrocyte Differentiation

Chondrocyte proliferation and differentiation maintain normal skeletal development and growth (Fig. 2.1). Chondrocytes near the

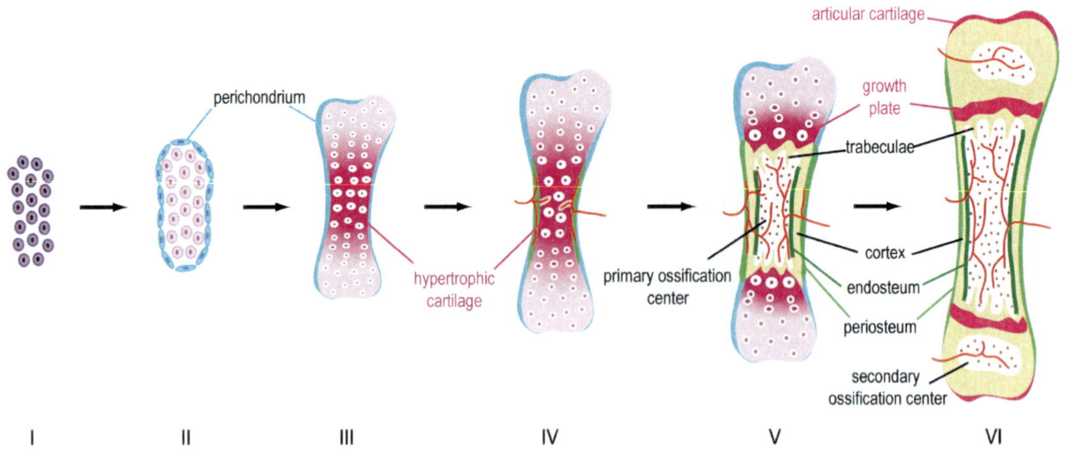

Figure 2.1. Stages of endochondral ossification. *I*: mesenchymal condensations; *II*: cartilage template; *III*: chondrocyte hypertrophy; *IV*: vascular invasion; *V*: formation of the primary ossification center; and *VI*: formation of the secondary ossification center and longitudinal growth.

periphery of the cartilage template proliferate, and, as they grow toward the center of the cartilage elements, they differentiate into prehypertrophic and hypertrophic chondrocytes, causing the template to grow, be vascularized, and ossified. During this process, hypertrophic cartilage is removed, whereas chondrocytes continue to be produced in the periarticular region. This coupling of proliferation and differentiation forms the growth plate and supports longitudinal bone growth. Successful coordination of this process requires the integration of signals derived from numerous sources by the intrinsic factors present in each cell type. Chondrocytes produce factors that regulate the progression of endochondral ossification, directly or in cooperation with other cell types. For example, hypoxia inducible factor 1 (HIF1) alpha and vascular endothelial growth factor A (VEGFA) found in chondrocytes are essential for cell survival and differentiation [75, 93]. Indian hedgehog (Ihh) in chondrocytes stimulates chondrocyte proliferation via the Ihh receptors Smo and Ptc-1 [58, 79]. Other factors that regulate chondrocyte proliferation are of the TGF-β family, including multiple isoforms of TGF-β and BMPs [62, 63, 74, 97]. These ligands and their receptors are expressed and active in chondrocytes and perichondrial cells (see Table 2.1). Members of the FGF family antagonize the proliferative effects of Ihh and BMPs primarily through the FGF receptor isoform FGFR3, expressed by the chondrocytes [72]. However, the ligand of FGFR3, FGF18, is expressed in perichondrial cells [70]. Other growth factor pathways act on the two cell populations that together permit functional paracrine FGF signaling. An example is Ihh that mediates some effects of both FGF and BMP signaling on chondrocyte proliferation (see next section) [62, 74].

The transition from proliferation to hypertrophy is controlled by chondrocyte-intrinsic and extrinsic signals. The transcription factors, Runx2 and Runx3, are upregulated in prehypertrophic and hypertrophic chondrocytes to regulate chondrocyte maturation via Ihh [29, 46, 82, 91]. As will be described subsequently, this transition is also under the control of the parathyroid hormone - related protein (PTHrP) receptor that is expressed in the prehypertrophic chondrocytes, specifically to prevent early maturation in response to its ligand PTHrP. PTHrP expression is mediated by a TGF-β and Ihh-responsive pathway in the perichondrium [3, 51, 52, 77]. In addition, hypertrophy is stimulated by BMP signaling, through either perichondrial cells or chondrocytes [49].

When chondrocytes become hypertrophic, they express genes that set up the steps leading to endochondral ossification [4, 17]. Hypertrophic chondrocytes secrete extracellular matrix components that allow matrix mineralization [48, 68], and, at the same time, produce matrix degrading enzymes that make cartilage removal possible; they thus induce terminal differentiation and cell death [19, 37, 38, 80]. Removal of hypertrophic cartilage when blood vessels enter and bring in matrix-resorbing cells requires VEGF, released by hypertrophic chondrocytes themselves [33].

2.3.2 Osteoblast Differentiation

Bone formation follows cartilage formation during endochondral ossification. Once chondrogenesis is initiated in the mesenchymal condensations, perichondrial cells at the periphery of the cartilage differentiate into osteoblasts. This initial step of osteogenesis is, as mentioned earlier, stimulated by high Wnt signaling in the perichondrium. This in turn induces the upregulation of *Runx2* and downregulation of *Sox9* to allow osteoblast differentiation [21]. Factors that act upstream of Runx2 to enhance osteoblast differentiation include Msx2, Satb2, and Bapx1 [25, 76, 84]. Factors that inhibit differentiation include Twist1 and Shn3 [7, 39, 44]. The transcription factor Osx is also required for bone formation [67] and, with Runx2, can directly induce the expression of osteoblast-specific genes, such as *osteocalcin* and *collagen type 1*. Both *Osx*- and *Runx2*-null mutant mice lack osteoblasts, but Runx2 is upstream of Osx in the transcriptional cascade [67]. Following the transition from osteochondroprogenitors to osteoblasts, another transcription factor, ATF4,

Table 2.1. Key factors regulating tissue interactions in skeletal development

Tissue/cell type	Genes	Effects on chondrocytes	Effects on osteoblasts–EC–OC
Cartilage/chondrocytes	*Sox9*	Promotes chondrogenesis, inhibits CH hypertrophy	Inhibits osteogenesis
	Runx2	Stimulates CH differentiation and hypertrophy	Indirectly stimulates OB differentiation via C
	Ihh/Smo/Ptc	Stimulates CH proliferation, regulates CH maturation	Stimulates OB differentiation
	Pthrp-r	Delays CH hypertrophy	
	Vegf	Promotes CH survival	Stimulates OB differentiation, recruits OC and EC
	Bmp2,3,4,5,7	Promotes CH proliferation and differentiation	Stimulates OB differentiation
	Fgfr1 and 3	Limits CH proliferation and differentiation	
	Mmp13	Degrades ECM, stimulates terminal differentiation	
	Tgf-β	Promotes chondrogenesis	
Perichondrium/osteoblasts	*Runx2*	Inhibits CH proliferation and hypertrophy	Stimulates OB differentiation
	Twist1	Favors CH hypertrophy	
	Fgf18	Inhibits CH proliferation and differentiation	Delays OB differentiation
	Smo/Ptc		Stimulates OB differentiation
	Pthrp	Decreases CH hypertrophy	
	Vegf		Stimulates OB differentiation, recruits OC and EC
	Bmp2,6,7	Stimulates CH proliferation, inhibits CH hypertrophy	
	Fgf7,8,17		
	Fgfr1 and 2		Delays OB differentiation
	Wnt5a	Promotes CH hypertrophy	Promotes ossification
	Mmp13		Remodel ECM, promotes OB differentiation
	Mt1-mmp		Promotes OB differentiation, inhibits mineralization
	Opg		Inhibits OC formation
	Rankl		Activates OC
	Tgf-β	Inhibits CH hypertrophy via PTHrP and FGF18	Promotes proliferation, Inhibits terminal OB differentiation, regulates OC differentiation
Blood vessels/EC	*Vegf-r*		Stimulates angiogenesis
Osteoclasts	*Mmp9*	Degrades ECM, stimulates CH terminal differentiation	Stimulates OB differentiation
	Rank		Activates OC
	EprhinB2		Stimulates OB differentiation
	Tgf-β		Regulates OC differentiation

C cartilage; *CH* chondrocytes; *OB* osteoblasts; *OC* osteoclasts; *EC* endothelial cells; *ECM* extracellular matrix.

plays a role in the transition to mature osteoblasts [89]. These transcription factors regulate osteoblast differentiation within the perichondrium to form the bone collar and regulate osteoblast differentiation in the cells in the primary ossification centers that form bone trabeculae in the metaphysis.

Many of the growth factors that regulate chondrocyte differentiation also direct osteoblast differentiation by regulating the expression and activity of this web of osteogenic transcription factors. For example, Runx2 integrates signals from FGF, integrin, BMP, TGF-β, and Wnt pathways through different mechanisms, including regulated Runx2 expression, phosphorylation, degradation, and interaction with transcriptional coactivators and corepressors. In this way, the cell intrinsic and extrinsic regulators of osteoblast differentiation determine the progression of osteoblast differentiation [40, 70, 74]. These regulatory networks are the target in both osteoblasts and chondrocytes of other tissue signals that interact with bone and cartilage during development.

2.4 Two-Way Interactions Between Cartilage and Bone

2.4.1 Tissue Manipulations Demonstrate the Interconnection Between Cartilage and Bone Development

The perichondrium plays a major role in the coordinated progression of endochondral ossification. This thin layer of cells, which surrounds the cartilage anlagen and persists around the cartilage, plays an important role in the paracrine regulation of chondrocyte proliferation and differentiation. Cartilage and perichondrium are closely associated during long bone development and secrete extracellular factors that can easily diffuse from one compartment to the other. This diffusion is essential, because ligands that are expressed exclusively by the perichondrium must signal through specific receptors in chondrocytes. This means that a functional signaling pathway requires both cell populations. The skeleton exploits this compartmentalization of ligand and receptor expression to provide additional levels of specificity and control for the many endocrine and paracrine pathways that impact endochondral ossification.

In parallel with genetic manipulations, classic approaches in embryology have revealed the important role of these tissue interactions in perichondrium and cartilage maturation. Culture of chick cartilage templates in the absence of the perichondrium showed that the perichondrium inhibits chondrocyte proliferation and hypertrophy [57]. Perichondrial removal also prevents terminal differentiation and delays vascular invasion of the hypertrophic cartilage [16] (Fig. 2.2), probably because the vascular network is established in the perichondrium before it can invade the hypertrophic cartilage (see below for the role of angiogenesis). Furthermore, skeletal elements without perichondrium cannot ossify normally, even when placed in a vascular environment that normally supports the replacement of cartilage by bone and bone marrow [16] (Fig. 2.2). Tissue recombination experiments with genetically labeled cells have shown that ossification is impaired because of the absence of osteoblast precursors that reside in the perichondrium [16]. Recombination of wild-type cartilage templates with a perichondrium from Rosa26-labeled mice can rescue ossification via Rosa26-labeled osteoblasts [16]. In parallel, these studies showed that stem cells derived from blood vessels do not give rise to osteoblasts, further supporting the role of the perichondrium as the primary source of osteoblasts [16]. Tissue manipulations have also helped to elucidate mechanisms of action of growth factors in the perichondrium. For example, TGF-β requires the presence of a perichondrium to fully inhibit chondrocyte hypertrophy [2, 66]. The perichondrium therefore is not only the source of osteoblasts that invade the hypertrophic cartilage to form metaphysis, but is also the source of signals that regulate osteogenesis and chondrogenesis [14, 16].

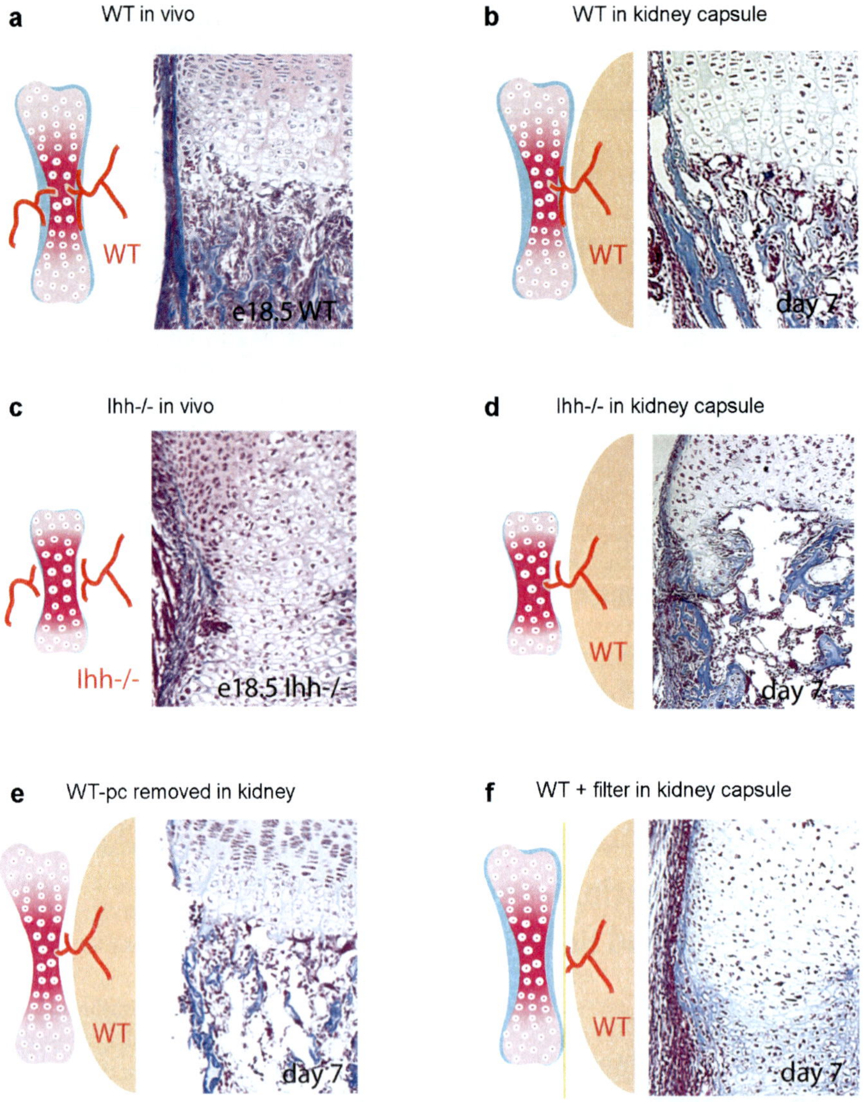

Figure 2.2. Tissue interactions required for endochondral ossification. (**a**) Normal bone development in vivo. (**b**) Normal development of wild-type skeletal elements is recapitulated after transplantation in wild-type kidney capsules. (**c**) Cartilage and perichondrial defects in $Ihh^{-/-}$ mutant mice prevent vascular invasion and ossification. (**d**) Partial rescue of endochondral ossification in $Ihh^{-/-}$ skeletal elements transplanted in wild-type kidney capsule that provides wild-type blood vessels. (**e**) Delayed vascular invasion and impaired ossification of skeletal elements stripped of the perichondrium and transplanted into wild-type kidney capsule. (**f**) Inhibition of vascular invasion and endochondral ossification in wild-type skeletal elements transplanted in the kidney capsule, but separated from the host vasculature by a filter [15, 16].

2.4.2 Signals Produced by Chondrocytes Influence Perichondrium Maturation and Osteoblast Differentiation

Signals from chondrocytes influence the maturation of perichondrium and the recruitment of perichondrial cells into matrix-synthetic osteoblasts. Some of these signals, such as Ihh, are produced only by chondrocytes, whereas others, such as BMP and FGF, are produced by many cell populations (see Table 2.1). In addition to inducing osteoblast differentiation via Ptc-1 and Smo expressed in osteoblast precursors, Ihh directs the location of osteoblast differentiation within the perichondrium [56]. This signal is required for osteoblast differentiation in the adjacent perichondrium and acts on ectopic cells within the proliferating zone, which express *Ihh* to induce osteoblast differentiation in the perichondrium [12, 13].

By regulating chondrocyte proliferation and differentiation, FGFs and BMPs influence osteoblast differentiation in the perichondrium indirectly. The effects of FGFs and BMPs on osteogenesis, are mediated in part by their ability to regulate the expression of *Ihh* in chondrocytes [62, 63, 74]. FGFs and BMPs originating from cartilage also can directly regulate osteoblast differentiation via their receptors expressed in the perichondrium [40, 70, 97]. As true for cartilage development, FGFs act by delaying and BMPs by enhancing osteoblast differentiation. FGFs regulate chondrocyte differentiation primarily through FGFR3, but in the perichondrium FGF action is mediated by FGFR1 and FGFR2. This makes it easier to differentiate the action of these growth factors on chondrocytes and osteoblasts [72]. However, the BMP receptors in cartilage and perichondrium are the same. Consequently, the effects of BMPs in the perichondrium are difficult to distinguish from their effects on cartilage, until the BMP receptors can be inactivated specifically in the perichondrium. Another difficulty in addressing the role of these growth factors in skeletal tissue is the functional redundancy among the members of the same family of molecules. As a result, mutations in FGFs or BMPs do not always induce skeletal phenotypes such as those described in Chap. 1 of this volume and elsewhere [27, 64, 78]. Some mutations, on the other hand, cannot be compensated for by other members of the same family, and because they cause early embryonic lethality, their effect on skeletal development cannot be assessed [65, 70].

2.4.3 Signals Originating from the Perichondrium Influence Chondrocyte Differentiation

The perichondrium expresses signaling molecules that, through several feedback loops, regulate osteoblast and chondrocyte differentiation and the organization of the growth plate. Many feedback loops require perichondrial cells as well as chondrocytes to be complete. A classic example is the expression of *PTHrP* by perichondrial cells in the periarticular region. PTHrP activates its receptors in proliferative and pre-hypertrophic chondrocytes, inducing the transition from proliferation to hypertrophy. The level of *PTHrP* expression is a net result of many interacting signaling pathways. *Ihh*, expressed by chondrocytes, induces *PTHrP* expression indirectly, by inducing the expression of *TGF-β2* in the perichondrium [3, 43, 52, 77, 86].

Another growth factor, FGF18, expressed in the perichondrium, plays a central role in the feedback loops regulating perichondrium–cartilage interactions. FGF18 and potentially other FGF family members originating from the perichondrium bind to FGFR3 and FGFR1 in chondrocytes to prevent chondrocyte proliferation and differentiation [20, 23, 70]. Induction of TGF-β expression by Ihh induces the perichondrial cell expression not only of PTHrP, but also of FGF18 [66]. PTHrP and FGF18, together, confer the inhibitory effects of TGF-β on hypertrophy, which are lost or severely reduced without input by the perichondrium [1, 24].

The BMP pathway also utilizes the combination of perichondrial cells and chondrocytes to exert its effects on cartilage. BMP2, 4, 5, and 7, expressed in the perichondrium, stimulate cartilage growth via their chondrocyte receptors [62, 63, 74, 97]. Wnt family members that are involved in early cell fate decisions, as discussed earlier, also play a role in perichondrium-mediated cartilage differentiation. For example, Wnt5a, produced by the perichondrium, regulates the transition from proliferating to prehypertrophic chondrocytes [35]. Here again, tissue-specific genetic deletions will help define the reciprocal roles of various growth factors on cartilage and perichondrium, doing so by deletion of the growth factor in a given tissue or its receptors and downstream targets.

2.5 Four-Way Interactions Among Cartilage, Bone, Blood Vessels, and Matrix-Resorbing Cells

2.5.1 Role of Angiogenesis

Angiogenesis is crucial in bone development. Before the initiation of skeletogenesis, blood vessels are distributed uniformly within the limb bud and then must regress for the occurrence of mesenchymal condensations [90]. This initial patterning of limb vasculature is directly under the influence of Sox9, which controls skeletal cell differentiation and *Vegf* expression in mesenchymal condensations [30]. Whether angiogenesis reciprocally plays a role in regulating mesenchymal condensations and early skeletogenesis is not yet established, but its role during the later stages of endochondral ossification is better understood. Maturation of perichondrium owing to factors secreted by adjacent differentiating chondrocytes and intrinsic osteogenic factors (see above) induces a first wave of angiogenesis within the perichondrium. Terminal differentiation of chondrocytes supports a second wave of angiogenesis for the formation of marrow cavity [19, 92, 94] (Fig. 2.1). The waves of angiogenesis are triggered by high levels of VEGFA, first in the perichondrium and then in the hypertrophic cartilage [94]. Invasion of the perichondrium and hypertrophic cartilage by blood vessels and matrix-resorbing cells initiates a new series of tissue interactions.

As is the case for cartilage–perichondrium interactions, tissue manipulations have helped identify the functions of the cell types involved in this process. For example, physically blocking the migration of the blood vessels inhibits cartilage removal and migration of osteoclasts and osteoblasts to form the primary ossification center [16] (Fig. 2.2). Blocking angiogenesis by inhibiting VEGF delays chondrocyte terminal differentiation, osteoblast differentiation, and osteoclast recruitment [16, 33]. VEGF is essential for coordination of the key steps of endochondral ossification, which involve chondrocyte differentiation, vascular invasion, recruitment of osteoclast, and osteoblast differentiation [92–94]. Another factor, Ihh, that plays a vital role in chondrocyte and osteoblast differentiation, is also involved in synchronizing angiogenesis with chondrogenesis and osteogenesis [15]. This concept was demonstrated by transplanting $Ihh^{-/-}$ skeletal elements into a wild-type vascular environment, where the recruitment of wild-type blood vessels can partially rescue the ossification defect. However, in this environment, $Ihh^{-/-}$ endothelial cells cannot survive; this indicates an intrinsic defect in angiogenesis combined with abnormal cartilage differentiation and a deficient perichondrium (Fig. 2.2) [15].

2.5.2 Role of Matrix-Resorbing Cells

A unique feature of long bone development is the transient nature of the cartilage templates that establish the shape and size of the future skeletal elements. These templates must be removed before the bones can fully ossify and before the bone marrow compartment is formed. Removal of cartilage templates and primary spongiosa is primarily due to the action of matrix-resorbing cells, including septoclasts and osteoclasts [28, 53]. Unlike the osteochondroprogenitor cells of the long bones, which are of mesenchymal origin, osteoclasts are derived from the monocyte/macrophage lineage of the hematopoietic progenitor cell population. Arriving by way of the vascular invasion of the cartilage template, osteoclasts degrade mineralized matrix by generating an acidic microenvironment that is rich in proteolytic enzymes such as cathepsin K. The degradation of the cartilaginous template is also supported by the action of many extracellular enzymes, such as MMPs and ADAMs, which are produced by hypertrophic chondrocytes, osteoblasts, and endothelial cells, as well as by osteoclasts [8, 22, 28, 80, 88].

In addition to removing mineralized matrix, osteoclasts and other matrix-resorbing cells release and activate latent growth factors that are sequestered within the cartilage and bone, and regulate vascularization, cell proliferation, and differentiation. Thus, matrix-resorbing cells are actively involved in the multitissue control of endochondral ossification. Osteoclasts release VEGF; this attracts blood vessels and acts on the adjacent perichondrium to stimulate osteoblast migration within the primary ossification center [5, 33, 73, 88]. Likewise, the inactivation of latent TGF-β by osteoclasts promotes recruitment and proliferation of osteochondroprogenitors to the sites of osteogenesis. In this way, osteoclasts play a central role in the initiation of osteogenesis, and by interacting with the osteoblasts, regulate bone formation and remodeling throughout life. Much is known about these signaling pathways in postnatal bone development and growth (see below), but less is understood about the interactions that occur during the early stages of endochondral ossification or how the migration of osteoclasts within the perichondrium triggers osteoblast differentiation.

2.6 Are These Tissue Interactions Maintained During Postnatal Life?

Bone continues to develop postnatally and many tissue interactions that take place in the developing skeleton remain active in the adult bone. Numerous studies have focused on bone remodeling in coordination with bone deposition. Osteoclast activation requires the production of receptor activator of nuclear factor kappa B ligand (RANKL) by osteoblasts, which binds to its receptor, RANK, on osteoclasts and their precursors [9]. More recently, ephrin ligands and receptors have been implicated as factors that mediate the bidirectional communication between osteoblasts and osteoclasts [96]. In addition, the transcriptional control of osteoblast differentiation is linked with the transcriptional control of osteoclastogenesis, as indicated by the genetic analyses of the AP1 family of proteins [44].

Interestingly, a number of molecules that play a role in long bone development during the embryonic stages are also involved in the cross-talk between osteoblasts and osteoclasts postnatally. Factors such as TGF-β can regulate both osteoblast and osteoclast function by the direct action on both cell types and by regulating osteoblast expression of osteoclast regulatory factors, like RANKL and osteoprotegrin (OPG) [1]. Likewise, BMP can act directly and indirectly to regulate osteoclast function [40–42, 71]. Other factors that regulate osteoclast activity do so via their actions on osteoblasts. While loss of Ihh signaling in mature osteoblasts via conditional inactivation of *Smo* prevents age-related bone loss, increased Ihh signaling in mice lacking *Ptch1* in mature osteoblasts is correlated with enhanced osteoblast differentiation and excessive bone remodeling [60, 69]. Ihh signaling acts primarily in osteoblasts to regulate osteoclast differentiation by controlling the expression of PTHrP and RANKL expression [60]. All the PTH and PTHrP actions on osteoclasts – which do not express PTH receptors – are mediated by the regulation of factors such as RANKL and OPG in osteoblasts and other cell types [61]. Disruption of these regulatory pathways has pathological consequences and can result in osteoporosis. Studying these tissue interactions in skeletal development has led to the development of a PTH-based therapy for osteoporosis, currently the only anabolic therapy. Many of the other pathways involved in skeletal development, including TGF-β, BMP, and Wnt, are now receiving attention as potential targets of anabolic therapies.

In the course of development of the bone marrow compartment, osteoblasts also interact with hematopoietic stem cells (HSCs) to regulate the hematopoietic niche and to initiate hematopoiesis [11, 36]. These interactions remain critical during postnatal life. Again, the key molecules that have been involved in various stages of bone development become essential in osteoblast–hematopoietic stem cell interactions. The Wnt signaling pathway that determines the cell fate decisions at the early condensation stage in the embryo and that subsequently plays a role in chondrocyte differentiation, is necessary to maintain hematopoietic stem cell quiescence and renewal [32]. Signaling through the BMP and PTH-PTHrP receptors continues after skeletogenesis and is essential for the regulation of hematopoietic stem cells by osteoblasts [10, 95].

In the adult, another level of complexity is the systemic regulation of bone mass via hormonal control [26, 55]. The skeleton plays a central role in regulating energy homeostasis and thereby affects many other tissues and organs, such as lipid metabolism and the central nervous system.

Finally, the process of bone development is recapitulated during skeletal regeneration. Although bone repair involves inflammatory cytokines and response to mechanical forces, the intrinsic regulation of chondrocyte and osteoblast differentiation is under the control of the same transcription factors and secreted molecules as in the course of development [31, 87]; interactions among cartilage, bone, osteoclasts, and blood vessels are critical to the process of bone healing [6, 18]. Mechanical forces have been shown to drive the fate of osteochondroprogenitors and to determine whether skeletal repair occurs by endochondral or intramembranous ossification [18, 83]. The mechanisms guiding these decisions remain unclear, but it is enticing to think that Wnt signaling may participate in this decision process, as it does in osteoblast/osteocyte development. Most of the growth factors involved in bone development are also implicated in bone repair, but the mechanisms by which these factors coordinate the multiple tissue interactions required for skeletal repair remain to be unraveled [47, 50, 59, 81, 85]. Considering that fracture repair is only successful in four of five cases, understanding the tissue interactions that control skeletal development and repair may improve the likelihood, quality, or speed of fracture repair.

2.7 Conclusion/Perspectives

As now known, cartilage and perichondrium development cannot be dissociated. The tight interactions between cartilage and perichondrium are particularly obvious at the molecular level, as several feedback loops are needed to regulate cell proliferation and differentiation. Moreover, many of these critical signaling pathways coordinate chondrogenesis and osteogenesis with angiogenesis and osteoclastogenesis. Thus, the differentiation of chondrocytes, osteoblasts, vascular cells, and matrix-resorbing cells is inseparable during skeletal development. Although cell differentiation on the whole can be recapitulated in vitro, the differentiation of one cell type in vivo is directly under the influence of adjacent cell types. To better understand these cellular and tissue interactions, animal models and genetic approaches can help define the role played by specific factors in cells and tissues. Animal models will continue to help elucidate defects in skeletal development and will be instrumental in the development of new treatments for skeletal repair and degenerative diseases such as osteoporosis.

References

1. Alliston T, Piek E, Derynck R (2008) TGF-β family signaling in skeletal development, maintenance, and disease. In: Derynck R, Miyazono K (eds) The TGF-β family. Cold Spring Harbor, Woodbury, pp 667–723
2. Alvarez J, Horton J, Sohn P, Serra R (2001) The perichondrium plays an important role in mediating the effects of TGF-beta1 on endochondral bone formation. Dev Dyn 221(3):311–321
3. Alvarez J, Sohn P, Zeng X, Doetschman T, Robbins DJ, Serra R (2002) TGFbeta2 mediates the effects of hedgehog on hypertrophic differentiation and PTHrP expression. Development 129(8):1913–1924
4. Amling M, Neff L, Tanaka S, Inoue D, Kuida K, Weir E, Philbrick WM, Broadus AE, Baron R (1997) Bcl-2 lies downstream of parathyroid hormone-related peptide in a signaling pathway that regulates chondrocyte maturation during skeletal development. J Cell Biol 136(1):205–213
5. Andersen TL, del Carmen Ovejero M, Kirkegaard T, Lenhard T, Foged NT, Delaisse JM (2004) A scrutiny of matrix metalloproteinases in osteoclasts: evidence for heterogeneity and for the presence of MMPs synthesized by other cells. Bone 35(5):1107–1119
6. Behonick DJ, Xing Z, Lieu S, Buckley JM, Lotz JC, Marcucio RS, Werb Z, Miclau T, Colnot C (2007) Role of matrix metalloproteinase 13 in both endochondral and intramembranous ossification during skeletal regeneration. PLoS ONE 2(11):e1150
7. Bialek P, Kern B, Yang X, Schrock M, Sosic D, Hong N, Wu H, Yu K, Ornitz DM, Olson EN, Justice MJ, Karsenty G (2004) A twist code determines the onset of osteoblast differentiation. Dev Cell 6(3):423–435
8. Boissy P, Lenhard TR, Kirkegaard T, Peschon JJ, Black RA, Delaisse JM, del Carmen Ovejero M (2003) An assessment of ADAMs in bone cells: absence of TACE activity prevents osteoclast recruitment and the formation of the marrow cavity in developing long bones. FEBS Lett 553(3):257–261
9. Boyle WJ, Simonet WS, Lacey DL (2003) Osteoclast differentiation and activation. Nature 423(6937): 337–342
10. Calvi LM, Adams GB, Weibrecht KW, Weber JM, Olson DP, Knight MC, Martin RP, Schipani E, Divieti P, Bringhurst FR, Milner LA, Kronenberg HM, Scadden DT (2003) Osteoblastic cells regulate the haematopoietic stem cell niche. Nature 425(6960):841–846
11. Chan CK, Chen CC, Luppen CA, Kim JB, Deboer AT, Wei K, Helms JA, Kuo CJ, Kraft DL, Weissman IL (2008) Endochondral ossification is required for haematopoietic stem-cell niche formation. Nature 457(7228):490–494
12. Chung UI, Lanske B, Lee K, Li E, Kronenberg H (1998) The parathyroid hormone/parathyroid hormone-related peptide receptor coordinates endochondral bone development by directly controlling chondrocyte differentiation. Proc Natl Acad Sci U S A 95(22): 13030–13035
13. Chung UI, Schipani E, McMahon AP, Kronenberg HM (2001) Indian hedgehog couples chondrogenesis to osteogenesis in endochondral bone development. J Clin Invest 107(3):295–304

14. Colnot C (2005) Cellular and molecular interactions regulating skeletogenesis. J Cell Biochem 95(4): 688–697
15. Colnot C, de la Fuente L, Huang S, Hu D, Lu C, St-Jacques B, Helms JA (2005) Indian hedgehog synchronizes skeletal angiogenesis and perichondrial maturation with cartilage development. Development 132(5):1057–1067
16. Colnot C, Lu C, Hu D, Helms JA (2004) Distinguishing the contributions of the perichondrium, cartilage and vascular endothelium to skeletal development. Dev Biol 269:55–69
17. Colnot C, Sidhu SS, Balmain N, Poirier F (2001) Uncoupling of chondrocyte death and vascular invasion in mouse galectin 3 null mutant bones. Dev Biol 229(1):203–214
18. Colnot C, Thompson Z, Miclau T, Werb Z, Helms JA (2003) Altered fracture repair in the absence of MMP9. Development 130(17):4123–4133
19. Colnot CI, Helms JA (2001) A molecular analysis of matrix remodeling and angiogenesis during long bone development. Mech Dev 100(2):245–250
20. Colvin JS, Bohne BA, Harding GW, McEwen DG, Ornitz DM (1996) Skeletal overgrowth and deafness in mice lacking fibroblast growth factor receptor 3. Nat Genet 12(4):390–397
21. Day TF, Guo X, Garrett-Beal L, Yang Y (2005) Wnt/beta-catenin signaling in mesenchymal progenitors controls osteoblast and chondrocyte differentiation during vertebrate skeletogenesis. Dev Cell 8(5): 739–750
22. Delaisse JM, Andersen TL, Engsig MT, Henriksen K, Troen T, Blavier L (2003) Matrix metalloproteinases (MMP) and cathepsin K contribute differently to osteoclastic activities. Microsc Res Tech 61(6): 504–513
23. Deng C, Wynshaw-Boris A, Zhou F, Kuo A, Leder P (1996) Fibroblast growth factor receptor 3 is a negative regulator of bone growth. Cell 84(6):911–921
24. Derynck R, Schneider RA, Piek E, Alliston T (2008) TGF-β family signaling in mesenchymal differentiation. In: Derynck R, Miyazono K (eds) The TGF-β family. Cold Spring Harbor, Woodbury. pp 613–655
25. Dobreva G, Chahrour M, Dautzenberg M, Chirivella L, Kanzler B, Farinas I, Karsenty G, Grosschedl R (2006) SATB2 is a multifunctional determinant of craniofacial patterning and osteoblast differentiation. Cell 125(5): 971–986
26. Ducy P, Amling M, Takeda S, Priemel M, Schilling AF, Beil FT, Shen J, Vinson C, Rueger JM, Karsenty G (2000) Leptin inhibits bone formation through a hypothalamic relay: a central control of bone mass. Cell 100(2):197–207
27. Dudley AT, Lyons KM, Robertson EJ (1995) A requirement for bone morphogenetic protein-7 during development of the mammalian kidney and eye. Genes Dev 9(22):2795–2807
28. Engsig MT, Chen Q, Vu TH, Pedersen A, Therdkidsen B, Lund LR, Henriksen T, Lenhard T, Foged NT, Werb Z, Delaisse J (2000) Matrix metalloproteinase 9 and vascular endothelial growth factor are essential for osteoclast recruitment into developing long bones. J Cell Biol 151(4):1–11
29. Enomoto H, Enomoto-Iwamoto M, Iwamoto M, Nomura S, Himeno M, Kitamura Y, Kishimoto T, Komori T (2000) Cbfa1 is a positive regulatory factor in chondrocyte maturation. J Biol Chem 275(12): 8695–8702
30. Eshkar-Oren I, Viukov SV, Salameh S, Krief S, Oh CD, Akiyama H, Gerber HP, Ferrara N, Zelzer E (2009) The forming limb skeleton serves as a signaling center for limb vasculature patterning via regulation of Vegf. Development 136(8):1263–1272
31. Ferguson C, Alpern E, Miclau T, Helms JA (1999) Does adult fracture repair recapitulate embryonic skeletal formation? Mech Dev 87(1–2):57–66
32. Fleming HE, Janzen V, Lo Celso C, Guo J, Leahy KM, Kronenberg HM, Scadden DT (2008) Wnt signaling in the niche enforces hematopoietic stem cell quiescence and is necessary to preserve self-renewal in vivo. Cell Stem Cell 2(3):274–283
33. Gerber HP, Vu TH, Ryan AM, Kowalski J, Werb Z, Ferrara N (1999) VEGF couples hypertrophic cartilage remodeling, ossification and angiogenesis during endochondral bone formation. Nat Med 5(6):623–628
34. Hall BK, Miyake T (2000) All for one and one for all: condensations and the initiation of skeletal development. Bioessays 22(2):138–147
35. Hartmann C, Tabin CJ (2000) Dual roles of Wnt signaling during chondrogenesis in the chicken limb. Development 127(14):3141–3159
36. Jacenko O, Ito S, Olsen BR (1996) Skeletal and hematopoietic defects in mice transgenic for collagen X. Ann N Y Acad Sci 785:278–280
37. Jimenez MJ, Balbin M, Alvarez J, Komori T, Bianco P, Holmbeck K, Birkedal-Hansen H, Lopez JM, Lopez-Otin C (2001) A regulatory cascade involving retinoic acid, Cbfa1, and matrix metalloproteinases is coupled to the development of a process of perichondrial invasion and osteogenic differentiation during bone formation. J Cell Biol 155(7):1333–1344
38. Jiménez MJ, Balbín M, López JM, Alvarez J, Komori T, López-Otín C (1999) Collagenase 3 is a target of Cbfa1, a transcription factor of the runt gene family involved in bone formation. Mol Cell Biol 19(6):4431–4442
39. Jones DC, Wein MN, Oukka M, Hofstaetter JG, Glimcher MJ, Glimcher LH (2006) Regulation of adult bone mass by the zinc finger adapter protein Schnurri-3. Science 312(5777):1223–1227
40. Kamiya N, Ye L, Kobayashi T, Lucas DJ, Mochida Y, Yamauchi M, Kronenberg HM, Feng JQ, Mishina Y (2008) Disruption of BMP signaling in osteoblasts through type IA receptor (BMPRIA) increases bone mass. J Bone Miner Res 23(12):2007-2017
41. Kamiya N, Ye L, Kobayashi T, Mochida Y, Yamauchi M, Kronenberg HM, Feng JQ, Mishina Y (2008) BMP signaling negatively regulates bone mass through sclerostin by inhibiting the canonical Wnt pathway. Development 135(22):3801–3811
42. Kaneda T, Nojima T, Nakagawa M, Ogasawara A, Kaneko H, Sato T, Mano H, Kumegawa M, Hakeda Y (2000) Endogenous production of TGF-beta is essential for osteoclastogenesis induced by a combination of receptor activator of NF-kappa B ligand and macrophage-colony-stimulating factor. J Immunol 165(8): 4254–4263
43. Karaplis AC, Luz A, Glowacki J, Bronson RT, Tybulewicz VL, Kronenberg HM, Mulligan RC (1994) Lethal skeletal dysplasia from targeted disruption of the parathyroid hormone-related peptide gene. Genes Dev 8(3):277–289

44. Karsenty G (2008) Transcriptional control of skeletogenesis. Annu Rev Genomics Hum Genet 9:183–196
45. Karsenty G, Wagner EF (2002) Reaching a genetic and molecular understanding of skeletal development. Dev Cell 2(4):389–406
46. Kim IS, Otto F, Zabel B, Mundlos S (1999) Regulation of chondrocyte differentiation by Cbfa1. Mech Devel 80(2):159–170
47. Kim JB, Leucht P, Lam K, Luppen C, Ten Berge D, Nusse R, Helms JA (2007) Bone regeneration is regulated by Wnt signaling. J Bone Miner Res 22(12):1913–1923
48. Kirsch T, Nah HD, Shapiro IM, Pacifici M (1997) Regulated production of mineralization-competent matrix vesicles in hypertrophic chondrocytes. J Cell Biol 137(5):1149–1160
49. Kobayashi T, Lyons KM, McMahon AP, Kronenberg HM (2005) BMP signaling stimulates cellular differentiation at multiple steps during cartilage development. Proc Natl Acad Sci U S A 102(50):18023–18027
50. Komatsu DE, Bosch-Marce M, Semenza GL, Hadjiargyrou M (2007) Enhanced bone regeneration associated with decreased apoptosis in mice with partial HIF-1alpha deficiency. J Bone Miner Res 22(3): 366–374
51. Kronenberg HM (2003) Developmental regulation of the growth plate. Nature 423(6937):332–336
52. Lanske B, Karaplis AC, Lee K, Luz A, Vortkamp A, Pirro A, Karperien M, Defize LHK, Ho C, Mulligan RC, Abou-Samra AB, Juppner H, Segre GV, Kronenberg HM (1996) PTH/PTHrP receptor in early development and Indian hedgehog-regulated bone growth. Science 273(5275): 663–666
53. Lee ER, Lamplugh L, Shepard NL, Mort JS (1995) The septoclast, a cathepsin B-rich cell involved in the resorption of growth plate cartilage. J Histochem cytochem 43(5):523–536
54. Lee ER, Lamplugh L, Shepard NL, Mort JS (1995) The septoclast, a cathepsin B-rich cell involved in the resorption of growth plate cartilage. J Histochem Cytochem 43(5):525–536
55. Lee NK, Sowa H, Hinoi E, Ferron M, Ahn JD, Confavreux C, Dacquin R, Mee PJ, McKee MD, Jung DY, Zhang Z, Kim JK, Mauvais-Jarvis F, Ducy P, Karsenty G (2007) Endocrine regulation of energy metabolism by the skeleton. Cell 130(3):456–469
56. Long F, Chung UI, Ohba S, McMahon J, Kronenberg HM, McMahon AP (2004) Ihh signaling is directly required for the osteoblast lineage in the endochondral skeleton. Development 131(6):1309–1318
57. Long F, Linsenmayer TF (1998) Regulation of growth region cartilage proliferation and differentiation by perichondrium. Development 125(6):1067–1073
58. Long F, Zhang XM, Karp S, Yang Y, McMahon AP (2001) Genetic manipulation of hedgehog signaling in the endochondral skeleton reveals a direct role in the regulation of chondrocyte proliferation. Development 128(24): 5099–5108
59. Maes C, Coenegrachts L, Stockmans I, Daci E, Luttun A, Petryk A, Gopalakrishnan R, Moermans K, Smets N, Verfaillie CM, Carmeliet P, Bouillon R, Carmeliet G (2006) Placental growth factor mediates mesenchymal cell development, cartilage turnover, and bone remodeling during fracture repair. J Clin Invest 116(5): 1230–1242
60. Mak KK, Bi Y, Wan C, Chuang PT, Clemens T, Young M, Yang Y (2008) Hedgehog signaling in mature osteoblasts regulates bone formation and resorption by controlling PTHrP and RANKL expression. Dev Cell 14(5):674–688
61. Miao D, He B, Jiang Y, Kobayashi T, Soroceanu MA, Zhao J, Su H, Tong X, Amizuka N, Gupta A, Genant HK, Kronenberg HM, Goltzman D, Karaplis AC (2005) Osteoblast-derived PTHrP is a potent endogenous bone anabolic agent that modifies the therapeutic efficacy of administered PTH 1–34. J Clin Invest 115(9): 2402–2411
62. Minina E, Kreschel C, Naski MC, Ornitz DM, Vortkamp A (2002) Interaction of FGF, Ihh/Pthlh, and BMP signaling integrates chondrocyte proliferation and hypertrophic differentiation. Dev Cell 3(3):439–449
63. Minina E, Wenzel HM, Kreschel C, Karp S, Gaffield W, McMahon AP, Vortkamp A (2001) BMP and Ihh/PTHrP signaling interact to coordinate chondrocyte proliferation and differentiation. Development 128(22):4523–4534
64. Moon AM, Boulet AM, Capecchi MR (2000) Normal limb development in conditional mutants of Fgf4. Development 127(5):989–996
65. Moon AM, Capecchi MR (2000) Fgf8 is required for outgrowth and patterning of the limbs. Nat Genet 26(4): 455–459
66. Mukherjee A, Dong SS, Clemens T, Alvarez J, Serra R (2005) Co-ordination of TGF-beta and FGF signaling pathways in bone organ cultures. Mech Dev 122(4):557–571
67. Nakashima K, Zhou X, Kunkel G, Zhang Z, Deng JM, Behringer RR, de Crombrugghe B (2002) The novel zinc finger-containing transcription factor osterix is required for osteoblast differentiation and bone formation. Cell 108(1):17–29
68. Nurminskaya M, Linsenmayer TF (1996) Identification and characterization of up-regulated genes during chondrocyte hypertrophy. Dev Dyn 206(3):260–271
69. Ohba S, Kawaguchi H, Kugimiya F, Ogasawara T, Kawamura N, Saito T, Ikeda T, Fujii K, Miyajima T, Kuramochi A, Miyashita T, Oda H, Nakamura K, Takato T, Chung UI (2008) Patched1 haploinsufficiency increases adult bone mass and modulates Gli3 repressor activity. Dev Cell 14(5):689–699
70. Ohbayashi N, Shibayama M, Kurotaki Y, Imanishi M, Fujimori T, Itoh N, Takada S (2002) FGF18 is required for normal cell proliferation and differentiation during osteogenesis and chondrogenesis. Genes Dev 16(7): 870–879
71. Okamoto M, Murai J, Yoshikawa H, Tsumaki N (2006) Bone morphogenetic proteins in bone stimulate osteoclasts and osteoblasts during bone development. J Bone Miner Res 21(7):1022–1033
72. Ornitz DM, Marie PJ (2002) FGF signaling pathways in endochondral and intramembranous bone development and human genetic disease. Genes Dev 16(12): 1446–1465
73. Ortega N, Behonick DJ, Colnot C, Cooper DN, Werb Z (2005) Galectin-3 is a downstream regulator of matrix metalloproteinase-9 function during endochondral bone formation. Mol Biol Cell 16(6):3028–3039
74. Pathi S, Rutenberg JB, Johnson RL, Vortkamp A (1999) Interaction of Ihh and BMP/Noggin signaling during cartilage differentiation. Dev Biol 209(2):239–253

75. Provot S, Zinyk D, Gunes Y, Kathri R, Le Q, Kronenberg HM, Johnson RS, Longaker MT, Giaccia AJ, Schipani E (2007) Hif-1alpha regulates differentiation of limb bud mesenchyme and joint development. J Cell Biol 177(3):451–464
76. Satokata I, Ma L, Ohshima H, Bei M, Woo I, Nishizawa K, Maeda T, Takano Y, Uchiyama M, Heaney S, Peters H, Tang ZQ, Maxson R, Maas R (2000) Msx2 deficiency in mice causes pleiotropic defects in bone growth and ectodermal organ formation. Nat Genet 24(4): 391–395
77. Serra R, Karaplis A, Sohn P (1999) Parathyroid hormone-related peptide (PTHrP)-dependent and -independent effects of transforming growth factor beta (TGF-beta) on endochondral bone formation. J Cell Biol 145(4): 783–794
78. Solloway MJ, Dudley AT, Bikoff EK, Lyons KM, Hogan BL, Robertson EJ (1998) Mice lacking Bmp6 function. Dev Genet 22(4):321–339
79. St-Jacques B, Hammerschmidt M, McMahon AP (1999) Indian hedgehog signaling regulates proliferation and differentiation of chondrocytes and is essential for bone formation. Genes Dev 13(16):2072–2086
80. Stickens D, Behonick DJ, Ortega N, Heyer B, Hartenstein B, Yu Y, Fosang AJ, Schorpp-Kistner M, Angel P, Werb Z (2004) Altered endochondral bone development in matrix metalloproteinase 13-deficient mice. Development 131(23): 5883–5895
81. Street J, Bao M, deGuzman L, Bunting S, Peale FV, Ferrara N, Steinmetz H, Hoeffel J, Cleland JL, Daugherty A, van Bruggen N, Redmond HP, Carano RA, Filvaroff EH (2002) Vascular endothelial growth factor stimulates bone repair by promoting angiogenesis and bone turnover. Proc Natl Acad Sci U S A 99(15): 9656–9661
82. Takeda S, Bonnamy JP, Owen MJ, Ducy P, Karsenty G (2001) Continuous expression of Cbfa1 in nonhypertrophic chondrocytes uncovers its ability to induce hypertrophic chondrocyte differentiation and partially rescues Cbfa1-deficient mice. Genes Dev 15(4): 467–481
83. Thompson Z, Miclau T, Hu D, Helms JA (2002) A model for intramembranous ossification during fracture healing. J Orthop Res 20(5):1091–1098
84. Tribioli C, Lufkin T (1999) The murine Bapx1 homeobox gene plays a critical role in embryonic development of the axial skeleton and spleen. Development 126(24): 5699–5711
85. Tsuji K, Bandyopadhyay A, Harfe BD, Cox K, Kakar S, Gerstenfeld L, Einhorn T, Tabin CJ, Rosen V (2006) BMP2 activity, although dispensable for bone formation, is required for the initiation of fracture healing. Nat Genet 38(12):1424–1429
86. Vortkamp A, Lee K, Lanske B, Segre GV, Kronenberg HM, Tabin CJ (1996) Regulation of rate of cartilage differentiation by Indian hedgehog and PTH-related protein. Science 273(5275):613–622
87. Vortkamp A, Pathi S, Peretti GM, Caruso EM, Zaleske DJ, Tabin CJ, (1998) Recapitulation of signals regulating embryonic bone formation during postnatal growth and in fracture repair. Mech Dev 71(1–2): 65–76
88. Vu TH, Shipley JM, Bergers G, Berger JE, Helms JA, Hanahan D, Shapiro SD, Senior RM, Werb Z (1998) MMP-9/gelatinase B is a key regulator of growth plate angiogenesis and apoptosis of hypertrophic chondrocytes. Cell 93(3):411–422
89. Yang X, Matsuda K, Bialek P, Jacquot S, Masuoka HC, Schinke T, Li L, Brancorsini S, Sassone-Corsi P, Townes TM, Hanauer A, Karsenty G (2004) ATF4 is a substrate of RSK2 and an essential regulator of osteoblast biology; implication for Coffin-Lowry syndrome. Cell 117(3):387–398
90. Yin M, Pacifici M (2001) Vascular regression is required for mesenchymal condensation and chondrogenesis in the developing limb. Dev Dyn 222(3):522–533
91. Yoshida CA, Yamamoto H, Fujita T, Furuichi T, Ito K, Inoue K, Yamana K, Zanma A, Takada K, Ito Y, Komori T (2004) Runx2 and Runx3 are essential for chondrocyte maturation, and Runx2 regulates limb growth through induction of Indian hedgehog. Genes Dev 18(8):952–963
92. Zelzer E, Glotzer DJ, Hartmann C, Thomas D, Fukai N, Soker S, Olsen BR (2001) Tissue specific regulation of VEGF expression during bone development requires Cbfa1/Runx2. Mech Dev 106(1–2):97–106
93. Zelzer E, Mamluk R, Ferrara N, Johnson RS, Schipani E, Olsen BR (2004) VEGFA is necessary for chondrocyte survival during bone development. Development 131(9): 2161–2171
94. Zelzer E, McLean W, Ng YS, Fukai N, Reginato AM, Lovejoy S, D'Amore PA, Olsen BR (2002) Skeletal defects in VEGF(120/120) mice reveal multiple roles for VEGF in skeletogenesis. Development 129(8): 1893–1904
95. Zhang J, Niu C, Ye L, Huang H, He X, Tong WG, Ross J, Haug J, Johnson T, Feng JQ, Harris S, Wiedemann LM, Mishina Y, Li L (2003) Identification of the haematopoietic stem cell niche and control of the niche size. Nature 425(6960):836–841
96. Zhao C, Irie N, Takada Y, Shimoda K, Miyamoto T, Nishiwaki T, Suda T, Matsuo K (2006) Bidirectional ephrinB2-EphB4 signaling controls bone homeostasis. Cell Metab 4(2):111–121
97. Zou H, Wieser R, Massagué J, Niswander L (1997) Distinct roles of type I bone morphogenetic protein receptors in the formation and differentiation of cartilage. Genes Dev 11(17):2191–2203

3. The Epiphyseal Growth Plate

H. Clarke Anderson[1] *and Irving M. Shapiro*

3.1 Introduction

"......the soul itself sits on a throne of nucleated cells, and flashes its mandates through skeins of glassy filaments which once were simple chains of vesicles."[2]

Bones elongate and children grow tall through the activities of a millimeter thin layer of cells wedged between the epiphyseal head and the diaphyseal shaft of the long bones. The form, function, and regulation of the activities of cells in this thin, transient, cartilaginous plate have fascinated scientists for a long time, and this growth plate is the focus of the studies reviewed in this chapter. A priori, it is important to acknowledge that apart from long bone, epiphyseal plate activity provides the mechanism of growth of almost all the osseous tissues of the human body. Moreover, other bone-related activities such as fracture repair share common pathways with those of chondrocytes located within the growth cartilage. Hence, an understanding of endochondral growth is relevant to bone elongation and repair, as well as systems that are central to cartilage formation, maturation and turnover.

The growth plate is a well-circumscribed tissue, but receives regulatory signals from the contiguous metaphyseal bone and the more distant articular cartilage. Moreover, as discussed in Chap. 2, the surrounding perichondrium regulates the activities of chondrocytes contained within the cartilage core. Superimposed on these signaling loops are cues from other organs undergoing somatic growth, contralateral bones, and from growth plates on the same bone, but in distant locations. How each of these signals is integrated into a common pathway to provide growth in a temporally and spatially controlled manner has not been fully elucidated. Nevertheless, our current understanding of cartilage physiology speaks to the extraordinary complexity of this tissue and its central role in the growth process.

Structure–function and regulatory studies of epiphyseal chondrocytes form the focus of this review, but it is the growth plate that is regarded as the important tissue for studies of the expression, regulation, and activity of many genes and proteins. One reason for the use of this transient tissue is that within the growth cartilage, one single cell type (a chondrocyte) undergoes terminal differentiation in a series of well-demarcated stages. These stage-specific changes include recruitment of precursor cells, followed by proliferation and maturation, to become terminally differentiated hypertrophic chondrocytes. In the

[1]This work was supported by NIH grants DE 010875 (IMS) and DE 013319 (I.M.S.), and DE05262 (HCA).

[2]The complete PG works of Oliver Wendell Holmes, Sr. by Oliver Wendell Holmes, Sr. (The Physician and Poet) (World eBook Library PGCC Collection) (http://www.WorldLibrary.net).

F. Bronner et al. (eds.), *Bone and Development*, Topics in Bone Biology 6,
DOI 10.1007/978-1-84882-822-3_3,

course of maturation and hypertrophy, a complex extracellular matrix is biosynthesized, vesicles are generated, and mineralization is induced. Subsequently, the differentiated cells exhibit an autophagic flux and eventually undergo apoptosis and die. Gene deletion, mutation, or overexpression can provide critical insights into the role of a specific transcript in the differentiation pathway. These findings can then be directly related to the cell function and animal locomotion, providing information of major interest to clinicians, developmental biologists, geneticists, biochemists, and cell and molecular biologists.

3.2 Growth Plate Architecture, Disposition, and Fusion

In 1844, Richard Owen noted that *"the seat of the active growth of the bone is in a cartilaginous crust at the ends of the diaphysis. When the epiphyses finally coalesce with the diaphysis, growth in the direction of the bone's axis is at one end."*[3] Owen's prescient comments concerning the function of the growth plate are directly relevant to mammalia. However, evaluation of the growth plate physiology across animal species indicates that there exist considerable functional and anatomical disparities: plates vary in shape, volume, number, fusion, disposition, and, following growth, in the extent of cartilage removal. In humans, the long bones – femur and tibia – have two growth plates that are located at the end of the bones. However, the small bones of the hands and feet – metacarpals and phalanges – have only a single (metapodial) epiphysis. Single center bones undergo longitudinal growth at one end only, whereas the growth plates of long bones generate growth at both ends. The level of coordination of growth rates in and between bones is extraordinary. Thus, in humans and many animals, the cells in the epiphyses of the proximal humerus stimulate much of the growth at the shoulder region, whereas the distal epiphyses of the ulna/radius generate growth of the wrist. The distal growth cartilage of the humerus and the proximal cartilage of the ulna/radius contribute little to overall bone growth [62, 141].

A detailed study comparing the growth plates across species has not been performed. In the 1940s and also later in the 1960s and 1970s, Haines [48] reported on the growth plate architecture of a number of animal species, including marsupials and lizards. Amphibia have the most extraordinary specialized epiphyseal cartilage. More recently, Felisbino and Carvalho [40] reported that the epiphyseal cartilage of the long bones of the bullfrog (*Rana catesbeiana*) terminated in a flared structure that enclosed an epiphyseal-like cartilage. The ovoid shape of this cartilage is probably functionally related to the frog's aerobic hopping gait, accompanied by the occasional gasp of "Ribit," rather than providing a mechanism for rapid growth. An extension of the diaphysis covered with periosteum separates the articular cartilage from the inner epiphyseal cartilage. Rozenblut et al. [108] noted that in the European water frog, the epiphyseal cartilages had an inner "metaphyseal" cartilage that plugged the end of the periosteal bone cylinder, but probably did not function in longitudinal growth. Rather, on the basis of the architecture of the tissue, the osteoblasts seem to be associated with the longitudinal growth mediated by the periosteum. Here, intramembranous bone formation promotes long-bone lengthening and the enclosed epiphyseal cartilage provides lateral growth, the reverse of what is seen in mammalian plates.

At the other end of the spectrum, and in stark contrast to both the amphibian and mammalian growth plate, is the avian physis, a greatly expanded structure, often 5–8 mm in thickness. Rather than exhibiting well-ordered columns of chondrocytes, the cells are arranged in an almost random fashion, with the entire tissue permeated by the vascular channels. This may explain the high rate of chondrocyte proliferation, the major mechanism for cartilage expansion. This level of specialization may be a response to the need that the bird has to grow rapidly, yet develop a specialized form of metaphyseal bone. Remarkably, a similar morphology exists in some dinosaurs. Barreto et al. [19] reported that the growth plate of the juvenile

[3] Lectures on the Comparative Anatomy and Physiology of the Vertebrate Animals: Delivered at the Royal College of Surgeons of England, in 1844, published by Longman, Brown, Green, and Longmans, 1846.

dinosaur, Maiasaura (Ornithischia: Hadrosauridae), was characterized by an extensive proliferative zone (PZ) and the invasion of vascular channels into the maturing cartilage. The authors noted that the architecture of the plate was not unlike that of the chicken!

In rodents, the rate and extent of chondrocytic hypertrophy are strongly correlated with the rate of bone elongation. With help of the data provided by Vanky et al. [134] on the relative size of each defined region of the growth cartilage in the mouse and knowledge of the duration of the average cell cycle, 36 h, similar to that in the rat [38], one can calculate that the total murine growth rate approximates 9.0 μm/h, with 80% of the growth due to chondrocyte hypertrophy.

When bone reaches its genetically determined length, longitudinal growth ceases and epiphyseal union takes place, defined by Haines [48] as *"beginning with the completion of the first mineralized bridge between epiphyseal and diaphyseal bone and ending with its replacement by bone and marrow."* In mammalia, the cartilage plate is resorbed and primary and secondary centers of ossification fuse. In birds, turtles, and crocodiles, a remnant of the cartilaginous plate remains throughout the life, and primary and secondary ossification centers remain separate. As a result, bones continue to grow slowly throughout life and animals can attain great length. Why does longitudinal bone growth cease? This had been assumed to be due to the physis fusing with the primary and secondary centers of ossification. Parfitt [99], using hand radiographs of a patient with pseudohypoparathyroidism, observed that growth had slowed several years before fusion occurred and has argued that "fusion is a marker of growth cessation, but not a determinant." From this perspective, *"growth cessation is the culmination of a progressive decline in the growth rate that begins years before fusion"* [17].

3.3 Detailed Anatomy and Cellular Dynamics of the Growth Plate

As mentioned earlier, growth plates at the ends of long bones constitute the site of longitudinal growth and the residua of the primary cartilaginous skeleton of vertebrate embryos (Fig. 3.1a). Figure 3.1b provides better cytologic detail of the proximal tibial growth plate from a 5-week-old rat. Growth plates are also present at primary growth sites in the skull, ribs, vertebra, and pelvis.

In the growing vertebrate animal, cells of the growth plate proliferate actively, undergoing division about every 48 h [44]. Microscopic examination of chondrocytes in the proliferative zone (PZ) of the growing rats (Fig. 3.1b) typically does not reveal cells undergoing classical mitosis, with chromosomes aligned on an equatorial plane. This suggests that division is extraordinarily fast or that the pattern of cell division is not classical. Still, cell division in the PZ has been confirmed with the aid of stains for dividing chromatin, e.g., tritiated thymidine, BRDU, or Ki 67/M1B-1 [39, 44, 62]. As shown in Fig. 3.1, the growth plate of a long bone can be divided into longitudinally oriented, stacked chondrocyte columns (Fig. 3.1).

The most superficial region of the upper tibial growth plate is that "reserve zone" or "resting zone" (RZ) (Fig. 3.1); it supplies stem-like cells that generate columnar clones of PZ chondrocytes [1].

In the PZ, the chondrocytes are aligned into vertical columns (rouleaux), with daughter cells lying beneath the mother cells. The PZ cells are flattened horizontally, like pancakes, and are stacked on top of each other to form the upper ends of the chondrocyte columns (Fig. 3.1). The rate of cell division in the PZ is rapid, especially in the embryo and during the immediate postnatal period. In humans, the linear growth rate in the fetus exceeds 100 cm/year. By birth, the growth rate drops to about 50 cm/year, and by age of 10 years, it is only about 5 cm/year. At puberty, there is a growth spurt [126]. Then, the growth plates "close" with no further linear growth.

In the hypertrophic zone (HZ), individual chondrocytes enlarge in circumference, but remain stacked in the vertical columns and are surrounded by increasing amounts of cartilage matrix (Fig. 3.1). The dividing line between PZ and HZ is indistinct, because there is no sharp transition point, as the chondrocytes in the lower PZ mature, differentiate, and actively synthesize

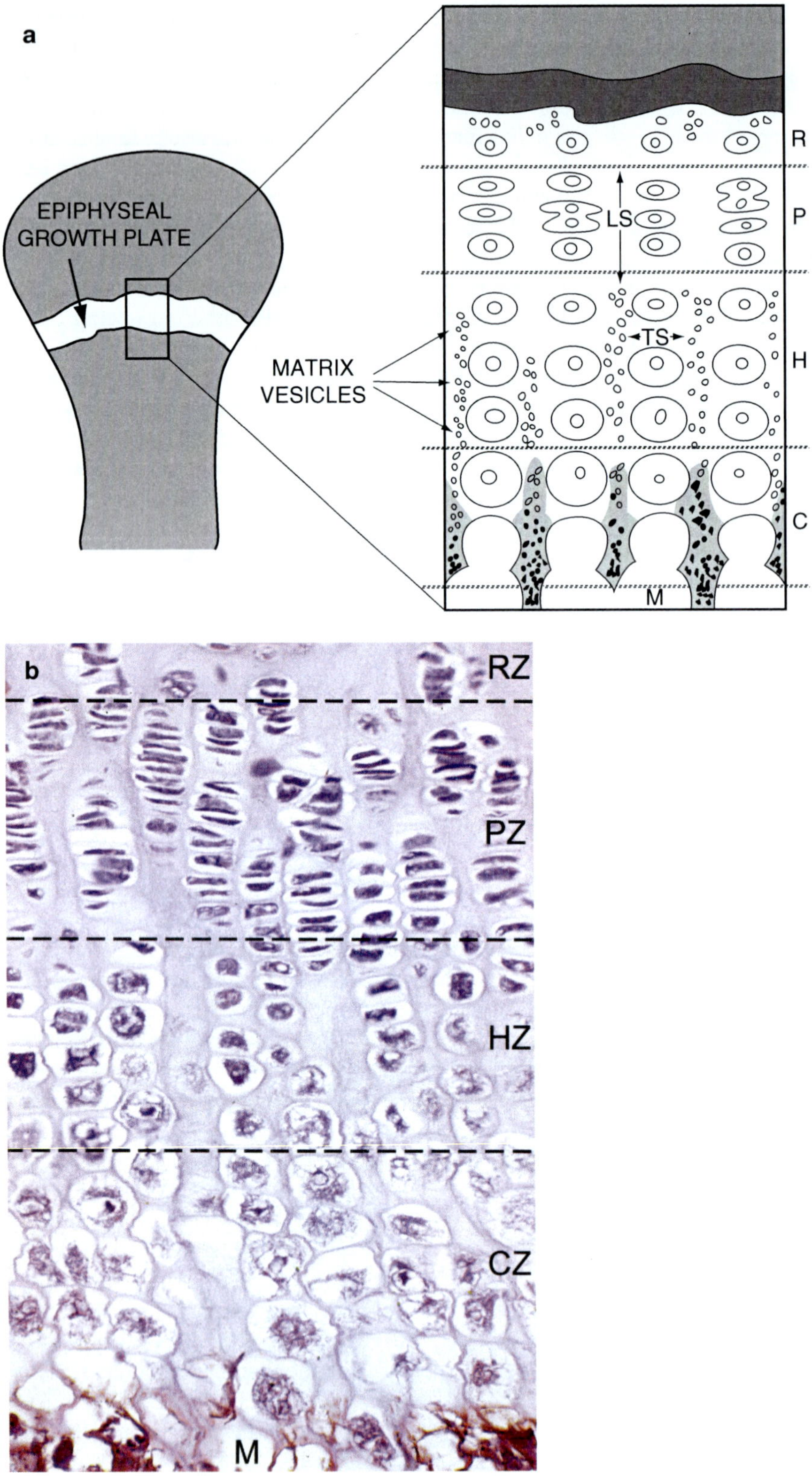
a
EPIPHYSEAL
GROWTH PLATE
R
LS
P
TS
H
MATRIX
VESICLES
C
M
b
RZ
PZ
HZ
CZ
M

and secrete matrix proteins, especially collagen type II and proteoglycans. Maturing HZ chondrocytes synthesize and secrete matrix protein with the aid of more cytoplasm and with an abundance of the rough endoplasmic reticulum and Golgi complexes.

The calcifying zone (CZ) is sometimes referred to as the lower hypertrophic zone because there is no sharp histological border between the upper HZ and the underlying CZ. It is in this region that mineralization takes place in the longitudinal septal cartilage matrix. The presence of mineral can therefore serve to distinguish the upper HZ from the CZ. The earliest indication of the beginning of mineralization is the detection by electron microscopy of needle-like crystals of hydroxyapatite (HA) that form in the sap of matrix vesicles (MVs) (Figs. 3.1a, 3.2, and 3.7a, below). Soon thereafter, mineralization self-propagates into the surrounding matrix, first to the longitudinal septa (where the MVs are concentrated), and then to the other parts of the cartilage matrix (see Figs. 3.1a, 3.2). In the lower CZ, most hypertrophic chondrocytes undergo apoptosis [38] by swelling or "oncosis" (Fig. 3.3) [80]. This presents a distinctive histological pattern unlike the more typical cell shrinking and nuclear condensation seen in the thymus and other tissues.

At the chondro-osseous junction, beneath the cartilaginous growth plate, ingrowing capillaries, osteoclasts, and septoclasts [74] from the underlying bony metaphysis erode and clear away the largely uncalcified transverse septa of the cartilage matrix, as well as the fragmentary remains of apoptotic chondrocytes. Septoclasts

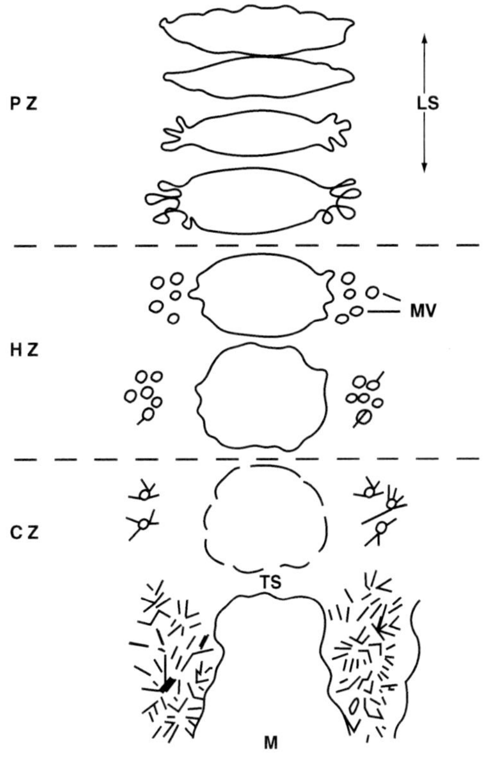

Figure 3.2. Successive stages of chondrocyte maturation and matrix vesicle (MV) budding from the lateral plasma membranes of the growth-plate chondrocytes in the lower proliferative zone (PZ) and upper hypertrophic zone (HZ). Needle-like hydroxyapatite crystal deposition begins within MVs of the hypertrophic zone (see Fig. 3.7a, b). Lower in the HZ, apatite crystals are released from the calcifying MVs. The apatite crystals self-nucleate and proliferate to form spherical mineral clusters in the calcified zone (CZ). These apatite clusters grow and ultimately fuse together in the CZ at its junction with the metaphysis (M). Capillaries, growing in from the metaphysis, penetrate the unmineralized transverse cartilage matrix septa (TS), while unresorbed, fully mineralized longitudinal septa project into the metaphysis, where they serve as a scaffold for the deposition of new bone matrix by in-growing osteoblasts. (Reprinted with permission from Front Biosci, 2005).

Figure 3.1. (**a**). Epiphyseal growth plate of a long bone, showing the site at which growth in length occurs. The growth plate is subdivided into the following anatomical regions: The reserve zone (R) at the top of the growth plate contains reserve stem cells that give rise to the underlying columns of chondrocytes. The proliferative zone (P) is a zone of active cell division where cell columns first appear, thus allowing the matrix to be anatomically subdivided into transverse matrix septa (TS) that separate cells within a column, and longitudinal septa (LS) that separate adjacent cell columns. The hypertrophic zone (H) contains enlarging chondrocytes, actively engaged in cartilage matrix synthesis and secretion. Calcifying matrix vesicles are released from the lateral edges of hypertrophic chondrocytes and accumulate in clusters in the longitudinal septa (LS). (Matrix vesicle-mediated calcification is discussed in detail in Sect. 3.6.) The calcifying zone (C) contains degenerating apoptotic chondrocytes. This is the level at which proliferating mineral spreads from the matrix vesicles radially outward to infiltrate the interstices of the longitudinal septal matrix. At the base of the growth plate lies the bony metaphysis (M) with small vessels that remove the uncalcified transverse matrix septa and degenerate cells, leaving calcified longitudinal septa on which osteoblasts from the marrow will deposit new bone (the primary spongiosa). (Reprinted from Anderson [9].) (**b**) Light microscopic section of the upper tibial growth plate of a growing, 5-week-old Sprague Dawley rat. Reserve zone (RZ), proliferative zone (PZ), hypertrophic zone (HZ), and calcifying zone (CZ) are designated. Calcification stained by alizarin red is seen in the longitudinal septa of the CZ just above a thin sample of the metaphysis (M), which lies beneath the lower edge of the CZ (hematoxylin and alizarin red stain, 1,800×).

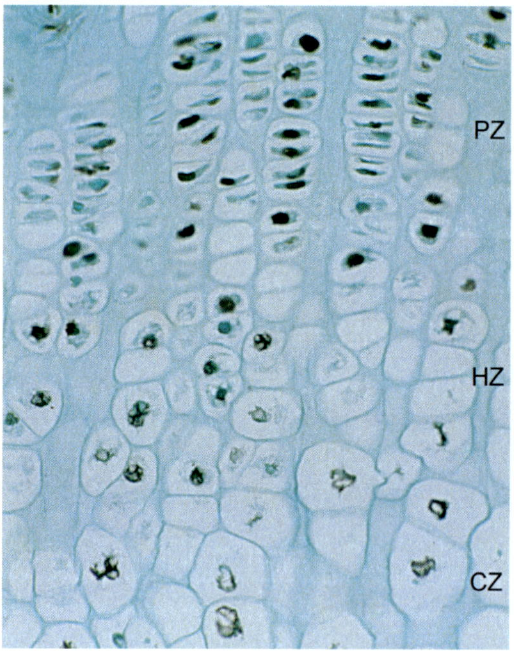

Figure 3.3. Rat growth plate, TUNEL-stained, showing black-staining nuclei in chondrocytes that undergo programmed cell death (apoptosis). Most hypertrophic zone (HZ) nuclei are in a later stage of apoptosis, with nuclei and cytoplasm showing hydropic swelling (oncosis), as well as TUNEL staining. Approximately 1/3 of lower proliferative zone (PZ) chondrocytes also stain black; this indicates that early apoptosis has already begun at this level (1,800×). (Reprinted with permission from Front Biosci, 2005).

can be distinguished from osteoclasts by being mononuclear, rich in cathepsin B, and by projecting a resorptive villus "finger" of the cytoplasm into the empty lacuna formerly occupied by an apoptotic terminal chondrocyte [74]. Vascular invasion is stimulated by several angiogenic factors released from the apoptotic chondrocytes, including vascular endothelial growth factor (VEGF) [45, 50] and basic fibroblast growth factor (FGF) [18]. VEGF is concentrated in isolated rat growth plate MVs [93]; MVs may therefore play a major morphogenetic role at the base of the growth plate by promoting the transition from cartilage to bone.

Following vascular invasion, new bone is generated at the surfaces of the unresorbed calcified cartilage of the persisting longitudinal septa. Bone is generated by ingrowing osteoblasts, derived from mesenchymal stromal (stem) cells of the adjacent marrow [83]. Shortly after its formation, the new bone of the metaphysis, with its inclusions of cartilage, is actively remodeled by ingrowing osteoclasts and osteoblasts to form the more durable and mechanically resistant lamellar bone of the endosteum.

3.4 Regulation of Growth Plate Development and Function

As with other body tissues, peptide, protein, and steroid hormones regulate the activities of cells in the growth plate. Hormones that have been linked to this activity include leptin, insulin-like growth factor (IGF), vitamin D metabolites, parathyroid hormone-related protein (PTHrP), thyroid hormone, sex steroids, and glucocorticoids. Apart from directly modifying chondrocyte activity, these molecules influence the effects of growth factors that regulate chondrocyte function. As a response to hormonal agents, chondrocytes or perichondrial cells express FGF, Indian hedgehog (IHH), bone morphogenetic proteins (BMP), transforming growth factor-beta (TGF-β), and VEGF; these molecules in turn modulate the chondrocyte activity in an autocrine or paracrine fashion. In a number of instances, activated chondrocytes upregulate the receptor expression, thereby enhancing the effects of hormones and local growth factors. The activity of cells is further modified by intracellular metabolic sensors, such as mTOR and AMP kinase (AMPK). Phosphorylation and dephosphorylation reactions transduce stimuli that influence the behavior of the activated cells, thereby amplifying or dampening extracellular and intracellular signals [59]. Not surprisingly, limited nutrient intake, decreased hypothalamic function, and genetic mutations in receptor structure can cause catastrophic changes in bone growth. Growth regulation is complex and depends on the concerted action of many types of molecules, as discussed in Chap. 2. Here, we focus on three major signaling loops: PTHrP–IHH, BMP-FGF, and growth hormone (GH)-leptin-IGF. Finally, the Wnt β-catenin signaling pathway will be discussed as an example of a powerful system that regulates chondrocyte hypertrophy, bone development, and growth.

Table 3.1. Factors that regulate chondrocyte proliferation

Factor	References
PTHrP	Kronenberg [69]
Bcl-2	Wang et al. [139]
IGF-1	van der Eerden et al. [133]
Wnt	Tanamura et al. [124]
T3	van der Eerden et al. [133]
FGF	Mancilla et al. [82]
Leptin	Gordeladze et al. [46]
BMPs	Anderson et al. [11]

See Table 3.1 for a summary of factors that regulate chondrocyte proliferation.

PTHrP promotes proliferation of chondrocytes of the lower RZ and PZ, and retards further differentiation into prehypertrophic and hypertrophic chondrocytes [70]. In the growth plate, PTHrP is synthesized by perichondrial cells, as well as RZ and PZ chondrocytes.

Probably, the most exquisite level of control is exerted by the PTHrP–IHH feedback loop, which was first described by Vortkamp et al. [136] (Fig. 3.4). The observation that PTHrP is a growth factor was surprising, because PTH is an anabolic hormone that has been linked to the hypercalcemia of malignancy. However, studies on transgenic and knockout animals indicated that both PTHrP and IHH were required for normal development and growth. Observations regarding the stage of the chondrocyte life cycle, which is sensitive to specific mutations or deletions, led to the understanding of the complex circuitry that regulates epiphyseal development and bone growth.

In a number of mammalian species, PTHrP, a molecule that shares extensive homology with PTH, is expressed by periarticular and perichondral cells, but not by cells in the cartilagenous plate. Chondrocytes have PTHrP receptors (PTHrPR), with the level of expression depending on the maturation state of the cell. In proliferative cells, the number of receptors is quite low, but their expression increases as the cells differentiate. The receptor, located on the outer aspect of the cells membrane, is a transmembrane G-protein coupled protein (patched) that activates downstream pathways, including PKA, IP3, and PKC.

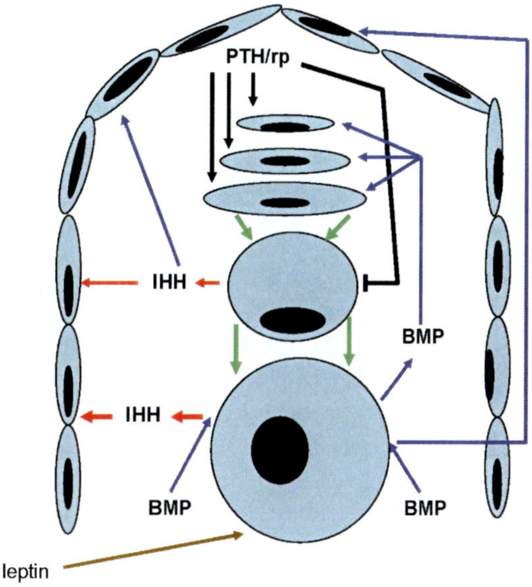

Figure 3.4. Regulation of chondrocyte proliferation and hypertrophy mediated by the interaction of IHH with PTHrP/PTH. IHH secreted by maturing chondrocytes diffuses into the periochondrial tissues and stimulates the expression of PTHrP/PTH by fibroblasts in the perichondrial and periarticular tissues. PTHrP/PTH diffuses back into the cartilage where it binds to its receptor and inhibits differentiation of the proliferating cells; at the same time, PTHrP/PTH promotes chondrocyte proliferation. In addition to the feed forward circuit, IHH is required for maintenance of chondrocyte proliferation. The maturing chondrocytes are inhibited by differentiation of BMPs, in particular BMP6. In an autocrine–paracrine fashion, chondrocytes can also secrete BMPs, which then serve to promote proliferation and may enhance PTHrP/PTH secretion by the periarticular chondrocytes.

In contrast to PTH/PTHrP, IHH is expressed by maturing, i.e., prehypertrophic and hypertrophic chondrocytes (Fig. 3.4). IHH is a highly conserved gene, present in most animals. As a morphogen, it binds to its receptor, a twelve-pass membrane protein called patched1 (membrane protein patched1). In the absence of IHH, patched1 seems to interact with Smo to form an inactive heteromeric-signaling complex. When the IHH ligand binds to patched1, the membrane complex undergoes a conformational change such that Smo is now free and can trigger the expression of a number of downstream target genes, including the transcription factor Gli1 and BMPs [96]. Also, as IHH levels are raised, patched1, serves as a sink for excess ligand, because its expression is a positive function of IHH. IHH and BMP signaling pathways can also interact with one another [90, 144].

Not surprisingly, there have been numerous attempts to relate the distribution of receptors and ligands to the regulation of chondrocyte differentiation in the growth plate. The most widely accepted model was put forward by Vortkamp et al. [136] and Kronenberg [70] and, notwithstanding many modifications, has been accepted by many investigators. The starting point for this model is the postmitotic maturing chondrocyte on its way to a fully developed hypertrophic cell. As these chondrocytes express IHH, they can bind to receptors on perichondrial and periosteal cells, as well as periarticular fibroblasts. By binding to its cognate receptor, patched1, IHH causes PTHrP expression. In turn, PTHrP, by diffusing into the plate and blocking differentiation, serves as a negative feedback function; in the periarticular regions, PTHrP stimulates continued proliferation. PTHrP also acts on osteoblasts and osteoclasts in the forming metaphysis, thereby enhancing bone formation and remodeling. The final feedback is mediated by hypertrophic chondrocytes that have escaped the maturation blockage; these cells downregulate IHH secretion and thus make terminal differentiation possible [61].

The long diffusion paths that ligands must travel to modulate the system present a major conceptual problem in relation to the regulatory loop discussed earlier. Conceptually, it would be easier if the ligands are bound to the receptors on the neighboring cells. In addition to the spatial considerations, temporal factors need to be built into the feedback circuit. For example, is inhibition of maturation a continuous or discontinuous process? If discontinuous, one can imagine that with a temporary arrest of inhibition, some cells escape the inhibitory signals and undergo terminal differentiation. Another factor to be considered is the effect of applied forces. The epiphysis is subject to considerable variations in tensile and compressive forces. Fluid flow within the cartilage plate would add flow to diffusion. Wu et al. [142] have demonstrated that cyclic mechanical stress induces IHH expression; Tanaka et al. [125] have reported that mechanical strain upregulates PTHrP expression. Possibly, night–day changes in tension and compression combined with the release of leptin and other regulatory factors may promote transport of the signal molecules (see also below).

On the basis of the preceding discussion, PTHrP is believed to drive chondrocyte proliferation, whereas IHH is considered as a powerful brake of the maturation pathway. Under- or over-activity of these two control systems may subsequently lead to epiphyseal dysfunction. For example, genetic deletion of PTHrP or PTH/PTHrPR results in a profound change in epiphyseal growth: The characteristic parallel columns of proliferating chondrocytes of the affected growth plate are atypical or even missing. Overexpression of PTHrP causes gross expansion of the proliferative region of the epiphysis. Mutations in the receptor expression also cause massive changes in the architecture of the cartilage; the phenotype can be lethal and has been likened to Blomstrand chondro-osteodystrophy. Point mutations in the gene that encodes the receptor disrupt normal epiphyseal growth in the mouse and are thought to be the cause of Jansen chondro-osteodystrophy in humans, a gross disturbance in the growth plate architecture that leads to a decrease in chondrocytic differentiation, resulting in limb shortening [60, 112].

Bcl-2 is a proto-oncogene protein that protects the growth-plate chondrocytes from terminal differentiation and apoptosis [139]. Bcl-2 is most concentrated in the cytoplasm of proliferative chondrocytes of the growth plate. It functions by forming inactivating heterocomplexes with Bax, a related proto-oncogene, which, if not inactivated, induces apoptosis of hypertrophic chondrocytes. In this way, Bcl-2 indirectly promotes the proliferative phase of growth plate chondrocytes (For more detail about the functions of BCl-2, see Sect. 3.9 below).

Wnts and β-catenin. In recent years, there has been intense interest in the role played by Wnts and β-catenin in the regulation of growth-plate development and function [29]. Wnts are one of the few evolutionarily conserved signal transduction pathways that serve a myriad of functions in almost all animal species, especially during development after birth and in the pathogenesis of the disease [47, 54]. Wnt signals are transduced in at least two distinct ways; the well-established or "canonical" Wnt/β-catenin

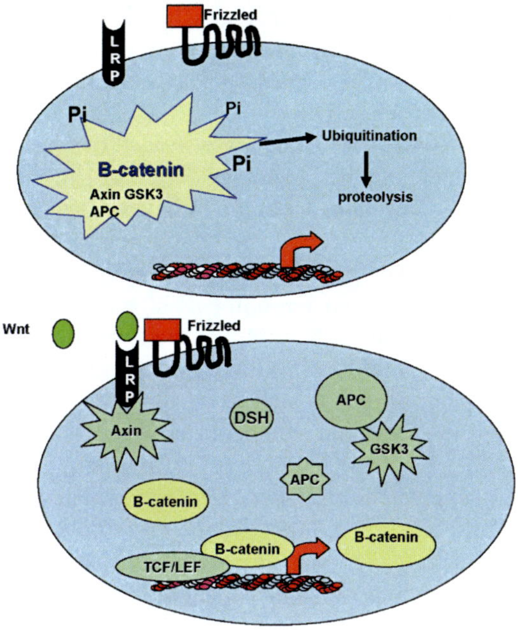

Figure 3.5. Schematic of Wnt signaling through the canonical pathway in maturing chondrocytes. *Top* figure shows that glycogen synthase kinase (GSK3β) is activated and phosphorylates β-catenin in the absence of Wnt. Hyperphosphorylated catenin is targeted for ubiquitination and undergoes degradation in the proteasome. *Bottom* figure shows that in the presence of Wnt, the protein binds to Frizzled and LRP 5/6 and induces phosphorylation of disheveled (DSH) which then inhibits GSK3β. In the hypophosphorylated state, the axin-SPC-GSK3β complex is not formed and β-catenin can travel to the nucleus where it serves as a coactivator with TCF/LEF transcription factors to regulate the expression of matrix metalloproteinases (MMP's), cyclins, and other target genes.

pathway (Fig. 3.5), and a β-catenin independent noncanonical pathway. In the nonstimulated state (canonical pathway), β-catenin interacts with APC and axin scaffold proteins and the macromolecular complex constitutes a substrate for glycogen synthase kinase (GSK3β) and casein kinase 1a (CK1a). This assembly enhances phosphorylation of β-catenin which, following ubiquination, undergoes proteolysis.

The membrane ligand for Wnt activation is the protein, Frizzled, and the coreceptors are the low-density lipoprotein receptor-related Lrp5 and Lrp6. Frizzled interacts with Wnt and activates the downstream Disheveled, to prevent phosphorylation of β-catenin. The protein then translocates to the nucleus where it interacts with the TCF/LEF family of the transcription factors to enhance the expression of target genes (Fig. 3.5). These genes include cyclin D1, c-myc, MMP-7, and MMP-26. To add to the complexity of the system, the noncanonical pathway is also active in chondrocytes. In chondrocytes, Wnt binds to Frizzled, which causes activation of PLC and release of intracellular calcium. Activation of calmodulin-dependent protein kinase II and PKC triggers a cellular response [71, 135]. Activation of rho GTPases results in dramatic changes in both cytoskeletal and microtubule systems.

It is now clear that the Wnt/β-catenin pathway is necessary for growth-plate development and endochondral ossification [3, 37, 55]. Activation of Wnt signaling in mature chondrocytes induces hypertrophy, matrix mineralization, and MMP-7, -9, and -13 production [124]. The canonical Wnt signaling pathway is regulated by autocrine and paracrine molecules that modify the binding of Wnt and Wnt receptors, as well as secreted Frizzled-related protein, which inhibits or dampens ligand-mediated signaling [37]. Andrade et al. [15] have shown that six Wnt family members are expressed in the growth plate. Of these, Wnt 2b, 4, and 10b signal through the canonical β-catenin pathway, whereas Wnt 5a, 5b, and 11 signal through the noncanonical pathway. Very surprisingly, the expression levels of proteins in the canonical and noncanonical pathways do not correlate significantly to explain the role of Wnt signaling in chondrocyte maturation and differentiation. When the cells achieve terminal differentiation status, there is a decrease in the expression that suggests that the Wnt proteins are of major importance early rather than later in the maturation process, possibly owing to the "overlapping or interacting roles in postnatal bone formation" [15]. However, mouse genetic studies indicate the importance of Wnt/β-catenin signaling in the progression of late differentiation stage of chondrocytes [3, 55]. In a recent study, Kerr et al. [63] found that GFP-Rac-1, together with Wnt/β-catenin, regulates chondrocyte maturation. Activation of Rac-1 increases chondrocyte cell volume and matrix metalloproteinase (MMP) generation – events that are associated with chondrocyte maturation; inhibition of Rac-1 stimulates proteoglycan production and proliferation, characteristics of the immature chondrocytes. These findings lend credence to the notion that the Wnt signaling pathway is of critical importance in chondrocyte maturation and growth-plate function. Wnt/β-catenin signaling also interacts with other regulatory signaling pathways, such as PTHrP and IHH, to control growth-plate structure and function [81, 92], but details of these complex interactions are not yet known.

FGF-BMP. One advantage of defining a regulatory loop is that it makes it possible to use the molecular circuitry to anchor and integrate the effects of other paracrine and autocrine growth factors. In addition to the PTH/PTHrP-IHH loop, BMPs (Fig. 3.4) and FGFs form a second series of regulatory proteins. However, whether the two loops integrate to form one super-loop is yet to be determined; it should be added that there is a good reason for believing that individual components of one system influence the activities of the other.

FGF is a member of the heparin-binding family of proteins, required for mesenchyme condensation and limb formation [95]. In humans, 22 isoforms serve as ligands for a family of five cognate membrane tyrosine kinase FGF receptors (FGFR1–5). As demonstrated by Krejci et al. [68], not all proteins are present in the cartilage. In embryonic human tissue, the predominant FGF isoforms are 1, 2, 17, and 19. In the postnatal plate, the perichondrium robustly expresses FGF 1, 2, 6, 7, 9, and 18; in the plate itself expression of FGF 2, 7, 18, and 22 is observed; the receptor proteins are FGFR1, 2, and 3 [73]. Loss of FGFR-3 expression in the growth plate causes elevated proliferation and hypertrophy and abnormal growth of long bones (see Chap. 1). Most authorities agree that FGFR-3 is a negative regulator of chondrocyte proliferation and, therefore, an important modulator of the terminally differentiated state.

More recent studies point to the importance of FGF18 in endochondral ossification. In mice, this isoform is expressed by cells in the perichondrium [33, 73]. Deletion of perichondrial FGF18 leads to a phenotype with decreased chondrocyte proliferation and differentiation, attributed to the absence of FGFR3 signaling. FGF18 also promotes VEGF expression in hypertrophic chondrocytes; this suggests that FGF18 is needed to bring about skeletal vascularization and subsequent recruitment of osteoblasts/osteoclasts [77]. Accordingly, the effects of FGF 18 may extend beyond the growth plate to integrate bone deposition and remodeling with growth-plate activities.

Like FGF, BMP signaling is needed to develop the hypertrophic phenotype (Fig. 3.4) [34, 146]. BMP 1–7 proteins are at their highest concentrations in the hypertrophic chondrocytes of the growth plate [11], with BMP-2 and -6 RNAs mostly in the hypertrophic cartilage, and BMP-7 predominant in the proliferating cartilage [94]. The BMP receptor (BMPRIA) is expressed in the perichondrium, as well as in the proliferating and hypertrophic chondrocytes, whereas other BMP receptors (BMPRIB, BMPRII, and ALK 2) are expressed throughout the growth plate [89]. Thus, the sites of BMPs and their receptors show considerable overlap in the growth plate, notwithstanding the fact that there is preferential expression in some regions.

A complicating factor is the presence of inhibitors of BMPs throughout the growth plate. These include fibrillins, heparan sulfate proteoglycans [56], mutated chondroitin-4-sulfotransferase [122], and the classic BMP inhibitors gremlin and chordin, plus inhibitory Smads 6 and 7 [16, 94]. Differential activity of these inhibitors influences and confounds the effects of FGF-BMP signaling.

The low levels of BMP signaling in the RZ are likely to maintain the cells in the RZ in a quiescent state [94]. In the maturing regions of the plate, BMP signaling may induce terminal differentiation. The question now is whether BMP-dependent signaling influences the activities of the other regulatory circuits discussed earlier. Minina et al. [90] showed that BMPs and IHH promote chondrocyte proliferation, whereas FGF independently inhibits proliferation, but influences the transit of chondrocytes to their terminally differentiated state. In this way, PTHrP and IHH, together with BMPs and FGF, form a feedback loop that regulates growth. Conceivably, signaling by the powerful and highly regulated BMP system is independent of the IHH-PTHrP circuit [67, 94], whereas FGF signaling may influence the IHH signaling pathway [144], because the IHH and FGF signaling pathways seem to act independently of each other in regulating the proliferative phase of the

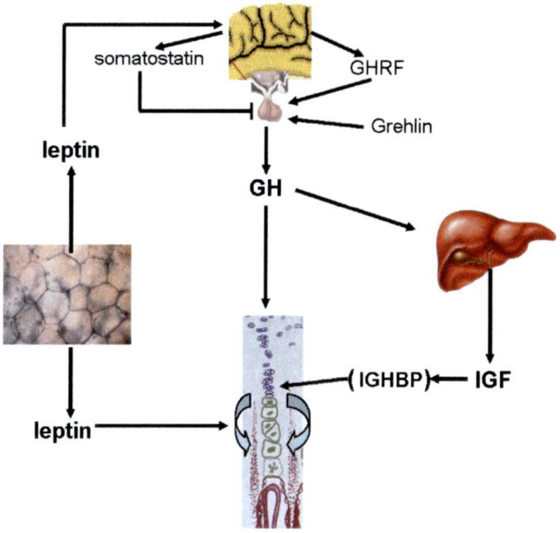

Figure 3.6. Regulation of chondrocyte maturation and epiphyseal growth by growth hormone (GH), insulin-like growth factor (IGF), and leptin. GH is secreted by secretor cells of the anterior pituitary gland. Secretion is modulated by hypothalamic proteins: promoted by growth hormone releasing factor (GHRF) and inhibited by somatostatin, Ghrelin, a gut hormone, and leptin, a hormone secreted by adipocytes. The hypothalamic proteins serve as GH secretogogues and act directly on the pituitary gland. In the liver, GH promotes the secretion of two IGF isoforms (IGF-I and IGF-II), which become bound to carrier protein (IGFBP). IGF, GH, and leptin act directly on the growth plate and promote chondrocyte proliferation and epiphyseal growth.

chondrocyte life cycle [88]. Even though these pathways exert effects that are independent of each other, it is likely that, because of redundancy, integration takes place through pathways not yet discovered.

IGF-1 is expressed by proliferating and prehypertrophic chondrocytes of the growth plate, as well as by the liver, and is activated by pituitary-generated GH. IGF-1 synthesis and secretion stimulates clonal expansion of PZ chondrocytes in an autocrine/paracrine manner (Fig. 3.6). GH/IGF-1 is critical for the adolescent growth spurt, and IGF-1-deficient mice show severe dwarfism. In the growth plate, IGF-1 stimulates chondrocyte proliferation and bone growth. Growth hormone and IGF are both required for normal growth in the child and adolescent. The major factors regulating IGF concentrations in serum are GH, nutritional intake, and thyroid hormones, and the latter stimulates GH secretion. Growth hormone resistance owing to mutations or deletion in the GH gene or receptor causes dwarfism (Laron syndrome).

Leptin (from the Greek *leptos*, thin) is a 16 kDa helical-rich protein that regulates satiety and energy expenditure. Leptin also regulates the activities of GH and IGF (Fig. 3.6) [131]. Cells in the growth plate express the leptin receptor and hypertrophic chondrocytes synthesize leptin. Once bound, leptin causes chondrocyte proliferation and expression of collagen types II and X to increase. It also induces an insulin-like growth factor isoform (IGF-1) and TGF-β. Osteoblasts express active leptin receptors that mediate signal transduction as indicated by the phosphorylation of Stat3 [75]. A single daily injection of leptin into mice that cannot synthesize leptin ($Ob(Lep)^{-/-}$) causes the long bone to become longer and denser [75]. Leptin stimulates osteoblast proliferation, promotes expression of the bone cell phenotype, and enhances osteoprogenitor cell maturation [131].

As leptin levels increase in obesity and the robustness of bone increases correspondingly, this hormone may serve to adjust bone density to load. Leptin also causes PTHrP to increase and IHH secretion to become inhibited. By acting on these two major components of the feedback loop, leptin effectively regulates the differentiation of epiphyseal chondrocytes.

Thyroid hormone (triiodothyronine, T3) promotes the recruitment of chondrocytes from the RZ to the PZ, and thus stimulates chondrocyte proliferation in the growth plate. T3 also promotes the differentiation of growth-plate chondrocytes [133]. This helps to account for the increased growth of long bones, as seen in young children with hyperthyroidism. However, hyperthyroidism ultimately leads to premature growth-plate fusion and short stature. As suggested earlier, thyroid hormone (T3) regulates Wnt/β-catenin that blocks chondrocyte hypertrophy and endochondral ossification. Nevertheless, postnatally, a T3-driven increase in Wnt/β-catenin signaling promotes growth-plate chondrocyte maturation and bone formation [124].

The main function of the FGF, especially of FGF-2 or basic FGF, is to control longitudinal bone growth by inhibiting PZ chondrocyte cell division [82]. It does this by the activation of the FGF receptors (FGFR1–4) that are localized in the chondrocytes. The activation brings about a marked decrease in PZ chondrocyte proliferation, along with a major reduction in the size of the HZ. In humans, activating mutations of the FGFR3 cause achondroplastic dwarfism [133]. Overexpression of FGF-2 causes an inhibition of the longitudinal growth of long bones, presumably by activating FGFR3 [30].

VEGF regulates angiogenesis, i.e., vascular ingrowth into the growth plate from the underlying metaphysis [42, 45]. It is most highly expressed in mature chondrocytes of the lower HZ, and when secreted by HZ chondrocytes, is targeted to its receptor, Flt, which is concentrated in the endothelial cells of the underlying metaphysis. VEGF is endothelial cell-specific. When inactivated *in vivo* by systemic administration of a soluble, decoy VEGF receptor, VEGF not only suppresses angiogenesis, but also impairs trabecular bone formation and the expansion of HZ of chondrocytes [45]. It is also involved in cell-survival mechanisms [2]. In some tissues, VEGF expression is regulated by hypoxia inducible factor (HIF)-1, a transcription factor that is expressed by cells of the growth plate (see section below). See Table 3.2 for a summary of factors regulating vascular ingrowth.

Several matrix metalloproteinases (MMPs) have been shown to promote angiogenesis at the base of the growth plate, especially MMP-3, -9, and -13 [49]. These MMPs are synthesized and secreted not only by lower hypertrophic and apoptotic chondrocytes of the growth plate, but also by the vascular endothelium of invading capillaries and nearby chondroclasts and osteoclasts [123]. Endothelial cell invasion of the cartilage matrix in the lower HZ is greatly aided by MMP digestion of the matrix collagen and proteoglycans [137]. MMP-9, in particular, may act directly on the microvessels of the metaphysis, causing them to invade and penetrate the adjacent cartilage matrix. MMP-9 may be the most important MMP, inasmuch as growth-plate vascularization and ossification are delayed in MMP-9-deficient mice and their growth plate becomes progressively longer, especially in the HZ [137]. For ways by which MMPs facilitate angiogenesis, refer to Rundhaug [109].

Table 3.2. Factors regulating vascular ingrowth

Factor	References
VEGF	Dai and Rabie [32]
MMP-3, -9, -13	Rundhaug [109]
Chondromodulin	Shukunami et al. [118]
Glucocorticoid	Smink et al. [120]
TGF-β	Alvarez et al. [5]
CTGF	Ivkovic et al. [57]

Chondromodulin inhibits angiogenesis in the growth plate, as do the thrombospondins-1 and -2, and the tissue inhibitors of metalloproteinases-2 and -3 [118].

Glucocorticoids are well-known inhibitors of growth-plate growth and vascularization. Prepubertal children treated with glucocorticoids exhibit general growth retardation [21]. In experimental animals, longitudinal bone growth is inhibited [17]. Glucocorticoids inhibit endochondral bone formation by (a) decreasing the PZ proliferation rate and height, (b) increasing the chondrocyte apoptosis rate in the HZ, and (c) interfering with normal vascularization at the base of the growth plate by inhibiting the expression of VEGF [120].

Transforming growth factor-beta (TGF-β) has multiple functions in the growth plate. It is most highly expressed in HZ [31], where, by enhancing PTHrP action [5], it inhibits hypertrophy and differentiation in the growth plate. Although vascular endothelial cells invading the growth plate from the underlying metaphysis are equipped with receptors for TGF-β [35], the mechanism of action of TGF-β on angiogenesis is not clear.

Connective tissue growth factor (CTGF) is prominently expressed in HZ chondrocytes of the postnatal growth plate. CTGF deficiency leads to skeletal dysmorphism, resulting from decreased chondrocyte proliferation and disoriented vascularization at the base of the growth plate [57]. CTGF binds to several growth and differentiation factors that regulate growth-plate development and endochondral bone formation, including the BMPs, TGFβ, and MMPs, as well as VEGF. CTGF-deficient mice not only have impaired vascularization at the base of the growth plate, but also lack aggrecan (proteoglycan) in the cartilage matrix; their chondrocyte columns are disoriented and the growth plates have diminished mechanical strength [57].

3.5 Mechanism of Growth-Plate Mineralization

The pattern of mineral initiation and propagation in the growth plate is spatially polarized, with mineral deposition occurring selectively in the longitudinal septa of the cartilage matrix at the lateral edges of the chondrocyte columns (Figs. 3.1a and 3.2) [6, 10]. The selective localization of the mineral in the longitudinal septal matrix is likely due to the fact that mineral-initiating MVs are deposited in the longitudinal septal matrix through polarized budding from the lateral edges of early HZ chondrocytes [26] (Fig. 3.2) and from the osteoid-facing surfaces of the osteoblasts during new bone formation [13].

The mechanism of MV-initiated biomineralization appears to be biphasic (Fig. 3.7). During Phase 1, Ca^{2+} and PO_4^{3-} become concentrated within MVs, generating hydroxyapatite (HA) crystals, often along the inner surfaces of the MV membrane (Fig. 3.7a). Ca^{2+} accumulation within MVs is promoted by Ca^{2+}-binding lipids of MVs, e.g., phosphatidyl serine, which is concentrated in MV membranes [101] and by Ca^{2+}-binding proteins, especially the annexins that are present in the MV sap [64].

Phosphate (PO_4^{3}) accumulation within and at the periphery of MVs is achieved by the activity of phosphatases, especially alkaline phosphatase, that are concentrated in and near the MV membrane (Fig. 3.7a) [4, 86]. Other phosphatases that are enriched in MVs and can promote Phase 1 mineral initiation include ATPase, adenosine monophosphoesterase (AMPase), and inorganic pyrophosphatase (PPiase). The primary action of these phosphatases is to hydrolyze the phosphate esters that are present in the extracellular fluid (ECF) and in the vesicle sap, thus releasing PO_4^{3-} (orthophosphate) for incorporation in the nascent $CaPO_4$ mineral. The PO_4 concentrating effect of the phosphatases is augmented by the action of a Na^- PO_4 cotransporter, with Na^+ released from the MV, in exchange for the entering PO_4^{3-} [91].

Phase 2 begins as the crystals pass through the MV membrane into the matrix of the longitudinal septa (Fig. 3.7b). Here, the HA crystals proliferate, with preformed crystals serving as templates or "nuclei," if adequate amounts of Ca^{2+} and PO_4^{3-} diffuse from the nearby blood vessels. As new, self-nucleated HA crystals aggregate, they form radial clusters that grow in size and fuse to form contiguous mineral deposits in the longitudinal septa of the lower hypertrophic (calcifying) zone of the growth plate (Fig. 3.2).

The speed and pattern of phase 2 mineralization are controlled by known and unknown

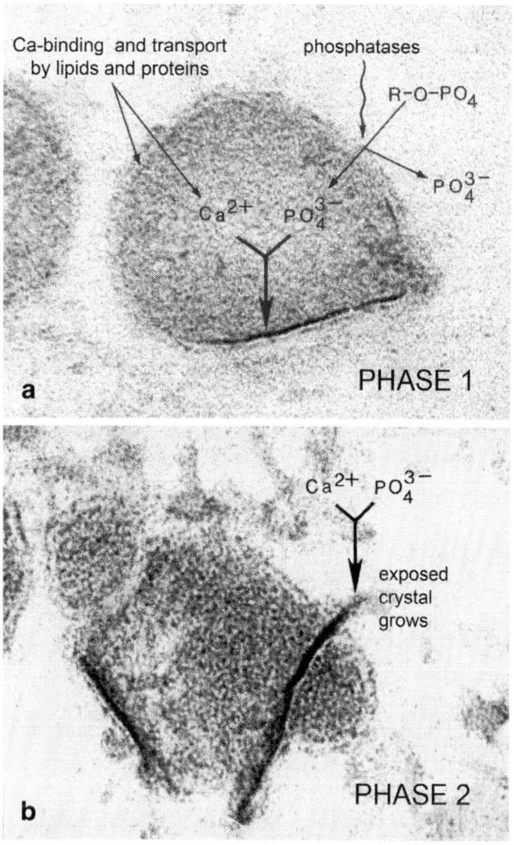

Figure 3.7. (**a**) Scheme for mineralization in matrix vesicles. During phase I, intravesicular calcium concentration is increased by its affinity for lipids and by Ca-binding proteins of the vesicle membrane and interior. Phosphatases, e.g., alkaline phosphatase, pyrophosphatase, or adenosine triphosphatase at the vesicle membrane, act on ester phosphate of the matrix or vesicle fluid to produce a local increase in PO_4 in the vicinity of the vesicle membrane. This in turn raises the intravesicular ionic product $(Ca^{2+}) \times (PO_4^{3-})$, resulting in initial deposition of $CaPO_4$ near the membrane. (**b**) As intravesicular crystals accumulate and grow, they are exposed to the extravesicular environment. Phase 2 begins with the exposure of preformed apatite crystals to extravesicular fluid, which in normal animals is supersaturated with respect to apatite, enabling further crystal nucleation to take place. Matrix vesicles pictured are in rat growth-plate cartilage. (Reprinted with permission from Anderson [7]).

factors outside the MVs. As pointed out earlier, the rate of mineral crystal growth depends on the diffusion of plasma Ca^{2+} and PO_4^{3-} ions to the ECF. However, their concentration in the ECF is not sufficient to initiate HA crystal formation. However, if HA crystals are released from MVs, the concentration of the two ions in the ECF is sufficient for HA to deposit on the crystals that then serve as templates [52]. In this process, matrix collagen (types I or II) plays a major role by nucleating and orienting newly formed HA crystals [72]. Factors that inhibit the rate of HA crystal proliferation include proteoglycans [27], osteocalcin [36], osteonectin [23], inorganic pyrophosphate (PPi) [41], and fetuin [111]. Mineralization inhibitors are important because they prevent the mineral from spreading to the tissues that do not normally calcify, e.g., the arteries in atherosclerosis or the weight-bearing joints in osteoarthritis [8].

3.6 Chondrocyte Metabolism Within the Growth Plate

The metabolism of the growth plate cartilage has been reviewed [117]. Because the life cycle of the chondrocyte is very short (1–3 days), its energy requirements are likely to be very high. The question that then arises is how the cell in the hypoxic confines of the growth plate can generate sufficient ATP from glycolysis to maintain membrane pumps, secrete a complex organic matrix, and activate mineral deposition. The answer to this fundamental question is that, unlike oxidative phosphorylation where the energy yield is high, but the rate is slow, the glycolytic pathway is very short and can deliver small amounts of ATP at a rate sufficient to meet the energy demands of the cell. Moreover, as the glycolytic pathway is the major energy conserving pathway in maturing chondrocytes, the O_2 needs are small. From this perspective, chondrocytes are exquisitely adapted to the avascular architecture of the growth plate.

While it is fairly obvious that the O_2 supply to the avascular plate must be low, till recently, evidence in support of this assumption has been limited. A derivative of metronidazole has been used to provide an index of the O_2 tension in situ and to demonstrate O_2 gradient in the growth plate, with the lowest O_2 concentrations (2–5%) in the core HZ [103, 116]. At the calcification front, the chondro-osseous junction sited closest to the metaphyseal blood vessels, the oxemic state of the chondrocytes would be higher than in the postmitotic core. Increased O_2 delivery is likely to favor osteoblast and osteoclast function, while possibly adversely influencing chondrocyte survival.

If there is a gradient in the tissue O_2 tension, how then does the cell adjust its metabolism to the oxemic state? Within the past decade, much has been learned about the mechanism by which the cells respond to changes in the local O_2 tension. Chondrocytes sense the local tension by the activities of sensor proteins, prolyl hydroxylases (PHDs) [130]. When activated, these oxoglutarate- and Fe^{2+}-dependent dioxygenases mediate hydroxylation of prolyl and asparagyl residues of the transcription protein, HIF. It has been shown that PHD isoenzymes are present in cultured chondrocytes and the growth plate itself [130]. Under normoxic conditions, the proline-hydroxylated form of HIF is recognized and bound to the von Hippel Lindau tumor suppressor protein (pVHL), an ubiquitin ligase. This complex is targeted to the proteasome for polyubiquitination and degradation [98]. However, when the pO_2 is low, there is a reduction in PHD activity, and pVHL-dependent ubiquitination is suppressed. Under this circumstance, HIF-1α translocates into the nucleus, binds to hypoxic responsive elements (HRE) on DNA, and promotes the transcription of specific target genes, many of which are concerned with the regulation of the glycolytic pathway. For example, HIF regulates the expression of PFK1, the pacemaker enzyme of glycolysis.

The question now arises as to whether HIF is expressed by cells in the growth cartilage. In an early study of the growth plate, it was shown that HIF was highly expressed in hypertrophic chondrocytes in situ and in culture [105, 130]. The functional importance of HIF was first demonstrated by Schipani et al. [113], who reported that mutant mice with conditionally inactivated HIF-1α gene exhibited profound changes in the cellular architecture of the growth plate. The number of hypertrophic cells was reduced, there was an increase in apoptotic cells in the proliferative and HZs, and the metaphysis was irregular and disorganized. The mechanism of these changes is as yet unknown, but it would not be unreasonable to assume that in the absence of HIF, many of the glycolytic genes remain inactivated, with the cell unable to promote glucose metabolism through anaerobic glycolysis. Moreover, as HIF regulates the activity of the genes linked to survival, many of the cells undergo premature apoptosis. Unlike the growth cartilage, the effect on the development of metaphyseal bone is not obvious. However, as the full development of the hypertrophic phenotype is linked closely with bone formation, a disturbance in epiphyseal function is likely to be transduced to cells at the chondro-osseous junction, with alterations in bone formation and resorption.

A few more words about the function of the HIF system (see Chap. 8) are warranted. Apart from upregulating glycolysis, HIF-1 slows the mitochondrial function, thereby decreasing the O_2 needs of the cell. In a series of recent studies, it was shown that HIF influenced energy generation at the mitochondrial level. In this case, rather than serving as a stimulatory function, HIF blocks the activity of the enzyme pyruvate dehydrogenase that converts pyruvate into acetyl CoA [119]. The enzyme is subject to control by both stimulatory factors (Ca^{2+}, insulin, etc.) and inhibitory reactions (phosphorylations), and serves as a control point that links glycolysis with the generation of mitochondrial energy (Fig. 3.8). In hypoxia, HIF stimulates a pyruvate dehydrogenase kinase to phosphorylate, and thereby to inhibit the pyruvate dehydrogenase. When this occurs, the rate of conversion of pyruvate to lactate by lactate dehydrogenase is raised. This reaction regenerates NAD and glycolysis is enhanced, further stabilizing the metabolism of the hypoxic cell. In summary, the low level of vascularization of the growth plate and the concomitant decrease in O_2 supply stabilize HIF. This in turn upregulates the enzymes involved in glycolysis, provides a source of reduced NAD, and downregulates O_{2-} consuming reactions at the mitochondrial level. On the basis of these findings, the PHD-HIF system must be viewed as a key regulator of chondrocyte metabolism.

It is noteworthy that a second HIF homolog, HIF-2, is present in the epiphyseal cartilage. This HIF isoform may serve as a cytoprotective function. Upregulation of HIF-2 lowers the level of reactive oxygen species (ROS) by enhancing the activities of the dismutating proteins, catalase and superoxide dismutase [28]. The low O_2 tension therefore seems to stabilize HIF-2 expression and raise the superoxide dismutase and catalase activities. The activity of both enzymes suppresses the generation of radicals in the cartilage and permits terminal differentiation.

3.7 Deletion of Chondrocytes from the Epiphyseal Growth Plate

Chondrocytes are deleted from the epiphysis by apoptosis, an activity process that, by deleting the cells from the cartilage, provides space for metaphyseal bone formation and growth. Apoptosis or programmed cell death – a process that has been conserved throughout evolution – removes unwanted or damaged cells from tissues [143]. In cartilage, the apoptotic event is marked by plasma membrane breaks, hydropic swelling [58], a dilated endoplasmic reticulum, and DNA fragmentation [43, 107].

It is generally agreed that there are two well-defined apoptotic signaling systems that regulate the induction of cell death (Fig. 3.8). A wide variety of stimuli activate the *intrinsic pathway* including hypoxia, redox-stress, and serum (growth factor) deprivation. In terminally differentiated chondrocytes, considerable emphasis has been placed on determining the role of the Bcl2 family of proteins in regulating the induction of the intrinsic pathway of apoptosis. Bcl2, Bcl XL, and Mc-l1 are inhibitors of apoptosis that preserve the voltage gradient across the inner membrane of the mitochondrion and prevent protein loss. In contrast, Bax and Bak create membrane pores and stimulate apoptosis. A third group of proteins, including Bad, Bid, NOXA, PUMA Bim, and BMF that have a conserved BH3-only domain, also enhance apoptosis. These proteins activate

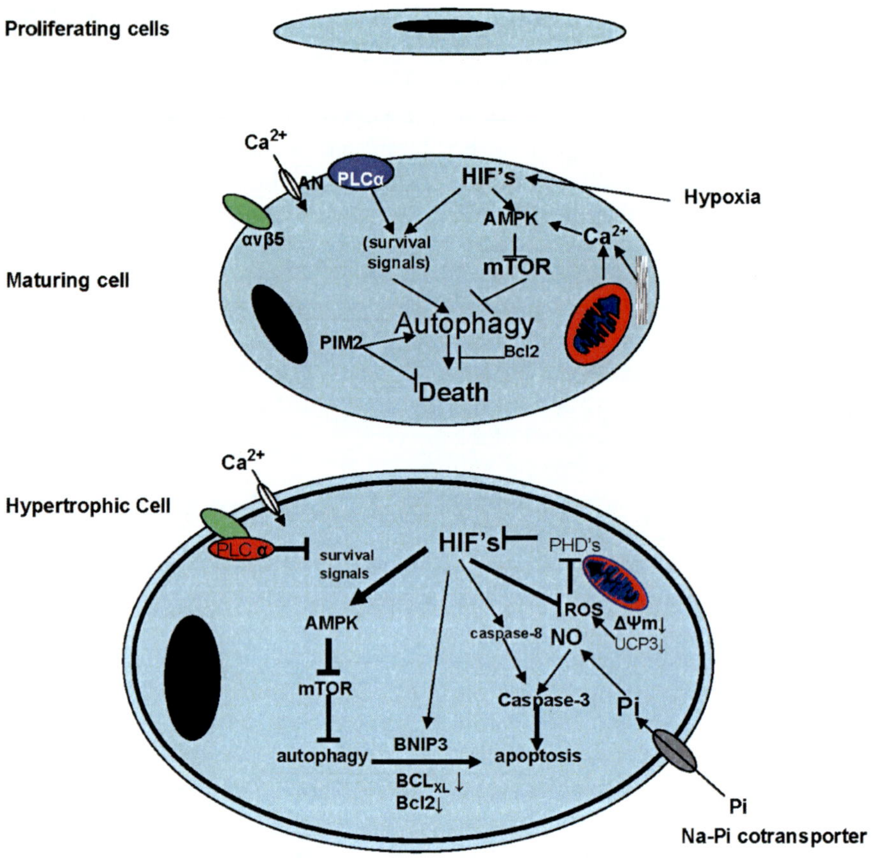

Figure 3.8. Events leading to autophagy and apoptosis in growth-plate chondrocytes. In maturing postmitotic chondrocytes, the low pO_2 of the growth plate causes expression of both HIF-1 and -2. HIF-1 promotes survival activity by upregulating anaerobic energy metabolism and autophagy. AMP kinase (AMPK) activity is increased by HIF-1 and by Ca^{2+} released from mitochondria, the endoplasmic reticulum, and possibly from tissue fluid via annexin channels. In addition to activating autophagic flux, PIM2, together with Bcl2, blocks apoptosis. In hypertrophic chondrocytes, an increase in HIF-1 activity and a decrease in HIF-2 activity result in the sustained activation of AMPK and an increase in the rate of autophagic flux. This increase is enhanced by an elevation in the generation of ROS owing to the decrease in both HIF-2 and UCP3 activity, which results in suppression of the PHD oxygen sensors and an elevation in HIB-1 activity. Furthermore, increased caspase-8 and NO generation, mediated by HIF-1 and Pi, results in caspase-3-mediated apoptosis. The hypertrophic cell is also sensitized to apoptogen challenges, mediated by the $CaxP_i$ ion pair. Sensitization is probably due to the HIF-1-mediated increase in the proapoptotic protein BNIP3 and the progression of autophagic flux.

apoptosis by binding prosurvival Bcl2 proteins and neutralizing their function [97].

When the pathway of apoptosis is stimulated, membrane potential is lost and a transient change in permeability of this mitochondrial membrane is generated, causing release of one or more proteins (cytochrome c and APAF-1). The presence of these proteins in the cytosol triggers the formation of an apoptosome, a macromolecular complex that recruits and binds pro-caspase 9. This multimeric enzyme complex then activates the executioner enzyme, pro-caspase-3. Once activated, this caspase cleaves the proteins within the cell and elicits changes that include cell shrinkage, nuclear condensation, and fragmentation of the organelles and membranes. Products of caspase hydrolysis can be engulfed by cells; this obviates problems that result from an inflammatory response.

In contrast to the intrinsic pathway, death ligands bind receptors on the cell membrane and trigger cell death. Common ligands include the TNF family of ligands including FASL, RANKL, BLYS/BAFF, and APO2L/TRAIL. Formation of a complex multimeric receptor at the plasma membrane (the DISC complex) binds pro-caspase-8 and activates it. This caspase can then activate caspase-3 directly or modulate the mitochondrial function, so as to release cytochrome c and form an apoptosome.

Which of these pathways regulates chondrocyte apoptosis and what is the activating molecule or condition? Because apoptosis represents a critical stage in the life cycle of the chondrocyte, there can be no simple answer. To stimulate apoptosis requires inputs from the local environment, interactions between the cells and late stage matrix components, responses to the presence of other cells at the chondro-osseous junction, and dependency on both hormonal and local (paracrine) factors. Moreover, there is accumulating evidence that it is the extrinsic pathway that serves as a regulatory system. It has been assumed that molecules released at the chondro-osseous junction promote cell death. When calcified, cartilage is being replaced by bone, the matrix molecules accumulate in the microenvironment of the terminally differentiated chondrocytes and, if active, could sensitize cells to apoptosis or induce it. Solubilization of apatite by osteoclasts (septoclasts) would cause Ca^{2+} and phosphate ion (Pi) concentration to become elevated locally and have an effect on the viability of hypertrophic chondrocytes.

Mansfield et al. [84] demonstrated that Pi can serve as an apoptogen, even if Ca^{2+} ions are absent. When the Pi level is low, a small rise in the medium Ca^{2+} concentration is sufficient to cause a marked increase in cell death, although the cation alone does not affect the apoptosis process. When the Pi concentration in the culture was raised to 3.0 mM from the normal serum Pi concentration of 2.0–2.5, an increase in the Ca^{2+} concentration from 1.8 to 2.8 mM caused a dramatic elevation in chondrocyte death. Moreover, irrespective of the medium Pi concentration, the presence of Ca^{2+} chelators inhibited chondrocyte apoptosis. Because it was not clear whether Pi-mediated apoptosis was receptor-mediated or linked to loading the treated cells with Pi, inhibitors were used to block Pi-Na cotransport. As a result, apoptosis was blocked [85]. Moreover, this transport system was sensitive to PTH and vitamin D, agents that modulate chondrocyte maturation and cartilage calcification [20]. In addition to being under humoral control, symport function also depends on the maturation status of the cell.

Apart from causing changes in the mitochondrial function, the ion-pair stimulated ROS generation by the hypertrophic chondrocytes. The elevation of intracellular Ca^{2+} and Pi caused hyperpolarization of mitochondria, as well as a rapid and extensive elevation in ROS levels. Analysis of the kinetics of release indicated that there was an initial lag phase after which the ROS levels increased sixfold before there was any evidence of apoptosis. Moreover, ROS generation was evident soon after the mitochondria became hyperpolarized and remained high for most of the hyperpolarization period [84, 106]. Evaluation of NO generation by ion pair-treated chondrocytes provided a new slant on the possible triggering mechanisms [128]. Pi caused an elevation in NO levels in concert with the activation of caspases and inhibition of mitochondrial function. Recently, Zhong et al. [145], evaluating the role of a prothrombin peptide fragment in apoptosis, noted that inhibition of iNOS-dependent NO generation, possibly involving PKC (see below), also prevented apoptosis in growth-plate chondrocytes. Teixeira et al. [127] showed that when NO synthesis was blocked, the mitochondrial membrane potential was maintained and apoptosis was inhibited. Moreover, the generation of NO leads to the depletion of intracellular thiols [129]. Chondrocyte maturation promotes activation of the apoptotic pathway; this causes ROS and NO generation to increase, leading to a loss of the mitochondrial membrane potential and a decrease in the intracellular thiols [115]. All these events enhance the sensitivity of chondrocytes to environmental apoptogens.

Details of the role played by members of the Bcl-2 gene family in regulating apoptosis has been provided by Oshima et al. [97], who identified a putative proapoptotic gene in the chondrocytes. When this gene was silenced, Pi-induced apoptosis was suppressed. Bnip3 expression increased with hypertrophic differentiation and during Pi-induced apoptosis in ATDC5 cells [97]. Knockdown of Bnip3 blocked Pi-induced apoptosis, whereas overexpression increased Pi-induced chondrocyte apoptosis. Knockdown of Bcl-xL promoted chondrocyte apoptosis. Bcl-xL is expressed uniformly in the growth plate, whereas Bnip3 expression is localized exclusively in the hypertrophic chondrocytes. To further explore the role of Bcl-xL, a chondrocyte-specific mouse mutant was generated. In these dwarf mice the HZ was markedly reduced because of increased apoptosis of the maturing chondrocytes. These studies confirm the pivotal role played by members of the Bcl2 family in regulating chondrocyte apoptosis and in impairing the anti-apoptotic function of Bcl-xL. Bnip3 expression therefore can be observed to determine the fate of the hypertrophic cells.

One drawback to the studies described above is that Pi was a necessary component of the culture system, and hence studies using cultured cells were confounded by the presence of this anion. Magne et al. [79] used the ATDC5 cell line that expresses the type III Na–Pi cotransporters to promote mineralization of the extracellular matrix without the addition of exogenous phosphate and confirmed that Pi accelerated chondrocyte terminal differentiation and, with Ca^{2+}, induced apoptosis and matrix mineralization. Magne et al. [79] speculated that the increase in intracellular Pi levels during maturation accelerates chondrogenic differentiation and, together with elevated levels of soluble Ca^{2+} in the HZ, induces apoptosis-dependent mineralization.

One further approach to assessing the validity of Pi as an inducer of apoptosis is to use *Hyp* mice, an animal with depressed blood Pi concentration, and a model of X-linked hypophosphatemia. Sabbagh et al. [110] showed that a low serum Pi is associated with a decrease in the number of apoptotic hypertrophic chondrocytes and an expansion of the growth plate. These findings strongly support the importance of Pi as a regulator of apoptosis in the growth plate and explain the expanded epiphysis in rickets, which is believed to be due to the retention of chondrocytes. Thus, it is circulating Pi, rather than locally deposited Pi, that is the key to hypertrophic chondrocyte apoptosis.

The changes in Bcl2 family members discussed earlier lend strong support to the notion that apoptosis is activated through the intrinsic pathway. However, this issue is far from settled. Pucci et al. [104] in a recent study of cultured chondrocytes found little evidence in support of apoptosome formation. If this is generally true, then it is conceivable that the intrinsic canonical pathway has undergone tissue-specific modification. A second pathway that may also regulate apoptosis links cell death with membrane receptor function and adhesion. It has been known for some time that when membrane receptor binding does not occur, a form of apoptosis called anoikis is triggered. These membrane receptors are critical for integrin-mediated outside-in signaling and for the activation of ligand-binding affinity (inside-out signaling). Two proteins are involved in the induction of apoptosis, the β5 cytoplasmic domain of αvβ5 and annexin V that bind to the activated form of PKC and trigger apoptosis [25, 114]. Building on this information, Wang and Kirsch [138] demonstrated that the balance between annexin V/β5 integrin and annexin V/PKCa plays a role in regulating growth-plate apoptosis, with annexin V binding to the active PKCa, stimulating apoptosis, and annexin V binding to B5 integrin, regulating the interactions between annexin V/β5 and annexin V/PKCa. What makes this observation particularly relevant to the growth plate is that both annexin V and β5 integrin are robustly expressed by the hypertrophic chondrocyte close to the chondro-osseous junction.

3.8 Chondrocyte Survival vs. Death: Induction of Autophagy

As discussed earlier, some terminally differentiated chondrocytes do not die by apoptosis. One alternate pathway is autophagy, a term used to denote a process in which the cell degrades the organelles, membranes, and isolated proteins. If the activity is not self-limiting, it results in total disintegration of the cell. Within the cell, autophagy is initiated by the formation of an isolation membrane that then sequesters cellular proteins in a vesicle or autophagosome, which then fuses with the lysosomes to form an autophagolysosome. Degradation of the enclosed macromolecules within the autophagolysosome generates amino acids and free fatty acids that are recycled to yield intracellular nutrients and energy. Twenty-seven genes encode autophagy-related (Atg) proteins [66]. These proteins are required for the formation of multiprotein complexes that include an autophagy-specific phosphatidylinositol 3-kinase (PI3K) assembly, as well as ubiquitin-like protein conjugates. Not surprisingly, the autophagic process is closely regulated by a number of proteins, including AMPK, HIF's, PIM2, and mTOR (mammalian target of rapamycin) kinase.

mTOR is a serine–threonine protein kinase that acts as a nutrient sensor and indirectly assesses the oxemic status of the cell [24]. The activated kinase represses autophagy. Hypoxia and the subsequent stabilization of HIF, together with nutrient depletion, inhibit mTOR activity. Both the events are permissive for autophagy [78]. Energy depletion also inhibits mTOR with suppression owing to the activation of AMPK [121]. This kinase is an energy sensor that is sensitive to the AMP level in the cell; its activity is dependent on a second enzyme, adenylate kinase [53].

AMPK activity influences glycolysis, glucose utilization, fatty acid synthesis, fatty acid oxidation, and lipolysis. Protein synthesis may also be influenced by AMPK, through modification of the activity elongation factor, EF-2. PIM2 is a serine–threonine kinase, which is robustly expressed in the cells of the growth plate, where it promotes autophagic flux by modulating the expression and organization of LC3 and Beclin-1, and by inhibiting the induction of apoptosis [22].

Autophagy has been identified with a non-apoptotic form of cell death (type II apoptosis) and dying cells frequently contain autophagic vacuoles. Yet, induction of autophagy may also promote cell survival. This prosurvival activity can be considered to be a biological strategy that permits survival during periods of nutrient deprivation, with degradation of membrane triglycerides and proteins providing the fuel to stoke mitochondrial ATP energy production, thereby extending cell longevity. How autophagy regulates chondrocyte death is important in relation to the normal tissue function and chondrocyte survival.

The fate of the differentiated cell is the result of the interaction between two groups of proteins: the autophagic ATG protein, Beclin-1, and the members of the Bcl-2 family of proteins. Beclin-1 was originally identified as a Bcl-2 interacting protein [100] that, by binding to Bcl-2, decreases the free concentration of this anti-apoptotic protein. This, in turn, increases the sensitivity of the cells to apoptogens [76]. In our view, the activation of autophagic flux would also depend on the niche conditions in the growth plate, regulated by the agents HIF-1, HIF-2, and AMPK, among others. The protein that serves as a nexus for inputs from HIF, AMPK, and other signaling pathways, such as Akt/PI3K, is mTOR [121]. Two other proteins mediate autophagic flux. PIM2, together with Bcl2, blocks apoptosis and UCP3, which, together with HIF-2, regulates ROS levels in the growth plate [140].

One can then ask how each of these enzymatic activities regulates autophagy/apoptosis. In hypertrophic chondrocytes, an increase in HIF-1 activity and a decrease in HIF-2 activity would sustain AMPK activation and increase the rate of autophagic flux. The increase in flux is enhanced by additional generation of ROS, which lowers HIF-2 and UCP3. As a result, the PHD oxygen sensors are suppressed and HIF-1 activity is raised. Conceivably, an HIF-1-and Pi-dependent increase in caspase-8 and NO generation also promotes caspase-3-mediated apoptosis.

To test whether autophagy promotes chondrocyte survival in the growth plate, Bohensky et al. [22] evaluated the in vivo expression of the two proteins that are characteristic of autophagy: Beclin-1 and LC3, a protein that condenses in the intracellular vesicles during autophagy. Suppression of Beclin increased BID cleavage and caspase-8 activation, and enhanced cell death; thus, expression of this autophagy gene enhanced chondrocyte survival. The authors commented that other members of the protein family, including Noxa, Bnip3, and BAD, may also be activated. The activation of caspase-8 was a novel finding and is related to the role of the extrinsic pathway of apoptosis. From a physiological perspective, autophagic signaling seems to enhance cell survival, especially during the later stages of terminal differentiation, when the cells are assailed by apoptotic stimuli.

In the same study [22], the linkage between hypoxia and survival was evaluated. Because HIF-1 maintained Beclin-1 levels, it seems to regulate at least one component of the autophagic pathway. It was concluded, therefore, that in the challenging microenvironment of the growth plate, HIF-1 maintains the viability of the proliferating and prehypertrophic chondrocytes until maturation is completed. Eventually, extended autophagic activity sensitizes terminally differentiated chondrocytes to local and intrinsic signals, resulting in apoptosis and deletion of cells from the growth plate. This release, in turn, accelerates cartilage replacement by bone and induces bone growth.

3.9 Diseases of the Growth Plate

Rickets occurs mostly in children whose growth plates are actively growing and is caused by a failure of mineralization in the growth plates and bones. The result is that bones grow poorly and bend, because poorly mineralized bones tend to bend when exposed to mechanical stress during normal activities. Breathing, for example, causes ribs to bend inward and, in rickets leads to development of a "pigeon breast," owing to compensatory outward bowing of the sternum. The retarded mineralization causes accumulation of unresorbed cartilage matrix and enlarged growth plates. The bones in rickets are also incompletely mineralized, a condition termed osteomalacia. Decreased mineralization of growth plates and bones, as seen in rickets, is owing to a variety of factors that cause lower Ca^{2+} and/or PO_4^{3-} in cartilage and bone. In children, hypocalcemia is typically caused by a deficiency of vitamin D leading to impaired calcium absorption.

Rickets and osteomalacia in adults are also due to hypophosphatemia. Even if plasma levels of Ca^{2+} are normal, bone mineralization is diminished in the presence of hypophosphatemia, which is often the result of excessive urinary excretion of PO_4^{3-} [102]. Pathologic causes of hypophosphatemia include decreased gastrointestinal PO_4 absorption and several hereditary forms of hyperphosphaturia [102].

Hypophosphatasia is a heritable form of rickets and/or osteomalacia that results from defects in the gene for alkaline phosphatase, an enzyme found in bones, liver, and kidneys, the so-called tissue nonspecific alkaline phosphatase (TNAP). TNAP promotes normal mineralization of the growth plate and newly formed bone [13]. Figure 3.9 compares the relative amount and distribution of mineral in normal cartilage and bone matrix with that from a TNAP-deficient growth plate and bone [14]. In hypophosphatasia, phase 1 of MV mineralization is not impeded by TNAP deficiency. Rather, the failure of mineralization in hypophosphatasia is mostly due to blocking of normal Phase 2 mineral propagation at the perimeter of TNAP-enriched MVs [12, 14].

Achondroplasia is the most common form of dwarfism in humans. As discussed in Chap. 1 of this volume, it is caused by mutations of the FGF receptor 3 gene (FGFR3) that cause functional overactivity of this receptor, resulting in slow chondrocyte proliferation and differentiation in the growth plate [51]. One of the several related mutations brings about a Gly 380 Arg amino acid substitution in the transmembrane domain of the FGFR3 receptor. Although achondroplasia is a dominant mutation, over 80% of the cases result from a new mutation of FGFR3, not carried in the parental genes. The bodily phenotype is characterized by shortened stature, owing to reduced growth in the growth plates of the long bones. The skull is enlarged and the forehead is bulging. The bones of the midface are small, because the size of the facial bones is a function of endochondral bone formation in the growth plates of the calvarium [51]. Growth plates throughout the body are disordered, with narrowed zones of proliferation and hypertrophy and disorganized chondrocyte columns. Horizontal bone trabeculae are prematurely deposited at the base of the growth plate. This seals the plate and prevents further growth.

Osteochondromas and *enchondromas* are benign tumors that arise from displaced chondrocytes that migrate out from the growth plate and/or its perichondrium [65, 87]. Osteochondromas are located primarily in or on the surface of the metaphyseal bone.

Osteochondromas are mushroom-like outgrowths that arise from the periosteal surface of the metaphysis, close to the perichondrium of the growth plate. A "cartilage cap" lies on top of an osteochondroma. It resembles a growth

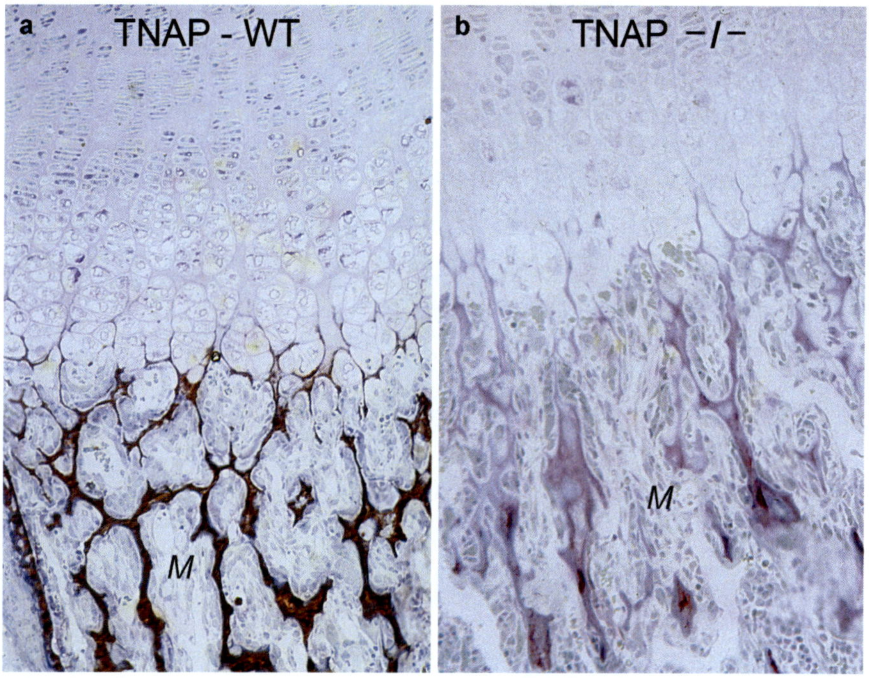

Figure 3.9. Alizarin red calcium stains for mineral in TNAP normal mouse tibial growth plate (**A**) vs. TNAP-deficient tibial growth plate (**B**). The TNAP-deficient tibias show a significant reduction in dark red alizarin-staining of calcium phosphate mineral deposits, in the calcified zone of the growth plate, and in the bone trabeculae of the underlying metaphysis (Modified from Anderson [14]) ((**A**) magnification 420×; (**B**) magnification 530×).

plate, is rotated 90°, and grows perpendicularly to the long axis of the bone, with hypertrophic chondrocytes in a layer closest to its base and proliferative chondrocytes near the surface. The bony base of the osteochondroma consists of an outer cortex with underlying cancellous bone; it resembles the normal metaphysis and is continuous with it [87]. The growth pattern of osteochondroma is like that of a displaced growth plate, growing at 90° from the longitudinal axis of the bone [132]. Almost all osteochondromas are benign and occur as solitary or multiple lesions in the hereditary multiple exostoses syndrome [132].

Enchondromas usually begin as benign cartilaginous neoplasms of childhood, arising from chondrocytes at the base of the growth plate. Chondrocytes of enchondromas do not undergo the rigidly controlled pattern of apoptosis and resorption seen in the growth plate, but form cartilaginous tumors in the metaphysis [87]. Hereditary multiple enchondromas result from deletion mutation(s) of the EXT1 or EXT2 gene. In patients with hereditary multiple enchondromatosis syndromes, there is a relatively high risk to develop chondrosarcoma [132].

3.10 Summary

The growth plate is a remarkable organ where structure reflects function to an exceptional degree. Thus, with chondrocytes in the growth plate, orientation at different levels reflects the state of cellular maturation and differentiation at that particular level. Partly because of this it has been possible to analyze and characterize, to a remarkable degree, the metabolic activity ongoing at a particular level, from conversion from stem cells, to proliferation, to differentiation (with matrix synthesis and initiation of mineralization), and finally to apoptosis. However, notwithstanding the advances in our knowledge of growth plate structure and function, an understanding of how growth plate chondrocytes interact with other, more distant tissues is far from complete. For example, little is known about the mechanisms by which growth plate chondrocytes communicate with cells of underlying bone, with distant growth plates, and with other cells of the body. Active current areas of research include growth plate interaction with adipose tissue (which produces leptin) and regulation of the growth plate by the neurotransmitter, serotonin. A challenge for the coming decade is to elucidate how these intraorgan signals are controlled and integrated.

References

1. Abad V, Meyers JL, Weise M, Gafni RI, Barnes KM, Nilsson O, Bacher JD, Baron J (2002) The role of the resting zone in growth plate chondrogenesis. Endocrinology 143:1851–1857
2. Agrawal A, Gajghate S, Smith H, Anderson DG, Albert TJ, Shapiro IM, Risbud MV (2008) Cited2 modulates hypoxia-inducible factor-dependent expression of vascular endothelial growth factor in nucleus pulposus cells of the rat intervertebral disc. Arthritis Rheum 58:3798–3808
3. Akiyama H, Lyons JP, Mori-Akiyama Y, Yang X, Zhang R, Zhang Z, Deng JM, Taketo MM, Nakamura T, Behringer RR, McCrea PD, de Crombrugghe B (2004) Interactions between Sox9 and beta-catenin control chondrocyte differentiation. Genes Dev 18:1072–1087
4. Ali SY, Sajdera SW, Anderson HC (1970) Isolation and characterization of calcifying matrix vesicles from epiphyseal cartilage. Proc Natl Acad Sci U S A 67:1513–1520
5. Alvarez J, Sohn P, Zeng X, Doetschman T, Robbins DJ, Serra R (2002) TGFbeta2 mediates the effects of hedgehog on hypertrophic differentiation and PTHrP expression. Development 129:1913–1924
6. Anderson HC (1969) Vesicles associated with calcification in the matrix of epiphyseal cartilage. J Cell Biol 41:59–72
7. Anderson HC (1978) Introduction to the second conference on matrix vesicle calcification, Metab Bone Dis Relat Res 1 83–87
8. Anderson HC (1983) Calcific diseases. A concept. Arch Pathol Lab Med 107:341–348
9. Anderson HC (1985) Normal biological mineralization. Role of cells, membranes and matrix vesicles. In: Rubin RP, Weiss GF, Putney JW Jr (eds) Calcium in biological systems. Pienum, New York, p 600
10. Anderson HC, Garimella R, Tague SE (2005) The role of matrix vesicles in growth plate development and biomineralization. Front Biosci 10:822–837
11. Anderson HC, Hodges PT, Aguilera XM, Missana L, Moylan PE (2000) Bone morphogenetic protein (BMP) localization in developing human and rat growth plate, metaphysis, epiphysis, and articular cartilage. J Histochem Cytochem 48:1493–1502
12. Anderson HC, Hsu HH, Morris DC, Fedde KN, Whyte MP (1997) Matrix vesicles in osteomalacic hypophosphatasia bone contain apatite-like mineral crystals. Am J Pathol 151:1555–1561
13. Anderson HC, Reynolds JJ (1973) Pyrophosphate stimulation of calcium uptake into cultured embryonic bones. Fine structure of matrix vesicles and their role in calcification. Dev Biol 34:211–227
14. Anderson HC, Sipe JB, Hessle L, Dhanyamraju R, Atti E, Camacho NP, Millan JL (2004) Impaired calcification around matrix vesicles of growth plate and bone in alkaline phosphatase-deficient mice. Am J Pathol 164:841–847
15. Andrade AC, Nilsson O, Barnes KM, Baron J (2007) Wnt gene expression in the post-natal growth plate: regulation with chondrocyte differentiation. Bone 40:1361–1369
16. Balemans W, Van Hul W (2002) Extracellular regulation of BMP signaling in vertebrates: a cocktail of modulators. Dev Biol 250:231–250
17. Baron J, Klein KO, Colli MJ, Yanovski JA, Novosad JA, Bacher JD, Cutler GB Jr (1994) Catch-up growth after glucocorticoid excess: a mechanism intrinsic to the growth plate. Endocrinology 135:1367–1371
18. Baron J, Klein KO, Yanovski JA, Novosad JA, Bacher JD, Bolander ME, Cutler GB Jr (1994) Induction of growth plate cartilage ossification by basic fibroblast growth factor. Endocrinology 135:2790–2793
19. Barreto C, Albrecht RM, Bjorling DE, Horner JR, Wilsman NJ (1993) Evidence of the growth plate and the growth of long bones in juvenile dinosaurs. Science 262:2020–2023
20. Berndt T, Kumar R (2007) Phosphatonins and the regulation of phosphate homeostasis. Annu Rev Physiol 69:341–359
21. Blodgett FM, Burgin L, Iezzoni D, Gribetz D, Talbot NB (1956) Effects of prolonged cortisone therapy on the statural growth, skeletal maturation and metabolic status of children. N Engl J Med 254:636–641
22. Bohensky J, Shapiro IM, Leshinsky S, Terkhorn SP, Adams CS, Srinivas V (2007) HIF-1 regulation of chondrocyte apoptosis: induction of the autophagic pathway. Autophagy 3:207–214
23. Boskey AL, Moore DJ, Amling M, Canalis E, Delany AM (2003) Infrared analysis of the mineral and matrix in bones of osteonectin-null mice and their wildtype controls. J Bone Miner Res 18:1005–1011
24. Brugarolas J, Lei K, Hurley RL, Manning BD, Reiling JH, Hafen E, Witters LA, Ellisen LW, Kaelin WG Jr (2004) Regulation of mTOR function in response to hypoxia by REDD1 and the TSC1/TSC2 tumor suppressor complex. Genes Dev 18: 2893–2904
25. Cardo-Vila M, Arap W, Pasqualini R (2003) Alpha v beta 5 integrin-dependent programmed cell death triggered by a peptide mimic of annexin V. Mol Cell 11:1151–1162

26. Cecil RNA, Anderson HC (1978) Freeze-fracture studies of matrix vesicle calcification in epiphyseal growth plate. Metab Bone Dis Relat Res 1:89–97
27. Chen CC, Boskey AL, Rosenberg LC (1984) The inhibitory effect of cartilage proteoglycans on hydroxyapatite growth. Calcif Tissue Int 36:285–290
28. Chen H, Shi H (2008) A reducing environment stabilizes HIF-2alpha in SH-SY5Y cells under hypoxic conditions. FEBS Lett 582:3899–3902
29. Chun JS, Oh H, Yang S, Park M (2008) Wnt signaling in cartilage development and degeneration. BMB Rep 41:485–494
30. Coffin JD, Florkiewicz RZ, Neumann J, Mort-Hopkins T, Dorn GW II, Lightfoot P, German R, Howles PN, Kier A, O'Toole BA et al (1995) Abnormal bone growth and selective translational regulation in basic fibroblast growth factor (FGF-2) transgenic mice. Mol Biol Cell 6:1861–1873
31. D'Angelo M, Billings PC, Pacifici M, Leboy PS, Kirsch T (2001) Authentic matrix vesicles contain active metalloproteases (MMP). A role for matrix vesicle-associated MMP-13 in activation of transforming growth factor-beta. J Biol Chem 276:11347–11353
32. Dai J, Rabie AB (2007) VEGF: an essential mediator of both angiogenesis and endochondral ossification. J Dent Res 86:937–950
33. Davidson D, Blanc A, Filion D, Wang H, Plut P, Pfeffer G, Buschmann MD, Henderson JE (2005) Fibroblast growth factor (FGF) 18 signals through FGF receptor 3 to promote chondrogenesis. J Biol Chem 280:20509–20515
34. De Luca F, Barnes KM, Uyeda JA, De-Levi S, Abad V, Palese T, Mericq V, Baron J (2001) Regulation of growth plate chondrogenesis by bone morphogenetic protein-2. Endocrinology 142:430–436
35. Dickson KM, Bergeron JJ, Philip A, O'Connor-McCourt M, Warshawsky H (2001) Localization of specific binding sites for 125I-TGF-beta1 to fenestrated endothelium in bone and anastomosing capillary networks in enamel organ suggests a role for TGF-beta1 in angiogenesis. Calcif Tissue Int 68:304–315
36. Ducy P, Geoffroy V, Karsenty G (1996) Study of osteoblast-specific expression of one mouse osteocalcin gene: characterization of the factor binding to OSE2. Connect Tissue Res 35:7–14
37. Enomoto-Iwamoto M, Kitagaki J, Koyama E, Tamamura Y, Wu C, Kanatani N, Koike T, Okada H, Komori T, Yoneda T, Church V, Francis-West PH, Kurisu K, Nohno T, Pacifici M, Iwamoto M (2002) The Wnt antagonist Frzb-1 regulates chondrocyte maturation and long bone development during limb skeletogenesis. Dev Biol 251:142–156
38. Farnum CE, Wilsman NJ (1989) Cellular turnover at the chondro-osseous junction of growth plate cartilage: analysis by serial sections at the light microscopical level. J Orthop Res 7:654–666
39. Farquharson C, Loveridge N (1990) Cell proliferation within the growth plate of long bones assessed by bromodeoxyuridine uptake and its relationship to glucose 6-phosphate dehydrogenase activity. Bone Miner 10:121–130
40. Felisbino SL, Carvalho HF (1999) The epiphyseal cartilage and growth of long bones in Rana catesbeiana. Tissue Cell 31:301–307
41. Fleisch H, Russell RG, Straumann F (1966) Effect of pyrophosphate on hydroxyapatite and its implications in calcium homeostasis. Nature 212:901–903
42. Garcia-Ramirez M, Toran N, Andaluz P, Carrascosa A, Audi L (2000) Vascular endothelial growth factor is expressed in human fetal growth cartilage. J Bone Miner Res 15:534–540
43. Garimella R, Bi X, Camacho N, Sipe JB, Anderson HC (2004) Primary culture of rat growth plate chondrocytes: an in vitro model of growth plate histotype, matrix vesicle biogenesis and mineralization. Bone 34:961–970
44. Gay CV, Leach RM (1985) Tritiated thymidine uptake in chondrocytes of chickens afflicted with tibial dyschondroplasia. Avian Dis 29:1224–1229
45. Gerber HP, Vu TH, Ryan AM, Kowalski J, Werb Z, Ferrara N (1999) VEGF couples hypertrophic cartilage remodeling, ossification and angiogenesis during endochondral bone formation. Nat Med 5:623–628
46. Gordeladze JO, Reseland JE (2003) A unified model for the action of leptin on bone turnover. J Cell Biochem 88:706–712
47. Gordon MD, Nusse R (2006) Wnt signaling: multiple pathways, multiple receptors, and multiple transcription factors. J Biol Chem 281:22429–22433
48. Haines RW (1975) The histology of epiphyseal union in mammals. J Anat 120:1–25
49. Hasky-Negev M, Simsa S, Tong A, Genina O, Monsonego Ornan E (2008) Expression of matrix metalloproteinases during vascularization and ossification of normal and impaired avian growth plate. J Anim Sci 86:1306–1315
50. Horner A, Bishop NJ, Bord S, Beeton C, Kelsall AW, Coleman N, Compston JE (1999) Immunolocalisation of vascular endothelial growth factor (VEGF) in human neonatal growth plate cartilage. J Anat 194 (pt 4):519–524
51. Horton WA, Hall JG, Hecht JT (2007) Achondroplasia. Lancet 370:162–172
52. Howell DS, Pita JC, Marquez JF, Madruga JE (1968) Partition of calcium, phosphate, and protein in the fluid phase aspirated at calcifying sites in epiphyseal cartilage. J Clin Invest 47:1121–1132
53. Hoyer-Hansen M, Jaattela M (2007) AMP-activated protein kinase: a universal regulator of autophagy? Autophagy 3:381–383
54. Huang H, He X (2008) Wnt/beta-catenin signaling: new (and old) players and new insights. Curr Opin Cell Biol 20:119–125
55. Hu H, Hilton MJ, Tu X, Yu K, Ornitz DM, Long F (2005) Sequential roles of Hedgehog and Wnt signaling in osteoblast development. Development 132:49–60
56. Irie A, Habuchi H, Kimata K, Sanai Y (2003) Heparan sulfate is required for bone morphogenetic protein-7 signaling. Biochem Biophys Res Commun 308:858–865
57. Ivkovic S, Yoon BS, Popoff SN, Safadi FF, Libuda DE, Stephenson RC, Daluiski A, Lyons KM (2003)

Connective tissue growth factor coordinates chondrogenesis and angiogenesis during skeletal development. Development 130:2779–2791
58. Jones RK, Searle RF, Stewart JA, Turner S, Bulmer JN (1998) Apoptosis, bcl-2 expression, and proliferative activity in human endometrial stroma and endometrial granulated lymphocytes. Biol Reprod 58:995–1002
59. Kahn BB, Alquier T, Carling D, Hardie DG (2005) AMP-activated protein kinase: ancient energy gauge provides clues to modern understanding of metabolism. Cell Metab 1:15–25
60. Karaplis AC, He B, Nguyen MT, Young ID, Semeraro D, Ozawa H, Amizuka N (1998) Inactivating mutation in the human parathyroid hormone receptor type 1 gene in Blomstrand chondrodysplasia. Endocrinology 139:5255–5258
61. Karperien M, Lanser P, de Laat SW, Boonstra J, Defize LH (1996) Parathyroid hormone related peptide mRNA expression during murine postimplantation development: evidence for involvement in multiple differentiation processes. Int J Dev Biol 40:599–608
62. Kember NF (1972) Comparative patterns of cell division in epiphyseal cartilage plates in the rat. J Anat 111:137–142
63. Kerr BA, Otani T, Koyama E, Freeman TA, Enomoto-Iwamoto M (2008) Small GTPase protein Rac-1 is activated with maturation and regulates cell morphology and function in chondrocytes. Exp Cell Res 314:1301–1312
64. Kirsch T (2005) Annexins – their role in cartilage mineralization. Front Biosci 10:576–581
65. Kitsoulis P, Galani V, Stefanaki K, Paraskevas G, Karatzias G, Agnantis NJ, Bai M (2008) Osteochondromas: review of the clinical, radiological and pathological features. In Vivo 22:633–646
66. Klionsky DJ, Cregg JM, Dunn WA Jr, Emr SD, Sakai Y, Sandoval IV, Sibirny A, Subramani S, Thumm M, Veenhuis M, Ohsumi Y (2003) A unified nomenclature for yeast autophagy-related genes. Dev Cell 5:539–545
67. Kobayashi T, Soegiarto DW, Yang Y, Lanske B, Schipani E, McMahon AP, Kronenberg HM (2005) Indian hedgehog stimulates periarticular chondrocyte differentiation to regulate growth plate length independently of PTHrP. J Clin Invest 115:1734–1742
68. Krejci P, Krakow D, Mekikian PB, Wilcox WR (2007) Fibroblast growth factors 1, 2, 17, and 19 are the predominant FGF ligands expressed in human fetal growth plate cartilage. Pediatr Res 61:267–272
69. Kronenberg HM (2006) PTHrP and skeletal development. Ann N Y Acad Sci 1068:1–13
70. Kronenberg HM (2007) The role of the perichondrium in fetal bone development. Ann N Y Acad Sci 1116:59–64
71. Kuhl M, Sheldahl LC, Park M, Miller JR, Moon RT (2000) The Wnt/Ca2 + pathway: a new vertebrate Wnt signaling pathway takes shape. Trends Genet 16:279–283
72. Landis WJ, Arsenault AL (1989) Vesicle- and collagen-mediated calcification in the turkey leg tendon. Connect Tissue Res 22:35–42; discussion 53–61
73. Lazarus JE, Hegde A, Andrade AC, Nilsson O, Baron J (2007) Fibroblast growth factor expression in the postnatal growth plate. Bone 40:577–586
74. Lee ER, Lamplugh L, Shepard NL, Mort JS (1995) The septoclast, a cathepsin B-rich cell involved in the resorption of growth plate cartilage. J Histochem Cytochem 43:525–536
75. Lee YJ, Park JH, Ju SK, You KH, Ko JS, Kim HM (2002) Leptin receptor isoform expression in rat osteoblasts and their functional analysis. FEBS Lett 528:43–47
76. Levine B, Sinha S, Kroemer G (2008) Bcl-2 family members: dual regulators of apoptosis and autophagy. Autophagy 4:600–606
77. Liu Z, Lavine KJ, Hung IH, Ornitz DM (2007) FGF18 is required for early chondrocyte proliferation, hypertrophy and vascular invasion of the growth plate. Dev Biol 302:80–91
78. Lum JJ, DeBerardinis RJ, Thompson CB (2005) Autophagy in metazoans: cell survival in the land of plenty. Nat Rev Mol Cell Biol 6:439–448
79. Magne D, Bluteau G, Faucheux C, Palmer G, Vignes-Colombeix C, Pilet P, Rouillon T, Caverzasio J, Weiss P, Daculsi G, Guicheux J (2003) Phosphate is a specific signal for ATDC5 chondrocyte maturation and apoptosis-associated mineralization: possible implication of apoptosis in the regulation of endochondral ossification. J Bone Miner Res 18:1430–1442
80. Majno G, Joris I (1995) Apoptosis, oncosis, and necrosis. An overview of cell death. Am J Pathol 146:3–15
81. Mak KK, Chen MH, Day TF, Chuang PT, Yang Y (2006) Wnt/beta-catenin signaling interacts differentially with Ihh signaling in controlling endochondral bone and synovial joint formation. Development 133:3695–3707
82. Mancilla EE, De Luca F, Uyeda JA, Czerwiec FS, Baron J (1998) Effects of fibroblast growth factor-2 on longitudinal bone growth. Endocrinology 139:2900–2904
83. Maniatopoulos C, Sodek J, Melcher AH (1988) Bone formation in vitro by stromal cells obtained from bone marrow of young adult rats. Cell Tissue Res 254:317–330
84. Mansfield K, Pucci B, Adams CS, Shapiro IM (2003) Induction of apoptosis in skeletal tissues: phosphate-mediated chick chondrocyte apoptosis is calcium dependent. Calcif Tissue Int 73:161–172
85. Mansfield K, Teixeira CC, Adams CS, Shapiro IM (2001) Phosphate ions mediate chondrocyte apoptosis through a plasma membrane transporter mechanism. Bone 28:1–8
86. Matsuzawa T, Anderson HC (1971) Phosphatases of epiphyseal cartilage studied by electron microscopic cytochemical methods. J Histochem Cytochem 19:801–808
87. Milgram JW (1983) The origins of osteochondromas and enchondromas. A histopathologic study. Clin Orthop Relat Res 264–284
88. Minina E, Kreschel C, Naski MC, Ornitz DM, Vortkamp A (2002) Interaction of FGF, Ihh/Pthlh, and BMP signaling integrates chondrocyte proliferation and hypertrophic differentiation. Dev Cell 3:439–449

89. Minina E, Schneider S, Rosowski M, Lauster R, Vortkamp A (2005) Expression of Fgf and Tgfbeta signaling related genes during embryonic endochondral ossification. Gene Expr Patterns 6:102–109
90. Minina E, Wenzel HM, Kreschel C, Karp S, Gaffield W, McMahon AP, Vortkamp A (2001) BMP and Ihh/PTHrP signaling interact to coordinate chondrocyte proliferation and differentiation. Development 128: 4523–4534
91. Montessuit C, Caverzasio J, Bonjour JP (1991) Characterization of a Pi transport system in cartilage matrix vesicles. Potential role in the calcification process. J Biol Chem 266:17791–17797
92. Nagayama M, Iwamoto M, Hargett A, Kamiya N, Tamamura Y, Young B, Morrison T, Takeuchi H, Pacifici M, Enomoto-Iwamoto M, Koyama E (2008) Wnt/beta-catenin signaling regulates cranial base development and growth. J Dent Res 87:244–249
93. Nahar NN, Missana LR, Garimella R, Tague SE, Anderson HC (2008) Matrix vesicles are carriers of bone morphogenetic proteins (BMPs), vascular endothelial growth factor (VEGF), and noncollagenous matrix proteins. J Bone Miner Metab 26:514–519
94. Nilsson O, Parker EA, Hegde A, Chau M, Barnes KM, Baron J (2007) Gradients in bone morphogenetic protein-related gene expression across the growth plate. J Endocrinol 193:75–84
95. Niswander L, Martin GR (1993) FGF-4 and BMP-2 have opposite effects on limb growth. Nature 361:68–71
96. Nusse R (1996) Patching up Hedgehog. Nature 384: 119–120
97. Oshima Y, Akiyama T, Hikita A, Iwasawa M, Nagase Y, Nakamura M, Wakeyama H, Kawamura N, Ikeda T, Chung UI, Hennighausen L, Kawaguchi H, Nakamura K, Tanaka S (2008) Pivotal role of Bcl-2 family proteins in the regulation of chondrocyte apoptosis. J Biol Chem 283:26499–26508
98. Pan Y, Mansfield KD, Bertozzi CC, Rudenko V, Chan DA, Giaccia AJ, Simon MC (2007) Multiple factors affecting cellular redox status and energy metabolism modulate hypoxia-inducible factor prolyl hydroxylase activity in vivo and in vitro. Mol Cell Biol 27:912–925
99. Parfitt AM (2002) Misconceptions (1): epiphyseal fusion causes cessation of growth. Bone 30:337–339
100. Pattingre S, Tassa A, Qu X, Garuti R, Liang XH, Mizushima N, Packer M, Schneider MD, Levine B (2005) Bcl-2 antiapoptotic proteins inhibit Beclin 1-dependent autophagy. Cell 122:927–939
101. Peress NS, Anderson HC, Sajdera SW (1974) The lipids of matrix vesicles from bovine fetal epiphyseal cartilage. Calcif Tissue Res 14:275–281
102. Pettifor JM (2008) What's new in hypophosphataemic rickets? Eur J Pediatr 167:493–499
103. Provot S, Schipani E (2007) Fetal growth plate: a developmental model of cellular adaptation to hypoxia. Ann N Y Acad Sci 1117:26–39
104. Pucci B, Adams CS, Fertala J, Snyder BC, Mansfield KD, Tafani M, Freeman T, Shapiro IM (2007) Development of the terminally differentiated state sensitizes epiphyseal chondrocytes to apoptosis through caspase-3 activation. J Cell Physiol 210: 609–615
105. Rajpurohit R, Koch CJ, Tao Z, Teixeira CM, Shapiro IM (1996) Adaptation of chondrocytes to low oxygen tension: relationship between hypoxia and cellular metabolism. J Cell Physiol 168:424–432
106. Rajpurohit R, Mansfield K, Ohyama K, Ewert D, Shapiro IM (1999) Chondrocyte death is linked to development of a mitochondrial membrane permeability transition in the growth plate. J Cell Physiol 179:287–296
107. Roach HI, Aigner T, Kouri JB (2004) Chondroptosis: a variant of apoptotic cell death in chondrocytes? Apoptosis 9:265–277
108. Rozenblut B, Ogielska M (2005) Development and growth of long bones in European water frogs (Amphibia: Anura: Ranidae), with remarks on age determination. J Morphol 265:304–317
109. Rundhaug JE (2005) Matrix metalloproteinases and angiogenesis. J Cell Mol Med 9:267–285
110. Sabbagh Y, Carpenter TO, Demay MB (2005) Hypophosphatemia leads to rickets by impairing caspase-mediated apoptosis of hypertrophic chondrocytes. Proc Natl Acad Sci U S A 102: 9637–9642
111. Schinke T, Amendt C, Trindl A, Poschke O, Muller-Esterl W, Jahnen-Dechent W (1996) The serum protein alpha2-HS glycoprotein/fetuin inhibits apatite formation in vitro and in mineralizing calvaria cells. A possible role in mineralization and calcium homeostasis. J Biol Chem 271:20789–20796
112. Schipani E, Kruse K, Juppner H (1995) A constitutively active mutant PTH-PTHrP receptor in Jansen-type metaphyseal chondrodysplasia. Science 268:98–100
113. Schipani E, Ryan HE, Didrickson S, Kobayashi T, Knight M, Johnson RS (2001) Hypoxia in cartilage: HIF-1alpha is essential for chondrocyte growth arrest and survival. Genes Dev 15:2865–2876
114. Schlaepfer DD, Jones J, Haigler HT (1992) Inhibition of protein kinase C by annexin V. Biochemistry 31:1886–1891
115. Shapiro IM, Adams CS, Freeman T, Srinivas V (2005) Fate of the hypertrophic chondrocyte: microenvironmental perspectives on apoptosis and survival in the epiphyseal growth plate. Birth Defects Res C Embryo Today 75:330–339
116. Shapiro IM, Mansfield KD, Evans SM, Lord EM, Koch CJ (1997) Chondrocytes in the endochondral growth cartilage are not hypoxic. Am J Physiol 272: C1134–C1143
117. Shapiro IM, Srinivas V (2007) Metabolic consideration of epiphyseal growth: survival responses in a taxing environment. Bone 40:561–567
118. Shukunami C, Oshima Y, Hiraki Y (2005) Chondromodulin-I and tenomodulin: a new class of tissue-specific angiogenesis inhibitors found in hypovascular connective tissues. Biochem Biophys Res Commun 333:299–307
119. Simon MC (2006) Coming up for air: HIF-1 and mitochondrial oxygen consumption. Cell Metab 3:150–151

120. Smink JJ, Buchholz IM, Hamers N, van Tilburg CM, Christis C, Sakkers RJ, de Meer K, van Buul-Offers SC, Koedam JA (2003) Short-term glucocorticoid treatment of piglets causes changes in growth plate morphology and angiogenesis. Osteoarthritis Cartilage 11:864–871
121. Srinivas V, Bohensky J, Shapiro IM (2009) Autophagy: a new phase in the maturation of growth plate chondrocytes is regulated by HIF, mTOR and AMP kinase. Cells Tissues Organs 189:88–92
122. Takada T, Katagiri T, Ifuku M, Morimura N, Kobayashi M, Hasegawa K, Ogamo A, Kamijo R (2003) Sulfated polysaccharides enhance the biological activities of bone morphogenetic proteins. J Biol Chem 278:43229–43235
123. Takahara M, Naruse T, Takagi M, Orui H, Ogino T (2004) Matrix metalloproteinase-9 expression, tartrate-resistant acid phosphatase activity, and DNA fragmentation in vascular and cellular invasion into cartilage preceding primary endochondral ossification in long bones. J Orthop Res 22:1050–1057
124. Tamamura Y, Otani T, Kanatani N, Koyama E, Kitagaki J, Komori T, Yamada Y, Costantini F, Wakisaka S, Pacifici M, Iwamoto M, Enomoto-Iwamoto M (2005) Developmental regulation of Wnt/beta-catenin signals is required for growth plate assembly, cartilage integrity, and endochondral ossification. J Biol Chem 280:19185–19195
125. Tanaka N, Ohno S, Honda K, Tanimoto K, Doi T, Ohno-Nakahara M, Tafolla E, Kapila S, Tanne K (2005) Cyclic mechanical strain regulates the PTHrP expression in cultured chondrocytes via activation of the $Ca2^{+}$ channel. J Dent Res 84:64–68
126. Tanner JM, Davies PS (1985) Clinical longitudinal standards for height and height velocity for North American children. J Pediatr 107:317–329
127. Teixeira CC, Ischiropoulos H, Leboy PS, Adams SL, Shapiro IM (2005) Nitric oxide-nitric oxide synthase regulates key maturational events during chondrocyte terminal differentiation. Bone 37: 37–45
128. Teixeira CC, Rajpurohit R, Mansfield K, Nemelivsky YV, Shapiro IM (2003) Maturation-dependent thiol loss increases chondrocyte susceptibility to apoptosis. J Bone Miner Res 18:662–668
129. Teixeira CC, Shapiro IM, Hatori M, Rajpurohit R, Koch C (1996) Retinoic acid modulation of glutathione and cysteine metabolism in chondrocytes. Biochem J 314(pt 1):21–26
130. Terkhorn SP, Bohensky J, Shapiro IM, Koyama E, Srinivas V (2007) Expression of HIF prolyl hydroxylase isozymes in growth plate chondrocytes: relationship between maturation and apoptotic sensitivity. J Cell Physiol 210:257–265
131. Thomas T, Martin A (2005) Bone metabolism and energy balance: role for leptin. Joint Bone Spine 72: 471–473
132. Tiet TD, Alman BA (2003) Developmental pathways in musculoskeletal neoplasia: involvement of the Indian hedgehog-parathyroid hormone-related protein pathway. Pediatr Res 53:539–543
133. van der Eerden BC, Karperien M, Wit JM (2003) Systemic and local regulation of the growth plate. Endocr Rev 24:782–801
134. Vanky P, Brockstedt U, Hjerpe A, Wikstrom B (1998) Kinetic studies on epiphyseal growth cartilage in the normal mouse. Bone 22:331–339
135. Veeman MT, Axelrod JD, Moon RTA (2003) second canon. Functions and mechanisms of beta-catenin-independent Wnt signaling. Dev Cell 5:367–377
136. Vortkamp A, Lee K, Lanske B, Segre GV, Kronenberg HM, Tabin CJ (1996) Regulation of rate of cartilage differentiation by Indian hedgehog and PTH-related protein. Science 273:613–622
137. Vu TH, Shipley JM, Bergers G, Berger JE, Helms JA, Hanahan D, Shapiro SD, Senior RM, Werb Z (1998) MMP-9/gelatinase B is a key regulator of growth plate angiogenesis and apoptosis of hypertrophic chondrocytes. Cell 93:411–422
138. Wang W, Kirsch T (2006) Annexin V/beta5 integrin interactions regulate apoptosis of growth plate chondrocytes. J Biol Chem 281:30848–30856
139. Wang Y, Toury R, Hauchecorne M, Balmain N (1997) Expression of Bcl-2 protein in the epiphyseal plate cartilage and trabecular bone of growing rats. Histochem Cell Biol 108:45–55
140. Watanabe H, Bohensky J, Freeman T, Srinivas V, Shapiro IM (2008) Hypoxic induction of UCP3 in the growth plate: UCP3 suppresses chondrocyte autophagy. J Cell Physiol 216:419–425
141. Wilsman NJ, Farnum CE, Leiferman EM, Fry M, Barreto C (1996) Differential growth by growth plates as a function of multiple parameters of chondrocytic kinetics. J Orthop Res 14:927–936
142. Wu Q, Zhang Y, Chen Q (2001) Indian hedgehog is an essential component of mechanotransduction complex to stimulate chondrocyte proliferation. J Biol Chem 276:35290–35296
143. Wyllie AH, Golstein P (2001) More than one way to go. Proc Natl Acad Sci U S A 98:11–13
144. Yoon BS, Lyons KM (2004) Multiple functions of BMPs in chondrogenesis. J Cell Biochem 93:93–103
145. Zhong M, Wike LJ, Ryaby JT, Carney DH, Boyan BD, Schwartz Z (2008) Thrombin peptide TP508 prevents nitric oxide mediated apoptosis in chondrocytes in the endochondral developmental pathway. Biochim Biophys Acta 1783:12–22
146. zur Nieden NI, Kempka G, Rancourt DE, Ahr HJ (2005) Induction of chondro-, osteo- and adipogenesis in embryonic stem cells by bone morphogenetic protein-2: effect of cofactors on differentiating lineages. BMC Dev Biol 5:1

4. Hedgehog Signaling in Growth Plate and Bone Development

Jean B. Regard, Kingston K. Mak, Joshua A. Gordon, and Yingzi Yang

4.1 Introduction

Genetic studies in *Drosophila melanogaster* first published in 1980 revealed mutations called "hedgehog" and "patched", named for the odd appearance of mutant fly embryos [89]. Since then, work from numerous groups studying many model organisms has come together to reveal what is currently called the Hedgehog (Hh) signaling pathway. Largely, though not completely, conserved from *Drosophila* to human, this pathway has been shown to be a master regulator of cell proliferation and differentiation, influencing many critical processes that range from early embryonic pattern formation to tissue homeostasis in adulthood. As might be expected for a network of such importance, dysregulation of this pathway has also been implicated in a broad spectrum of human diseases, including many varieties of neoplasia and a number of congenital malformations [41, 86].

Hh is a secreted morphogen that can form a gradient over many cell diameters to affect the basic cellular behavior, including proliferation, differentiation, and survival. While *Drosophila* has a single Hh gene, the family has been expanded to three in vertebrates: Sonic Hedgehog (Shh), Indian Hedgehog (Ihh), and Desert Hedgehog (Dhh). Vertebrate Hhs have both distinct and overlapping expression patterns and functions. Dhh expression is restricted to gonads, where it regulates spermatogenesis, and to peripheral neurons, where it regulates the nerve sheath formation [7, 92]. Shh and Ihh are more widely expressed and have sometimes overlapping and often distinct roles that are determined by their expression patterns. For example, while Shh and Ihh play redundant roles in the regulation of left/right asymmetry and cardiac morphogenesis [122], only Shh is expressed in the zone of polarizing activity (ZPA) and is important for anterior–posterior patterning of the limb bud [99, 101].

In particular, Hh signaling has emerged as one of the most important and extensively studied pathways in bone development and homeostasis. Understanding this pathway's role in skeletal tissues is paramount to making advances in both basic and translational bone research, and may hold clues toward therapeutic development. In this chapter, we will focus on vertebrate Hh signaling in bone, covering the basic mechanisms of signaling, roles in skeletal development and disease, and its emerging importance in adult bone homeostasis. Special emphasis will be placed on in vivo findings using mouse genetics, where both gain-of-function and loss-of-function approaches have been important in understanding the physiological significance of this pathway.

F. Bronner et al. (eds.), *Bone and Development*, Topics in Bone Biology 6,
DOI 10.1007/978-1-84882-822-3_4,

4.2 The Hedgehog Signaling Pathway

All Hh proteins are first generated as ~45 kDa proproteins that undergo extensive posttranslational modification prior to secretion (Fig. 4.1a). Hh proteins contain a catalytic C-terminal region responsible for autoproteolytic cleavage to produce the N-terminal 19 kDa active form. During proteolysis, a cholesterol moiety is attached to the newly formed C-terminus of Hh proteins [96]. Hh is further modified by skinny hedgehog, an acyl-transferase, which adds a palmitate residue to the N-terminus [11, 93]. These modifications result in a truncated, dually lipid-modified, fully active Hh that is secreted from cells and forms a gradient across several cell diameters, allowing a graded response by the receiving cells. The precise mechanisms by which these lipid modifications regulate secretion and gradient formation are not fully understood. Cholesterol modification is associated with linking Hh to the cell membrane and regulating its release from cells, whereas palmitoylation is thought to allow higher order Hh complexes to form, thus enabling long-range signaling [11, 13, 18, 26, 97, 112]. Extensive investigation has revealed that Hh requires specific proteins for secretion and passage through the extracellular space. Dispatched (Disp), a 12-transmembrane-containing protein with significant homology to Patched (Ptch) (see below), is required for the release of lipid-modified Hh [8, 68]. The movement of Hh through the extracellular space is also regulated. The glypicans Dally and Dally-like, as well as enzymes known to be involved in heparan sulfate proteoglycan (HSPG) synthesis (Tout-Velu/EXT-1), regulate Hh diffusion [5, 20, 95, 116].

Upon reaching the sensing cell, Hh binds to Ptch, which, like Disp, contains 12 transmembrane domains (Fig. 4.1c). Hh binding to Ptch relieves the inhibition of Smoothened (Smo) by Ptch, which is a 7-transmembrane-containing protein required for signaling [102, 110]. Hh binding to Ptch is also modulated by a number of coreceptors and regulators [including Hedgehog interacting protein (HIP), megalin, growth arrest specific-1 (GAS-1), and Ihog/CDO] that participate in cell surface binding of Hh ligands [16, 58, 63, 75–77, 81, 118]. Apart from acting as a receptor, Ptch also mediates endocytosis and lysosomal degradation of Hh [39, 108]. The mechanism of Smo inhibition by Ptch remains unknown, although it appears to be catalytic in nature [102].

Once Smo is activated, it transmits the Hh signal through altered processing of Glioblastoma (Gli) proteins (Fig. 4.1c) [66]. Gli1, Gli2, and Gli3 are zinc finger transcription factors and mammalian homologs of the *Drosophila* cubitus interruptus (Ci) protein [113]. Mammalian Glis have both overlapping and distinct activities [3, 4, 74, 113]. The processing and function of Gli3 most closely resembles that of Ci. In the absence of Hh, Gli3 is processed to form a shortened repressor form (Gli-R) that inhibits transcription of Hh target genes (Fig. 4.1b). In the presence of Hh, Gli3 persists in a full-length activator form (Gli-A) that accumulates in the nucleus and activates the transcription of Hh target genes (Fig. 4.1c). Gli2, like Gli3, can become a repressor, but is thought to exist in the pathway mostly as an activator. Gli1 lacks the sites required for processing and exists only in the activator form [3]. Gli1 itself is a Hh target, and induces and amplifies the expression of Hh targets, but is not strictly required for Hh signaling [91].

Hh signal transduction from Smo on the cell surface to the activation of Ci/Gli proteins is incompletely understood and some aspects are not conserved from *Drosophila* to vertebrates [111]. In the fly, Hh signaling inhibition requires a kinesin-like protein Costal2(Cos2), which tethers Ci and allows Ci, after phosphorylation by several kinases, including protein kinase A and casein kinase 1α, to generate the Ci repressor form [43, 67]. In mammals, divergence at the level of Smo, Cos2, and supressor of fused (Su(Fu)) have been documented; Cos2 and its homologs are not genetically required for Gli processing and Su(Fu) plays a critical role [77, 111, 112]. Also, in vertebrates, primary cilia have emerged as cell structures required for Hh signaling. Primary cilia are microtubule-based organelles that protrude from the basal body. Genetic ablation of components important for the formation or maintenance of the cilia leads to Hh signaling deficiencies [4, 37, 38, 59, 61, 82]. In the absence of Hh, Ptch1, Gli2, and Gli3 are present in primary

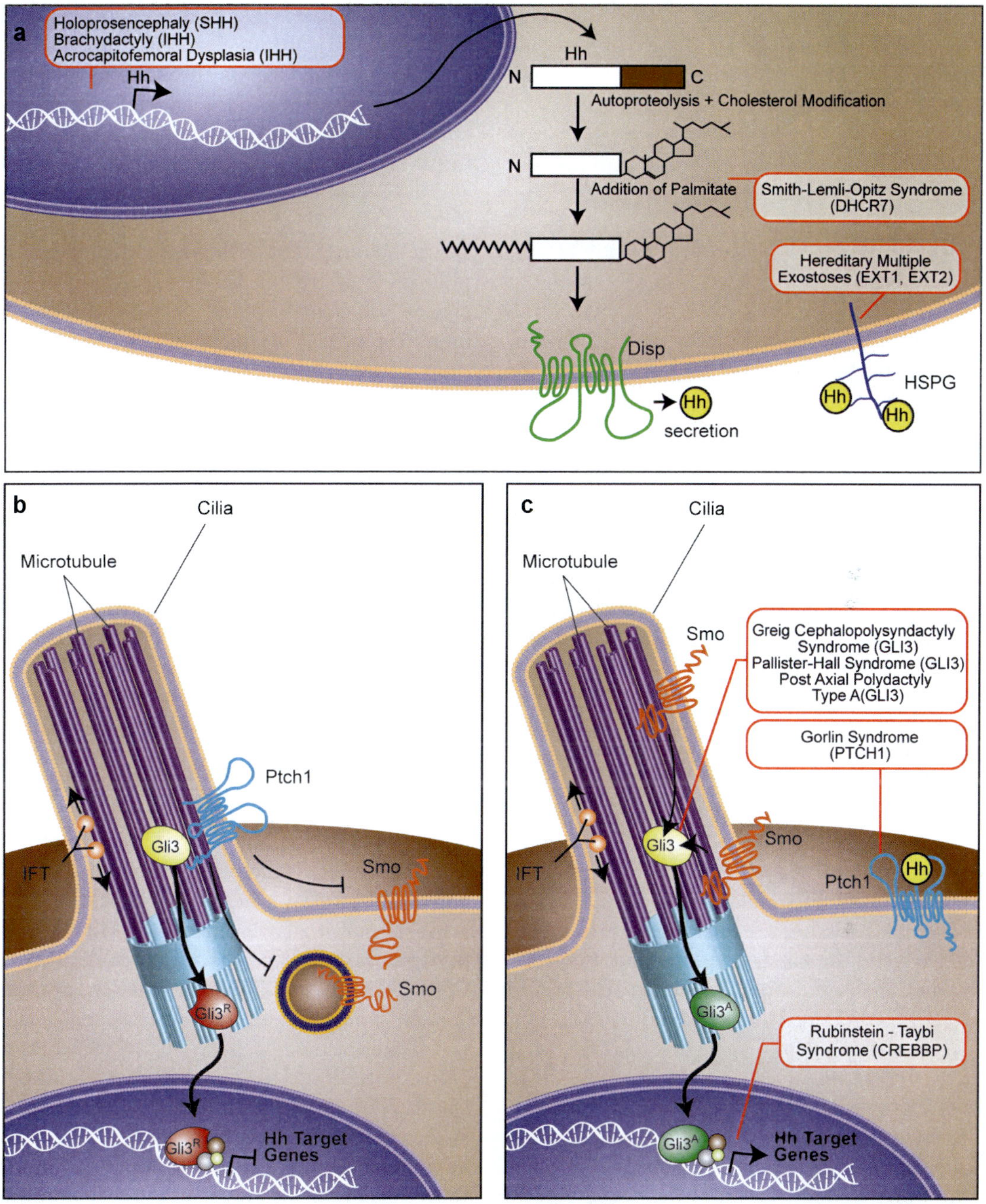

Figure 4.1. (**a**) Following translation, Hedgehog (Hh) undergoes a round of autoproteolysis and a cholesterol moiety is covalently added to the C-terminus; subsequently, Hh is palmitoylated on the N-terminus. These lipid modifications are required for proper morphogen gradient formation. Dispatched (Disp) is important for the release of lipid-modified Hh, so that heparan sulfate proteoglycans (HSPG) can bind Hh and affect its diffusion. (**b**) In the absence of Hh, Patched 1 (Ptch1) is present in primary cilia. It excludes the presence of Smoothened (Smo) and suppresses its function. Gli3 is proteolytically cleaved to generate the repressor form (Gli3R) that translocates to the nucleus and suppresses the expression of Hh target genes. (**c**) When present, Hh binds to Ptch1 and relieves Smo suppression. Ptch1 migrates away from and Smo migrates to the cilia. Gli3 is converted to a full-length activator form (Gli3A) that translocates to the nucleus and activates the expression of Hh target genes. Numerous cofactors exist, which play roles in multiple aspects of Hh secretion and signaling. A number of genetic syndromes are caused by mutations within this pathway (*red boxes*).

cilia, but Smo is excluded [31]. As Hh binds to Ptch1, Ptch1 is removed from the cilia and Smo becomes localized to the cilia. This process activates the Hh pathway [19, 37, 51].

4.3 Hh in Human Genetics/ Patterning

The importance of Hh signaling in human development is underscored by the number of congenital malformation syndromes caused by mutations at various pathway steps. The syndromes overlaid in Fig. 4.1 illustrate the sites of these mutations.

Mutations in Shh lead to holoprosencephaly (HPE) [MIM 236100], a common developmental defect that is characterized by the failure of the prosencephalon (embryonic forebrain) to form two distinct cerebral hemispheres. Craniofacial defects also associated with HPE include cleft palate, single maxillary incisor, and hypoterolism, or, in the most extreme cases, cyclopia [100].

Brachydactyly type A-1 [MIM 112500] or acrocapitofemoral dysplasia [MIM 607778] can be caused by mutations in IHH. Brachydactylyl type A-1 is an autosomal dominant, mild skeletal dysplasia confined mostly to shortened middle phalanges and decreased stature [28, 62, 123]. Acrocapitofemoral dysplasia is transmitted as an autosomal recessive, characterized by cone-shaped epiphyses in the hands and hips, and premature epimetaphyseal fusion that result in early growth arrest and shortened limbs and stature [32].

Smith–Lemli–Opitz syndrome (SLOS) [MIM 270400] is an autosomal recessive disorder caused by mutations in the gene encoding 7-dehydrocholesterol reductase (DHCR7), an enzyme that catalyzes the conversion of 7-dehydrocholesterolis to cholesterol [25, 107]. Decreased cholesterol modification of Shh leading to altered Shh secretion was initially thought to underlie these defects, but more recent data suggest that the defect may be the inability of the cells to respond to Hh [18, 53]. Developmental abnormalities associated with SLOS include microcephaly, upturned nose, micrognathia, cleft palate, short thumbs, reduced stature, syndactyly, and postaxial polydactyly.

Multiple exostoses, types 1 and 2 [MIM 133700/133701], are autosomal-dominant disorders characterized by bony protuberances called exostoses or osteochondromas that arise in the epiphyseal growth plates [21]. Mutations causing these disorders have been linked to EXT1 and EXT2, which encode glycosyltransferases required for HSPG formation. These genes constrain the range of the Hh gradient. A hypomorphic allele of Ext1 in the reverse expands the area of Hh signaling and delays chondrocyte hypertrophy [54]. As mentioned earlier, mutations of the *Drosophila* ortholog of Ext, Tout-Velu, also cause abnormal diffusion of Hh. In the fly, however, loss of Tout-Velu function causes decreased Hh diffusion [5].

Gorlin syndrome [MIM 109400], also known as nevoid basal cell carcinoma syndrome, is due to mutations in Ptch1. Gorlin syndrome is inherited in an autosomal-dominant fashion and is caused by haploinsufficiency of Ptch1, leading to ectopic activation of the Hh pathway [29]. Apart from developing numerous basal cell carcinomas, Gorlin syndrome patients present with macrocephaly with frontal bossing, hypertelorism, increased stature, calcification of the falces, axial skeleton anomalies, cystic bone lesions, and polydactyly [29].

Interestingly, mutations in GLI3 lead to three overlapping, yet distinct, disorders: Greig cephalopolysyndactyly syndrome (GCPS) [MIM 175700] [114], Pallister–Hall syndrome (PHS) [MIM 146510] [45], and postaxial polydactyly type A (PAP-A) [MIM 174200] [98]. GCPS is characterized by polydactyly, syndactyly, and craniofacial abnormalities, including macrocephaly and hypertelorism. Translocations, deletions, and point mutations causing loss of Gli3 function have been associated with GCPS and are thought to be due to haploinsufficiency. Autosomal-dominant PHS is caused by frameshift and nonsense mutations that lead to constitutive expression of the repressor form of GLI3. Skeletal manifestations of PHS include polydactyly, syndactyly, and an upturned nose. PAP-A phenotypes are largely restricted to postaxial polydactyly.

Rubinstein–Taybi syndrome (RTS) [MIM 600140] is an autosomal-dominant disorder caused by haploinsufficiency of the CREB binding protein (CREBBP; P300; CBP), a coactivator of Gli3 [2, 94]. There are distinctive facial features associated with RTS, such as hypoplastic maxilla with narrow palate, prominent beaked nose, large anterior fontanel, microcephaly, as well as short stature, broad thumbs/first toes, delayed ossification, axial skeleton abnormalities, and to a lesser extent, syndactyly and polydactyly.

Saethre–Chotzen syndrome (SCS) [MIM 101400], also known as acrocephalosyndactyly type III, is an autosomal-dominant disorder characterized by premature fusion of the cranial structures, prominent beaked nose, broad thumbs/first toes, hypertelorism, ossification defects, brachydactyly, syndactyly, and decreased stature. SCS is caused by mutations in the TWIST1 gene that encodes a basic helix-loop-helix transcription factor that antagonizes the function of another basic helix-loop-helix transcription factor, dHAND2 [24]. DHand2 regulates limb patterning by controlling Shh expression and inhibiting Gli3 expression in the posterior limb [12, 23, 104].

4.4 Hh in Skeletal Patterning and Craniofacial Development

As craniofacial development is covered in Chap. 12, the contribution of Hh signaling to craniofacial development will only be briefly described in this chapter.

Shh plays a critical role in patterning the axial skeleton. It is expressed in the notochord and floorplate of the neural tube and specifies the ventral-medial portion of somites to become sclerotome [15]. This in turn gives rise to the vertebrae and ribs. In Shh-null mice, the entire vertebral column is absent and only a few ribs are formed partially [15]. Shh is a potent mitogen in presomitic mesoderm (PSM) explants, and, via Gli2 and Gli3, promotes the formation of sclerotome [9, 15, 22]. Shh induces expression of the transcription factors Sox9 and Nkx3.2. This renders PSM sensitive to bone morphogenic proteins (BMPs) and allows differentiation of chondrocytes and the axial skeleton development [83, 84, 120].

As reflected by the many human syndromes associated with altered digit formation/identity, Shh is a major regulator of limb patterning, but the mechanism by which Shh patterns limbs is under active debate. The embryonic primordium of the limb, the limb bud, is initiated as an outgrowth of the lateral plate mesoderm covered by a sheath of ectoderm. Cells originating in the somites also migrate into the limb, adding to the mesenchyme already present and forming the full complement of cells that participate in limb development. Proper skeletal patterning requires the interaction of many precisely orchestrated signaling pathways that form a set of anatomical features along three axes: ventro-dorsal, anterior–posterior (A–P), and proximo-distal (P–D). Shh is expressed in the ZPA in the posterior portion of the early limb and plays a critical role in patterning these tissues along the A–P axis. Shh also has an indirect role in P–D outgrowth and patterning (Fig. 4.2). In particular, Shh regulates the digit number and identity [106]. If a piece of tissue from the ZPA or if beads soaked in Shh are transplanted to the anterior limb bud, digits are duplicated as a mirror image of the original set of the digits [99, 106]. The limbs of Shh-null mice contain only the most anterior digit; this demonstrates an essential role in A-P axis formation [14]. Similarly, when limbs are treated with cyclopamine (an Hh antagonist) after gradient formation, only the most anterior digit forms properly. Lack of the repressor and activator forms of Gli3 protein or removal of both Gli3 and Shh results in unpatterned supernumerary digits. This indicates that Shh regulates the digit number and identity by controlling the balance of Gli3 repressor and activator forms [60, 105].

Early models of limb patterning suggested that ZPA-derived Shh regulates digit formation in a concentration- and time-dependent manner, with higher or longer doses of Shh specifying the formation of more posterior digits in a dose-dependent manner [117]. Indeed, cells derived from the ZPA contribute significantly to the posterior digits [30]. Current evidence suggests a model in which the anterior-most digit 1 (the “thumb”) is formed independently of Shh. Digits 2 and 3 form with only low Shh activity; the most posterior digits 4 and 5 are formed

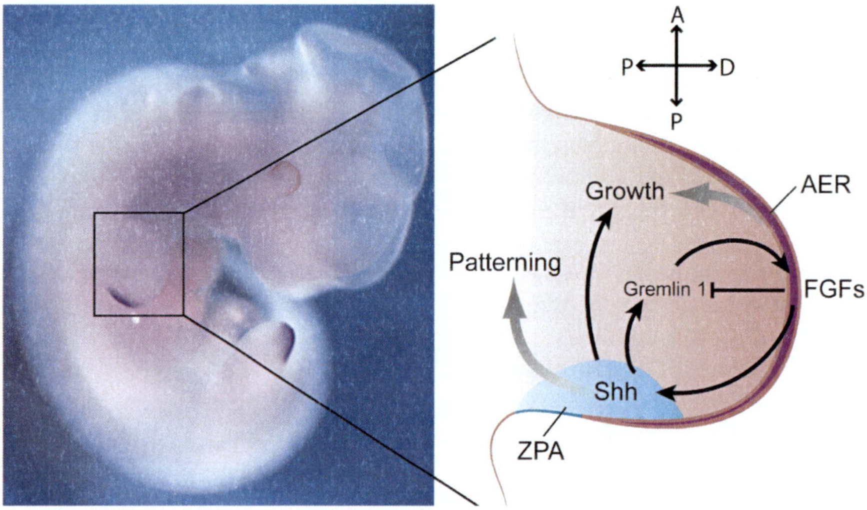

Figure 4.2. The function of sonic hedgehog in limb patterning. In situ hybridization experiments reveal that sonic hedgehog (Shh) is expressed in the zone of polarizing activity (ZPA) in the limb bud of a mouse embryo at 10.5 dpc (*left image*, courtesy of Derek Gildea). Shh plays a direct role in regulating limb patterning along the anterior–posterior (A–P) axis and an indirect role in regulating growth along the proximal–distal (P–D) axis (*right*). Shh positively regulates the expression of Gremlin1 that, through inhibition of BMP signaling, permits the expression of fibroblast growth factor (FGF) 4/8 in the apical ectodermal ridge (AER). FGFs, in turn, promote continued expression of Shh from the ZPA, thus forming a positive feedback loop critical to regulate limb patterning and growth.

from cells that witness the highest levels of Shh [30]. Decreases in the amount of Shh produced in the ZPA also have an effect on the posterior digits; this highlights the importance of a spatiotemporal gradient of Hh in limb patterning.

Recent work suggests that current models are incomplete and previous data should be reinterpreted. Shh, in addition to specifying digits, also expands the digit progenitor cells. It therefore has a critical role in integrating growth and patterning [109, 124]. In the chick developing limb, ectopic Shh induces *N-myc* and *CyclinD2* expression, and cyclopamine treatment reduces the number of mesenchymal cells in S-phase; Shh therefore also controls proliferation [109]. In contrast to the loss of posterior digits that is associated with the disruption of Shh signaling, inhibition of proliferation only leads to a decrease in the anterior digits, with digit progenitor cells forming posterior structures. Interestingly, when cell division recovers, Shh expression from the ZPA is maintained for longer duration. This suggests that the proliferative state of limb mesenchyme may feed back to the ZPA to maintain Shh expression [109]. Removal of a floxed allele of Shh from the mouse limb bud at various stages of development with the aid of an inducible Cre system [124] leads to the progressive loss of digits and a reduced mitotic index, as it does in the chick. If the role of Shh is to specify the posterior digits, then later removal of Shh should lead to a gradual loss of digits, with the direction from the posterior toward the anterior end. Instead of the predicted sequential order of digit loss (5-4-3-2), Zhu et al. [124] witnessed an alternating pattern of 3-5-2-4. The first digit lost on removal of Shh was digit 3 (the middle digit), not digit 5 (the "pinkie"), as had been predicted. Digit formation followed the order of 4-2-5-3. Therefore, it is the last digit to form that is the first digit to be lost when Hh signaling is reduced. Digit location alone may not be sufficient to define digit identity, but these findings are further evidence that our understanding of Shh in patterning the limb is far from complete.

Apart from regulating A–P axis formation and patterning, Shh also affects P–D limb outgrowth. Shh plays an indirect role in maintaining the apical ectodermal ridge (AER), a key regulator of P–D limb growth and patterning. Shh induces the expression of Gremlin1 that blocks the BMP signaling and maintains the integrity of the AER [10, 48, 57]. FGFs expressed in the AER, in turn, control the proliferation of limb bud mesenchymal cells along the P–D axis and also feed back to the ZPA to maintain Shh expression [87, 88].

Shh also is expressed in the ectoderm of the frontonasal prominence, where it regulates the craniofacial patterning and development [33, 35]. Neural crest cells (NCCs), a population of multipotent progenitor cells, arise from the border between the neural and nonneural ectoderm early in development [27]. A subset of NCCs migrates to the frontonasal prominence and first pharyngeal arch to give rise to the craniofacial skeletal structures. In mice null for Shh, facial features are unidentifiable and most craniofacial bones are absent [15]. Blocking Shh function in the head region of the developing chick leads to an increase in NCC apoptosis and a loss of some cranial structures [1, 34]. In the mouse, removal of Smo from NCCs similarly leads to decreased proliferation, increased apoptosis, and a dramatic loss of most of the NCC-derived craniofacial structures, though the NCCs themselves appear to form correctly [42]. Thus, Shh is neither essential in specifying NCCs, nor in driving migration, but is required for the correct proliferation and differentiation of NCCs within the craniofacial region.

4.5 Ihh in Endochondral Bone Formation

As discussed in Chap. 2, bone formation during embryonic development occurs by two processes: intramembranous ossification and endochondral ossification. During intramembranous ossification, mesenchymal progenitor cells differentiate into osteoblasts that secrete bone matrix without forming cartilage first. This is the process through which mandibles and flat bones of the skull develop. Endochondral ossification, on the other hand, occurs in most other parts of the body. During endochondral ossification, mesenchymal progenitor cells differentiate into chondrocytes to form a cartilage mold of the future bone. In the developing cartilage, chondrocytes sequentially go through a tightly controlled program of proliferation and differentiation, and eventually exit the cell cycle and become hypertrophic. Osteoblasts and blood vessels subsequently invade the hypertrophic cartilaginous region and replace it with trabecular bone.

Shh has emerged as a master regulator of early embryonic pattern formation and craniofacial morphogenesis, but Ihh is the key regulator of endochondral bone growth and ossification. As mesenchymal cells condense to initiate chondrocyte differentiation during endochondral bone formation, *Ihh* is first expressed in the newly differentiated chondrocytes [6, 40, 115]. Later, in the formed cartilage, *Ihh* expression becomes restricted to postmitotic prehypertrophic and early hypertrophic chondrocytes, in which the parathyroid hormone/parathyroid hormone-related peptide receptor 1 (*Pthr1*) is also expressed at high levels. The critical role played by Ihh in regulating the balance of chondrocyte proliferation and hypertrophy via parathyroid hormone-related peptide (PTHrP) expression was first reported by Vortkamp et al. [115]. In chick embryos, ectopic expression of Ihh in the developing long bone cartilage led to upregulated *Pthrp* expression and a severe delay in the progression from proliferating chondrocytes to hypertrophic chondrocytes. The phenotype resulting from this process was the opposite to the accelerated chondrocyte hypertrophy observed in mice lacking PTHrP or Pthr1; this indicates that PTHrP and Ihh form a negative regulatory feedback loop [46, 56]. The mechanism by which Ihh expressed in the prehypertrophic chondrocytes regulates *Pthrp* expression in the periarticular joint region is still not known. It is noteworthy that hypomorphic mutations in a heparan sulfate producing glycosyltransferase, exostosin 1 (EXT1), lead to expanded regions of Ihh signaling and delayed chondrocyte hypertrophy. This may mean that Ihh regulates PTHrP directly [54]. The Ihh/PTHrP loop then acts as a sensor within the growth plate to regulate the pace of chondrocyte hypertrophy (Fig. 4.3). As chondrocytes leave the PTHrP signaling domain and undergo hypertrophy, it is the newly differentiated, postmitotic, prehypertrophic chondrocytes that produce Ihh. Enhanced chondrocyte hypertrophy therefore will lead to more Ihh production which, acting as a negative feedback signal, will slow down further chondrocyte hypertrophy by keeping chondrocytes in the proliferating state. In turn, this is the result of upregulating PTHrP expression in the periarticular region. This negative feedback loop is critical for the balance between growth and ossification.

Studies with Ihh-null mice have complemented the overexpression studies described earlier and have significantly enhanced our understanding of the role played by Ihh in skeletal development. Skeletal elements that lack Ihh regulation are in the correct position, but are dramatically reduced in size. They are even smaller than PTHrP or Pthr1-null mice [46, 56, 101]. The dramatic reduction in size of the proliferating zone and the acceleration of chondrocyte hypertrophy owing to loss of PTHrP expression, along with the action of *Ptch1* in proliferating chondrocytes, suggests that Ihh also regulates chondrocyte proliferation directly, independently of PTHrP.

When both Ihh and PTHrP are removed from mouse embryos, the double mutant mice are identical with Ihh null mice, but are more affected than PTHrP-null mice. PTHrP may therefore mediate a subset of Ihh activity [47]. Interestingly, a ligand-independent, constitutively activated form of (Pthr1*) is capable of rescuing the PTHrP$^{-/-}$ phenotype. This has provided an opportunity to explore the PTHrP-independent functions of Ihh. When the Pthr1* mice are bred into the Ihh$^{-/-}$ background, it results in Ihh$^{-/-}$;Pthr1* mouse embryos that have shortened long bones, similar to those in the Ihh$^{-/-}$ mice [47]. These findings can be interpreted as indicating that PTHrP signaling prevents premature chondrocyte hypertrophy in the absence of Ihh signaling, but that chondrocyte proliferation is also regulated by Ihh signaling, independently of PTHrP.

The direct effects of Ihh signaling on chondrocyte proliferation have been further explored by conditional removal of Smo from mouse chondrocytes in vivo (Smo^{Chon}) [65]. Smo^{Chon} mice have normal onset of chondrocyte hypertrophy, normal expression of markers of chondrocyte hypertrophy, reduced PTHrP expression in chondrocytes, but increased periarticular PTHrP expression. Thus, in contrast to Ihh-null mice, loss of Hh signaling only in the chondrocytes does not seem to interfere with the progression of chondrocyte hypertrophy. Smo^{Chon} limbs are shorter, however, and showed decreased chondrocyte proliferation, similar to that seen in Ihh-null mice. Conversely, ectopic expression of either Ihh or a constitutively active form of Smo in chondrocytes leads to increased proliferation.

One of the most striking features of Ihh-null mice is their lack of osteoblast differentiation and bone formation [101]. Ihh signaling inhibits the generation of the Gli3 repressor form. In Gli3$^{-/-}$;Ihh$^{-/-}$ embryos, many of the PTHrP-dependent and -independent chondrocyte phenotypes that are absent in Ihh$^{-/-}$ embryos are present again. However, endochondral bone still fails to form in Gli3$^{-/-}$;Ihh$^{-/-}$ mice [55]. Ihh is required for osteoblast differentiation by inducing expression of Runx2, a transcription factor required to establish the osteoblast lineage [64]. The expressions of *Ptch1* and *Gli1*, the transcriptional targets of Ihh signaling, are particularly robust in perichondral regions. This indicates that perichondral cells are a major target of Ihh signaling [64]. Upregulated Hh signaling increases osteoblastic marker expression and induces ectopic bone [50, 85]. However, when Hh signaling is lost by removing Smo from perichondral cells, bone collar formation is completely abolished, as is the development of primary spongiosa [102]. This demonstrates that Hh signaling is needed to enable the mesenchymal progenitor cells to differentiate into the osteoblast lineage. Gli3 mediates the effect of Ihh in cartilage development largely by suppressing Gli3 in repressor form, so that the Gli3 in activator form can bring about osteoblast differentiation. As the levels of Hh that are needed to block Gli3R processing are lower than those required to stimulate Gli3A [44], low levels of Hh signaling can maintain normal cartilage development, but higher levels are needed for osteoblast differentiation.

The requirement for Ihh does not appear to be absolute, inasmuch as osteoblasts still form in the intramembranous bones of the skull of Ihh$^{-/-}$ mice, and limbs of Ihh$^{-/-}$ can still form bone when transplanted to the renal capsule [17, 101]. Conceivably, Hh signaling activity may still be present in the Ihh$^{-/-}$ skull and Ihh$^{-/-}$ limb. How Hh signaling drives osteoblast formation

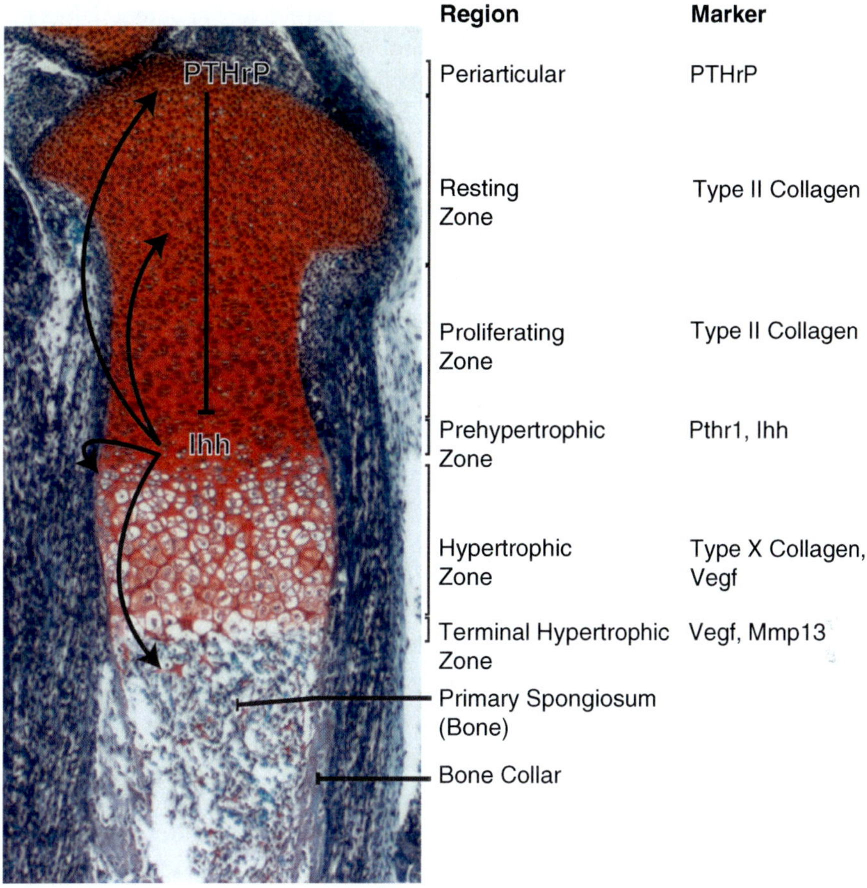

Figure 4.3. Growth plate structure and regulation by Indian hedgehog. *Ihh* is expressed by postmitotic prehypertrophic and early hypertrophic chondrocytes and regulates multiple aspects of endochondral ossification. Ihh controls proliferation of chondrocytes in the resting/proliferating zones. Ihh also signals to the periarticular region and positively regulates PTHrP expression. PTHrP subsequently feeds back to the prehypertrophic zone, inhibiting chondrocyte hypertrophy. This forms an Ihh/PTHrP negative feedback loop that acts as a sensor within the growth plate to regulate the pace of chondrocyte hypertrophy. Ihh also signals to the perichondrium and newly formed bone to promote osteoblast differentiation.

remains to be determined, but interactions with Wnt and BMP pathways may be important [36, 64, 119]. Through a poorly defined mechanism, Ihh also controls vascular invasion and maintenance in long bones. Loss of Ihh causes abnormal blood vessel positioning surrounding the hypertrophic cartilage and delayed angiogenesis. Subsequently, these blood vessels regress and disappear and do not support persistence or expansion of the ossification centers [17].

Many signaling pathways, such as FGF, BMP, and canonical Wnt signaling, function upstream or downstream of Hh signaling. The relationships between these pathways are cell context-dependent. For instance, canonical Wnt and Hh signaling interact distinctly to control osteoblast differentiation, chondrocyte proliferation, hypertrophy, survival, and synovial joint formation in the developing endochondral bone [110]. From β-catenin loss-of-function and Hh gain-of-function double-mutants studies, canonical Wnt signaling is known to be required for osteoblast differentiation downstream of Hh signaling. However, in chondrocyte survival, canonical Wnt signaling is required upstream of Hh signaling to inhibit chondrocyte apoptosis. Yet, Hh signaling also inhibits chondrocyte hypertrophy and synovial joint formation independently of canonical Wnt signaling. FGF signaling is required upstream of Hh signaling to regulate the onset of chondrocyte hypertrophy, but acts independently of Hh signaling in regulating terminal chondrocyte hypertrophy and proliferation [79]. BMP and Ihh signals act in parallel to induce chondrocyte proliferation [80], but BMP may mediate Hh signaling activity in regulating synovial joint development [72]. Thus, the interaction of these pathways involves complicated networks with multiple levels of crosstalk that are essential for proliferation and differentiation of chondrocytes and osteoblasts.

Ihh also plays a role in maintaining the postnatal growth plate. Loss of Ihh signaling activity later in life through either pharmacologic blockade or genetic removal leads to premature loss of the growth plate and short stature. Administering a small molecule hedgehog antagonist (HhAntag) to 10-day-old mice causes a rapid and permanent disruption of the growth plate within 2 days, leading to a decrease in chondrocyte proliferation, inducing premature hypertrophy and disrupting long bone development so that the limbs are markedly shortened [49]. Maeda et al. [70], using the genetic cre/lox system, removed Ihh from chondrocytes in neonates. This leads to reduced *Pthrp* expression, premature chondrocyte hypertrophy, and abnormal mineralization of the growth plate and joints [70].

Within a week of tamoxifen treatment, the growth plate disappears and limbs shorten. However, autonomous downregulation of Hh signaling in postnatal chondrocytes using the same tamoxifen-inducible Cre line and a floxed allele of Smo leads to delayed hypertrophy and reduced mineralization [73]. The discrepancies between these two studies can be explained by the difference in PTHrP expression levels. In the postnatal cartilage, PTHrP expression is progressively weaker when compared with that in the embryonic cartilage. In addition, only periarticular cells and the upper layer of articular chondrocytes are competent to express low levels of PTHrP. Thus, loss of Ihh leads to reduced PTHrP expression in both periarticular cells and the upper layer of articular chondrocytes and subsequent premature chondrocyte hypertrophy. In contrast, cell autonomous reduction of Hh signaling takes place only in the cartilage, including the chondrocytes deep in the joint cartilage and the growth plates, and will not downregulate PTHrP expression in periarticular cells. It is therefore apparent that in this case, the role of Ihh in promoting chondrocyte hypertrophy independently of PTHrP dominates over its PTHrP-dependent role. As a result, chondrocyte hypertrophy is delayed.

As is the case for the $Ihh^{-/-}$ mouse phenotype [101], loss of chondrocyte-derived Ihh in neonates leads to reduced osteoblast differentiation and function, including a loss of trabeculation and reduced bone mineral density in the metaphyseal region [70]. Similarly, inhibition of Hh signaling with HhAntag diminishes osteoblast proliferation and function, and causes bone formation to be reduced [49]. Ohba et al. [90] administered the Smo antagonist cyclopamine to 8-week-old mice for 1 month and witnessed a mild decrease in bone mineral density, with reduced trabeculation, decreased bone deposition, and fewer osteoblasts. Surprisingly, sustained upregulation of Hh signaling in osteoblasts leads to severe osteopenia. This suggests that bone formation and bone resorption are both subject to regulation by the Hh signaling pathway.

4.6 Hh in Joint Formation

Hh signaling also plays a key role in synovial joint and articular cartilage formation. Both an increase and decrease in Hh activation lead to abnormal joint formation. A striking feature of the Ihh null mice is the failure to segment and form joints, with multiple joints remaining partially fused [101]. In the distal chick wing, retroviral-induced misexpression of either Shh or Ihh leads to a loss of interphalangeal joints and misexpression of *gdf-5*, a BMP family member [78]. Similarly, ectopic activation of the Hh pathway in mouse chondrocytes leads to joint cartilage fusions. Overexpression of either Ihh or Shh under the control of the Col2a1-promoter leads to misformed, fused, or missing joints of the elbow and phalanges [52, 80, 103]. Cell autonomous upregulation of the Hh pathway in cartilage by selectively removing Ptch1 in chondrocytes also leads to joint fusions and mineralization within the joints [72]. Consistent with the report by Minina et al. [80], BMPs are upregulated in the joint region when Ptch1 is removed. As BMP signaling inhibits synovial joint formation, it is likely that BMPs, in regulating this process, mediate the activity of Hh signaling.

Removal of either Ptch1 or Smo alters joint cartilage maintenance in postnatal cartilage [73]. Inasmuch as PTHrP expression levels in the joint cartilage and in periarticular cells of mutants are dramatically reduced in the postnatal cartilage, it is apparent that Hh signaling promotes chondrocyte hypertrophy around the second ossification center, whereas reduced Hh signaling decreases chondrocyte hypertrophy in this region. These findings indicate that Hh signaling is critical for postnatal cartilage homeostasis and that unduly high levels of Hh signaling may constitute a risk factor for osteoarthritis.

4.7 Hh in Skeletal Homeostasis

The effects of activating Hh signaling on adult bone homeostasis have recently been explored [71, 90]. Because Ptch1 suppresses Smo function, its removal leads to ligand-independent activation of Hh signaling [72]. Genetic gain- and loss-of-function experiments in postnatal bone, by conditionally removing Ptch1 or Smo alleles from mature osteoblasts, have uncovered novel roles of Hh signaling in bone homeostasis [71, 121]. Removing Ptch1 from mature osteoblasts (referred to hereafter as $Ptch1^{MOb}$) in mice results in skeletal features reminiscent of Gorlin syndrome, including frontal bossing, large calvaria, and hypertelorism. In these mice, cortical and trabecular bone mass decreased dramatically, yet osteoblast differentiation increased. Ohba et al. [90] studied mice that were globally heterozygous for Ptch1 (referred to hereafter as $Ptch1^{+/-}$), and observed an increase in bone mass, along with an increase in osteoblasts differentiation. In vivo, both of the mutant-strains exhibited an increase in the number of osteoblasts and accelerated bone deposition. The major difference between these two mutants lies in osteoclast differentiation. The long bones of $Ptch1^{+/-}$ mice contained ~50% more osteoclasts than controls, whereas those of $Ptch1^{MOb}$ mice exhibited a 3+-fold increase. In both the mutants, loss of Ptch1 in osteoblasts increased the expression of receptor activator of NF-B (*Rankl*) and induced osteoclastogenesis [71, 90]. However, osteoblasts from $Ptch1^{+/-}$ mice induced only a doubling of osteoclast formation, whereas those from $Ptch1^{MOb}$ mice induced an eightfold increase. Bone turnover in both the strains increased, but because of the much greater increase in bone resorption in the $Ptch1^{MOb}$ mice, they developed osteopenia.

Blocking Hh signaling in mice using a floxed allele of Smo (referred to hereafter as Smo^{MOb}) showed a complimentary phenotype. Smo^{MOb} mice have reduced *PTHrP* and *Rankl* expression and fewer osteoclasts. Very interestingly, 1-year-old, but not 3-month-old Smo^{MOb} mice exhibit increased trabecular bone mass and cortical thickness [71]. Additional experiments [71] have made it evident that Hh signaling controls *PTHrP* expression in osteoblasts, as it does in cartilage development. PTHrP signaling in osteoblasts mediates Hh signaling that promotes *Rankl* expression. It does so by activating protein kinase A (PKA) and its target transcription factor, the cAMP responsive element-binding protein (CREB). This is consistent with the earlier finding that sustained PTH infusion leads to increased bone resorption [69]. Thus, Hh signaling controls bone homeostasis by regulating the temporal and spatial expression of *PTHrP*. Hh signaling decreases progressively as the osteoblasts mature and move further away from the growth plates. With this progressive loss of Hh signaling activity, *PTHrP* expression is gradually reduced in maturing osteoblasts, and as a result, the ability of osteoblasts to induce osteoclast differentiation is reduced. Therefore, for normal bone maintenance and remodeling, Hh signaling must be kept low in mature osteoblasts to ensure low *PTHrP* expression and to prevent excessive osteoclast formation. In contrast to its role in embryonic endochondral bone formation, Hh signaling plays an opposite role in postnatal bone formation and resorption. Therefore, careful manipulation of the enhancing and inhibiting roles of Hh signaling may be beneficial for osteoporosis treatment.

Acknowledgments

We thank Julia Fekecs and Darryl Leja for their help in creating the figures.

References

1. Ahlgren SC, Bronner-Fraser M (1999) Inhibition of sonic hedgehog signaling in vivo results in craniofacial neural crest cell death. Curr Biol 9:1304–1314
2. Akimaru H, Chen Y, Dai P, Hou DX, Nonaka M, Smolik SM, Armstrong S, Goodman RH, Ishii S (1997) Drosophila CBP is a co-activator of cubitus interruptus in hedgehog signalling. Nature 386:735–738
3. Aza-Blanc P, Lin HY, Ruiz i Altaba A, Kornberg TB (2000) Expression of the vertebrate Gli proteins in Drosophila reveals a distribution of activator and repressor activities. Development 127:4293–4301
4. Bai CB, Stephen D, Joyner AL (2004) All mouse ventral spinal cord patterning by hedgehog is Gli dependent and involves an activator function of Gli3. Dev Cell 6:103–115
5. Bellaiche Y, The I, Perrimon N (1998) Tout-velu is a Drosophila homologue of the putative tumour suppressor EXT-1 and is needed for Hh diffusion. Nature 394:85–88
6. Bitgood MJ, McMahon AP (1995) Hedgehog and Bmp genes are coexpressed at many diverse sites of cell-cell interaction in the mouse embryo. Dev Biol 172: 126–138
7. Bitgood MJ, Shen L, McMahon AP (1996) Sertoli cell signaling by Desert hedgehog regulates the male germline. Curr Biol 6:298–304
8. Burke R, Nellen D, Bellotto M, Hafen E, Senti KA, Dickson BJ, Basler K (1999) Dispatched, a novel sterol-sensing domain protein dedicated to the release of cholesterol-modified hedgehog from signaling cells. Cell 99:803–815
9. Buttitta L, Mo R, Hui CC, Fan CM (2003) Interplays of Gli2 and Gli3 and their requirement in mediating Shh-dependent sclerotome induction. Development 130: 6233–6243
10. Capdevila J, Tsukui T, Rodriquez Esteban C, Zappavigna V, Izpisua Belmonte JC (1999) Control of vertebrate limb outgrowth by the proximal factor Meis2 and distal antagonism of BMPs by Gremlin. Mol Cell 4:839–849
11. Chamoun Z, Mann RK, Nellen D, von Kessler DP, Bellotto M, Beachy PA, Basler K (2001) Skinny hedgehog, an acyltransferase required for palmitoylation and activity of the hedgehog signal. Science 293: 2080–2084
12. Charite J, McFadden DG, Olson EN (2000) The bHLH transcription factor dHAND controls Sonic hedgehog expression and establishment of the zone of polarizing activity during limb development. Development 127: 2461–2470
13. Chen MH, Li YJ, Kawakami T, Xu SM, Chuang PT (2004) Palmitoylation is required for the production of a soluble multimeric Hedgehog protein complex and long-range signaling in vertebrates. Genes Dev 18:641–659
14. Chiang C, Litingtung Y, Harris MP, Simandl BK, Li Y, Beachy PA, Fallon JF (2001) Manifestation of the limb prepattern: limb development in the absence of sonic hedgehog function. Dev Biol 236:421–435
15. Chiang C, Litingtung Y, Lee E, Young KE, Corden JL, Westphal H, Beachy PA (1996) Cyclopia and defective axial patterning in mice lacking Sonic hedgehog gene function. Nature 383:407–413
16. Chuang PT, McMahon AP (1999) Vertebrate Hedgehog signalling modulated by induction of a Hedgehog-binding protein. Nature 397:617–621
17. Colnot C, de la Fuente L, Huang S, Hu D, Lu C, St-Jacques B, Helms JA (2005) Indian hedgehog synchronizes skeletal angiogenesis and perichondrial maturation with cartilage development. Development 132:1057–1067
18. Cooper MK, Wassif CA, Krakowiak PA, Taipale J, Gong R, Kelley RI, Porter FD, Beachy PA (2003) A defective response to Hedgehog signaling in disorders of cholesterol biosynthesis. Nat Genet 33:508–513
19. Corbit KC, Aanstad P, Singla V, Norman AR, Stainier DY, Reiter JF (2005) Vertebrate Smoothened functions at the primary cilium. Nature 437: 1018–1021
20. Dasgupta U, Dixit BL, Rusch M, Selleck S, The I (2007) Functional conservation of the human EXT1 tumor suppressor gene and its Drosophila homolog tout velu. Dev Genes Evol 217:555–561
21. Duncan G, McCormick C, Tufaro F (2001) The link between heparan sulfate and hereditary bone disease: finding a function for the EXT family of putative tumor suppressor proteins. J Clin Invest 108:511–516
22. Fan CM, Porter JA, Chiang C, Chang DT, Beachy PA, Tessier-Lavigne M (1995) Long-range sclerotome induction by sonic hedgehog: direct role of the amino-terminal cleavage product and modulation by the cyclic AMP signaling pathway. Cell 81:457–465
23. Fernandez-Teran M, Piedra ME, Kathiriya IS, Srivastava D, Rodriguez-Rey JC, Ros MA (2000) Role of dHAND in the anterior-posterior polarization of the limb bud: implications for the Sonic hedgehog pathway. Development 127:2133–2142
24. Firulli BA, Krawchuk D, Centonze VE, Vargesson N, Virshup DM, Conway SJ, Cserjesi P, Laufer E, Firulli AB (2005) Altered Twist1 and Hand2 dimerization is associated with Saethre-Chotzen syndrome and limb abnormalities. Nat Genet 37:373–381
25. Fitzky BU, Witsch-Baumgartner M, Erdel M, Lee JN, Paik YK, Glossmann H, Utermann G, Moebius FF (1998) Mutations in the Delta7-sterol reductase gene in patients with the Smith–Lemli–Opitz syndrome. Proc Natl Acad Sci U S A 95:8181–8186
26. Gallet A, Rodriguez R, Ruel L, Therond PP (2003) Cholesterol modification of hedgehog is required for

trafficking and movement, revealing an asymmetric cellular response to hedgehog. Dev Cell 4:191–204
27. Gammill LS, Bronner-Fraser M (2003) Neural crest specification: migrating into genomics. Nat Rev Neurosci 4:795–805
28. Gao B, Guo J, She C, Shu A, Yang M, Tan Z, Yang X, Guo S, Feng G, He L (2001) Mutations in IHH, encoding Indian hedgehog, cause brachydactyly type A-1. Nat Genet 28:386–388
29. Gorlin RJ (2004) Nevoid basal cell carcinoma (Gorlin) syndrome. Genet Med 6:530–539
30. Harfe BD, Scherz PJ, Nissim S, Tian H, McMahon AP, Tabin CJ (2004) Evidence for an expansion-based temporal Shh gradient in specifying vertebrate digit identities. Cell 118:517–528
31. Haycraft CJ, Banizs B, Aydin-Son Y, Zhang Q, Michaud EJ, Yoder BK (2005) Gli2 and Gli3 localize to cilia and require the intraflagellar transport protein polaris for processing and function. PLoS Genet 1:e53
32. Hellemans J, Coucke PJ, Giedion A, De Paepe A, Kramer P, Beemer F, Mortier GR (2003) Homozygous mutations in IHH cause acrocapitofemoral dysplasia, an autosomal recessive disorder with cone-shaped epiphyses in hands and hips. Am J Hum Genet 72:1040–1046
33. Helms JA, Kim CH, Hu D, Minkoff R, Thaller C, Eichele G (1997) Sonic hedgehog participates in craniofacial morphogenesis and is down-regulated by teratogenic doses of retinoic acid. Dev Biol 187:25–35
34. Hu D, Helms JA (1999) The role of sonic hedgehog in normal and abnormal craniofacial morphogenesis. Development 126:4873–4884
35. Hu D, Marcucio RS, Helms JA (2003) A zone of frontonasal ectoderm regulates patterning and growth in the face. Development 130:1749–1758
36. Hu H, Hilton MJ, Tu X, Yu K, Ornitz DM, Long F (2005) Sequential roles of Hedgehog and Wnt signaling in osteoblast development. Development 132:49–60
37. Huangfu D, Anderson KV (2005) Cilia and Hedgehog responsiveness in the mouse. Proc Natl Acad Sci U S A 102:11325–11330
38. Huangfu D, Liu A, Rakeman AS, Murcia NS, Niswander L, Anderson KV (2003) Hedgehog signalling in the mouse requires intraflagellar transport proteins. Nature 426:83–87
39. Incardona JP, Lee JH, Robertson CP, Enga K, Kapur RP, Roelink H (2000) Receptor-mediated endocytosis of soluble and membrane-tethered Sonic hedgehog by Patched-1. Proc Natl Acad Sci U S A 97:12044–12049
40. Iwasaki M, Le AX, Helms JA (1997) Expression of Indian hedgehog, bone morphogenetic protein 6 and gli during skeletal morphogenesis. Mech Dev 69: 197–202
41. Jacob L, Lum L (2007) Deconstructing the hedgehog pathway in development and disease. Science 318:66–68
42. Jeong J, Mao J, Tenzen T, Kottmann AH, McMahon AP (2004) Hedgehog signaling in the neural crest cells regulates the patterning and growth of facial primordia. Genes Dev 18:937–951
43. Jia J, Tong C, Wang B, Luo L, Jiang J (2004) Hedgehog signalling activity of Smoothened requires phosphorylation by protein kinase A and casein kinase I. Nature 432:1045–1050
44. Jiang J, Hui CC (2008) Hedgehog signaling in development and cancer. Dev Cell 15:801–812
45. Kang S, Graham JM Jr, Olney AH, Biesecker LG (1997) GLI3 frameshift mutations cause autosomal dominant Pallister-Hall syndrome. Nat Genet 15:266–268
46. Karaplis AC, Luz A, Glowacki J, Bronson RT, Tybulewicz VL, Kronenberg HM, Mulligan RC (1994) Lethal skeletal dysplasia from targeted disruption of the parathyroid hormone-related peptide gene. Genes Dev 8:277–289
47. Karp SJ, Schipani E, St-Jacques B, Hunzelman J, Kronenberg H, McMahon AP (2000) Indian hedgehog coordinates endochondral bone growth and morphogenesis via parathyroid hormone related-protein-dependent and -independent pathways. Development 127:543–548
48. Khokha MK, Hsu D, Brunet LJ, Dionne MS, Harland RM (2003) Gremlin is the BMP antagonist required for maintenance of Shh and Fgf signals during limb patterning. Nat Genet 34:303–307
49. Kimura H, Ng JM, Curran T (2008) Transient inhibition of the Hedgehog pathway in young mice causes permanent defects in bone structure. Cancer Cell 13:249–260
50. Kinto N, Iwamoto M, Enomoto-Iwamoto M, Noji S, Ohuchi H, Yoshioka H, Kataoka H, Wada Y, Yuhao G, Takahashi HE, Yoshiki S, Yamaguchi A (1997) Fibroblasts expressing Sonic hedgehog induce osteoblast differentiation and ectopic bone formation. FEBS Lett 404:319–323
51. Kiprilov EN, Awan A, Desprat R, Velho M, Clement CA, Byskov AG, Andersen CY, Satir P, Bouhassira EE, Christensen ST, Hirsch RE (2008) Human embryonic stem cells in culture possess primary cilia with hedgehog signaling machinery. J Cell Biol 180:897–904
52. Kobayashi T, Soegiarto DW, Yang Y, Lanske B, Schipani E, McMahon AP, Kronenberg HM (2005) Indian hedgehog stimulates periarticular chondrocyte differentiation to regulate growth plate length independently of PTHrP. J Clin Invest 115:1734–1742
53. Koide T, Hayata T, Cho KW (2006) Negative regulation of Hedgehog signaling by the cholesterogenic enzyme 7-dehydrocholesterol reductase. Development 133: 2395–2405
54. Koziel L, Kunath M, Kelly OG, Vortkamp A (2004) Ext1-dependent heparan sulfate regulates the range of Ihh signaling during endochondral ossification. Dev Cell 6:801–813
55. Koziel L, Wuelling M, Schneider S, Vortkamp A (2005) Gli3 acts as a repressor downstream of Ihh in regulating two distinct steps of chondrocyte differentiation. Development 132:5249–5260
56. Lanske B, Karaplis AC, Lee K, Luz A, Vortkamp A, Pirro A, Karperien M, Defize LH, Ho C, Mulligan RC, Abou-Samra AB, Juppner H, Segre GV, Kronenberg HM (1996) PTH/PTHrP receptor in early development

and Indian hedgehog-regulated bone growth. Science 273:663–666
57. Laufer E, Nelson CE, Johnson RL, Morgan BA, Tabin C (1994) Sonic hedgehog and Fgf-4 act through a signaling cascade and feedback loop to integrate growth and patterning of the developing limb bud. Cell 79:993–1003
58. Lee CS, Buttitta L, Fan CM (2001) Evidence that the WNT-inducible growth arrest-specific gene 1 encodes an antagonist of sonic hedgehog signaling in the somite. Proc Natl Acad Sci U S A 98:11347–11352
59. Lei Q, Zelman AK, Kuang E, Li S, Matise MP (2004) Transduction of graded Hedgehog signaling by a combination of Gli2 and Gli3 activator functions in the developing spinal cord. Development 131:3593–3604
60. Litingtung Y, Dahn RD, Li Y, Fallon JF, Chiang C (2002) Shh and Gli3 are dispensable for limb skeleton formation but regulate digit number and identity. Nature 418:979–983
61. Liu A, Wang B, Niswander LA (2005) Mouse intraflagellar transport proteins regulate both the activator and repressor functions of Gli transcription factors. Development 132:3103–3111
62. Liu M, Wang X, Cai Z, Tang Z, Cao K, Liang B, Ren X, Liu JY, Wang QK (2006) A novel heterozygous mutation in the Indian hedgehog gene (IHH) is associated with brachydactyly type A1 in a Chinese family. J Hum Genet 51:727–731
63. Liu Y, Liu C, Yamada Y, Fan CM (2002) Growth arrest specific gene 1 acts as a region-specific mediator of the Fgf10/Fgf8 regulatory loop in the limb. Development 129:5289–5300
64. Long F, Chung UI, Ohba S, McMahon J, Kronenberg HM, McMahon AP (2004) Ihh signaling is directly required for the osteoblast lineage in the endochondral skeleton. Development 131:1309–1318
65. Long F, Zhang XM, Karp S, Yang Y, McMahon AP (2001) Genetic manipulation of hedgehog signaling in the endochondral skeleton reveals a direct role in the regulation of chondrocyte proliferation. Development 128:5099–5108
66. Lum L, Beachy PA (2004) The Hedgehog response network: sensors, switches, and routers. Science 304: 1755–1759
67. Lum L, Zhang C, Oh S, Mann RK, von Kessler DP, Taipale J, Weis-Garcia F, Gong R, Wang B, Beachy PA (2003) Hedgehog signal transduction via Smoothened association with a cytoplasmic complex scaffolded by the atypical kinesin, Costal-2. Mol Cell 12:1261–1274
68. Ma Y, Erkner A, Gong R, Yao S, Taipale J, Basler K, Beachy PA (2002) Hedgehog-mediated patterning of the mammalian embryo requires transporter-like function of dispatched. Cell 111:63–75
69. Ma YL, Cain RL, Halladay DL, Yang X, Zeng Q, Miles RR, Chandrasekhar S, Martin TJ, Onyia JE (2001) Catabolic effects of continuous human PTH (1–38) in vivo is associated with sustained stimulation of RANKL and inhibition of osteoprotegerin and gene-associated bone formation. Endocrinology 142: 4047–4054
70. Maeda Y, Nakamura E, Nguyen MT, Suva LJ, Swain FL, Razzaque MS, Mackem S, Lanske B (2007) Indian Hedgehog produced by postnatal chondrocytes is essential for maintaining a growth plate and trabecular bone. Proc Natl Acad Sci U S A 104:6382–6387
71. Mak KK, Bi Y, Wan C, Chuang PT, Clemens T, Young M, Yang Y (2008) Hedgehog signaling in mature osteoblasts regulates bone formation and resorption by controlling PTHrP and RANKL expression. Dev Cell 14:674–688
72. Mak KK, Chen MH, Day TF, Chuang PT, Yang Y (2006) Wnt/beta-catenin signaling interacts differentially with Ihh signaling in controlling endochondral bone and synovial joint formation. Development 133:3695–3707
73. Mak KK, Kronenberg HM, Chuang PT, Mackem S, Yang Y (2008) Indian hedgehog signals independently of PTHrP to promote chondrocyte hypertrophy. Development
74. Marigo V, Johnson RL, Vortkamp A, Tabin CJ (1996) Sonic hedgehog differentially regulates expression of GLI and GLI3 during limb development. Dev Biol 180:273–283
75. McCarthy RA, Barth JL, Chintalapudi MR, Knaak C, Argraves WS (2002) Megalin functions as an endocytic sonic hedgehog receptor. J Biol Chem 277:25660–25667
76. McLellan JS, Yao S, Zheng X, Geisbrecht BV, Ghirlando R, Beachy PA, Leahy DJ (2006) Structure of a heparin-dependent complex of Hedgehog and Ihog. Proc Natl Acad Sci U S A 103:17208–17213
77. McLellan JS, Zheng X, Hauk G, Ghirlando R, Beachy PA, Leahy DJ (2008) The mode of Hedgehog binding to Ihog homologues is not conserved across different phyla. Nature
78. Merino R, Macias D, Ganan Y, Economides AN, Wang X, Wu Q, Stahl N, Sampath KT, Varona P, Hurle JM (1999) Expression and function of Gdf-5 during digit skeletogenesis in the embryonic chick leg bud. Dev Biol 206:33–45
79. Minina E, Kreschel C, Naski MC, Ornitz DM, Vortkamp A (2002) Interaction of FGF, Ihh/Pthlh, and BMP signaling integrates chondrocyte proliferation and hypertrophic differentiation. Dev Cell 3:439–449
80. Minina E, Wenzel HM, Kreschel C, Karp S, Gaffield W, McMahon AP, Vortkamp A (2001) BMP and Ihh/PTHrP signaling interact to coordinate chondrocyte proliferation and differentiation. Development 128:4523–4534
81. Morales CR, Zeng J, El Alfy M, Barth JL, Chintalapudi MR, McCarthy RA, Incardona JP, Argraves WS (2006) Epithelial trafficking of Sonic hedgehog by megalin. J Histochem Cytochem 54:1115–1127
82. Motoyama J, Milenkovic L, Iwama M, Shikata Y, Scott MP, Hui CC (2003) Differential requirement for Gli2 and Gli3 in ventral neural cell fate specification. Dev Biol 259:150–161
83. Murtaugh LC, Chyung JH, Lassar AB (1999) Sonic hedgehog promotes somitic chondrogenesis by altering the cellular response to BMP signaling. Genes Dev 13:225–237
84. Murtaugh LC, Zeng L, Chyung JH, Lassar AB (2001) The chick transcriptional repressor Nkx3.2 acts downstream of Shh to promote BMP-dependent axial chondrogenesis. Dev Cell 1:411–422

85. Nakamura T, Aikawa T, Iwamoto-Enomoto M, Iwamoto M, Higuchi Y, Pacifici M, Kinto N, Yamaguchi A, Noji S, Kurisu K, Matsuya T (1997) Induction of osteogenic differentiation by hedgehog proteins. Biochem Biophys Res Commun 237:465–469
86. Nieuwenhuis E, Hui CC (2005) Hedgehog signaling and congenital malformations. Clin Genet 67:193–208
87. Niswander L, Jeffrey S, Martin GR, Tickle C (1994) A positive feedback loop coordinates growth and patterning in the vertebrate limb. Nature 371:609–612
88. Niswander L, Tickle C, Vogel A, Booth I, Martin GR (1993) FGF-4 replaces the apical ectodermal ridge and directs outgrowth and patterning of the limb. Cell 75:579–587
89. Nusslein-Volhard C, Wieschaus E (1980) Mutations affecting segment number and polarity in Drosophila. Nature 287:795–801
90. Ohba S, Kawaguchi H, Kugimiya F, Ogasawara T, Kawamura N, Saito T, Ikeda T, Fujii K, Miyajima T, Kuramochi A, Miyashita T, Oda H, Nakamura K, Takato T, Chung UI (2008) Patched1 haploinsufficiency increases adult bone mass and modulates Gli3 repressor activity. Dev Cell 14:689–699
91. Park HL, Bai C, Platt KA, Matise MP, Beeghly A, Hui CC, Nakashima M, Joyner AL (2000) Mouse Gli1 mutants are viable but have defects in SHH signaling in combination with a Gli2 mutation. Development 127:1593–1605
92. Parmantier E, Lynn B, Lawson D, Turmaine M, Namini SS, Chakrabarti L, McMahon AP, Jessen KR, Mirsky R (1999) Schwann cell-derived Desert hedgehog controls the development of peripheral nerve sheaths. Neuron 23:713–724
93. Pepinsky RB, Zeng C, Wen D, Rayhorn P, Baker DP, Williams KP, Bixler SA, Ambrose CM, Garber EA, Miatkowski K, Taylor FR, Wang EA, Galdes A (1998) Identification of a palmitic acid-modified form of human Sonic hedgehog. J Biol Chem 273:14037–14045
94. Petrij F, Giles RH, Dauwerse HG, Saris JJ, Hennekam RC, Masuno M, Tommerup N, van Ommen GJ, Goodman RH, Peters DJ et al (1995) Rubinstein–Taybi syndrome caused by mutations in the transcriptional co-activator CBP. Nature 376:348–351
95. Pons S, Marti E (2000) Sonic hedgehog synergizes with the extracellular matrix protein vitronectin to induce spinal motor neuron differentiation. Development 127:333–342
96. Porter JA, Ekker SC, Park WJ, von Kessler DP, Young KE, Chen CH, Ma Y, Woods AS, Cotter RJ, Koonin EV, Beachy PA (1996) Hedgehog patterning activity: role of a lipophilic modification mediated by the carboxy-terminal autoprocessing domain. Cell 86:21–34
97. Porter JA, Young KE, Beachy PA (1996) Cholesterol modification of hedgehog signaling proteins in animal development. Science 274:255–259
98. Radhakrishna U, Wild A, Grzeschik KH, Antonarakis SE (1997) Mutation in GLI3 in postaxial polydactyly type A. Nat Genet 17:269–271
99. Riddle RD, Johnson RL, Laufer E, Tabin C (1993) Sonic hedgehog mediates the polarizing activity of the ZPA. Cell 75:1401–1416
100. Roessler E, Belloni E, Gaudenz K, Jay P, Berta P, Scherer SW, Tsui LC, Muenke M (1996) Mutations in the human Sonic Hedgehog gene cause holoprosencephaly. Nat Genet 14:357–360
101. St-Jacques B, Hammerschmidt M, McMahon AP (1999) Indian hedgehog signaling regulates proliferation and differentiation of chondrocytes and is essential for bone formation. Genes Dev 13:2072–2086
102. Taipale J, Cooper MK, Maiti T, Beachy PA (2002) Patched acts catalytically to suppress the activity of Smoothened. Nature 418:892–897
103. Tavella S, Biticchi R, Morello R, Castagnola P, Musante V, Costa D, Cancedda R, Garofalo S (2006) Forced chondrocyte expression of sonic hedgehog impairs joint formation affecting proliferation and apoptosis. Matrix Biol 25:389–397
104. te Welscher P, Fernandez-Teran M, Ros MA, Zeller R (2002) Mutual genetic antagonism involving GLI3 and dHAND prepatterns the vertebrate limb bud mesenchyme prior to SHH signaling. Genes Dev 16:421–426
105. te Welscher P, Zuniga A, Kuijper S, Drenth T, Goedemans HJ, Meijlink F, Zeller R (2002) Progression of vertebrate limb development through SHH-mediated counteraction of GLI3. Science 298:827–830
106. Tickle C, Summerbell D, Wolpert L (1975) Positional signalling and specification of digits in chick limb morphogenesis. Nature 254:199–202
107. Tint GS, Irons M, Elias ER, Batta AK, Frieden R, Chen TS, Salen G (1994) Defective cholesterol biosynthesis associated with the Smith–Lemli–Opitz syndrome. N Engl J Med 330:107–113
108. Torroja C, Gorfinkiel N, Guerrero I (2004) Patched controls the Hedgehog gradient by endocytosis in a dynamin-dependent manner, but this internalization does not play a major role in signal transduction. Development 131:2395–2408
109. Towers M, Mahood R, Yin Y, Tickle C (2008) Integration of growth and specification in chick wing digit-patterning. Nature 452:882–886
110. van den Heuvel M, Ingham PW (1996) Smoothened encodes a receptor-like serpentine protein required for hedgehog signalling. Nature 382:547–551
111. Varjosalo M, Li SP, Taipale J (2006) Divergence of hedgehog signal transduction mechanism between Drosophila and mammals. Dev Cell 10:177–186
112. Varjosalo M, Taipale J (2008) Hedgehog: functions and mechanisms. Genes Dev 22:2454–2472
113. Von Ohlen T, Lessing D, Nusse R, Hooper JE (1997) Hedgehog signaling regulates transcription through cubitus interruptus, a sequence-specific DNA binding protein. Proc Natl Acad Sci U S A 94:2404–2409
114. Vortkamp A, Gessler M, Grzeschik KH (1991) GLI3 zinc-finger gene interrupted by translocations in Greig syndrome families. Nature 352:539–540
115. Vortkamp A, Lee K, Lanske B, Segre GV, Kronenberg HM, Tabin CJ (1996) Regulation of rate of cartilage differentiation by Indian hedgehog and PTH-related protein. Science 273:613–622
116. Yan D, Lin X (2008) Opposing roles for glypicans in Hedgehog signalling. Nat Cell Biol 10:761–763

117. Yang Y, Drossopoulou G, Chuang PT, Duprez D, Marti E, Bumcrot D, Vargesson N, Clarke J, Niswander L, McMahon A, Tickle C (1997) Relationship between dose, distance and time in Sonic Hedgehog-mediated regulation of anteroposterior polarity in the chick limb. Development 124:4393–4404
118. Yao S, Lum L, Beachy P (2006) The ihog cell-surface proteins bind Hedgehog and mediate pathway activation. Cell 125:343–357
119. Yuasa T, Kataoka H, Kinto N, Iwamoto M, Enomoto-Iwamoto M, Iemura S, Ueno N, Shibata Y, Kurosawa H, Yamaguchi A (2002) Sonic hedgehog is involved in osteoblast differentiation by cooperating with BMP-2. J Cell Physiol 193:225–232
120. Zeng L, Kempf H, Murtaugh LC, Sato ME, Lassar AB (2002) Shh establishes an Nkx3.2/Sox9 autoregulatory loop that is maintained by BMP signals to induce somitic chondrogenesis. Genes Dev 16: 1990–2005
121. Zhang M, Xuan S, Bouxsein ML, von Stechow D, Akeno N, Faugere MC, Malluche H, Zhao G, Rosen CJ, Efstratiadis A, Clemens TL (2002) Osteoblast-specific knockout of the insulin-like growth factor (IGF) receptor gene reveals an essential role of IGF signaling in bone matrix mineralization. J Biol Chem 277:44005–44012
122. Zhang XM, Ramalho-Santos M, McMahon AP (2001) Smoothened mutants reveal redundant roles for Shh and Ihh signaling including regulation of L/R asymmetry by the mouse node. Cell 105:781–792
123. Zhu G, Ke X, Liu Q, Li J, Chen B, Shao C, Gong Y (2007) Recurrence of the D100N mutation in a Chinese family with brachydactyly type A1: evidence for a mutational hot spot in the Indian hedgehog gene. Am J Med Genet A 143A:1246–1248
124. Zhu J, Nakamura E, Nguyen MT, Bao X, Akiyama H, Mackem S (2008) Uncoupling Sonic hedgehog control of pattern and expansion of the developing limb bud. Dev Cell 14:624–632

5. Role of microRNA in Skeleton Development

Ben Gradus and Eran Hornstein

5.1 What Are miRNAs?

5.1.1 miRNA Genes and Their Genomic Organization

miRNAs are single-stranded RNAs of ~22 nucleotides that repress protein expression at a posttranscriptional level through base pairing, usually with the 3′ untranslated region (3′ UTR) of the target mRNA [1, 5, 75]. Since the discovery of the founding members of the miRNA family, lin-4 and let-7 [37, 64, 81], hundreds of miRNA genes have been identified. Many of these are independent transcriptional units that do not differ much from other protein-coding genes in recruiting transcription factors and RNA polymerase II for their transcription. miRNA genes may have promoter-enhancing regulatory sequences upstream – however, about half of miRNA genes are embedded within the introns of protein-coding genes. This omits the need for independent transcriptional regulatory elements and results in coupled transcriptional control, i.e., where the miRNA is coexpressed with the gene that codes for the protein. Posttranscriptional processing of miRNA precursors is then conducted in concert with the splicing of the mRNA that codes for the given protein.

5.1.2 Posttranscriptional Processing of miRNAs

miRNAs are subject to extensive posttranscriptional processing, essential for their functional maturation. Inside the nucleus, "microprocessing" refers to the cleavage of a primary miRNA precursor (pri-miRNA), which initially may be dozens of kilobases long. The resulting RNA stem-and-loop structure is about 70 nucleotides long and is known as the "pre-miRNA" hairpin. Often, a pri-miRNA is in fact a polycistron genetic element that harbors a few miRNA hairpins. The microprocessor is a multiprotein complex that contains the RNaseIII-containing protein Drosha, with cofactors such as DGCR8 and p68. The microprocessor is a prerequisite for the biosynthesis of most miRNAs [3, 8, 25, 67]. After microprocessing, the pre-miRNA hairpin is exported from the nucleus by Exportin-5 [47, 86] and is subject to further cleavage by the RNaseIII-containing protein Dicer [31, 38]. This yields a mature miRNA, which is a ~22nt single-stranded RNA oligonucleotide. The mature miRNA is then loaded onto the RNA-induced silencing complex (RISC), which endows it with repressive capacity. As perturbation of the single Dicer gene in the vertebrate genome inactivates the miRNA function, this approach often is used as an experimental loss-of-function strategy to

F. Bronner et al. (eds.), *Bone and Development*, Topics in Bone Biology 6,
DOI 10.1007/978-1-84882-822-3_5,

uncover the role of the miRNA pathway [15, 23, 27, 32, 33, 83].

5.1.3 miRNA Regulation of the Target Genes

The mature miRNA inside the RISC provides target specificity, whereas the Argonaute proteins provide catalytic activity [49, 59]. Argonaute proteins deadenylate and decap the mRNAs that are undergoing miRNA-dependent destabilization [7, 53], whereas other mechanisms provide translational repression [13, 14]. Together, RISC-dependent translational repression and RISC-dependent mRNA decay constitute the two dominant mechanisms by which miRNAs modulate gene expression [4, 44, 68, 82].

How do miRNAs confer target specificity? The discovery of the first miRNA, lin-4, established the principle of partial sequence complementation [37, 81]. Later, comparative genomic tools characterized the general rules for target recognition [9, 19, 34, 40, 41]. These studies uncovered the importance of a minimal "seed" sequence that is only 7–8 nucleotides long, located at the 5′ end of the miRNA. Some miRNA-target pairs do not follow these rules, exhibiting virtually perfect complementarity of the miRNA:target pair [28, 84, 85] or seedless 3′-compensatory sites. In the latter, insufficient 5′ pairing is compensated for by strong pairing to the miRNA 3′ region [9, 26].

5.1.4 miRNAs as Regulators of Development

The function of the first miRNA, discovered by Ambros et al. [37], was to regulate the cell-fate decisions in the development of the nematode, *Caenorhabditis elegans*. Since then, a large body of work has indicated that miRNAs play a role in the development and regulation of many embryological processes [10, 11, 80]. These inferences have derived support from the striking spatial expression patterns observed for many miRNAs in the embryos of multiple species [17, 74, 79] and from the bioinformatic studies that showed that developmental genes are significantly enriched with miRNA-binding sites at their 3′ UTR [40, 62, 70, 88].

5.2 Introduction to Bone Development and Mesenchymal Stem Cells

The developmental process that initiates bone organogenesis (reviewed in [35] and the preceding volumes of this book series) starts when mesenchymal cells respond to specific cues to form condensations. These mesenchymal condensations in turn give rise to bone through direct (intramembranous) osteoblast differentiation, similar to that for the flat bones of the skull. In bones derived through the endochondral ossification pathway, mesenchymal condensations give rise to chondrocytes that subsequently produce cartilage by the secretion of a defined extracellular matrix. The cartilage shapes the mold for endochondral bone and is later replaced by osteoblasts in a highly regulated process, as described in Chap. 2. Chondrocytes proliferate and further differentiate into a hypertrophic stage, whereby they direct the mineralization of their surrounding matrix, attract blood vessels, and induce osteoblast differentiation. These osteoblasts invade the cartilage, replace the chondrocytes in an organized fashion, and secrete bone matrix or osteoid.

Mesenchymal stem cells (MSCs) are multipotent cells that arise from the mesenchyme during development. In vitro, they can proliferate and differentiate into several cell types, such as osteoblasts, myocytes, adipocytes, or chondrocytes. Signaling pathways that regulate skeletal tissue formation, in vivo and in cultured MSCs, include Hedgehog, Wnt, fibroblast growth factors (FGF), and bone morphogenetic proteins (BMP) signaling. Specific pathways are activated by a secreted ligand and induce an intracellular cascade. These signals activate a specific transcriptional program, in which miRNAs also are embedded. This chapter will discuss miRNA involvement in bone development on the basis of mouse and zebrafish experiments and in vitro studies of MSCs.

5.3 Mouse Models of Dicer-Dependent Inactivation of miRNA Activity in the early Limb Mesenchyme and the Growth Plate

Conditional loss of Dicer function provides a good, entry-level model to evaluate the role of the miRNA pathway in vivo. The Tabin and Kronenberg groups were able to show that miRNAs are involved in limb development, using a set of Cre deletions and a Dicer conditional allele [27, 33]. The role of miRNAs, downstream of the Dicer, was evaluated using early onset prx1-Cre, expressed throughout the limb mesenchyme. Loss of Dicer activity results in massive cell death; this suggests that miRNA activity is important in repressing unwanted apoptosis in early limb mesenchyme, possibly through regulation of FGF signaling [27]. Loss of Dicer expression also blocks the synthesis of miR-196 in the hind limb, needed upstream of Hoxb8 expression [28]. The apoptosis observed in the prx1-Cre; Dicer model is consistent with the reports that indicate that a Dicer model is involved in other organs, in the sense that apoptosis emerges as a common consequence of inactivation of master regulators of miRNA synthesis. However, the early limb-bud model is significantly different from the later effect of Dicer in differentiated chondrocytes, where loss of miRNA activity owing to a Dicer conditional allele recombining with a Col2a1-Cre deletion does not induce apoptosis. A likely interpretation is therefore that miRNAs are no longer essential for chondrocyte survival after differentiation has occurred. Nonetheless, the loss of miRNA function in growth-plate chondrocytes causes decreased proliferation and enhanced differentiation into hypertrophy [33]. The combination of precocious maturation and decreased proliferation results in a smaller chondrocyte pool, a reduction in the number of columnar proliferating chondrocytes, and a reduction in bone width. Altogether, these changes subsequently lead to a smaller skeleton [33], but the molecular mechanism by which miRNA affects chondrocyte proliferation and differentiation is not well understood. To study if stimulation of hypertrophy in the Dicer model perturbs Ihh/PTHrP signaling, Kobayashi et al. [33] evaluated Hh signaling through the detection of Patched1 mRNA levels, a readout of Hh activity. If patched1 expression is not affected, then accelerated hypertrophic differentiation is probably downstream of Hh signaling or resides in an independent pathway. The authors, therefore, crossed a constitutively active PTHrP receptor allele onto the background of the Col2a1-Cre; Dicer mice. As this allele also failed to rescue the Dicer phenotype, it was concluded that the involvement of miRNAs resides outside of the Ihh/PTHrP signaling pathway [33]. Consequently, the Prx1-Cre; Dicer and Col2a1-Cre; Dicer models are still without a mechanistic explanation for the observed phenotype. Two pathways, FGF and BMP, regulate chondrocyte proliferation and differentiation at the growth plate, and thus may be important for a better understanding of the Dicer phenotype. In addition, deregulation of miRNA function affects BMP and FGF signaling, as discussed later in this chapter.

5.4 Evaluation of miRNA Function in the Signaling Pathway that leads to Bone development

5.4.1 miRNAs in Hh Signaling

Hedgehog signaling through the function of the morphogen Sonic Hedgehog (Shh) is pivotal in early limb development, and in regulating bone development through Indian Hedgehog (Ihh). In the early limb bud, upstream of the activation of Shh, miR-196 is a hind limb-specific repressor of the Shh inducer, Hoxb8. This provides the hind limb with a safeguard mechanism to inhibit unwanted Hoxb8 expression [28, 71].

Another miRNA, miR-214, may be involved in hedgehog signaling during muscle development in zebra fish [22, 42]. When miR-214 is knocked down, fish embryos exhibit "U-shaped" somites and a ventrally curved body axis. This defect is typically associated with perturbation of Hh signaling in cell-type specification of somite musculature. These experiments uncovered that suppressor of fused (Sufu) and dispatched-2 (Disp2) are targets of miR-214 [22, 42]. The Sufu and Disp2 3′ UTRs are regulated in vivo by misexpression of miR-214; in turn, the miR-214 knockdown phenotype can be rescued by simultaneous repression of Sufu or Disp2 [22, 42]. Modulating the activity of Sufu and Disp2 by miR-214 may therefore provide a means to fine-tune cell response to Hh signaling. However, these observations should be substantiated by genetic studies in a mouse model before the relevance of miR-214 as a component of Hh signaling in zebra fish is extrapolated to mammals. The need for further evaluation is underscored by the initial characterization of the mouse knockout of the miR-214 gene, that does not seem to lead to a simple hedgehog signaling phenocopy [78].

5.4.2 miR-214 Functions in Hh and Twist Signaling

miR-214 is intriguing not only because of its possible role as a regulator of Hh signaling, but also because it is regulated by Twist, a transcription factor involved in osteoblast differentiation [58]. Twist haploinsufficiency causes Saethre–Chotzen syndrome, a disorder characterized by craniosynostosis, facial dysmorphism, and preaxial polydactyly [30] (see Chap. 1 in this volume). However, how Twist regulates bone development is not understood. Twist is engaged in Hh signaling through regulation of Gli transcription factors [57, 77], and therefore, may regulate Hh signaling in more than one way (Fig. 5.1). Interestingly, a 7.9-kb noncoding transcript, contained within an intron of the mouse Dynamin3 (Dnm3) gene, was recently discovered downstream of Twist [39, 46, 78]. This noncoding gene, Dnm3os, is the primary precursor (pri-miRNA) of miR-214 and of another miRNA,

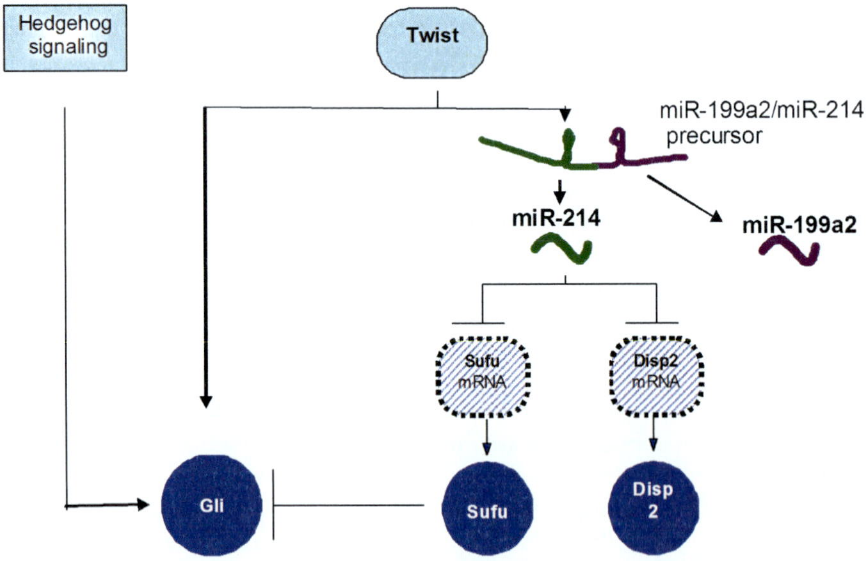

Figure 5.1. miRNA are intertwined through the Twist and Hh signaling pathways during bone development. Twist controls Hh signaling directly through the regulation of Gli-family protein expression [57, 77]. Twist may also be affecting Hh signaling in a miRNA-dependent fashion, because it activates the transcription of the miR-199a2/miR-214 precursor (*purple* and *green*, respectively) [39, 78]. Processing of this miRNA precursor pair results in the formation of a mature miR-214 form (*green*), which represses the expression of Sufu and Disp2 mRNA (*dashed boxes*), at least in some contexts [22, 42]. Downregulation of Sufu allows for Gli activation, because Sufu is a posttranslational repressor of Gli expression.

miR-199a2 (Fig. 5.1). This indicates that the transcription of these miRNAs is regulated by the transcription factor Twist [39, 78]. Dnm3os knockout mice are viable, but exhibit skeletal abnormalities, including craniofacial hypoplasia, defects in dorsal neural arches, and malformation of the vertebral spinous processes. Together, these observations suggest that one or both miRNAs embedded inside the Dnm3os precursor are involved in bone development. If miR-214 is indeed a Hh component, its knockout should be phenocopying recognized Hh mutants. At present, however, it is difficult to know whether the relatively subtle bone defects in the miR-214/mir-199a2 knockout mouse reflect attenuation of Hh signaling [78]. As two miRNA genes have been deleted, it is a challenge to determine which part of the phenotype is downstream of miR-214, and what is the consequence of the miR-199a2 knockout. If additional characterization of the miR-214/miR-199a2 knockout would reveal if these miRNAs are indeed the fine-tuning genes involved in Hh signaling, this would magnify the importance of miRNA in functioning as the genetic modifiers and molecular "fine-tuners" [6, 29].

If Twist regulates Gli transcription factors [57, 77], and if miR-214 is in fact involved in mammalian Hh signaling, this implies that Twist would regulate Gli protein expression, probably by regulating their transcription; at the same time, Twist may also target other Hh components indirectly through the activation of the miRNA gene (Fig. 5.1).

5.4.3 miRNAs Are Tightly Linked to BMP Signaling

BMPs are members of the transforming growth factor beta (TGF beta) superfamily that activate transcriptional programs for lineage determination. Their effectors are Smad proteins that play a central role in intracellular signaling. When a BMP ligand is bound to its receptor, a cascade is initiated, which leads to phosphorylation and activation of the receptor-regulated Smads (Smad 1/5/8), which form heteromeric complexes with their cofactor, Smad4. They then translocate into the nucleus and regulate the transcription of various target genes.

BMP2 treatment of C2C12 mesenchymal cells induces osteoblast differentiation, concomitantly with the repression of an alternative myocytic fate. In the course of BMP2-induced osteogenesis, the expression levels of many miRNAs change, becoming downregulated. The downregulated miRNAs are thought to target components of multiple osteogenic pathways. Conceivably, the downregulation of the miRNAs paves the way for the upregulation of osteogenic genes. In this context, it may be useful to look at the two roles played by the muscle-specific miR-133 in myocyte and osteoblast differentiation. In myocyte differentiation, miR-133 is upregulated downstream of the transcription factors myogenin, MyoD, SRF, and Mef2 [12, 45, 63]. In osteoblast differentiation, the myocyte-specific RNA, miR-133, targets Runx2, an early BMP response gene that is essential for bone formation. Similarly, miR-135 targets Smad5, a key transducer of the BMP2 osteogenic signal. miR-133 and miR-135, together, inhibit the differentiation of osteoprogenitors by attenuating Runx2 and Smad5 expression [43]. miR-133 and miR-135 may therefore function as safeguards against the activation of the osteoblastic program in differentiating muscle cells. In the absence of miR-133, committed myogenic progenitors are more likely to respond to pro-osteoblastic signals. BMP-2 imposes transcriptional repression of miR-133; this process seems to be a prerequisite for osteoblast fate selection. Indeed, failure to downregulate miR-133, as when it is experimentally overexpressed, restrains the BMP2-induced Runx2 and the upregulation of Smad5 [43]. It appears, therefore, that BMP2 can commit mesenchymal cells to the osteoblast lineage, not only by the direct activation of the pro-osteoblastic programs, but also by inhibiting the expression of miRNAs that promote a different sibling cell fate (Fig. 5.2).

miR-125b is another miRNA gene that is expressed in MSCs and acts as a repressor of osteoblastic differentiation. Introduction of BMP-4 downregulates miR-125b expression, thereby enabling osteoblast differentiation. Conversely, overexpression of miR-125b inhibits BMP-4-induced osteoblast differentiation [54]. Thus, it is possible that miR-125b, miR-135, and miR-133 play a role in maintaining the progenitor state or in reinforcing an alternative (myocyte) fate for cultured MSCs. This probably helps in conferring

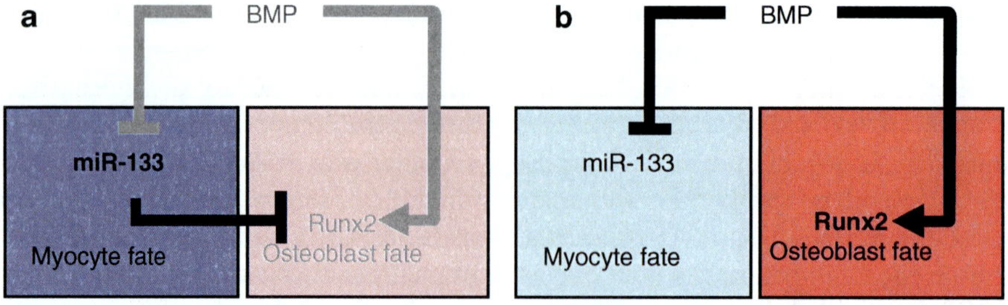

Figure 5.2. The choice of a particular cell fate is reinforced by miRNA activity. (**a**) When a promyocytic program is activated in mesenchymal stem cells, the myocyte-specific miR-133 represses Runx2 expression, to insure that the sibling, osteoblast cell fate is not induced. (**b**) The expression of miR-133 is transcriptionally repressed by BMP signals, promoting a coherent osteoblast differentiation program [43]. BMP commits mesenchymal cells into the osteoblast lineage by direct activation of pro-osteoblast programs, and by inhibiting miRNAs that promote an alternative, sibling cell fate. This interpretation is consistent with a more general view of miRNA function as genes that confer robustness to the genetic program by safeguarding against the expression of unwanted genes [16, 23, 24, 28, 70].

robust transitions between different cell fates. When those miRNAs are taken away, the transition becomes fuzzy and there is a bigger chance for the emergence of ill-defined, ambiguous fates. This interpretation is consistent with the general view that miRNAs function to confer robustness to the genetic program and safeguard against the expression of unwanted genes [16, 23, 24, 28, 29, 70].

However, there is more to the BMP/Smad pathway with miRNA activity. For example, miRNAs may act as upstream regulators of Smad1 expression [48] and as downstream target of Smad1 activity. Intriguingly, Smad1 is involved in the regulation of miRNA processing, downstream of BMP signaling [18]. It appears that Smad1, a transcription factor, interacts with the Drosha/DGCR8/p68 microprocessor complex and is a cofactor of Drosha, required for efficient post-transcriptional microprocessing of a subset of miRNAs. Thus, Smad1-dependent maturation facilitates microprocessing of the miRNA primary precursor (Fig. 5.3). Smad1 proteins control Drosha-mediated miRNA maturation [18], which should be further evaluated in vivo and in processes other than smooth muscle differentiation. Currently, Smad1 appears to be the first protein that endows tissue specificity to post-transcriptional regulation of miRNA expression. Moreover, Smad1 is unique in that it provides sequence specificity that affects some, but not all, miRNAs [18]. Finally, Smad1-dependent, post-transcriptional regulation of miRNAs responds to BMP and TGF-beta signaling; miRNAs, therefore, may be effectors of BMP signaling. miR-21 is one miRNA whose expression correlates with TGF-beta signaling in tumors [61], probably as a result of Smad1-dependent microprocessing [18]. miR-21 is highly expressed in osteosarcomas [36] and osteoblasts (Gradus and Hornstein, unpublished 2010). It may therefore be worthwhile to explore whether miR-21, by inducing BMP/TGF-beta signaling, plays a role in bone development.

5.4.4 miRNA and FGF Signaling

Regulation of chondrocyte proliferation and hypertrophic differentiation by BMPs is balanced by the antagonistic signal of FGF [50, 60, 87] (see Chap. 6 of this volume). The importance of FGF is brought out by FGF receptor 3 mutations leading to inherited human dwarfism syndromes, e.g., achondroplasia (see Chap. 1 of this volume). The Sprouty proteins, spry1 and spry2, regulate the ERK-mediated signaling downstream of the FGF receptor. The expression of spry1 and spry2 is repressed by miR-21; this upregulates the ERK signaling in cardiomyocytes [65, 73]. spry4, another homolog expressed with spry1 and spry2 in developing bone, may also contain an miR-21 binding site [40]. Thus, miR-21 emerges as a gene that can regulate the intensity of FGF signaling through its regulation of spry1, spry2, and possibly spry4.

In limb buds lacking Dicer activity, FGF signaling is reduced, whereas spry2 expression is upregulated [27]. Moreover, the massive apoptosis observed in Dicer limb buds is due to spry2 upregulation, because spry2 is known to induce

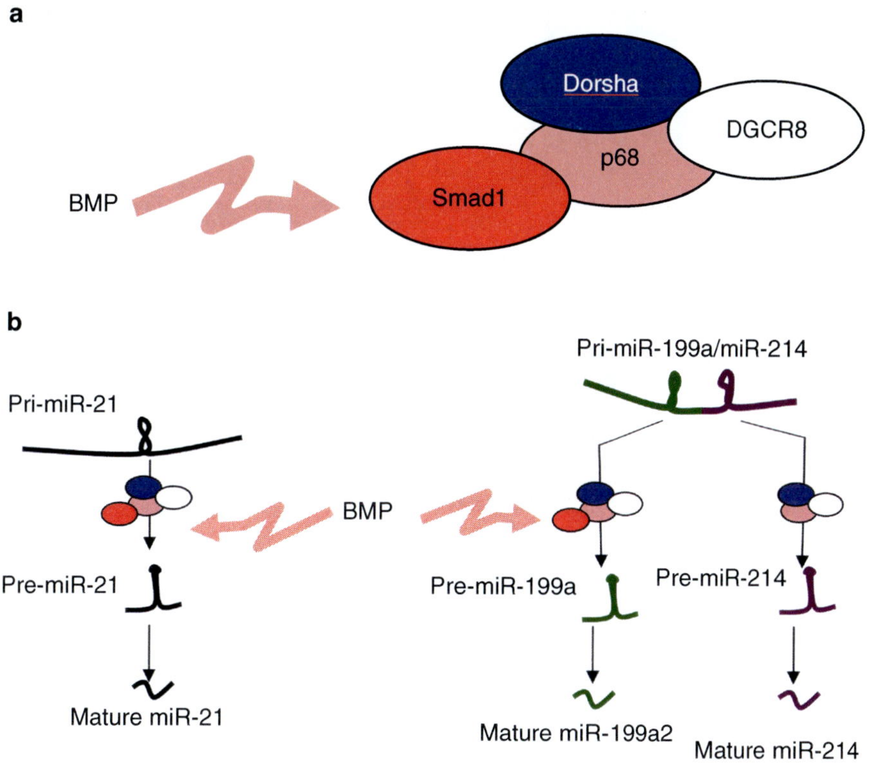

Figure 5.3. Smad1 is a context-specific regulator of miRNA maturation, downstream of BMP signaling. (**a**) Smad1 (*red*) is a cofactor of the microprocessor protein complex along with p68, Drosha, and DGCR8, whose activity is modulated by BMP signaling (*red lightning*) [18]. (**b**) This complex facilitates the maturation of at least two pre-miRNAs: miR-21 (*black*) and miR-199a2 (*green*) from their longer, pri-miRNA, precursor. miR-214 (*purple*) that is derived from the same transcript as miR-199a2, is not as sensitive to Smad1 posttranscriptional regulation [18].

programed cell death [27, 52]. As miR-21 is expressed in the limb bud [28, 33] and acts upstream of the spry genes, the elevated spry2 levels in the Dicer-null limb bud may reflect inactivation of miR-21. miR-21 may also act downstream of Smad1 in the growth plate [18]. If that is true, then miR-21 can mediate BMP signaling and affect the regulation of FGF levels. miR-21-dependent regulation of spry in the growth plate may therefore have the role of coordinating the contra-regulatory BMP and FGF signals (Fig. 5.4).

5.4.5 The Cartilage-Specific miR-140 and its Role in PDGF Signaling

In recent years, a number of miRNAs have attracted interest with respect to osteoblast and chondrocyte differentiation. One of these, miR-140, has a striking chondrocyte-specific expression pattern [17, 74, 79], with a potential role in cartilage differentiation [56, 74]. At the molecular level, one role of miR-140 may be to repress histone deacetylase 4 (HDAC4), known to be important for bone development as a repressor of chondrocyte hypertrophy [76]. Multiple binding sites for miR-140 on HDAC4 3′ UTR are conserved in the vertebrate gene products, and miR-140 and HDAC4 interact with one another [74]. If substantiated by in vivo studies, miRNA may turn out to play a role in regulating chondrocyte hypertrophic differentiation.

In zebra fish, miR-140 is important in cranial cartilage development, functioning as a modulator of the platelet derived growth factor (PDGF) pathway. In vertebrate species, migratory cranial neural crest cells can differentiate into several cell types, including chondrocytes that populate and establish craniofacial structures. A migratory

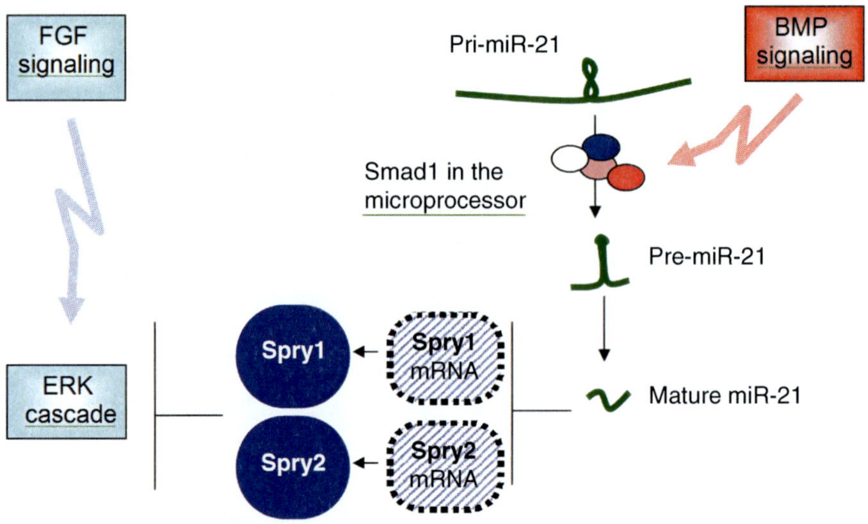

Figure 5.4. The microprocessing of miR-21 (*green*) requires Smad1 (*red*) function within the microprocessor complex and BMP signaling (*dashed red lightning*). Mature miR-21 represses the expression of sprouty genes (spry1, spry2, *dashed blue squares*), which are intracellular negative regulators of FGF-ERK signaling (*blue lightning*). Thus, miR-21 may act as an intermediary factor downstream of BMP signaling in the regulation of FGF levels. This may provide a means to coordinate the contra-regulatory BMP and FGF signals in the growth plate.

stream of neural crest cells that generate the roof of the mouth express PDGF receptor alpha (pdgfrα), and are subject to PDGF signaling that modulates the migration of these cranial neuronal crest cells along typical trajectories [2, 20].

The pdgfrα transcript 3′ UTR contains a binding site for miR-140, which downregulates the protein levels in vivo [20]. Introduction of ectopic miR-140 into fish embryos has resulted in the repression of pdgfrα expression. Morphologically, a range of facial defects results, including clefting of the crest-derived cartilage that develops in the roof of the larval mouth. These defects are similar to that in the mouse pdgfrα gene knockout [55, 66, 69, 72]. This reinforces the interpretation that pdgfrα is the major component affected by miR-140 overexpression [20]. Conversely, miR-140 morpholino knockdown in fish elevates the pdgfrα protein levels, yet, takes the PDGF signaling off balance, so that excessive neural crest cells accumulated around the optic stalk, a source of the ligand. As the binding sites for miR-140 in the 3′ UTR of pdgfrα are conserved across vertebrate species, and because the pdgfr knockout mice are reminiscent of the miRNA defect, mir-140 may play a similar role in other vertebrates.

5.5 An Integrative Model for miRNA Activity in Limb Development

In summary, miRNAs constitute a large group of posttranscriptional regulators whose fuller involvement in the development is likely to be known in the coming years. miRNAs are interwoven in specific pathways related to bone development. Conditional loss of Dicer function has provided insight into miRNA function in vivo [27, 33], but the transition from this model to deciphering the role of specific miRNAs is complicated. One important result from the work of Kobayashi et al. [33] is that miRNAs involved in the development of Col2a1 descendent are not a part of Ihh/PTHrP signaling. In this connection, it is worth noting the role of miRNAs in BMP signaling, as this pathway is downstream of or in parallel with the Ihh pathway. miRNAs interact with BMP signals at many levels. BMP/Smad signaling regulates proliferation and hypertrophic differentiation of the chondrocytes [50]. Ihh and BMP signaling together regulate the level of chondrocyte proliferation, thereby pushing the chondrocytes out of the PTHrP signaling range. A drop in BMP signaling leads to smaller skeletal elements, because proliferation is decreased and hypertrophy is accelerated. This outcome is reminiscent of the Dicer phenotype [51]. Based on the evidence that supports a close interaction of miRNAs with the BMP/Smad signaling network, we suggest that this network may be significantly involved in bone development. We also predict that BMP-related miRNAs explain at least part of the Dicer phenotypes; other miRNAs involved in the proliferation may contribute to regulating the size of the skeletal components.

Understanding the impact of miRNAs in embryonic development is still in its infancy. However, the wealth of resources currently utilized to assess function will lead to a fuller picture. Knowing how individual miRNAs are integrated in the pathways that regulate osteoblast and chondrocyte differentiation will lead to better understanding of how genetic networks bring about normal development and what diseases result from perturbing their expression.

Acknowledgment

The work at the Hornstein lab is supported by research grants from the JDRF, IDF, BIRAX, the Benoziyo Center for Neurological Disease, the Estate of Flourence Blau and the Wolfson Family Charitable trust for miRNA work at the Weizmann Institute.

References

1. Ambros V (2004) The functions of animal microRNAs. Nature 431:350–355
2. Andrae J, Gallini R, Betsholtz C (2008) Role of platelet-derived growth factors in physiology and medicine. Genes Dev 22:1276–1312
3. Babiarz JE, Ruby JG, Wang Y, Bartel DP, Blelloch R (2008) Mouse ES cells express endogenous shRNAs, siRNAs, and other microprocessor-independent, Dicer-dependent small RNAs. Genes Dev 22:2773–2785
4. Baek D, Villen J, Shin C, Camargo FD, Gygi SP, Bartel DP (2008) The impact of microRNAs on protein output. Nature 455:64–71
5. Bartel DP (2004) MicroRNAs: genomics, biogenesis, mechanism, and function. Cell 116:281–297
6. Bartel DP, Chen CZ (2004) Micromanagers of gene expression: the potentially widespread influence of metazoan microRNAs. Nat Rev Genet 5:396–400
7. Behm-Ansmant I, Rehwinkel J, Doerks T, Stark A, Bork P, Izaurralde E (2006) mRNA degradation by miRNAs and GW182 requires both CCR4:NOT deadenylase and DCP1:DCP2 decapping complexes. Genes Dev 20: 1885–1898
8. Berezikov E, Chung WJ, Willis J, Cuppen E, Lai EC (2007) Mammalian mirtron genes. Mol Cell 28:328–336
9. Brennecke J, Stark A, Russell RB, Cohen SM (2005) Principles of microRNA-target recognition. PLoS Biol 3:e85
10. Bushati N, Cohen SM (2007) microRNA functions. Annu Rev Cell Dev Biol 23:175–205
11. Carrington JC, Ambros V (2003) Role of microRNAs in plant and animal development. Science 301:336–338
12. Chen JF, Mandel EM, Thomson JM, Wu Q, Callis TE, Hammond SM et al (2006) The role of microRNA-1 and microRNA-133 in skeletal muscle proliferation and differentiation. Nat Genet 38:228–233
13. Chendrimada TP, Finn KJ, Ji X, Baillat D, Gregory RI, Liebhaber SA et al (2007) MicroRNA silencing through RISC recruitment of eIF6. Nature 447:823–828
14. Chu CY, Rana TM (2006) Translation repression in human cells by microRNA-induced gene silencing requires RCK/p54. PLoS Biol 4:e210
15. Cobb BS, Nesterova TB, Thompson E, Hertweck A, O'Connor E, Godwin J et al (2005) T cell lineage choice and differentiation in the absence of the RNase III enzyme Dicer. J Exp Med 201:1367–1373
16. Cohen SM, Brennecke J (2006) Developmental biology. Mixed messages in early development. Science 312:65–66
17. Darnell DK, Kaur S, Stanislaw S, Davey S, Konieczka JH, Yatskievych TA et al (2007) GEISHA: an in situ hybridization gene expression resource for the chicken embryo. Cytogenet Genome Res 117:30–35
18. Davis BN, Hilyard AC, Lagna G, Hata A (2008) SMAD proteins control DROSHA-mediated microRNA maturation. Nature 454:56–61
19. Doench JG, Sharp PA (2004) Specificity of microRNA target selection in translational repression. Genes Dev 18:504–511
20. Eberhart JK, He X, Swartz ME, Yan YL, Song H, Boling TC et al (2008) MicroRNA Mirn140 modulates Pdgf signaling during palatogenesis. Nat Genet 40:290–298
21. Flynt AS, Lai EC (2008) Biological principles of microRNA-mediated regulation: shared themes amid diversity. Nat Rev Genet 9:831–842
22. Flynt AS, Li N, Thatcher EJ, Solnica-Krezel L, Patton JG (2007) Zebrafish miR-214 modulates Hedgehog signaling to specify muscle cell fate. Nat Genet 39:259–263
23. Giraldez AJ, Cinalli RM, Glasner ME, Enright AJ, Thomson JM, Baskerville S et al (2005) MicroRNAs regulate brain morphogenesis in zebrafish. Science 308:833–838
24. Giraldez AJ, Mishima Y, Rihel J, Grocock RJ, Van Dongen S, Inoue K et al (2006) Zebrafish MiR-430 promotes deadenylation and clearance of maternal mRNAs. Science 312: 75–79

25. Gregory RI, Chendrimada TP, Shiekhattar R (2006) MicroRNA biogenesis: isolation and characterization of the microprocessor complex. Methods Mol Biol 342:33–47
26. Grimson A, Farh KK, Johnston WK, Garrett-Engele P, Lim LP, Bartel DP (2007) MicroRNA targeting specificity in mammals: determinants beyond seed pairing. Mol Cell 27:91–105
27. Harfe BD, McManus MT, Mansfield JH, Hornstein E, Tabin CJ (2005) The RNaseIII enzyme Dicer is required for morphogenesis but not patterning of the vertebrate limb. Proc Natl Acad Sci U S A 102:10898–10903
28. Hornstein E, Mansfield JH, Yekta S, Hu JK, Harfe BD, McManus MT et al (2005) The microRNA miR-196 acts upstream of Hoxb8 and Shh in limb development. Nature 438:671–674
29. Hornstein E, Shomron N (2006) Canalization of development by microRNAs. Nat Genet 38(suppl):S20–S24
30. Howard TD, Paznekas WA, Green ED, Chiang LC, Ma N, Ortiz de Luna RI et al (1997) Mutations in TWIST, a basic helix-loop-helix transcription factor, in Saethre-Chotzen syndrome. Nat Genet 15:36–41
31. Hutvagner G, Zamore PD (2002) A microRNA in a multiple-turnover RNAi enzyme complex. Science 297:2056–2060
32. Kanellopoulou C, Muljo SA, Kung AL, Ganesan S, Drapkin R, Jenuwein T et al (2005) Dicer-deficient mouse embryonic stem cells are defective in differentiation and centromeric silencing. Genes Dev 19:489–501
33. Kobayashi T, Lu J, Cobb BS, Rodda SJ, McMahon AP, Schipani E et al (2008) Dicer-dependent pathways regulate chondrocyte proliferation and differentiation. Proc Natl Acad Sci U S A 105:1949–1954
34. Krek A, Grun D, Poy MN, Wolf R, Rosenberg L, Epstein EJ et al (2005) Combinatorial microRNA target predictions. Nat Genet 37:495–500
35. Kronenberg HM (2003) Developmental regulation of the growth plate. Nature 423:332–336
36. Landgraf P, Rusu M, Sheridan R, Sewer A, Iovino N, Aravin A et al (2007) A mammalian microRNA expression atlas based on small RNA library sequencing. Cell 129:1401–1414
37. Lee RC, Feinbaum RL, Ambros V (1993) The *C. elegans* heterochronic gene lin-4 encodes small RNAs with antisense complementarity to lin-14. Cell 75:843–854
38. Lee Y, Jeon K, Lee JT, Kim S, Kim VN (2002) MicroRNA maturation: stepwise processing and subcellular localization. EMBO J 21:4663–4670
39. Lee YB, Bantounas I, Lee DY, Phylactou L, Caldwell MA, Uney JB (2008) Twist-1 regulates the miR-199a/214 cluster during development. Nucleic Acids Res 37(1):123–128
40. Lewis BP, Burge CB, Bartel DP (2005) Conserved seed pairing, often flanked by adenosines, indicates that thousands of human genes are microRNA targets. Cell 120:15–20
41. Lewis BP, Shih IH, Jones-Rhoades MW, Bartel DP, Burge CB (2003) Prediction of mammalian microRNA targets. Cell 115:787–798
42. Li N, Flynt AS, Kim HR, Solnica-Krezel L, Patton JG (2008) Dispatched Homolog 2 is targeted by miR-214 through a combination of three weak microRNA recognition sites. Nucleic Acids Res 36:4277–4285
43. Li Z, Hassan MQ, Volinia S, van Wijnen AJ, Stein JL, Croce CM et al (2008) A microRNA signature for a BMP2-induced osteoblast lineage commitment program. Proc Natl Acad Sci U S A 105:13906–13911
44. Lim LP, Lau NC, Garrett-Engele P, Grimson A, Schelter JM, Castle J et al (2005) Microarray analysis shows that some microRNAs downregulate large numbers of target mRNAs. Nature 433:769–773
45. Liu N, Williams AH, Kim Y, McAnally J, Bezprozvannaya S, Sutherland LB et al (2007) An intragenic MEF2-dependent enhancer directs muscle-specific expression of microRNAs 1 and 133. Proc Natl Acad Sci U S A 104:20844–20849
46. Loebel DA, Tsoi B, Wong N, Tam PP (2005) A conserved noncoding intronic transcript at the mouse Dnm3 locus. Genomics 85:782–789
47. Lund E, Guttinger S, Calado A, Dahlberg JE, Kutay U (2004) Nuclear export of microRNA precursors. Science 303:95–98
48. Luzi E, Marini F, Sala SC, Tognarini I, Galli G, Brandi ML (2008) Osteogenic differentiation of human adipose tissue-derived stem cells is modulated by the miR-26a targeting of the SMAD1 transcription factor. J Bone Miner Res 23:287–295
49. Meister G, Landthaler M, Patkaniowska A, Dorsett Y, Teng G, Tuschl T (2004) Human Argonaute2 mediates RNA cleavage targeted by miRNAs and siRNAs. Mol Cell 15:185–197
50. Minina E, Kreschel C, Naski MC, Ornitz DM, Vortkamp A (2002) Interaction of FGF, Ihh/Pthlh, and BMP signaling integrates chondrocyte proliferation and hypertrophic differentiation. Dev Cell. 3:439–449
51. Minina E, Wenzel HM, Kreschel C, Karp S, Gaffield W, McMahon AP et al (2001) BMP and Ihh/PTHrP signaling interact to coordinate chondrocyte proliferation and differentiation. Development 128:4523–4534
52. Minowada G, Jarvis LA, Chi CL, Neubuser A, Sun X, Hacohen N et al (1999) Vertebrate Sprouty genes are induced by FGF signaling and can cause chondrodysplasia when overexpressed. Development 126:4465–4475
53. Mishima Y, Giraldez AJ, Takeda Y, Fujiwara T, Sakamoto H, Schier AF et al (2006) Differential regulation of germline mRNAs in soma and germ cells by zebrafish miR-430. Curr Biol 16:2135–2142
54. Mizuno Y, Yagi K, Tokuzawa Y, Kanesaki-Yatsuka Y, Suda T, Katagiri T et al (2008) miR-125b inhibits osteoblastic differentiation by down-regulation of cell proliferation. Biochem Biophys Res Commun 368:267–272
55. Morrison-Graham K, Schatteman GC, Bork T, Bowen-Pope DF, Weston JA (1992) A PDGF receptor mutation in the mouse (Patch) perturbs the development of a non-neuronal subset of neural crest-derived cells. Development 115:133–142
56. Nicolas FE, Pais H, Schwach F, Lindow M, Kauppinen S, Moulton V et al (2008) Experimental identification of microRNA-140 targets by silencing and overexpressing miR-140. RNA 14:2513–2520
57. O'Rourke MP, Soo K, Behringer RR, Hui CC, Tam PP (2002) Twist plays an essential role in FGF and SHH signal transduction during mouse limb development. Dev Biol 248:143–156

58. O'Rourke MP, Tam PP (2002) Twist functions in mouse development. Int J Dev Biol 46:401–413
59. Okamura K, Ishizuka A, Siomi H, Siomi MC (2004) Distinct roles for Argonaute proteins in small RNA-directed RNA cleavage pathways. Genes Dev 18:1655–1666
60. Ornitz DM, Marie PJ (2002) FGF signaling pathways in endochondral and intramembranous bone development and human genetic disease. Genes Dev 16:1446–1465
61. Qian B, Katsaros D, Lu L, Preti M, Durando A, Arisio R et al (2008) High miR-21 expression in breast cancer associated with poor disease-free survival in early stage disease and high TGF-beta1. Breast Cancer Res Treat 117(1):131–140
62. Rajewsky N, Socci ND (2004) Computational identification of microRNA targets. Dev Biol 267:529–535
63. Rao PK, Kumar RM, Farkhondeh M, Baskerville S, Lodish HF (2006) Myogenic factors that regulate expression of muscle-specific microRNAs. Proc Natl Acad Sci U S A 103:8721–8726
64. Reinhart BJ, Slack FJ, Basson M, Pasquinelli AE, Bettinger JC, Rougvie AE et al (2000) The 21-nucleotide let-7 RNA regulates developmental timing in *Caenorhabditis elegans*. Nature 403:901–906
65. Sayed D, Rane S, Lypowy J, He M, Chen IY, Vashistha H et al (2008) MicroRNA-21 targets Sprouty2 and promotes cellular outgrowths. Mol Biol Cell 19:3272–3282
66. Schatteman GC, Morrison-Graham K, van Koppen A, Weston JA, Bowen-Pope DF (1992) Regulation and role of PDGF receptor alpha-subunit expression during embryogenesis. Development 115:123–131
67. Seitz H, Zamore PD (2006) Rethinking the microprocessor. Cell 125:827–829
68. Selbach M, Schwanhausser B, Thierfelder N, Fang Z, Khanin R, Rajewsky N (2008) Widespread changes in protein synthesis induced by microRNAs. Nature 455:58–63
69. Soriano P (1997) The PDGF alpha receptor is required for neural crest cell development and for normal patterning of the somites. Development 124:2691–2700
70. Stark A, Brennecke J, Bushati N, Russell RB, Cohen SM (2005) Animal MicroRNAs confer robustness to gene expression and have a significant impact on 3′UTR evolution. Cell 123:1133–1146
71. Stratford TH, Kostakopoulou K, Maden M (1997) Hoxb-8 has a role in establishing early anterior-posterior polarity in chick forelimb but not hindlimb. Development 124:4225–4234
72. Tallquist MD, Soriano P (2003) Cell autonomous requirement for pdgfralpha in populations of cranial and cardiac neural crest cells. Development 130:507–518
73. Thum T, Gross C, Fiedler J, Fischer T, Kissler S, Bussen M et al (2008) MicroRNA-21 contributes to myocardial disease by stimulating MAP kinase signalling in fibroblasts. Nature 456:980–984
74. Tuddenham L, Wheeler G, Ntounia-Fousara S, Waters J, Hajihosseini MK, Clark I et al (2006) The cartilage specific microRNA-140 targets histone deacetylase 4 in mouse cells. FEBS Lett 580:4214–4217
75. Valencia-Sanchez MA, Liu J, Hannon GJ, Parker R (2006) Control of translation and mRNA degradation by miRNAs and siRNAs. Genes Dev 20:515–524
76. Vega RB, Matsuda K, Oh J, Barbosa AC, Yang X, Meadows E et al (2004) Histone deacetylase 4 controls chondrocyte hypertrophy during skeletogenesis. Cell 119:555–566
77. Villavicencio EH, Yoon JW, Frank DJ, Fuchtbauer EM, Walterhouse DO, Iannaccone PM (2002) Cooperative E-box regulation of human GLI1 by TWIST and USF. Genesis 32:247–258
78. Watanabe T, Sato T, Amano T, Kawamura Y, Kawamura N, Kawaguchi H et al (2008) Dnm3os, a non-coding RNA, is required for normal growth and skeletal development in mice. Dev Dyn 237(12):3738–3748
79. Wienholds E, Kloosterman WP, Miska E, Alvarez-Saavedra E, Berezikov E, de Bruijn E et al (2005) MicroRNA expression in zebrafish embryonic development. Science 309:310–311
80. Wienholds E, Plasterk RH (2005) MicroRNA function in animal development. FEBS Lett 579:5911–5922
81. Wightman B, Ha I, Ruvkun G (1993) Posttranscriptional regulation of the heterochronic gene lin-14 by lin-4 mediates temporal pattern formation in *C. elegans*. Cell 75:855–862
82. Wu L, Belasco JG (2008) Let me count the ways: mechanisms of gene regulation by miRNAs and siRNAs. Mol Cell 29:1–7
83. Yang WJ, Yang DD, Na S, Sandusky GE, Zhang Q, Zhao G (2005) Dicer is required for embryonic angiogenesis during mouse development. J Biol Chem 280:9330–9335
84. Yekta S, Shih IH, Bartel DP (2004) MicroRNA-directed cleavage of HOXB8 mRNA. Science 304:594–596
85. Yekta S, Tabin CJ, Bartel DP (2008) MicroRNAs in the Hox network: an apparent link to posterior prevalence. Nat Rev Genet 9:789–796
86. Yi R, Qin Y, Macara IG, Cullen BR (2003) Exportin-5 mediates the nuclear export of pre-microRNAs and short hairpin RNAs. Genes Dev 17:3011–3016
87. Yoon BS, Pogue R, Ovchinnikov DA, Yoshii I, Mishina Y, Behringer RR et al (2006) BMPs regulate multiple aspects of growth-plate chondrogenesis through opposing actions on FGF pathways. Development 133:4667–4678
88. Zhao Y, Samal E, Srivastava D (2005) Serum response factor regulates a muscle-specific microRNA that targets Hand2 during cardiogenesis. Nature 436:214–220

6. FGF/FGFR Signaling in Skeletal Dysplasias

Pierre J. Marie

6.1 Introduction

Fibroblast growth factor (FGF) signaling plays an important role during endochondral and intramembranous bone development. The identification of skeletal abnormalities induced by genetic mutations in FGF receptors (FGFR) that induce chondrodysplasias and craniosynostosis in humans has provided major insights into the role of FGF/FGFR signaling in the control of cartilage and bone formation. This chapter summarizes the role of FGF/FGFR signaling in cellular and molecular mechanisms in chondrogenesis in the growth plate and in osteogenesis in cranial bone. The chapter also describes what is known about the pathological processes that have resulted in skeletal dysplasias owing to FGR mutations.

6.2 FGF Signaling in the Growth Plate

The epiphyseal growth plate consists of several cellular zones (Fig. 6.1). In the proximal resting zone, cells give rise to proliferating chondrocytes that are located in the proliferating zone. These cells differentiate into prehypertrophic chondrocytes and then become mature hypertrophic chondrocytes. Close to the metaphyseal area, hypertrophic chondrocytes undergo apoptosis. Chondrocyte proliferation, differentiation, and death in the growth plate are tightly controlled by FGF/FGFR signaling [101]. The FGF family includes 22 molecules that signal by activating four distinct receptors (FGFR1–4) with different isoforms [32]. However, a limited number of FGFs and FGFR are expressed in endochondral bone. FGF2 and FGF9 are expressed in chondrocytes, but their function in cartilage formation is not known, because deletion of FGF2 or FGF9 does not lead to abnormal cartilage in mice [17, 18, 89]. FGF7, FGF8, FGF17, and FGF18 are expressed in the perichondrium [73, 97, 134]. In contrast to FGF7, FGF8 and FGF17 do not regulate chondrogenesis in vivo [41, 83, 133], whereas FGF18 plays an important role in chondrogenesis control, as discussed below.

FGFs activate FGFRs, the key regulators of endochondral bone growth [99]. FGFR1 is expressed in prehypertrophic and hypertrophic chondrocytes, whereas FGFR3 is expressed in the resting and proliferating zones [7, 26, 103]; this implies a role in the regulation of chondrocyte proliferation and differentiation. FGF18 signals to FGFR1 in hypertrophic chondrocytes and to FGFR1 or FGFR2 in the perichondrium (Fig. 6.1). Activated FGFR1 signaling in vivo suppresses growth-plate chondrocyte mitogenesis; this results in achondroplasia-like dwarfism

F. Bronner et al. (eds.), *Bone and Development*, Topics in Bone Biology 6,
DOI 10.1007/978-1-84882-822-3_6, © Springer-Verlag London Limited 2010

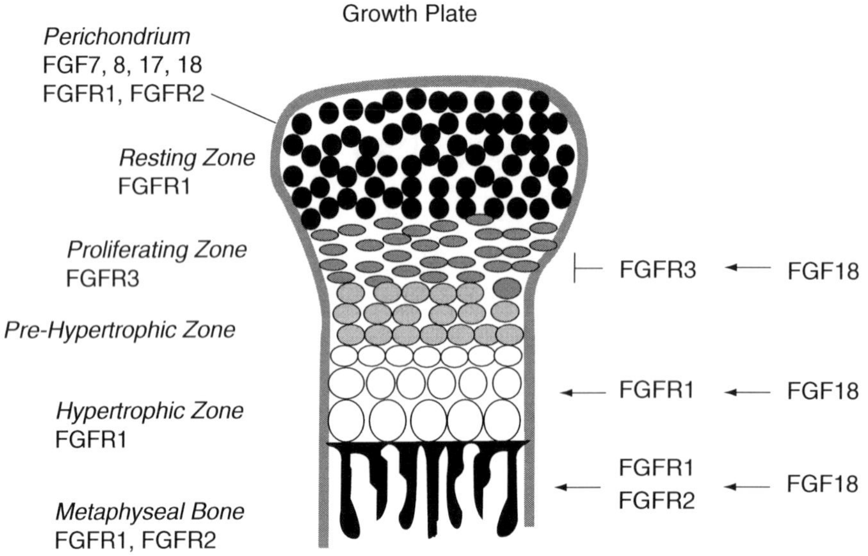

Figure 6.1. FGF/FGFR signaling in the growth plate. Several FGFs and FGFRs are expressed differently in the zones of the growth plate. FGF18 interaction with FGFR3 leads to growth arrest in proliferating chondrocytes. FGFR1 and FGFR2 regulate chondrocyte and osteoblast differentiation in the hypertrophic zone and metaphyseal regions, respectively.

[127]. FGF18, by activating FGFR3c in the chondrocytes [35], causes limited chondrocyte proliferation [22, 29, 100] by direct signaling events [116]. Activated FGFR3 reduces chondrocyte cell proliferation in mice [27]; FGFR-3$^{-/-}$ mice show excessive long bone growth associated with increased chondrocyte proliferation [16, 68, 95]. In addition to regulating chondrocyte proliferation, FGF18 regulates skeletal vascularization and recruitment of osteoblasts to the metaphysis by regulating VEGF expression [73]. Consistent with its important role in chondrogenesis, FGF18 expression is closely regulated in chondrocytes. It is upregulated by the inhibition of glycogen synthase kinase 3. The latter is an important mediator of Wnt signaling and reflects the link between Wnt signaling and FGF signaling in the course of endochondral bone development [57]. FGF18 expression is transcriptionally upregulated by Runx2, which in turn is induced by Wnt signaling [108].

Activation of FGFR3 in chondrocytes induces nuclear translocation of STAT1 and the expression of the cell-cycle inhibitor p21 [44, 117, 124] that inhibits cell growth. Furthermore, FGFR3-mediated signaling through STAT1 induces cell death in chondrocytes [63] (Fig. 6.1). FGF18 may also act on chondrocytes indirectly by modulating bone morphogenetic protein (BMP) signaling. FGF18 suppresses the induction of noggin, a BMP antagonist [107]. Conversely, BMP pathways inhibit FGF signaling in the growth plate [84, 137]. This indicates multiple interactions between FGF and BMP signaling pathways in modulating proliferation and differentiation of chondrocytes. FGFR3 signaling may also control chondrocytes indirectly through downregulation of Ihh and BMP4 in the growth plate [93]. Interestingly, a recent report indicates that chondrocyte-specific activation of FGFR3 in mice induces premature synchondrosis closure and fusion of ossification centers through a MAPK-dependent BMP pathway; this suggests a role for BMP signaling in the fusion of ossification centers and decreased endochondral bone growth brought about by the activation of FGFR3 in chondrocytes [82]. These reports make obvious the complicated regulation needed to balance proliferation and differentiation of chondrocytes, and the important role played by FGF signaling during endochondral development.

6.3 Implication of FGF/FGFR Signaling in Chondrodysplasias

The importance of FGF signaling in chondrogenesis was brought out by evidence that FGFR3 genetic mutations result in chondrodysplasias [99, 132]. The first finding was that a point mutation in the transmembrane domain of FGFR3 is involved in achondroplasia, the most common genetic form of human dwarfism with devastating effects on skeletal development (Fig. 6.2a) [113, 119]. Other forms of skeletal dysplasias related to FGFR3 have been identified, including hypochondroplasia [4] and thanatophoric dysplasia [114, 115, 125, 126]. In achondroplasia, point mutation in the transmembrane domain of FGFR3 activates the receptor in the absence of ligand [69, 88, 94, 131]. In thanatophoric dysplasia type 1, two substitutions in the extracellular domain of FGFR3 result in ligand-insensitive constitutive activation of FGFR3, whereas in thanatophoric dysplasia type 2, a substitution in the FGFR3 tyrosine kinase domain results in ligand-sensitive hyperactivation of the receptor [94] as a result of stabilization of a non-inhibitory conformation of the kinase regulatory loop [86]. Attenuation of FGFR through ubiquitination or internalization may also induce chondrocyte abnormalities in chondrodysplasias. Activating mutations in FGFR3 in achondroplasia increase the stability of the receptor through disruption of Cbl-mediated ubiquitination and lysosomal degradation of FGFR3, notwithstanding excessive ubiquitination. This amplifies the FGFR3 signal [5, 13, 70, 88]. Consistent with the findings is the increase in FGFR3 and STAT1 expression in growth plates and cultured chondrocytes from patients with achondroplasia and thanatophoric dysplasia [25, 64].

Activated FGFR3 signaling acts on several cellular mechanisms that are involved in achondroplasia and thanatophoric dysplasias. As described earlier, FGFR3 is an important signaling molecule that negatively regulates chondrogenesis [9, 129]. Overexpression of activated FGFR-3 reduces chondrocyte cell proliferation in mice [48, 68, 93, 118], whereas FGFR3 mutations increase abnormal signaling activity [45, 70] to activate STATs and upregulate cell-cycle inhibitors [68, 123]. This occurrence indicates that STAT1 mediates inhibition of endochondral growth by mutant FGFR3. FGFR3 mutants also activate ERK1/2 MAPK signaling [71]. It is not surprising, therefore, that

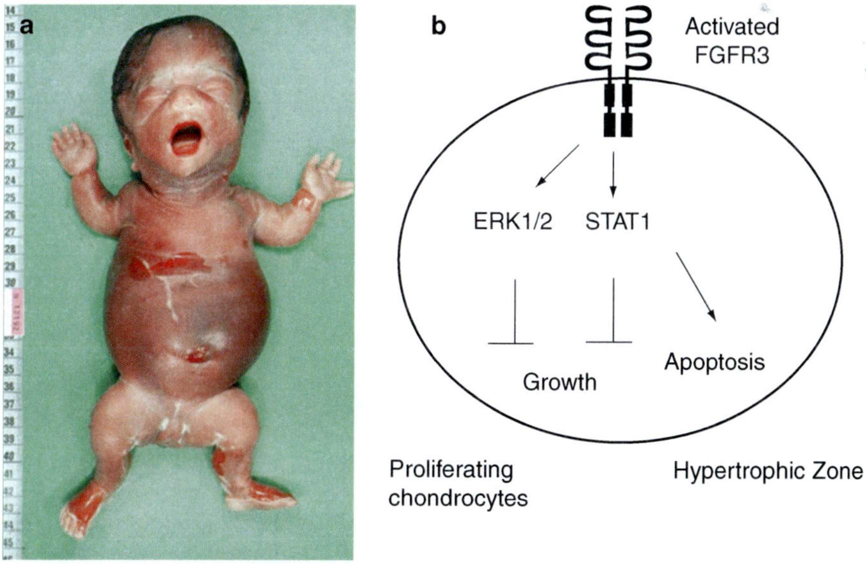

Figure 6.2. (**a**) Severe skeletal deformities in a patient with achondroplasia (courtesy of Dr. M. LeMerrer, Inserm U781, Hopital Necker, Paris, France). (**b**) Abnormal FGF/FGFR signaling induced by FGFR3 mutations in the growth plate. Activating FGFR3 mutations in achondroplasia activate ERK1/2 and STAT1, which in turn cause growth arrest in proliferating chondrocytes and apoptosis in the hypertrophic zone.

when the MAPK pathway is inhibited, achondroplasia induced by FGFR3 activation can be overcome [135]. Constitutive activation of MEK1 in chondrocytes inhibits chondrocyte differentiation [92]; this suggests that FGFR3 signaling inhibits chondrocyte differentiation through the MAPK pathway and inhibits chondrocyte proliferation through the STAT1 pathway (Fig. 6.2b).

A limited number of downstream targets of FGFR3 signaling in chondrocytes have been identified. Snail1, a transcriptional effector, is upregulated by activated FGFR3; this in turn represses chondrocyte differentiation in thanatophoric dysplasia [23]. Phosphorylation of pRb family members and Akt may also help to regulate chondrocyte proliferation by FGFR3 [62, 106]. In vitro, FGF signaling inhibits proliferation of chondrocytes by the inhibition of Rb and p107, both of which mediate cell growth [62]. FGF signaling also interacts with Wnt signaling in chondrocyte regulation. Wnt signaling induces FGF18 expression [108] and may thereby inhibit chondrocyte proliferation [12, 30, 46, 122]. Wnt-induced inhibition of chondrocyte proliferation is abrogated in FGFR-3 null mice [57]; this points to a role for Wnt signaling in chondrogenesis inhibition due to FGFR3 signaling. FGFR3 signaling may also have indirect effects on chondrocytes, by affecting hedgehog signaling and BMP4 expression [93]. A FGFR3 mutation downregulates Ihh/PTHrP signals in a mouse model of thanatophoric dysplasia type 1 [10], but this may not apply to human chondrodysplasias because Ihh/PTHrP expression is normal in human achondroplasias or thanatophoric dysplasia types 1 or 2 [19].

FGFR3 activation in human chondrocytes induces cell apoptosis. Chondrocytes from patients with thanatophoric dysplasia show increased PLCγ-activated STAT1, resulting in an increase in the Bax/Bcl-2 ratio and apoptosis [43, 63]. Interestingly, IGF-1 treatment prevents apoptosis induced by FGFR3 mutation by activating PI3K and MAPK pathways [60]. In summary, FGFR3 activation in chondrodysplasias induces abnormalities in chondrocyte proliferation, differentiation, and life span by activation of specific signaling pathways (Fig. 6.2b). These findings may lead to developing targeted therapeutics in achondroplasia [2].

6.4 FGF Signaling in Cranial Bone

Cranial bones are formed by intramembranous ossification and expand during development, but do not fuse at the junction with other cranial bones; this allows skull expansion during growth [15, 91, 98, 110]. The junction between calvarial bones, called suture, allows for separation between two membrane bones. Most cells surrounding the suture are mesenchymal cells, a minority of which differentiate into preosteoblasts and mature osteoblasts that form the bone. When bone is the formed, most osteoblasts become osteocytes or bone-lining cells, but some die by apoptosis (Fig. 6.3).

Rodent studies have shown that suture cells are subject to regulation by multiple factors, including transforming growth factor β BMPs, FGFs, and Wnt proteins [98, 110]. FGF/FGFR signaling plays a major role in cranial suture development [21]. The mesenchymal splice variant of FGFR2 (FGFr2IIIc) is expressed in early mesenchymal condensates and later in sites of intramembranous ossification where it interacts with FGF18 [33, 35]. During cranial bone development, FGF18 is expressed in mesenchymal cells and differentiating osteoblasts [97], whereas FGFR1 and FGFR2 are expressed in preosteoblasts and osteoblasts [26, 51, 54, 59, 87], and FGFR2 expression is associated with endogenous FGF2 expression [109, 111] (Fig. 6.3).

In cranial bone, FGF signaling is a positive regulator of osteogenesis. In vitro, FGF2, 9, and

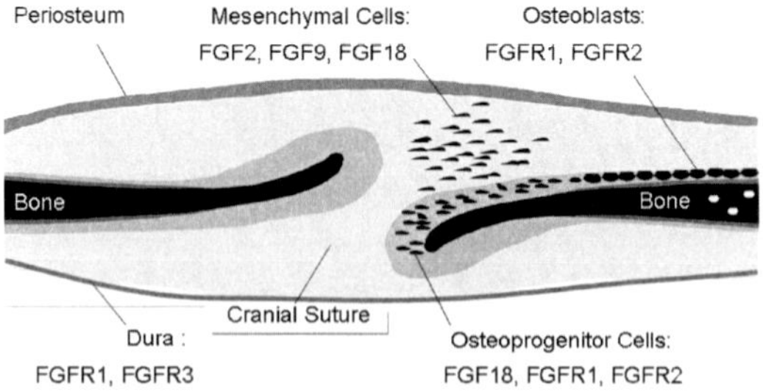

Figure 6.3. FGF/FGFR signaling in the cranial suture. FGF interactions with FGFRs in suture cells regulate the balance between osteoblast proliferation differentiation and survival thereby maintaining the cranial suture.

18 upregulate the replication of calvarial cells [8, 24, 120] and promote osteogenic differentiation [51]. Sustained treatment with FGF2 promotes replication and differentiation of cranial osteoblasts in vitro [24]. Bone formation in FGF2-deficient mice is therefore decreased [89] and if FGF2 biological activity is blocked, cranial osteogenesis is prevented in vivo [39, 90]. FGF18 also stimulates osteoblast proliferation and differentiation in vivo [97], whereas cranial suture closure and ossification are delayed in FGF18-deficient mice [97, 72].

FGFRs are important regulators of osteoblastogenesis. In vivo studies have shown that FGFR1 regulates osteoblasts at different stages of maturation, whereas FGFR3 regulates the activation of more differentiated osteoblasts [53]. Mice that conditionally lack FGFR2 or harbor mutations in the mesenchymal splice form of FGFR2 develop skeletal dwarfism, with decreased osteoblast proliferation and bone mineral density [33, 140]. FGF signaling also controls osteoblast apoptosis, inducing apoptosis in differentiated osteoblasts in vitro [24] and increased apoptosis in mouse calvaria [77, 81]. Thus, FGF/FGFR signaling regulates osteoblastogenesis at all stages of the osteoblast lineage (Fig. 6.3).

Several signaling pathways induced by FGF/FGFR activation have been identified in osteoblasts, including ERK1/2, protein kinase C (PKC), Src, and PI3K/Akt [49, 79]. When these signaling pathways are activated, many genes involved in osteogenesis are expressed, from the osteoprogenitor cell to the end of osteoblast life. In cranial bone, FGFs regulate osteoblast function indirectly by interaction with BMP signaling [59]; this suggests that BMP signaling regularly plays a role in cranial suture fusion. FGF2 and FGFR2 inhibit the expression of the BMP antagonist, noggin, in the patent cranial suture. This results in increased BMP4 activity and suture fusion [130]. FGF2 also promotes BMP2 during cranial bone development by causing Runx2 levels to increase [14]. It is therefore likely that the biological activities of FGFs in bone not only depend on the balance between FGF and FGFR, but also on the activity of other signaling molecules, including BMPs.

6.5 Implication of FGF/FGFR Signaling in Craniosynostosis

The role of FGFR signaling in craniosynostosis has been made clear by multiple lines of genetic evidence. Missense gain-of-function mutations in FGFR1–3 induce premature fusion of one or more cranial sutures in about 1 over 2,500 live births, causing over 100 skeletal disorders including Apert, Crouzon, and other syndromes [52, 61, 132]. The molecular mechanisms that contribute to FGFR gain-of-functions mutations include constitutive (ligand-independent) activation [38, 76, 96, 104, 112] or ligand-dependent activation of FGFRs [1, 50, 102, 138, 139]. This emphasizes the complexity of the molecular mechanisms that result in the activation of FGFRs inducing craniosynostosis [85]. The phenotype induced by the activating FGFR mutations in cranial suture cells has been determined in vitro and in vivo. In Apert craniosynostosis, the most severe syndrome, activated FGFR2, clearly induces acceleration of osteoblast differentiation in human cranial osteoblasts and premature cranial suture ossification (Fig. 6.4). This

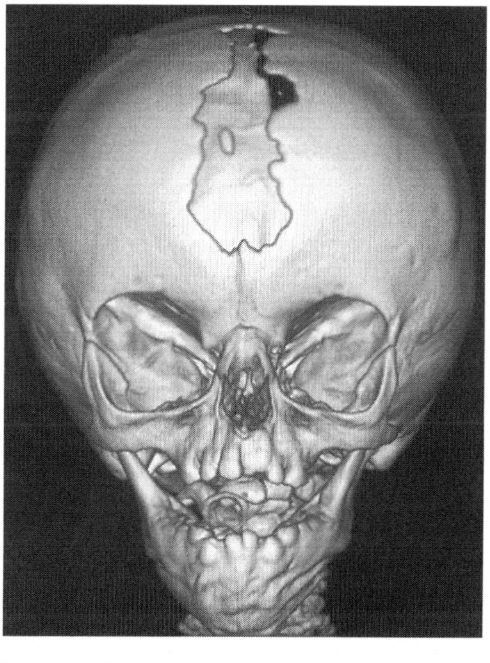

Figure 6.4. Premature suture fusion in a young patient with Apert syndrome (courtesy of Drs. Arnaud and Renier, Hopital Necker-Enfants Malades, Paris, France).

leads to increased subperiosteal osteogenesis in the cranial suture (reviewed in [80]) and results from an increased expression of osteoblast genes, induced by activated FGFR2. These include alkaline phosphatase, type I collagen, and osteocalcin [36, 66, 75, 124]. These studies provide important insights into the molecular mechanisms that play a role in the premature cranial suture fusion in craniosynostosis. FGFR mutations in mice lead to results similar to what happens to humans, i.e., premature fusion of cranial sutures, but the cellular phenotype in mice and humans is not the same [79]. In mice, Apert or Crouzon FGFR2 mutations stimulate calvarial cell proliferation, but inhibit osteoblast differentiation and mineralization [77, 78, 105]. FGFR1 or FGFR2 activating mutations in mice may or may not increase osteoblast proliferation and differentiation [11, 128, 136, 141]. This variation may be due to the variable effects of FGFR mutations on different sutures or the effect of FGFR mutations on osteoblasts at different stages of maturation [132]. Apart from these variable effects, matrix deposition increases and suture closure accelerates [42].

Several signaling pathways induced by FGFR gain-of-function mutations are involved in craniosynostosis (Fig. 6.5). Initial studies in human mutant osteoblasts have shown that Apert FGFR2 mutations activate PLC gamma and its downstream effector PKC alpha; this leads to increased osteoblast gene expression [36,66]. Apert FGFR2 mutations also induce Cbl-mediated downregulation of the two Src family members, Lyn and Fyn, in human osteoblasts; this contributes to premature osteoblast differentiation ([56]; Fig. 6.5). Inhibition of MEK-ERK signaling inhibits craniosynostosis induced by Apert FGFR2 mutation in mouse models. Therefore, ERK activation may play a pathogenic role in mouse craniosynostosis [58, 121].

Another important mechanism in craniosynostosis is FGFR2 downregulation induced by FGFR2 mutations. Apert FGFR2 mutations induce Cbl-mediated FGFR2 degradation by the proteasome in Apert osteoblasts [65], thereby increasing osteoblast differentiation (Fig. 6.5). This observation is consistent with the decreased expression of FGFR2 in Crouzon syndrome [6]. Activated FGFR2 also showed increased binding

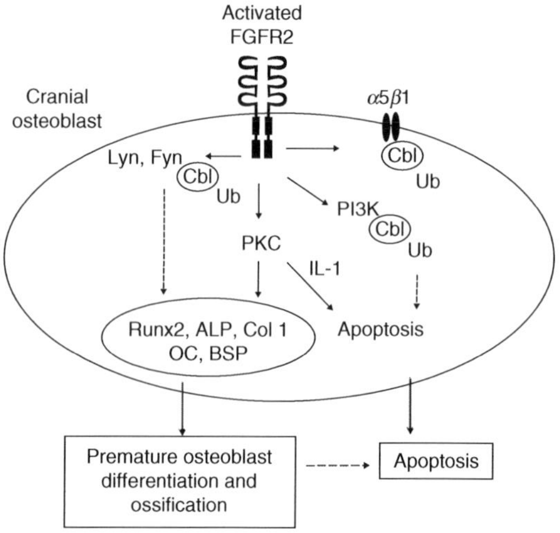

Figure 6.5. Signaling and phenotype induced by FGFR2 mutations in cranial osteoblasts in Apert craniosynostosis. Apert FGFR2 mutations activate PKC activity, which in turn upregulates osteoblast gene expression and osteogenesis, thus causing premature cranial ossification. FGFR2 mutations also induce Cbl-mediated Src (Lyn Fyn) proteasome degradation; this promotes osteoblast differentiation in mutant human cranial osteoblasts. FGFR2 activation results in PI3K and α5 integrin ubiquitination and proteasome degradation, causing cell survival to decrease. Another mechanism involves PKC-mediated IL1-dependent activation of caspases, resulting in the apoptosis of more mature osteoblasts.

to the adaptor protein FRS2 [47], which is involved in the negative feedback mechanism that is induced by FGFR stimulation [34]. Uncoupling between the docking protein FRS2 alpha and activated Crouzon-like FGFR2c mutant can prevent Crouzon-like craniosynostosis induced by activated FGFR2 in mice [34]. These findings emphasize the role of FRS2 alpha in the attenuation of signals in osteoblasts induced by FGFR activation, and the important role of role of Cbl and FRS2 alpha in the attenuation of signals induced by FGFR2 activation.

Some progress has been made in the identification of genes that act downstream of activated FGFR signaling in craniosynostosis. Runx2, an essential transcription factor involved in osteoblastogenesis, is a target gene for activated FGFR signaling. In human cranial osteoblasts, FGFR2 upregulates Runx2 expression [40]. Consistent with this observation is that activating FGFR1 and FGFR2 mutations increase Runx2 expression in mouse and human osteoblasts [3, 31, 121]. Conversely, disruption of FGFR2IIIc, the mesenchymal splice variant of FGFR2, decreases the transcription of Runx2 and thereby retards ossification [33]. This suggests that FGFR2-induced Runx2 expression may contribute to the accelerated osteoblast differentiation in craniosynostosis. Other transcription factors such as Sox2 may also be involved in FGFR2-induced craniosynostosis in mice [78]. Interestingly, Apert or Crouzon FGFR2 mutations downregulate some Wnt target genes in mice [78]. Microarray analysis of patent sutures in children with craniosynostosis has shown that other genes are upregulated during suture fusion [20]. However, whether these genes are actually implicated in expressing the phenotype induced by FGFR mutations has not been determined. Interactions between several signaling molecules, some not yet identified, probably contribute to premature osteoblast differentiation and cranial suture ossification.

Activated FGFR signaling in human and mouse models of craniosynostosis also causes osteoblast apoptosis. Apoptosis is a normal occurrence in suture development and is essential for eliminating osteoblasts when differentiation is complete [37]. Apert and Crouzon activating FGFR2 mutations promote apoptosis in mature osteoblasts in mouse and human genetic models [11, 14, 74]. In Apert syndrome, activation of osteoblast apoptosis is mediated by PKC activation and increased IL-1 and Fas, caspase-8, and Bax/Bcl-2 levels [67]. Moreover, FGFR2 activation in this syndrome reduces osteoblast matrix attachment. This results from Cbl-mediated recruitment, ubiquitination, and proteasome degradation of the $\alpha 5$ integrin. The subsequent reduction in cell attachment triggers caspase-dependent apoptosis through Bax/Bcl-2 and activation of the cascade-9-caspase-3-cascade [55]. Additionally, activated FGFR2 in Apert syndrome induces Cbl-mediated PI3K ubiquitination and proteasome degradation. These cause a decrease in the survival of more mature osteoblasts ([28]; Fig. 6.5). This effect of activated FGFR2 signaling on osteoblast apoptosis may appear surprising, given the overall positive effect of mutant FGFR on bone formation. However, the increased apoptosis induced by activated FGFR2 in mature osteoblasts may be necessary to compensate for the accelerated osteoblast differentiation induced by FGFR2 signaling. It is evident that in craniosynostosis, activated FGFR signaling has a complicated, maturation-dependent effect on osteoblastogenesis and cranial ossification.

6.6 Conclusion and Perspectives

In the course of the last decade, cellular, molecular, and genetic approaches have led to better understanding of the regulatory role of FGF/FGFR signaling in endochondral and cranial ossification. Analysis of the skeletal and cellular phenotypes induced by FGFR mutations in mouse models and in children bearing FGFR mutations has improved our knowledge of the pathogenesis of chondrodysplasias and craniosynostosis. Genetic and functional studies have identified cellular and molecular pathways that are targeted by activated FGF/FGFR signaling and involved in the development of skeletal dysplasias. This has led to the concept that antagonists of FGFR or downstream signaling pathways may prevent skeletal dysplasias induced by FGFR mutations in mice. This constitutes an important step toward therapy.

More work is needed to identify the precise role of FGFRs and their ligands in regulating cell proliferation, differentiation, and apoptosis during endochondral and cranial ossification in humans. Moreover, studies are needed to identify the role of signaling pathways in the abnormal chondroblast and osteoblast phenotypes induced by FGFR mutations. The sequence of genes induced by activated FGFR signaling and implicated in the pathogenesis of human skeletal dysplasias needs to be identified. This may add new information about the pathogenesis of human skeletal dysplasias and lead to novel therapeutic approaches.

Acknowledgments

The work of the author on this subject was supported by INSERM and has been awarded by the French Academy of Medicine (2008).

References

1. Anderson J, Burns HD, Enriquez-Harris P, Wilkie AOM, Heath JK (1998) Apert syndrome mutations in fibroblast growth factor receptor 2 exhibit increased affinity for FGF ligand. Hum Mol Gen 7:1475–1483
2. Aviezer D, Golembo M, Yayon A (2003) Fibroblast growth factor receptor-3 as a therapeutic target for achondroplasia-genetic short limbed dwarfism. Curr Drug Targets 4:353–365
3. Baroni T, Carinci P, Lilli C, Bellucci C, Aisa MC, Scapoli L, Volinia S, Carinci F, Pezzetti F, Calvitti M, Farina A, Conte C, Bodo M (2005) P253R fibroblast growth factor receptor-2 mutation induces RUNX2 transcript variants and calvarial osteoblast differentiation. J Cell Physiol 202:524–535
4. Bellus GA, McIntosh I, Smith EA, Aylesworth AS, Kaitila I, Horton WA, Greenhaw GA, Hecht JT, Francomano CA (1995) A recurrent mutation in the tyrosine kinase domain of fibroblast growth factor receptor 3 causes hypochondroplasia. Nat Genet 10: 357–359
5. Bonaventure J, Horne WC, Baron R (2007) The localization of FGFR3 mutations causing thanatophoric dysplasia type I differentially affects phosphorylation processing and ubiquitination of the receptor FEBS J 274:3078–3093. Erratum in: FEBS J 274(15):4008
6. Bresnick S, Schendel S (1995) Crouzon disease correlates with low fibroblast growth factor receptor activity in stenosed cranial sutures. J Craniofac Surg 6:245–250
7. Britto JA, Evans RD, Hayward RD, Jones BM (2001) From genotype to phenotype: the differential expression of FGF, FGFR, and TGFbeta genes characterizes human cranioskeletal development and reflects clinical presentation in FGFR syndromes, Plast Reconstr Surg 108:2026–2039
8. Canalis E, Centrella M, McCarthy T (1988) Effects of basic fibroblast growth factor on bone formation in vitro. J Clin Invest 81:1572–1577
9. Chen L, Adar R, Yang X, Monsonego EO, Li C, Hauschka PV, Yayon A, Deng CX (1999) Gly369Cys mutation in mouse FGFR3 causes achondroplasia by affecting both chondrogenesis and osteogenesis. J Clin Invest 104:1517–1525
10. Chen L, Li C, Qiao W, Xu X, Deng CA (2001) Ser(365)--> Cys mutation of fibroblast growth factor receptor 3 in mouse downregulates Ihh/PTHrP signals and causes severe achondroplasia. Hum Mol Genet 10:457–465
11. Chen L, Li D, Li C, Engel A, Deng CX (2003) A Ser252Trp [corrected] substitution in mouse fibroblast growth factor receptor 2 (Fgfr2) results in craniosynostosis Bone 33:169–178. Erratum in: Bone (2005)37:876
12. Chimal-Monroy J, Montero JA, Gañan Y, Macias D, Garcia-Porrero JA, Hurle JM (2002) Comparative analysis of the expression and regulation of Wnt5a Fz4 and Frzb1 during digit formation and in micromass cultures. Dev Dyn 224:314–320
13. Cho JY, Guo C, Torello M, Lunstrum GP, Iwata T, Deng C, Horton WA (2004) Defective lysosomal targeting of activated fibroblast growth factor receptor 3 in achondroplasia. Proc Natl Acad Sci U S A 101: 609–614
14. Choi KY, Kim HJ, Lee MH, Kwon TG, Nah HD, Furuichi T, Komor T, Nam SH, Kim YJ, Kim HJ, Ryoo HM (2005) Runx2 regulates FGF2-induced Bmp2 expression during cranial bone development. Dev Dyn 233:115–121
15. Cohen MM Jr (2005) Perspectives on craniosynostosis. Am J Med Genet A 136:313–326
16. Colvin JS, Bohne BA, Harding DG, McEwen DG, Ornitz, DM (1996) Skeletal overgrowth and deafness in mice lacking fibroblast growth factor receptor 3. Nat Genet 12:390–397
17. Colvin JS, Green RP, Schmahl J, Capel B, Ornitz D.M (2001) Male-to-female sex reversal in mice lacking fibroblast growth factor 9. Cell 104:875–889
18. Colvin JS, White A, Pratt SJ, Ornitz DM (2001) Lung hypoplasia and neonatal death in Fgf9-null mice identify this gene as an essential regulator of lung mesenchyme. Development 128:2095–2106
19. Cormier S, Delezoide AL, Benoist-Lasselin C, Legeai-Mallet L, Bonaventure J, Silve C (2002) Parathyroid hormone receptor type 1/Indian hedgehog expression is preserved in the growth plate of human fetuses affected with fibroblast growth factor receptor type 3 activating mutations. Am J Pathol 161:1325–1335
20. Coussens AK, Wilkinson CR, Hughes IP, Morris CP, van Daal A, Anderson PJ, Powell BC (2007) Unravelling the molecular control of calvarial suture fusion in children with craniosynostosis. BMC Genomics 8:458
21. Dailey L, Ambrosetti D, Mansukhani A, Basilico C (2005) Mechanisms underlying differential responses to FGF signaling. Cytokine Growth Factor Rev 16:233–247
22. Davidson D, Blanc A, Filion D, Wang H, Plut P, Pfeffer G, Buschmann MD, Henderson JE (2005) Fibroblast growth factor (FGF) 18 signals through FGF receptor 3 to promote chondrogenesis. J Biol Chem 280:20509–20515
23. de Frutos CA, Vega S, Manzanares M, Flores JM, Huertas H, Martíz-Frí ML, Nieto MA (2007) Snail1 is a transcriptional effector of FGFR3 signaling during chondrogenesis and achondroplasias. Dev Cell 13:872–883
24. Debiais F, Graulet AM, Marie PJ (1998) Fibroblast growth factor-2 differently affects human neonatal calvaria osteoblastic cells depending on the stage of cell differentiation. J Bone Miner Res 13:645–654
25. Delezoide AL, Lasselin-Benoist C, Legeai-Mallet L, Brice P, Senée V, Yayon A, Munnich A, Vekemans M, Bonaventure J (1997) Abnormal FGFR 3 expression in cartilage of thanatophoric dysplasia fetuses. Hum Mol Genet 6:1899–1906
26. Delezoide, AL, Benoist-Lasselin, C, Legeai-Mallet, L, Le Merrer, M, Munnich, A, Vekemans M, Bonaventure J (1998) Spatio-temporal expression of FGFR1, 2 and 3 genes during human embryo-fetal ossification. Mech Dev 77:19–30
27. Deng C, Wynshaw-Boris A, Zhou F, Kuo A, Leder P (1996) Fibroblast growth factor receptor 3 is a negative regulator of bone growth. Cell 84:911–921
28. Dufour C, Guenou H, Kaabeche K, Bouvard D, Sanjay A, Marie PJ (2008) FGFR2-Cbl interaction in lipid rafts triggers attenuation of PI3K/Akt signaling and osteoblast survival. Bone 42:1032–1039

29. Ellsworth JL, Berry J, Bukowski T, Claus J, Feldhaus A, Holderman S, Holdren MS, Lum KD, Moore EE, Raymond F, Ren H, Shea P, Sprecher C, Storey H, Thompson DL, Waggie K, Yao L, Fernandes RJ, Eyre DR, Hughes SD (2002) Fibroblast growth factor-18 is a trophic factor for mature chondrocytes and their progenitors Osteoarth Cart 10:308–320. Erratum in: Osteoarth Cart (2002)10:826
30. Enomoto-Iwamoto M, Kitagaki J, Koyama E, Tamamura Y, Wu C, Kanatani N, Koike T, Okada H, Komori T, Yoneda T, Church V, Francis-West PH, Kurisu K, Nohno T, Pacifici M, Iwamoto M (2002) The Wnt antagonist Frzb-1 regulates chondrocyte maturation and long bone development during limb skeletogenesis. Dev Biol 251:142–156
31. Eswarakumar VP, Horowitz MC, Locklin R, Morriss-Kay GM, Lonai P (2004) A gain-of-function mutation of Fgfr2c demonstrates the roles of this receptor variant in osteogenesis. Proc Natl Acad Sci U S A 101:12555–12560
32. Eswarakumar VP, Lax I, Schlessinger J (2005) Cellular signaling by fibroblast growth factor receptors. Cytokine Growth Factor Rev 16:139–149
33. Eswarakumar VP, Monsonego-Ornan E, Pines M, Antonopoulou I, Morriss-Kay GM, Lonai P (2002) The IIIc alternative of Fgfr2 is a positive regulator of bone formation. Development 129:3783–3793
34. Eswarakumar VP, Ozcan F, Lew ED, Bae JH, Tome F, Booth CJ, Adams DJ, Lax I, Schlessinger J (2006) Attenuation of signaling pathways stimulated by pathologically activated FGF-receptor 2 mutants prevents craniosynostosis. Proc Natl Acad Sci U S A 103: 18603–18608
35. Eswarakumar VP, Schlessinger J (2007) Skeletal overgrowth is mediated by deficiency in a specific isoform of fibroblast growth factor receptor 3. Proc Natl Acad Sci U S A 104:3937–3942
36. Fragale A, Tartaglia M, Bernardini S, Michela Di Stasi AM, Di Rocco C, Velardi F, Teti A, Battaglia PA, Migliacco S (1999) Decreased proliferation and altered differentiation in osteoblasts from genetically and clinically distinct craniosynostotic disorders. Am J Pathol 154:1465–1477
37. Fromigué O, Modrowski D, Marie PJ (2005) Apoptosis in membranous bone formation: role of fibroblast growth factor and bone morphogenetic protein signaling. Crit Rev Eukaryot Gene Expr 15:75–92
38. Galvin BD, Hart KC, Meyer AN, Webster MK, Donoghue DJ (1996) Constitutive receptor activation by Crouzon syndrome mutations in fibroblast growth factor receptor (FGFR)2 and FGFR2/Neu chimeras. Proc Natl Acad Sci U S A 93:7894–7899
39. Greenwald JA, Mehrara BJ, Spector JA, Warren SM, Fagenholz PJ, Smith LE, Bouletreau PJ, Crisera FE, Ueno H, Longaker MT (2001) *In vivo* modulation of FGF biological activity alters cranial suture fate. Am J Pathol 158:441–452
40. Guenou H, Kaabeche K, Mee SL, Marie PJ (2005) A role for fibroblast growth factor receptor-2 in the altered osteoblast phenotype induced by Twist haploinsufficiency in the Saethre-Chotzen syndrome. Hum Mol Genet 14:1429–1439
41. Guo L, Degenstein L, Fuchs E (1996) Keratinocyte growth factor is required for hair development but not for wound healing. Genes Dev 10:165–175
42. Hajihosseini MK, Wilson S, De Moerlooze L, Dickson C (2001) A splicing switch and gain-of-function mutation in FgfR2-IIIc hemizygotes causes Apert/Pfeiffer-syndrome-like phenotypes. Proc Natl Acad Sci U S A 98:3855–3860
43. Harada D, Yamanaka Y, Ueda K, Nishimura R, Morishima T, Seino Y, Tanaka H (2007) Sustained phosphorylation of mutated FGFR3 is a crucial feature of genetic dwarfism and induces apoptosis in the ATDC5 chondrogenic cell line via PLCgamma-activated STAT1. Bone 41:273–281
44. Hart KC, Robertson SC, Donoghue DJ (2001) Identification of tyrosine residues in constitutively activated fibroblast growth factor receptor 3 involved in mitogenesis Stat activation and phosphatidylinositol 3-kinase activation. Mol Biol Cell 12:931–942
45. Hart KC, Robertson SC, Kanemitsu MY, Meyer AN, Tynan JA, Donoghue DJ (2000) Transformation and Stat activation by derivatives of FGFR1, FGFR3, and FGFR4. Oncogene 19:3309–3320
46. Hartmann C, Tabin CJ (2000) Dual roles of Wnt signaling during chondrogenesis in the chicken limb. Development 127:3141–3159
47. Hatch NE, Hudson M, Seto ML, Cunningham ML, Bothwell M (2006) Intracellular retention degradation and signaling of glycosylation-deficient FGFR2 and craniosynostosis syndrome-associated FGFR2 C278F. J Biol Chem 281:27292–27305
48. Henderson JE, Naski MC, Aarts MM, Wang D, Cheng L, Goltzman D, Ornitz DM (2000) Expression of FGFR3 with the G380R achondroplasia mutation inhibits proliferation and maturation of CFK2 chondrocytic cells. J Bone Miner Res 15:155–165
49. Hurley MM, Naski MC, Marie PJ (2007) Fibroblast growth factor (FGF) and FGF receptor families in bone. In: Bilezikian, Raisz LG, Rodan GA (eds) Principles of bone biology, 3rd edn. Academic Press, San Diego
50. Ibrahimi OA, Eliseenkova AV, Plotnikov AN, Yu K, Ornitz DM, Mohammadi M (2001) Structural basis for fibroblast growth factor receptor 2 activation in Apert syndrome. Proc Natl Acad Sci U S A 98:7182–7187
51. Iseki S, Wilkie AOM, Heath JK, Ishimaru T, Eto K, aMorrisskay GM (1997) Fgfr2 and osteopontin domains in the developing skull vault are mutually exclusive and can be altered by locally applied FGF2. Development 124:3375–3384
52. Jabs EW (1998) Toward understanding the pathogenesis of craniosynostosis through clinical and molecular correlates. Clin Genet 53:79–86
53. Jacob AL, Smith C, Partanen J, Ornitz DM (2006) Fibroblast growth factor receptor 1 signaling in the osteo-chondrogenic cell lineage regulates sequential steps of osteoblast maturation. Dev Biol 296:315–318
54. Johnson D, Iseki S, Wilkie AO, Morriss-Kay GM (2000) Expression patterns of Twist and Fgfr1 -2 and -3 in the developing mouse coronal suture suggest a key role for Twist in suture initiation and biogenesis. Mech Dev 91:341–345

55. Kaabeche K, Guenou G, Bouvard D, Didelot N, Listrat A, Marie PJ (2005) Cbl-mediated ubiquitination of alpha 5 integrin subunit mediates fibronectin-dependent osteoblast detachment and apoptosis induced by FGFR2 activation. J Cell Sci 118:1223–1232
56. Kaabeche K, Lemonnier J, Le Mee S, Caverzasio J, Marie PJ (2004) Cbl-mediated degradation of Lyn and Fyn induced by constitutive fibroblast growth factor receptor-2 activation supports osteoblast differentiation. J Biol Chem 279:36259–36267
57. Kapadia, RM, Guntur, AR, Reinhold, MI, Naski, MC (2005) Glycogen synthase kinase 3 controls endochondral bone development: contribution of fibroblast growth factor 18. Dev Biol 285:496–507
58. Kim HJ, Lee MH, Park HS, Park MH, Lee SW, Kim SY, Choi JY, Shin HI, Kim HJ, Ryoo HM (2003) Erk pathway and activator protein 1 play crucial roles in FGF2-stimulated premature cranial suture closure. Dev Dyn 227:335–346
59. Kim HJ, Rice DP, Kettunen PJ, Thesleff I (1998) FGF-BMP- and Shh-mediated signaling pathways in the regulation of cranial suture morphogenesis and calvarial bone development. Development 125:1241–1251
60. Koike M, Yamanaka Y, Inoue M, Tanaka H, Nishimura R, Seino Y (2003) Insulin-like growth factor-1 rescues the mutated FGF receptor 3 (G380R) expressing ATDC5 cells from apoptosis through phosphatidylinositol 3-kinase and MAPK. J Bone Miner Res 18:2043–2051
61. Lajeunie E, Catala M, Renier D (1999) Craniosynostosis: from a clinical description to an understanding of bone formation of the skull. Childs Nerv Syst 15:676–680
62. Laplantine E, Rossi F, Sahni M, Basilico C, Cobrinik D (2002) FGF signaling targets the pRb-related p107 and p130 proteins to induce chondrocyte growth arrest. J Cell Biol 158:741–750
63. Legeai-Mallet L, Benoist-Lasselin C, Delezoide A L, Munnich A, Bonaventure J, (1998) Fibroblast growth factor receptor 3 mutations promote apoptosis but do not alter chondrocyte proliferation in thanatophoric dysplasia J Biol Chem 273:13007–13014
64. Legeai-Mallet L, Benoist-Lasselin C, Munnich A, Bonaventure J (2004) Overexpression of FGFR3 Stat1 Stat5 and p21Cip1 correlates with phenotypic severity and defective chondrocyte differentiation in FGFR3-related chondrodysplasias. Bone 34:26–36
65. Lemonnier J, Delannoy P, Hott M, Lomri A, Modrowski D, Marie PJ (2000) The Ser252Trp fibroblast growth factor receptor-2 (FGFR-2) mutation induces PKC-independent downregulation of FGFR-2 associated with premature calvaria osteoblast differentiation. Exp Cell Res 256:158–167
66. Lemonnier J, Hay E, Delannoy P, Lomri A, Modrowski D, Caverzasio J, Marie PJ (2001) Role of N-cadherin and protein kinase C in osteoblast gene activation induced by the S252W fibroblast growth factor receptor 2 mutation in Apert craniosynostosis. J Bone Miner Res 16:832–845
67. Lemonnier J, Haÿ E, Delannoy Ph, Fromigué O, Lomri A, Modrowski M, Marie PJ (2001) Increased osteoblast in Apert craniosynostosis: Role of protein kinase C and interleukin-1. Am J Pathol 158:1833–1842
68. Li C, Chen L, Iwata T, Kitagawa M, Fu XY, Deng CX (1999) A Lys644Glu substitution in fibroblast growth factor receptor 3 (FGFR3) causes dwarfism in mice by activation of STATs and ink4 cell cycle inhibitors. Hum Mol Genet 8:35–44
69. Li Y, Mangasarian K, Mansukhani A, Basilico C (1997) Activation of FGF receptors by mutations in the transmembrane domain. Oncogene 14:1397–1406
70. Lievens PM, Mutinelli C, Baynes D, Liboi E (2004) The kinase activity of fibroblast growth factor receptor 3 with activation loop mutations affects receptor trafficking and signaling. J Biol Chem 279(41): 43254–43260
71. Lievens PM, Roncador A, Liboi EK (2006) 644E/M FGFR3 mutants activate Erk1/2 from the endoplasmic reticulum through FRS2 alpha and PLC gamma-independent pathways. J Mol Biol 357:783–792
72. Liu Z, Xu J, Colvin JS, Ornitz DM (2002) Coordination of chondrogenesis and osteogenesis by fibroblast growth factor 18. Genes Dev 16:859–869
73. Liu, Z, Lavine, KJ, Hung, IH, Ornitz, D M (2007) FGF18 is required for early chondrocyte proliferation, hypertrophy and vascular invasion of the growth plate. Dev Biol 302:80–91
74. Lomri A, Lemonnier J, Delannoy P, Marie PJ (2001) Identification of genes induced by the Ser252Trp FGFR-2 Apert mutation in osteoblasts using atlas human expression arrays: evidence for increased expression of PKCα IL-1αand RhoA GTPase. J Bone Miner Res 164:705–712
75. Lomri A, Lemonnier J, Hott M, de Perseval N, Lajeunie E, Munnich A, Renier D, Marie PJ (1998) Increased calvaria cell differentiation and bone matrix formation induced by fibroblast growth factor receptor-2 mutations in Apert syndrome. J Clin Invest 101:1310–1317
76. Mangasarian K, Li Y, Mansukhani A, Basilico C (1997) Mutation associated with Crouzon syndrome causes ligand-independent dimerization and activation of FGF receptor-2. J Cell Physiol 172:117–125
77. Mansukhani A, Bellosta P, Sahni M, Basilico C (2000) Signaling by fibroblast growth factors (FGF) and fibroblast growth factor receptor 2 (FGFR2)-activating mutations blocks mineralization and induces apoptosis in osteoblasts. J Cell Biol 149:1297–1308
78. Mansukhani A, Ambrosetti D, Holmes G, Cornivelli L, Basilico C (2005) Sox2 induction by FGF and FGFR2 activating mutations inhibits Wnt signaling and osteoblast differentiation. J Cell Biol 168:1065–1076
79. Marie PJ (2003) Fibroblast growth factor signaling controlling osteoblast differentiation. Gene 316:23–32
80. Marie PJ, Kaabeche K, Guenou H (2008) Roles of FGFR2 and Twist in human craniosynostosis: insights from genetic mutations in cranial osteoblasts. Front Oral Biol 12:144–159
81. Mathijssen IM, van Leeuwen JP, Vermeij-Keers C (2000) Simultaneous induction of apoptosis collagen type I expression and mineralization in the developing

coronal suture following FGF4 and FGF2 application. J Craniofac Genet Dev Biol 20:127–136
82. Matsushita T, Wilcox WR, Chan YY, Kawanami A, Bükülmez H, Balmes G, Krejci P, Mekikian PB, Otani K, Yamaura I, Warman ML, Givol D, Murakami S (2009) FGFR3 promotes synchondrosis closure and fusion of ossification centers through the MAPK pathway. Hum Mol Genet 18:227–240
83. Meyers EN, Lewandoski M, Martin, GR (1998) An Fgf8 mutant allelic series generated by Cre- and Flp-mediated recombination. Nat Genet 18:136–141
84. Minina E, Wenzel HM, Kreschel C, Karp S, Gaffield W, McMahon AP, Vortkamp A (2001) BMP and Ihh/PTHrP signaling interact to coordinate chondrocyte proliferation and differentiation. Development 128:4523–4534
85. Mohammadi M, Olsen SK, Ibrahimi OA (2005) Structural basis for fibroblast growth factor receptor activation. Cytokine Growth Factor Rev 16:107–137
86. Mohammadi M, Schlessinger J, Hubbard SR (1996) Structure of the FGF receptor tyrosine kinase domain reveals a novel autoinhibitory mechanism. Cell 86: 577–587
87. Molteni A, Modrowski D, Hott M, Marie PJ (1999) Differential expression of fibroblast growth factor receptor-1 -2 and -3 and syndecan-1 -2 and -4 in neonatal rat mandibular condyle and calvaria during osteogenic differentiation in vitro. Bone 24:337–347
88. Monsonego-Ornan E, Adar R, Feferman T, Segev O, Yayon A (2000) The transmembrane mutation G380R in fibroblast growth factor receptor 3 uncouples ligand-mediated receptor activation from down-regulation. Mol Cell Biol 20:516–522
89. Montero A, Okada Y, Tomita M, Ito M, Tsurukami H, Nakamura T, Doetschman T, Coffin JD, Hurley MM (2000) Disruption of the fibroblast growth factor-2 gene results in decreased bone mass and bone formation. J Clin Invest 105:1085–1093
90. Moore R, Ferretti P, Copp A, Thorogood P (2002) Blocking endogenous FGF-2 activity prevents cranial osteogenesis. Dev Biol 243:99–114
91. Morriss-Kay GM, Wilkie AO (2005) Growth of the normal skull vault and its alteration in craniosynostosis: insights from human genetics and experimental studies. J Anat 207:637–653
92. Murakami S, Balmes G, McKinney S, Zhang Z, Givol D, de Crombrugghe BC (2004) Constitutive activation of MEK1 in chondrocytes causes Stat1-independent achondroplasia-like dwarfism and rescues the Fgfr3-deficient mouse phenotype Genes Dev 18:290–305
93. Naski MC, Colvin JS, Coffin JD, Ornitz DM (1998) Repression of hedgehog signaling and BMP4 expression in growth plate cartilage by fibroblast growth factor receptor 3. Development 125:4977–4988
94. Naski MC, Wang Q, Xu J, Ornitz DM (1996) Graded activation of fibroblast growth factor receptor 3 by mutations causing achondroplasia and thanatophoric dysplasia. Nat Genet 13:233–237
95. Naski, MC, Ornitz, DM (1998) FGF signaling in skeletal development. Front Biosci 3:D781–DD94
96. Neilson KM, Friesel RE (1995) Constitutive activation of fibroblast growth factor receptor-2 by a point mutation associated with Crouzon syndrome. J Biol Chem 270:26037–26040
97. Obayashi N, Shibayama M, Kurotaki Y, Imanishi M, Fujimori T, Itoh N (2002) FGF 18 is required for normal cell proliferation and differentiation during osteogenesis and chondrogenesis. Genes Dev 16:870–879
98. Opperman LA (2000) Cranial sutures as intramembranous bone growth sites Dev Dyn 219:472–485
99. Ornitz D, Marie PJ (2002) FGF signaling pathways in endochondral and intramembranous bone development and human genetic disease. Genes Dev 16:1446–1465
100. Ornitz DM (2001) Regulation of chondrocyte growth and differentiation by fibroblast growth factor receptor 3. Novartis Found Symp 232:63–76
101. Ornitz DM (2005) FGF signaling in the developing endochondral skeleton. Cytokine Growth Factor Rev 16:205–213
102. Park WJ, Meyers GA, Li X, Theda C, Day D, Orlow SJ, Jones MC, Jabs EW (1995) Novel FGFR2 mutations in Crouzon and Jackson-Weiss syndromes show allelic heterogeneity and phenotypic variability. Hum Mol Genet 4:1229–1233
103. Peters KG, Werner S, Chen G, William LT (1992) Two FGF receptor genes are differentially expressed in epithelial and mesenchymal tissues during limb formation and organogenesis in the mouse. Development 114:233–243
104. Plotnikov AN, Hubbard SR, Schlessinger J, Mohammadi M (2000) Crystal structures of two FGF-FGFR complexes reveal the determinants of ligand-receptor specificity. Cell 101:413–434
105. Ratisoontorn C, Fan GF, McEntee K, Nah HD (2003) Activating (P253R C278F) and dominant negative mutations of FGFR2: differential effects on calvarial bone cell proliferation differentiation and mineralization. Connect Tissue Res 44(suppl 1):292–297
106. Raucci A, Laplantine E, Mansukhani A, Basilico C (2004) Activation of the ERK1/2 and p38 mitogen-activated protein kinase pathways mediates fibroblast growth factor-induced growth arrest of chondrocytes. J Biol Chem 279:1747–1756
107. Reinhold MI, Abe M, Kapadia RM, Liao Z, Naski MC (2004) FGF18 represses noggin expression and is induced by calcineurin. J Biol Chem 279:38209–38219
108. Reinhold MI, Naski, MC (2007) Direct interactions of Runx2 and canonical Wnt signaling induce FGF18. J Biol Chem 282:3653–3663
109. Rice DP, Aberg T, Chan YS, Tang ZQ, Kettunen PJ, Pakarinen L, Maxson RE, Thesleff I (2000) Integration of FGF and TWIST in calvarial bone and suture development. Development 127:1845–1855
110. Rice DP, Rice R (2008) Locate condense differentiate grow and confront: developmental mechanisms controlling intramembranous bone and suture formation and function. Front Oral Biol 12:22–40
111. Rice DP, Rice R, Thesleff I (2003) Fgfr mRNA isoforms in craniofacial bone development. Bone 33:14–27

112. Robertson SC, Meyer AN, Hart KC, Galvin BD, Webster MK, Donoghue DJ (1998) Activating mutations in the extracellular domain of the fibroblast growth factor receptor 2 function by disruption of the disulfide bond in the third immunoglobulin-like domain. Proc Natl Acad Sci U S A 95:4567–4572
113. Rousseau F, Bonaventure J, Legeal-Mallet L, Pelet A, Rozet J-M, Maroteaux P, Le Merrer M, Munnich A (1994) Mutations in the gene encoding fibroblast growth factor receptor-3 in achondroplasia. Nature 371:252–254
114. Rousseau F, el Ghouzzi V, Delezoide AL, Legeai-Mallet L, Le Merrer M, Munnich A, Bonaventure J (1996) Missense FGFR3 mutations create cysteine residues in thanatophoric dwarfism type I (TD1). Hum Mol Genet 5:509–512
115. Rousseau F, Saugier P, Le Merrer M, Munnich A, Delezoide AL, Maroteaux P, Bonaventure J, Narcy F, Sanak M (1995) Stop codon FGFR3 mutations in thanatophoric dwarfism type 1. Nat Genet 10:11–12
116. Rozenblatt-Rosen O, Mosonego-Ornan E, Sadot E, Madar-Shapiro L, Sheinin Y, Ginsberg D, Yayon A (2002) Induction of chondrocyte growth arrest by FGF: transcriptional and cytoskeletal alterations. J Cell Sci 115:553–562
117. Sahni M, Ambrosetti DC, Mansukhani A, Gertner R, Levy D, Basilico C (1999) FGF signaling inhibits chondrocyte proliferation and regulates bone development through the STAT-1 pathway. Genes Dev 13:1361–1366
118. Segev O, Chumakov I, Nevo Z, Givol D, Madar-Shapiro L, Sheinin Y, Weinreb M, Yayon A (2000) Restrained chondrocyte proliferation and maturation with abnormal growth plate vascularization and ossification in human FGFR-3(G380R) transgenic mice. Hum Mol Genet 9:249–258
119. Shiang R, Thompson L M, Zhu, Y-Z, Church DM, Fielder TJ, Bocian M, Winokur S T, Wasmuth JJ (1994) Mutations in the transmembrane domain of FGFR3 cause the most common genetic form of dwarfism, achondroplasia. Cell 78:335–342
120. Shimoaka T, Ogasawara T, Yonamine A, Chikazu D, Kawano H, Nakamura K, Itoh N, Kawaguchi H (2002) Regulation of osteoblast, chondrocyte, and osteoclast functions by fibroblast growth factor (FGF)-18 in comparison with FGF-2 and FGF-10. J Biol Chem 277:7493–7500
121. Shukla V, Coumoul X, Wang RH, Kim HS, Deng CX (2007) RNA interference and inhibition of MEK-ERK signaling prevent abnormal skeletal phenotypes in a mouse model of craniosynostosis. Nat Genet 39:1145–1150
122. Stott NS, Jiang TX, Chuong CM (1999) Successive formative stages of precartilaginous mesenchymal condensations in vitro: modulation of cell adhesion by Wnt-7A and BMP-2. J Cell Physiol 180:314–324
123. Su WC, Kitagawa M, Xue N, Xie B, Garofalo S, Cho J, Deng C, Horton WA, Fu XY (1997) Activation of Stat1 by mutant fibroblast growth-factor receptor in thanatophoric dysplasia type II dwarfism. Nature 386:288–292
124. Tanimoto Y, Yokozeki M, Hiura K, Matsumoto K, Nakanishi H, Matsumoto T, Marie PJ, Moriyama K (2004) A soluble form of fibroblast growth factor receptor 2 (FGFR2) with S252W mutation acts as an efficient inhibitor for the enhanced osteoblastic differentiation caused by FGFR2 activation in Apert syndrome. J Biol Chem 279:45926–45934
125. Tavormina PL, Rimoin DL, Cohn DH, Zhu YZ, Shiang R, Wasmuth JJ (1995) Another mutation that results in the substitution of an unpaired cysteine residue in the extracellular domain of FGFR3 in thanatophoric dysplasia type I. Hum Mol Genet 4:2175–2177
126. Tavormina PL, Shiang R, Thompson LM, Zhu Y, Wilkin DJ, Lachman RS, Wilcox WR, Rimoin DL, Cohn DH, Wasmuth JJ (1995) Thanatophoric dysplasia (types I and II) caused by distinct mutations in fibroblast growth factor receptor 3. Nat Genet 9:321–328
127. Wang Q, Green RP, Zhao G, Ornitz DM (2001) Differential regulation of endochondral bone growth and joint development by FGFR1 and FGFR3 tyrosine kinase domains Development 2128:3867–3876
128. Wang Y, Xiao R, Yang F, Karim BO, Iacovelli AJ, Cai J, Lerner CP, Richtsmeier JT, Leszl JM, Hill CA, Yu K, Ornitz DM, Elisseeff J, Huso DL, Jabs EW (2005) Abnormalities in cartilage and bone development in the Apert syndrome FGFR2(+/S252W) mouse. Development 132:3537–3548
129. Wang YC, Spatz MK, Kannan K, Hayk H, Avivi A, Gorivodsky M, Pines M, Yayon A, Lonai P, Givol D (1999) A mouse model for achondroplasia produced by targeting fibroblast growth factor receptor 3. Proc Natl Acad Sci U S A 96:4455–4460
130. Warren SM, Brunet LJ, Harland RM, Economides AN, Longaker MT (2003) The BMP antagonist noggin regulates cranial suture fusion. Nature 422:625–629
131. Webster MK, Donoghue DJ (1996) Constitutive activation of fibroblast growth factor receptor 3 by the transmembrane domain point mutation found in achondroplasia EMBO J 15:520–527
132. Wilkie AO (2005) Bad bones, absent smell, selfish testes: the pleiotropic consequences of human FGF receptor mutations Cytokine Growth Factor Rev 16: 187–203
133. Xu J, Lawshe A, MacArthur CA, Ornitz DM (1999) Genomic structure, mapping, activity and expression of fibroblast growth factor 17. Mech Dev 83:165–178
134. Xu JS, Liu, ZH, Ornitz, DM (2000) Temporal and spatial gradients of Fgf8 and Fgf17 regulate proliferation and differentiation of midline cerebellar structures. Development 127:1833–1843
135. Yasoda A, Komatsu Y, Chusho H, Miyazawa T, Ozasa A, Miura M, Kurihara T, Rogi T, Tanaka S, Suda M, Tamura N, Ogawa Y, Nakao K (2004) Overexpression of CNP in chondrocytes rescues achondroplasia through a MAPK-dependent pathway. Nat Med 10:80–86
136. Yin L, Du X, Li C, Xu X, Chen Z, Su N, Zhao L, Qi H, Li F, Xue J, Yang J, Jin M, Deng C, Chen L (2008) A Pro253Arg mutation in fibroblast growth factor receptor 2 (Fgfr2) causes skeleton malformation mimicking human Apert syndrome by affecting both chondrogenesis and osteogenesis. Bone 42:631–643

137. Yoon BS, Pogue R, Ovchinnikov DA, Yoshii I, Mishina Y, Behringer RR, Lyons K M (2006) BMPs regulate multiple aspects of growth-plate chondrogenesis through opposing actions on FGF pathways. Development 133:4667–4678
138. Yu K, Herr AB, Waksman G, Ornitz DM (2000) Loss of fibroblast growth factor receptor 2 ligand-binding specificity in Apert syndrome. Proc Natl Acad Sci U S A 97:14536–14541
139. Yu K, Ornitz DM (2001) Uncoupling fibroblast growth factor receptor 2 ligand binding specificity leads to Apert syndrome-like phenotypes. Proc Natl Acad Sci U S A 98:3641–3643
140. Yu K, Xu J, Liu Z, Sosic D, Shao J, Olson EN, Towler DA, Ornitz DM (2003) Conditional inactivation of FGF receptor 2 reveals an essential role for FGF signaling in the regulation of osteoblast function and bone growth Development 130:3063–3074
141. Zhou YX, Xu X, Chen L, Li C, Brodie SG, Deng C X (2000) A Pro250Arg substitution in mouse Fgfr1 causes increased expression of Cbfal and premature fusion of calvarial sutures. Hum Mol Genet 12:2001–2008

7. The Role of Hypoxia-Induced Factors

Ernestina Schipani and Richa Khatri

7.1 Hypoxia and the Hif Family of Transcription Factors

The definition of "physiologically" normoxic conditions for either embryonic or adult cells varies significantly. The vast majority of adult normal tissues function at oxygen (O_2) levels between 2 and 9%, with ambient air at 21% O_2 [135]. Bone marrow, cartilage, kidney medulla, and thymus, on the other hand, can exist at 1% O_2 or lower [135]. In general, when O_2 tension reaches below 2%, this condition is considered to be moderate hypoxia. When O_2 tension goes below 0.5%, hypoxia is considered severe. Hypoxia is not only a pathophysiological component of many human disorders, including cancer and ischemic diseases, but is also a critical factor in fetal development and differentiation [21, 39, 82]. Before the circulatory system is established, mammalian development proceeds in a relatively low O_2 environment of about 3% [100, 120]. Moreover, studies that have utilized small-molecule hypoxia markers have shown the existence of specific regions of moderate to severe hypoxia in the developing embryos [21, 82].

Hypoxia-inducible factor-1 (Hif-1), a ubiquitously expressed transcription factor, is a major regulator of cellular adaptation to hypoxia [14, 38, 65, 88, 130] (Fig. 7.1). It is a heterodimeric DNA-binding complex that consists of two basic helix-loop-helix (bHLH) proteins of the PER/ARNT/SIM (PAS) subfamily, Hif-1α and Hif-1β [155]. Hif-1α and Hif-1β mRNAs are ubiquitously expressed [160]. In general, alpha-class members of the PAS subfamily respond to environmental signals, whereas beta-class molecules aid in targeting the heterodimer to their nuclear targets [45]. In the Hif-1 system, Hif-1α is activated when O_2 levels drop below 5%; its activity increases as O_2 tension decreases [18, 58, 60, 99, 112, 156] (Fig. 7.1). On the other hand, Hif-1β (also known as aryl hydrocarbon nuclear translocator or ARNT) is nonoxygen responsive. Upon heterodimerization with Hif-1α, the complex Hif-1α/Hif-1β binds to a specific sequence RCGTG, the hypoxia response element (HRE), and transactivates the target genes containing HREs [67] (Fig. 7.1).

Hif-1α does not directly sense variations in O_2 tension [19]; a class of 2-oxoglutarate-dependent and Fe^{2+}-dependent dioxygenases are the O_2 sensors [112] (Fig. 7.1). Two types of O_2 sensors are involved in Hif-1α action, namely, prolyl-hydroxylase domain proteins (PHDs) and asparaginyl hydroxylase. PHDs hydroxylate two prolyl residues (P402 and P564) in the Hif-1α region referred to as the O_2-dependent degradation domain (ODDD) [7]. This modification occurs in normoxic conditions and mediates the binding of the von Hippel–Lindau tumor suppressor

F. Bronner et al. (eds.), *Bone and Development*, Topics in Bone Biology 6,
DOI 10.1007/978-1-84882-822-3_7, © Springer-Verlag London Limited 2010

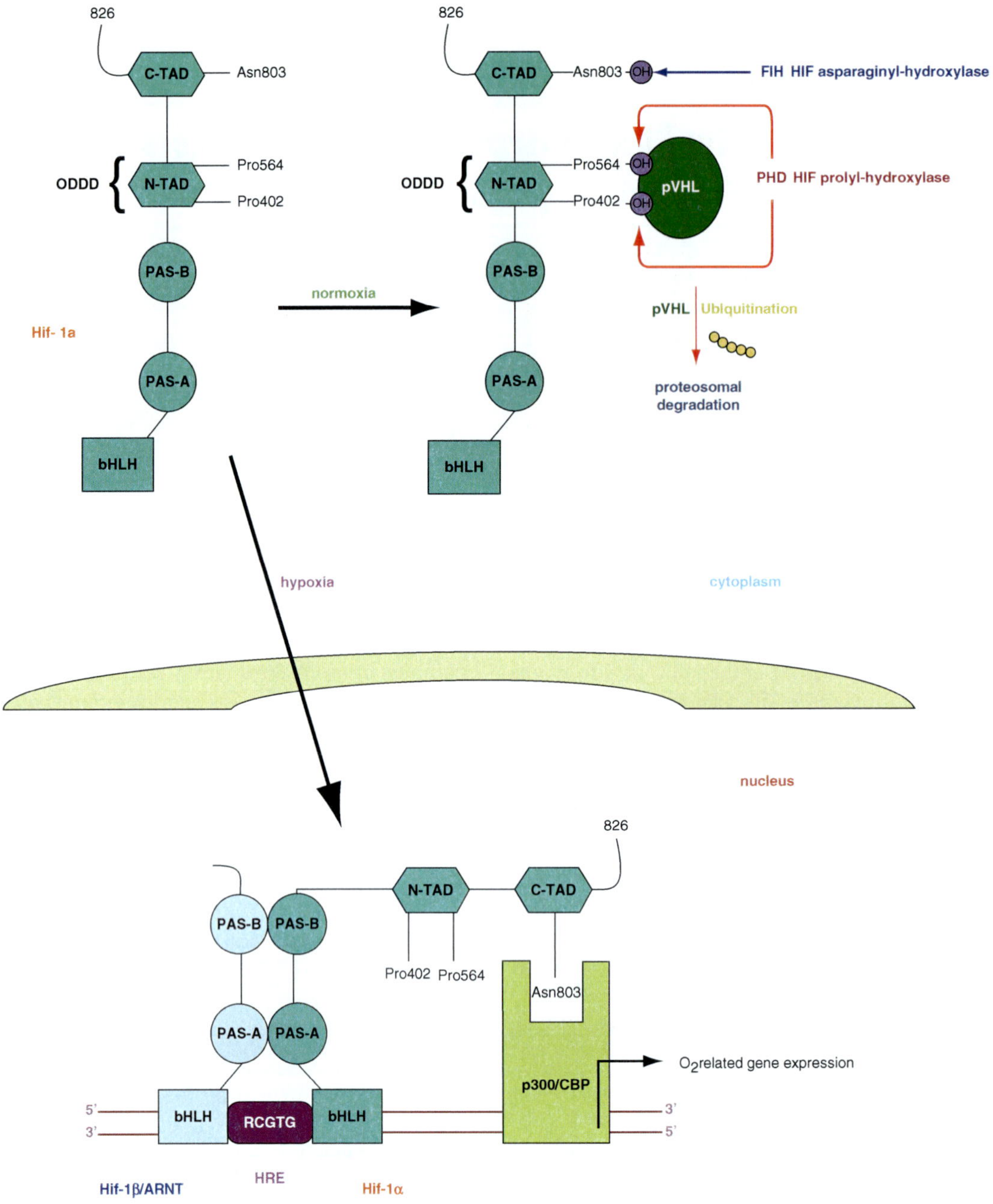

Figure 7.1. Hif-1α, its posttranslational modifications, and interacting proteins. For details, see text.

protein (pVHL), which is an E3 ubiquitin ligase, to Hif-1α (Fig. 7.1). Hif-1α is then marked with polyubiquitin chains and targeted for degradation by the proteasome (Fig. 7.1). In well-oxygenated tissues, where O_2 tension is higher than 5%, Hif-1α displays one of the shortest half-lives (<5 min) among the cellular proteins. Conversely, as described earlier, under hypoxic conditions, the activity of the PHDs is largely impaired and proline hydroxylation cannot occur. As a result, Hif-1α protein accumulates and this initiates a multi-step pathway that includes nuclear translocation of Hif-1α, dimerization with its partner Hif-1β, recruitment of transcriptional coactivators, and binding to HREs within the promoters of hypoxia-responsive genes [68] (Fig. 7.1). The second type of O_2 sensor is an asparaginyl hydroxylase, also called factor inhibiting Hif (FIH) [80]. This enzyme hydroxylates an asparagine residue (N803) in the carboxy-terminal transcriptional activation domain (C-TAD) of Hif-1α (Fig. 7.1). This covalent modification blocks C-TAD interaction with transcriptional co-activators, such as p300 and CBP. Thus, the two O_2 sensors, PHD and FIH, by regulating the destruction and activation of Hif-1α, respectively, ensure the repression of the Hif-1α pathway in well-oxygenated cells. As PHDs have lower affinity for O_2 and 2-oxyglutarate than FIH, they may be inactivated in vivo at O_2 values that still maintain FIH activity, yet keep C-TAD under repression [112]. Consistent with this model, two classes of Hif-1α-dependent genes have been reported, which are sensitive and nonsensitive to FIH [112]. According to the model, stabilization of Hif-1α alone may not be adequate to regulate genes that are both Hif-1α-dependent and FIH-sensitive.

pVHL, made up of 213 amino acids, is expressed in most tissues and cells [48]. Heterozygous missense mutations of the *VHL* gene are probably the cause of the von Hippel–Lindau syndrome [66, 115], a disease characterized by a dominant predisposition to develop pheochromocytomas and highly vascular tumors of the kidney, the central nervous system, and the retina [66, 115]. Tumorigenesis results from the loss or inactivation of the wild-type allele [66, 115]. The importance of VHL for proteolysis of Hif-1α is underscored by the finding that cells lacking a functional pVHL cannot degrade this transcription factor; as a result, Hif-1α accumulates [66, 115].

Stimuli other than hypoxia also cause Hif proteins to accumulate in normoxic cells, but the molecular mechanisms are not yet understood [168].

To date, more than 100 putative Hif-1α target genes have been identified [8, 43, 84, 162]. They are involved in biological processes including energy metabolism, angiogenesis, erythropoiesis, cell survival, apoptosis, and pH regulation [43, 97]. Mouse embryos lacking Hif-1α exhibit multiple morphological defects as early as embryonic day E8.5, and die in utero by E11 [25, 59, 121]. Hif-1α is also a strong promoter of tumor growth [38, 130]. Hypoxia and Hif-1α play a role in tumor development and progression, and they are responsible, at least in part, for the resistance of malignant lesions to radiation therapy [114]. Some highly malignant tumors exist in a severe hypoxic microenvironment, and inhibition of Hif-1α is currently being explored as a therapeutic approach [20]. Interestingly, genes associated with cell death, such as BNip3, a member of the Bcl-2 family of proapoptotic proteins [137], can also be induced by Hif-1 [11]. On the whole, however, Hif-1α promotes survival of hypoxic cells.

Two isoforms of Hif-1α have been characterized: Hif-2α and Hif-3α [42]. Hif-1α and Hif-2α have similar protein structure and undergo the same oxygen-dependent proteolysis. This may mean that they function redundantly, at least in some settings [108]. However, the pattern of expression of Hif-2α is restricted to blood vessels, lung, kidney, interstitial cells, liver, and neural crest [161], whereas Hif-1α is expressed in all cells. Moreover, mice that are null for Hif-1α die at early stages of embryonic development, but mice deficient in Hif-2α survive until mid-to-late gestation, or depending on the strain, until birth [17, 24, 25, 59, 109, 121, 126, 148]. The two isoforms, therefore, seem to have distinct developmental functions. Lastly, some genes are activated by both Hif-1α and Hif-2α, whereas others are preferentially activated by one or the other [55, 116, 157]. For a comprehensive review of the roles played by Hif-1α and Hif-2α in embryonic development and differentiation, see reference [135].

Hif-3α is not closely related to Hif-1α and Hif-2α [159]. Alternative splicing of the Hif-3α gene produces at least six different isoforms [98], one of which is an inhibitory protein that contains the N-terminal bHLH and PAS domains, yet lacks the C-TAD [96]. This protein acts as a negative regulator of Hif-mediated gene expression.

ARNT is constitutively expressed and is insensitive to changes in O_2 levels. Two homologs, ARNT2 and ARNT3, or bMAL are components of O_2-independent pathways [13, 70].

7.1.1 Hifs and Energy Metabolism

Hif-1α promotes cell survival in hypoxic conditions by a variety of mechanisms. Some involve regulation of glucose metabolism. In aerobic conditions, glucose is converted to pyruvate in the cytoplasm. Pyruvate then enters the tricarboxylic acid (TCA) cycle and oxidative phosphorylation takes place in the mitochondria [159]. Louis Pasteur was the first to record that O_2-deprived cells convert more glucose to lactate than cells in the normoxic cultures. This is the so-called "Pasteur effect." Induction of the Pasteur effect depends on Hif-1α that upregulates glucose transporters such as Glut1, glycolytic enzymes that stimulate ATP production by anaerobic glycolysis such as phosphoglycero-kinase 1 (PGK1), and the enzyme lactic dehydrogenase that converts pyruvate to lactate [59, 127, 128]. Moreover, Hif-1α inhibits mitochondrial oxidative phosphorylation by diminishing pyruvate entry into the TCA cycle [73, 106], at the same time upregulating expression of pyruvate dehydrogenase kinase, an enzyme that phosphorylates and inhibits pyruvate dehydrogenase. By preventing conversion of pyruvate to acetyl CoA, pyruvate cannot enter the TCA cycle [73]. Interestingly, Hif-1α also modulates the differential expression of cytochrome c oxidase 4 (COX4) isoforms, COX4-1 and COX4-2. It does so by activating the transcription of the genes that encode COX4-2 and LON. The latter is a mitochondrial protease that degrades COX4-1 [33]. This enables optimal mitochondrial respiration in hypoxia [159]. Paradoxically, cells under hypoxia are subject to oxidative stress and release of reactive oxygen species (ROS) [33]. By inhibiting the entry of pyruvate into the mitochondria, Hif-1α attenuates not only the mitochondrial respiration, even though its efficiency is improved, but also diminishes ROS production in hypoxic cells [33]. Lastly, Hif-1α regulates intracellular pH. In anaerobic glycolysis, lactic acid accumulates in the cytosol which is extruded with the help of Hif-1α. Hif-1α regulates the expression of the monocarboxylate transporter (MCT) 4 of the H^+/lactate cotransporter family [117, 152] and the Na^+/H^+ exchanger (NHE)1 [117].

Notably, Hif-2α does not significantly affect glucose metabolism, a further indication that Hif-1α and Hif-2α do not have the same targets [55].

7.1.2 Hifs and Angiogenesis

Both Hif-1α and Hif-2α are important modulators of angiogenesis, an essential process in normal development, as well as in pathological conditions such as cancer. Hif-1α is required for proper vascularization of the mouse embryo [121]. Hypoxia and Hifs induce expression of vascular endothelial growth factor A (VEGF-A) and other proangiogenic factors [35].

VEGF-A is a homodimeric glycoprotein of 45 kDA, which belongs to the dimeric cysteine-knot growth factor super-family. VEGF-A is a major regulator of angiogenesis and is also a most potent angiogenic factor [32, 171]. The mouse VEGF-A gene encodes at least three isoforms (VEGF120, VEGF164, and VEGF188) that arise via alternative splicing [54, 149]. In contrast to the two other isoforms, VEGF120 does not bind the extracellular matrix component heparan sulfate, an important signaling proteoglycan [23, 119]. VEGF-A may have a survival function in hematopoietic stem cells, acting through an internal autocrine loop [36].

A role of VEGF-A as a critical mediator of the survival action of Hif-1α is still under investigation. Paradoxically, in Hif-1α null embryos, VEGF-A expression is increased, not reduced, and vascular regression appears to be secondary to mesenchymal cell death, rather than to VEGF-A deficiency [25, 78].

7.1.3 Hifs and Autophagy

Hypoxia and Hif-1α, but not Hif-2α, modulate the autophagic process. Autophagy is lysosomal-dependent and is activated in numerous stress conditions. In autophagy, cells digest their cytoplasm and organelles; this provides macromolecules for energy generation and helps the cells to survive [63, 85, 134]. The term autophagy was introduced by deDuve, who discovered lysosomes, and provided the first evidence that lysosomes are involved in autophagy. Autophagy is linked to a variety of conditions of health and disease, including development and differentiation, cancer, tissue degeneration, and infections.

Autophagy can be differentiated into two classes: "microautophagy" and "macroautophagy" [85].

Microautophagy involves the direct engulfment of cytoplasm by the lysosomes; macroautophagy refers to the formation of a double-membrane vesicle that contains portions of cytoplasm and subsequently fuses to the lysosome. Autophagy is essential in mitochondrial homeostasis; moreover, the autophagic process, which is also triggered by endoplasmic reticulum (ER) stress, is required to counterbalance the expansion of ER during the unfolded protein response (UPR) [6, 164]. Autophagy can promote either survival, or if prolonged, can lead to death [134]. Hypoxia triggers autophagy and promotes cell survival with the aid of mechanisms that may involve Hif-1α [5, 107, 150, 172]. The hypoxic stress is also a trigger of UPR [31]. This could be a mechanism by which hypoxia leads to autophagy.

7.2 Hifs and Chondrocytes

Skeletal development depends on two mechanisms, intramembranous and endochondral [69]. In the first, mesenchymal cells develop directly into osteoblasts and form the flat bones of the skull. The second, accounting for the development of most other bones, involves a two-stage mechanism, whereby chondrocytes form a matrix template, the growth plate, which is then replaced by bone. During endochondral bone development, growth-plate chondrocytes undergo well-ordered and controlled phases of cell proliferation, maturation, and death. Proliferative chondrocytes synthesize collagen type II and form a columnar layer. They then stop proliferating and differentiate into postmitotic hypertrophic cells. Hypertrophic chondrocytes predominantly express type-X collagen and mineralize their surrounding matrix. Differentiation is followed by death of hypertrophic chondrocytes, followed by blood vessel invasion, and finally, by replacement of the cartilaginous matrix with bone.

The fetal growth plate is unique among mesenchymal tissues, because it is avascular and requires an angiogenic switch for bone to replace it. Consistent with its avascularity and differing from what is observed in a postnatal setting [132], the fetal growth plate contains a hypoxic central region [125]. The presence and degree of hypoxia in mammalian fetal cartilage can be made evident by injecting EF5, a marker for bioreductive activity, into pregnant female mice at various gestational times. EF5 reacts with cytoplasmic proteins in hypoxic cells; these adducts can be detected with a specific antibody [81, 92]. By this analysis, the fetal chondrocytic growth plate has been shown to bind to EF5, with no binding detected in the surrounding soft tissues. The most hypoxic chondrocytes are in the round proliferative layer near the joint space, in the center of the columnar proliferative layer and in the upper portion of the hypertrophic zone (Fig. 7.2) [125]. The EF5 findings document a gradient of oxygenation, from the proliferative to the hypertrophic zone, as well as from the outer to the inner region of the fetal growth plate. The high rate of O_2 diffusion to the mineralized hypertrophic layer may be the reason for the hypoxic condition of the early hypertrophic chondrocytes, even though they are located near the blood vessels of the primary spongiosa [125].

7.2.1 Hif-1α and Chondrocyte Survival

The analysis of genetically modified mice has demonstrated that Hif-1α is essential for endochondral bone development. No such role has been documented for Hif-2α.

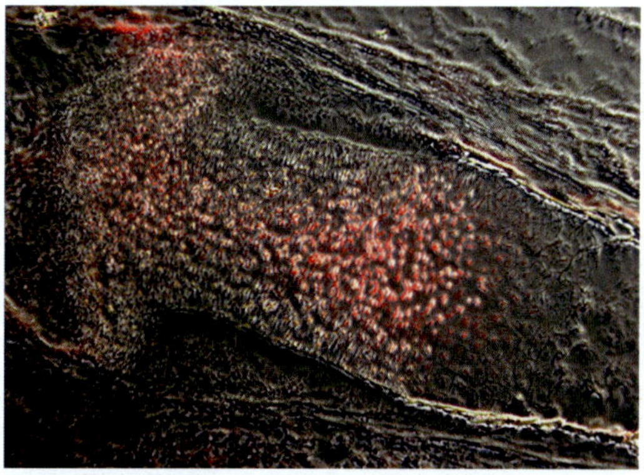

Figure 7.2. Histological section of the proximal epiphysis of an E15.5 mouse tibia. Staining with the marker of hypoxia, EF5 (*red signal*), shows that in an E15.5 mouse tibia growth plate, the round proliferative layer, the center of the columnar layer, and the upper hypertrophic zone are highly hypoxic (*red signal*), whereas, consistent with extensive vascularization of the primary spongiosa, the late hypertrophic chondrocytes are not hypoxic. (Reprinted from Schipani et al. [125], with the permission of Cold Spring Harbor Laboratory Press).

With the aid of a Cre-loxP conditional knockout strategy in which the Cre recombinase is driven by a fragment of the collagen type II promoter (Col2a1-Cre) and a floxed Hif-1α allele, it has been possible to demonstrate the critical and nonredundant role of Hif-1α in endochondral bone development [125]. As chondrocytes null for Hif-1α (Col2a1-Cre; Hif-1α$^{f/f}$) undergo massive cell death, particularly in the center of the developing growth plate, Hif-1α is essential for the survival of hypoxic chondrocytes in vivo [125] (Fig. 7.3). Death of cells at the center of the developing growth plate is not preceded by ectopic hypertrophy [125]. This suggests that chondrocyte death secondary to lack of Hif-1α is different at the molecular level from chondrocyte apoptosis that precedes blood vessel invasion and replacement of cartilage with bone.

Hif-1α is essential for hypoxic chondrocytes, but whether downstream mediators assure Hif-1α survival of chondrocytes is unknown. Hif-1α may regulate energy metabolism. The mRNA that encodes PGK1, a key enzyme of anaerobic glycolysis, is strikingly upregulated in the fetal growth plate [125], whereas PGK1 mRNA expression is reduced to background levels in the Col2a1-Cre; Hif-1α$^{f/f}$ growth plate [125]. These findings indicate that in the absence of Hif-1α, anaerobic glycolysis is impaired and hypoxic chondrocytes cannot maintain adequate ATP levels. The more severe hypoxia of Hif-1α–null chondrocytes [125] may be owing to the greater O_2 consumption by their mitochondria, inasmuch as Hif-1α inhibits mitochondrial activity.

Hif-1α may promote survival of hypoxic chondrocytes by upregulating VEGF-A. In the fetal growth plate, VEGF-A is expressed in late hypertrophic chondrocytes, where it is critical for blood vessel invasion and replacement of cartilage by bone [37, 94, 153, 167, 169, 170]. It is also expressed, although at a considerably lower level, in the center of the proliferative and upper hypertrophic layers, i.e., in the hypoxic zones of the growth plate [111, 169]. VEGF-A expression in the "hypoxic" domain of the growth plate is Hif-1α-dependent [111] [26, 110]. On the basis of these findings, VEGF-A may well be a downstream mediator of the survival function of Hif-1α. Consistent with this inference is that the universal knockout of VEGF164 and VEGF120 and the conditional knockout of all three VEGF-A isoforms leads to chondrocyte death in the center of the proliferative layer and in the upper hypertrophic zone of the fetal growth plate [95, 169, 171]. Although the degree of death is lower than what is observed in the Hif-1α-deficient growth plates, the conditional knockout of all three VEGF isoforms clearly mimics what happens in the Hif-1α–deficient growth plates [98, 173]. Paradoxically, VEGF-A expression is upregulated in viable chondrocytes adjacent to the area of cell death in the Hif-1α-deficient growth plate [125]. The question therefore remains open as to whether VEGF-A is a critical downstream effector of the Hif-1α survival function. VEGF-A binds to and activates two tyrosine kinase receptors, VEGFR1 (Flt-1) and VEGFR2 (KDR/Flk-1), which regulate both physiological and pathological angiogenesis

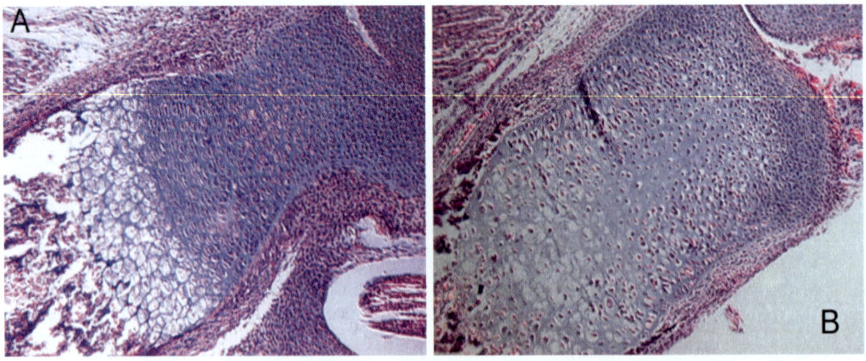

Figure 7.3. Histological sections of the distal epiphysis of newborn control (**a**) and Col2a1-Cre; Hif-1α$^{f/f}$ (**b**) mouse tibias stained with H & E. The center of the mutant growth plate is dramatically hypocellular as a consequence of massive central cell death. (Reprinted from Schipani et al. [125], with the permission of Cold Spring Harbor Laboratory Press).

[133]. Interestingly, fetal growth-plate chondrocytes neither express VEGFR2 nor VEGFR1; however, neuropilin-1 and 2, which are coreceptors for VEGF164 ligand, and VEGFR3, which does not bind VEGF-A, are present in chondrocytes.

Autophagy is another survival mechanism adopted by Hif-1α in hypoxic cells [129]. Chondrocyte death secondary to lack of Hif-1α may involve the autophagic pathway, inasmuch as accumulation of autophagic proteins such as Beclin1 in chondrocytes is a function of Hif-1α, at least in vitro [9]. Moreover, the lysosomal-dependent process of autophagy functions in growth-plate chondrocytes [131]. Therefore, chondrocyte survival in a hypoxic environment may indeed involve upregulation of the autophagic process.

7.2.2 Hif-1α and Chondrocyte Proliferation

Studies of gain-of-function mutations of the Hif-1α-mediated pathway in chondrocytes have shown that this transcription factor also modulates chondrocyte proliferation. Mice that lack pVHL in chondrocytes are viable, though severely dwarfed [111]. They have increased Hif-1α transcriptional activity in cartilage and their pVHL-deficient growth plates are remarkably hypocellular, with the chondrocyte proliferation rate markedly decreased. This inhibition is reversed in the Col2a1-Cre; Hif-1α^{f}/^{f}; VHL^{f}/^{f} double-mutant mice that lack both VHL and Hif-1α. Therefore, Hif-1α accumulation suppresses chondrocyte proliferation. Lack of VHL reduces cell proliferation in an in vitro fibrosarcoma model [93]. Moreover, in fetal growth plates deficient in Hif-1α, the proliferation rate of viable chondrocytes is strikingly increased [125]. Finally, hypoxia leads to cell cycle arrest in the G1/S phase, at least in part through upregulation of Hif-1α transcriptional activity [41]. Recent work has suggested that Hif-1α induces expression of cyclin kinase inhibitors by antagonizing c-Myc [77]. In VHL-deficient growth plates, the expression of the cyclin kinase inhibitor, p57, is increased [111], whereas the cyclin kinase inhibitors, p21 and p27, are elevated in the VHL-null fibrosarcoma model [41]. Additionally, cyclin G2, a cell cycle inhibitor, is upregulated by hypoxia [113, 162]; this indicates that modulation of cyclin G2 expression may be an additional tool used by the hypoxia/VHL/Hif-1α pathway to control cell proliferation.

7.2.3 Hifs and Chondrocyte Differentiation

An essential and specific function of chondrocytes is to synthesize extracellular matrix, whose two principal components are proteoglycans and collagens [72]. Hypoxia and Hifs increase cartilaginous matrix and thus drive mesenchymal cells to differentiate into chondrocytes. Growth plates of Col2a1-Cre; VHL^{f}/^{f} mice have more matrix in-between cells [111]; moreover, hypoxia leads to a Hif-1α-dependent increase in collagen type II protein in monolayer culture of mouse primary chondrocytes [110]. Embryonic mesenchymal condensations, which exclude blood vessels, are highly hypoxic and express Hif-1α in both limb bud and axial skeleton [3, 113]. Moreover, hypoxia-inducible reporter mice (5XHRE-LacZ reporter) show activation of the reporter in mesenchymal condensations [113]. Lastly, in conditional knockout mice (Prx1-Cre; Hif-1α^{f}/^{f}), whose Hif-1α is inactivated in limb-bud mesenchyme, Hif-1α stimulates mesenchymal cells to differentiate into chondrocytes [3, 113]. Prx1 is a homeobox gene that is expressed predominantly in mesenchyme [147]. Prx1-Cre mice express Cre recombinase largely in limb-bud mesenchyme, starting from E9.5, before any condensation forms [91]. Analysis of Prx1-Cre; Hif-1α^{f}/^{f} has shown that Hif-1α is not required for the formation of precartilaginous condensations [3, 113], but has a nonredundant and critical role in the differentiation of mesenchymal cells into chondrocytes. Lack of Hif-1α in limb-bud mesenchyme causes a remarkable delay in cartilage formation [3, 113], and the findings were confirmed in vitro [3, 118, 163]. The findings demonstrate the positive role of Hif-1α in chondrocyte differentiation and establish its essential role in endochondral bone development.

The role of hypoxia and Hif-1α in cell differentiation is tissue-specific, because Hif-1α maintains stem cells in an undifferentiated state [47, 62, 64, 87, 123, 135], inhibits differentiation of mesenchymal cells into osteoblasts, adipocytes, and myocytes [124, 135, 165, 166], and yet stimulates the differentiation of trophoblastic cells and dopaminergic neurons and chondrocytes [28, 101, 135, 143].

Regulation of posttranslational modification of collagens, with hydroxylation of collagen prolines, in particular, is one modality by which Hif-1α regulates chondrocyte differentiation. Prolyl-4-hydroxylases I and II (P4HaI and P4HaII) are the enzymes responsible for generating 4-hydroxyprolines in the collagens; these are essential for the formation of triple-helical collagens. P4Has are $\alpha_2\beta_2$ tetramers [103]; the α subunit contains the major portion of the catalytic site [103]. Because more β subunit than α subunit is produced [103], enzymatic activity is limited by the abundance of the α subunit. Two isoforms of α have been characterized, namely I and II, which form the P4HaI and P4HaII tetramers, respectively [103]. The $\alpha I_2\beta_2$ tetramer (P4HaI) is the main enzyme form in most cell types and tissues, whereas at least 70% of the total prolyl-4-hydroxylase activity in cultured mouse chondrocytes is due to the $\alpha II_2\beta_2$ (P4HaII) enzyme. In mouse cartilage, it amounts to about 80% [4]. The P4HaII is also the main enzyme form in capillary endothelial cells [4]. P4HaI and II require Fe^{2+}, 2-oxoglutarate, and O_2 for their enzymatic activity [103], with ascorbate required to maintain the iron ions in their biologically active Fe^{2+} form. P4Has have much lower Km for O_2 than the PHDs, which trigger Hif-1α degradation (20 vs. 250, respectively) [52]. This indicates that P4Has require a minimal amount of O_2 for proper function, i.e., they still function enzymatically at low O_2 levels [54]. The α subunits of P4HaI and P4HaII are targets of hypoxia in chondrocytes and other cell types in a Hif-1α-dependent fashion [44, 53, 113, 145]. Proper accumulation of extracellular matrix is not only essential for organ development, but also promotes cell differentiation and survival through specific cell–matrix interactions [30, 144]. Hif-1α may thus operate as a survival and differentiation factor in chondrocytes, improving the efficiency of posttranslational modifications of collagen type II and, in doing so, promote the formation of a proper extracellular matrix. A defect in posttranslational hydroxylation of collagens leads to a decrease in extracellular matrix and an increase in underhydroxylated collagens. This in turn may trigger a UPR [105, 151, 173] and may be a cause of the delayed chondrogenesis in mice that lack Hif-1α in limb-bud mesenchyme. The positive effect of Hif-1α on matrix accumulation in chondrocytes is consistent with the role of hypoxia in promoting fibrosis in pathological conditions [51].

Hypoxia and Hif-1α may also modulate chondrogenesis by upregulating expression of Sox9 [3, 118], a master regulator of chondrogenesis [2, 56, 83, 136]. In mouse bone marrow stromal (ST2) cells, in particular, hypoxia brings about an increase in nuclear accumulation of Hif-1α and Sox9 transcription [118]. Similar findings have been reported in limb-bud micromass cultures [3], but not in primary chondrocytes or ex vivo metatarsal explants [113].

On the basis of a teratoma model in which Hif-2α had been knocked into the Hif-1α locus, Hif-2α may have a role in chondrocyte differentiation and chondrogenesis [26]. Hif-2α is also elevated during chondrocyte differentiation, but no role in endochondral bone development has yet been reported [140].

7.2.4 Hif-1α and Joint Development

Hif-1α protein and VEGF-A mRNA are particularly abundant in the highly hypoxic developing joints, possibly because the avascular perichondrium surrounding them is thickened [113]. Even after the joint space has formed, articular chondrocytes are significantly more hypoxic than the rest of the cartilage [113]. Lack of Hif-1α in limb-bud mesenchyme delays joint development, without altering the thickening of the perichondrium [3, 113]. Thickening of the perichondrium, therefore, precedes joint formation and is likely to be critical for joint development.

GDF5, Wnt14, and Noggin are essential regulators of joint development [12, 46, 50, 74, 141]. Interestingly, microarray experiments have shown that brief exposure to 1% O_2 does not induce GDF5, Wnt14, or Noggin mRNA expression in ex vivo metatarsal explants [113]. This finding indicates that these factors are not a direct, transcriptional target of Hif-1α. Similar results were obtained with primary chondrocytes briefly cultured in hypoxic conditions [113]. Inasmuch as chondrogenesis and joint formation are tightly coupled [76], the delay of early chondrogenesis, secondary to the lack of Hif-1α, may impair joint formation. However, because of the pronounced expression of Hif-1α in the prospective joint, the delayed joint formation associated with loss of Hif-1α may not be the only consequence of a delay in early chondrogenesis.

7.2.5 Articular surface chondrocytes and Hifs

Like the fetal growth plate, articular cartilage is also an avascular tissue, which depends on synovial fluid diffusion for its metabolic needs [40]. Hypoxia upregulates the expression of cartilage matrix genes in human articular chondrocytes [102]. With the aid of RNA interference, it has been shown that Hif-2α, not Hif-1α, is necessary for Sox9 induction of key cartilage genes in articular surface chondrocytes [79]. Moreover, low O_2 enhances chondrogenesis of mesenchymal stem cells (MSCs) in vitro. These stem cells may be candidates for cell-based articular cartilage repair, involving a mechanism that utilizes Hif-2α rather than Hif-1α [71]. Nevertheless, the role played by Hif-2α in the developing articular surface chondrocytes is as yet uncertain.

7.3 Hif-1s and Osteoblasts

7.3.1 Hifs in Bone Modeling and Remodeling

Hypoxia is also responsible for coupling angiogenesis and bone formation. Osteoblasts, like other oxygen-sensitive cells, express components of the Hif-1 pathway. Studies in the late 1990s have shown that hypoxia is a potent stimulator of VEGF-A mRNA expression in osteoblastic cells [139]. More recently, manipulation of the Hif-1α pathway in osteoblasts has led to overproduction of VEGF-A and a dramatic increase of bone [158] (Fig. 7.4). Mutant mice that lack VHL in fully differentiated osteoblasts (ΔVHL) and thus overexpress Hifs, have a strikingly increased bone volume. Conversely, lack of Hif-1α in osteoblasts (ΔHif-1α) negatively impacts bone volume.

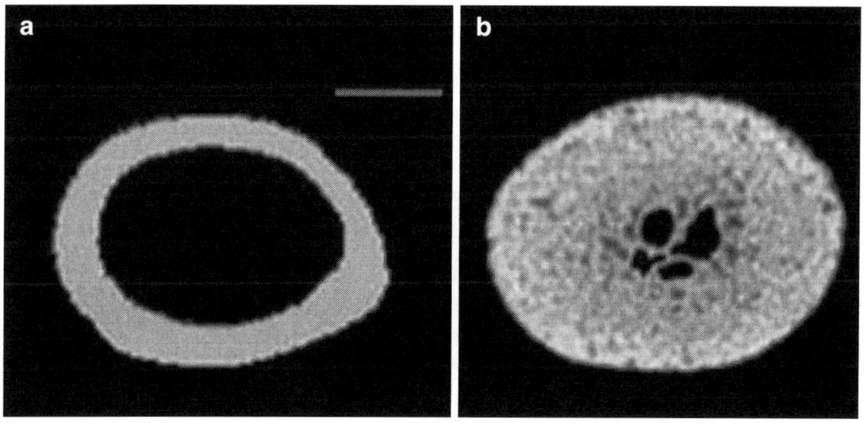

Figure 7.4. MicroCT of 6-week-old control (**a**) and ΔVHL (**b**) femurs; cross-sections are shown. Lack of VHL in osteoblasts results in dramatic increase in bone volume. Reprinted with permission from Wang et al. [158], with permission from the American Society for Clinical Investigation).

Moreover, bone formation in ovariectomized ΔHif-1α female mice is significantly more reduced than in ovariectomized wild-type mice [90]. The amount of bone in both ΔVHL and ΔHif-1α mice is directly proportional to the amount of skeletal vasculature. This suggests that regulation of bone mass in these mutants may be secondary to regulation of VEGF-A and angiogenesis. Consistent with this idea, VEGF-A mRNA expression is upregulated in trabecular bone of ΔVHL mice. In addition, in an ex vivo assay, ΔVHL metatarsals exhibit a dramatic increase in endothelial sprouting, which is entirely reversed by pre-incubation with an anti-VEGF neutralizing antibody. However, the putative mechanisms responsible for coupling angiogenesis to osteogenesis in both ΔVHL and ΔHif-1α mice remain to be determined. It has been proposed that the vascular setting provides a true niche for pericytic MSC-like cells and could be a source of osteoprogenitors or MSCs with osteogenic potential [122]. Thus, the VEGF-dependent increase in angiogenesis observed in ΔVHL mice leads to more bone by providing a larger pool of MSCs.

However, VEGF-A has also been reported to be critical for osteoblast differentiation. In particular, mice that express only the VEGF120 isoform exhibit both delayed invasion of the vessels into the primary ossification center and altered osteoblastic differentiation in vitro [170].

Interestingly, hypoxia per se is an inhibitor of osteoblast differentiation in vitro [124], which further suggests that the dramatic increase in bone volume in mice lacking pVHL in osteoblasts is not a cell-autonomous effect, but is rather secondary to the increase in blood vessels.

Numerous factors other than hypoxia stabilize Hif activity and increase VEGF-A expression in osteoblasts; an example is insulin-like growth factor (IGF) I. In human osteoblast-like cells, IGF-I induces a rapid, threefold increase in VEGF-A mRNA [1]. This is accompanied by an increase in Hif-2α protein without a corresponding change in Hif-2α mRNA expression [1]. IGF-I also stimulates phosphorylation of Akt, which is abolished by pretreating the cells with the phosphatidylinositol-3 kinase (PI3K) inhibitor, LY294002. Treatment with this inhibitor also significantly reduced Hif-2 α accumulation and induction of VEGF mRNA expression by IGF-1. Thus, IGF-1 appears to induce VEGF-A expression in osteoblasts by increasing the accumulation of Hif-2α protein in a PI3K-dependent fashion [1]. These findings highlight a potential role for Hif-2α in osteoblasts, that needs to be documented in vivo.

Interestingly, manipulation of Hif levels in osteoblasts does not noticeably influence the formation of the flat bones of the skull. The calvarial bones are formed through an intramembranous process, in which mesenchymal cells differentiate directly into osteoblasts without an intermediate avascular cartilaginous template. It is possible that signals from cranial sutures and/or from the dura induce the angiogenesis necessary for intramembranous ossification. This would explain the lack of blood vessel and bone phenotypes in the skull of ΔVHL- and ΔHif-1α-mutant mice.

7.3.2 Hifs in Bone Regeneration and Repair

Angiogenesis is essential for bone repair. It has been proposed that at fracture sites mechanical loading stimuli, along with hypoxia that results when the vascular and nutrient supply is interrupted, initiate the events that lead to bone repair [29]. If angiogenesis is delayed, chondrocytic cells, rather than osteoblasts, make up the healing tissue. This suggests that Hifs play a role in allocating mesenchymal lineage during repair [22].

Distraction osteogenesis (DO) is valuable for examining the cellular mechanisms that couple angiogenesis and bone formation during repair and regeneration. In DO, intramembranous bone formation is induced by the application of an external fixation device that applies gradual mechanical distraction across an osteotomy [57]. This procedure leads to a close temporal and spatial relationship between bone formation and vascular proliferation [29]. DO has also been used to investigate the role of Hif-1α in bone healing. In ΔVHL mice, loss of VHL at sites of DO is accomplished by increases in Hif-1α protein, in VEGF-A mRNA and protein, and in endothelial cells, leading to more blood vessels and more dense woven bone [154]. At DO sites in ΔHif-1α mice, the opposite takes place, namely deficient angiogenesis and delayed bone consolidation

[154]. Additionally, the mRNA and protein expressions of VEGF-A and osteoblast markers Runx2, alkaline phosphatase (ALP), and osteocalcin (OC) are decreased, but increased in ΔVHL [89]. Perhaps not surprisingly, desferrioxamine (DFO), a small molecule that, when administered directly into the distraction gap blocks the PHD activity and thus elevates Hif-1α, can improve healing in a manner virtually identical to that seen when Hif-1α is activated [154]. These studies provide proof for the principle that a therapeutic approach that modulates the Hif pathway may speed bone healing.

Numerous studies have highlighted the role of VEGF-A receptor signaling in bone repair and regeneration. Both receptors, which have different affinities for the VEGF-A ligands [16], are expressed by osteoblasts [49, 142]. During normal DO, both VEGFR1 and VEGFR2 and all three VEGF-A isoform mRNAs are induced. Moreover, inhibition of VEGF-A activity in the distraction gap by antibody blockade of VEGFR1 and VEGFR2 leads to a dramatic decrease in bone formation and a smaller number of blood vessels [61].

7.4 Hifs and Osteoclasts

Bone development demands a continuous supply of bone-resorbing osteoclasts, cells that are derived from the monocyte lineage and are multinucleated. Experimental evidence in favor of a role of Hif-1α as a survival factor for osteoclasts has been reported recently. Mice that lack the transcription factor Fra2 or are impaired in leukemia inhibitory factor (LIF) signaling display giant osteoclasts, and their bone marrow is highly hypoxic. This lack of oxygen may be the consequence of a placental defect that at the same time causes Hif-1α protein to accumulate in the bone [10]. Formation of tartrate-resistant acid phosphatase (TRAP) positive cells from fetal liver progenitors is significantly augmented by hypoxia [10]. These findings suggest that hypoxia together with Hif-1α favor formation, activity, and survival of multinucleated osteoclasts.

When the mouse leukemic monocyte cell line RAW 264.7 is exposed to hypoxia, the expression of the osteoclast markers of calcitonin receptors and cathepsin K is increased and their differentiation into TRAP-positive osteoclast-like cells is favored [138]. Hypoxia also positively modulates osteoclastogenesis in vitro because the supporting osteoblastic stroma releases IGFII [34]. Lastly, cultured monocyte-derived osteoclasts upregulate the Hif pathway in hypoxic conditions [75].

VEGF-A regulates osteoclastic differentiation, migration, and activity. Cells of the monocyte lineage express VEGFR1, and VEGF-A can substitute for M-CSF as a costimulator to support osteoclastogenesis in the presence of the receptor activator for nuclear factor kappa-B ligand (RANKL) [75, 104]. Moreover, osteoclasts stimulate angiogenesis by producing a variety of proangiogenic factors [15, 146]. These findings are in line with the well-known antiangiogenic properties of antiresorptive agents such as bisphosphonates [15], and with the findings that macrophages that share the same lineage with osteoclasts, express numerous proangiogenic factors [86]. Macrophage survival and activity in pathological settings such as inflammation are Hif-1α-dependent [27].

7.5 Summary

This chapter has highlighted the critical role of hypoxia and Hif-1α in cartilage development and bone modeling, remodeling, and regeneration. It will now be important to identify molecular mechanisms that mediate the complex and multifaceted action of this transcription factor in chondrocytes, osteoblasts, and osteoclasts. Identifying these mechanisms will significantly expand our understanding of normal cellular adaptation to hypoxia as well as bone and cartilage homeostasis.

References

1. Akeno N, Robins J, Zhang M, Czyzyk-Krzeska MF, Clemens TL (2002) Induction of vascular endothelial growth factor by IGF-I in osteoblast-like cells is mediated by the PI3K signaling pathway through the hypoxia-inducible factor-2alpha. Endocrinology 143:420–425

2. Akiyama H, Chaboissier MC, Martin JF, Schedl A, de Crombrugghe B (2002) The transcription factor Sox9 has essential roles in successive steps of the chondrocyte differentiation pathway and is required for expression of Sox5 and Sox6. Genes Dev 16:2813–2828
3. Amarilio R, Viukov S, Sharir A, Eshkar-Oren I, Johnson R, Zelzer E (2007) Hif1alpha regulation of Sox9 is necessary to maintain differentiation of hypoxic prechondrogenic cells during early chondrogenesis. Development 134:3917–3928
4. Annunen P, Autio-Harmainen H, Kivirikko K (1998) The novel type II prolyl 4-hydroxylase is the main enzyme form in chondrocytes and capillary endothelial cells, whereas the type I predominates in most cells. J Biol Chem 273:5989–5992
5. Azad MB, Chen Y, Henson ES, Cizeau J, McMillan-Ward E, Israels SJ, Gibson SB (2008) Hypoxia induces autophagic cell death in apoptosis-competent cells through a mechanism involving BNIP3. Autophagy 4:195–204
6. Bernales S, McDonald KL, Walter P (2006) Autophagy counterbalances endoplasmic reticulum expansion during the unfolded protein response. PLoS Biol 4:e423
7. Berra E, Benizri E, Ginouves A, Volmat V, Roux D, Pouyssegur J (2003) HIF prolyl-hydroxylase 2 is the key oxygen sensor setting low steady-state levels of HIF-1alpha in normoxia. EMBO J 22:4082–4090
8. Bishop T, Lau K, Epstein A, Kim S, Jiang M, O'Rourke D, Pugh C, Gleadle J, Taylor M, Hodgkin J, Ratcliffe P (2004) Genetic analysis of pathways regulated by the von Hippel-Lindau tumor suppressor in *Caenorhabditis elegans*. PLoS Biol 2:e289
9. Bohensky J, Shapiro I, Leshinsky S, Terkhorn S, Adams C, Srinivas V (2007) HIF-1 regulation of chondrocyte apoptosis: induction of the autophagic pathway. Autophagy 3:207–214
10. Bozec A, Bakiri L, Hoebertz A, Eferl R, Schilling AF, Komnenovic V, Scheuch H, Priemel M, Stewart CL, Amling M, Wagner EF (2008) Osteoclast size is controlled by Fra-2 through LIF/LIF-receptor signalling and hypoxia. Nature 454:221–225
11. Bruick R (2000) Expression of the gene encoding the proapoptotic Nip3 protein is induced by hypoxia. Proc Natl Acad Sci U S A 97:9082–9087
12. Brunet LJ, McMahon JA, McMahon AP, Harland RM (1998) Noggin, cartilage morphogenesis, and joint formation in the mammalian skeleton. Science 280: 1455–1457
13. Bunger MK, Wilsbacher LD, Moran SM, Clendenin C, Radcliffe LA, Hogenesch JB, Simon MC, Takahashi JS, Bradfield CA (2000) Mop3 is an essential component of the master circadian pacemaker in mammals. Cell 103:1009–1017
14. Bunn HF, Poyton RO (1996) Oxygen sensing and molecular adaptation to hypoxia. Physiol Rev 76:839–885
15. Cackowski F, Roodman G (2007) Perspective on the osteoclast: an angiogenic cell? Ann N Y Academ Sci 1117:12–25
16. Carano RA, Filvaroff EH (2003) Angiogenesis and bone repair. Drug Discov Today 8:980–989
17. Carmeliet P, Dor Y, Herbert J, Fukumura D, Brusselmans K, Dewerchin M, Neeman M, Bono F, Abramovitch R, Maxwell P, Koch CJ, Ratcliffe P, Moons L, Jain RK, Collen D, Keshet E (1998) Role of HIF-1alpha in hypoxia mediated apoptosis, cell proliferation and tumour angiogenesis. Nature 394:485–490
18. Chan D, Suthphin P, Denko N, Giaccia A (2002) Role of prolyl hydroxylation in oncogenically stabilized hyoxia-inducible factor-1alpha. J Biol Chem 277:40112–40117
19. Chan D, Sutphin P, Yen S, Giaccia A (2005) Coordinate regulation of the oxygen-dependent degradation domains of hypoxia-inducible factor 1 alpha. Mol Cell Biol 25:6415–6426
20. Chan DA, Krieg AJ, Turcotte S, Giaccia AJ (2007) HIF gene expression in cancer therapy. Meth Enzymol 435:323–345
21. Chen EY, Fujinaga M, Giaccia AJ (1999) Hypoxic microenvironment within an embryo induces apoptosis and is essential for proper morphological development. Teratology 60:215–225
22. Choi I, Ahn J, Chung C, Cho T (2000) Vascular proliferation and blood supply during distraction osteogenesis: a scanning electron microscopic observation. J Orthop Res 18:698–705
23. Cohen T, Gitay-Goren H, Sharon R, Shibuya M, Halaban R, Levi B, Neufeld G (1995) VEGF121, a vascular endothelia growth factor (VEGF) isoform lacking heparin binding ability, requires cell-surface heparan sulfates for efficient binding to the VEGF receptors of human melanoma cells. J Biol Chem 270:11322–11326
24. Compernolle V, Brusselmans K, Acker T, Hoet P, Tjwa M, Beck H, Plaisance S, Dor Y, Keshet E, Lupu F, Nemery B, Dewerchin M, Van Veldhoven P, Plate K, Moons L, Collen D, Carmeliet P (2002) Loss of HIF-2alpha and inhibition of VEGF impair fetal lung maturation, whereas treatment with VEGF prevents fatal respiratory distress in premature mice. Nat Med 8:702–710
25. Compernolle V, Brusselmans K, Franco D, Moorman A, Dewerchin M, Collen D, Carmeliet P (2003) Cardia bifida, defective heart development and abnormal neural crest migration in embryos lacking hypoxia-inducible factor -1alpha. Cardiovascular Res 60:569–579
26. Cramer T, Schipani E, Johnson R, Swodoba B, Pfander D (2004) Expression of VEGF isoforms by epithelial chondrocytes during low-oxygen tension is Hif-1alpha dependent. Osteoarthr Cartil 12:433–439
27. Cramer T, Yamanishi Y, Clausen B, Forster I, Pawlinski R, Mackman N, Haase V, Jaenisch R, Corr M, Nizt V, Firestein G, Gerber H, Ferrara N, Johnson R (2003) Hif-1alpha is essential for myeloid cell-mediated inflammation. Cell 112:645–657
28. Dahl KC, Fryer B, Mack F, Compernolle V, Maltepe E, Adelman D, Carmeliet P, Simon M (2005) Hypoxia-inducible factors 1alpha and 2alpha regulate trophoblast differentiation. Mol Cell Biol 25:10479–10491
29. Danis A (2001) Mechanism of bone lengthening by the Ilizarov technique. Bull Mem Acad R Med Belg 156: 107–112
30. Egerbacher M, Haeusler G (2003) Integrins in growth plate cartilage. Pediatr Endocrinol Rev 1:2–8

31. Feldman DE, Chauhan V, Koong AC (2005) The unfolded protein response: a novel component of the hypoxic stress response in tumors. Mol Cancer Res 3:597–605
32. Ferrara N, Gerber H, LeCouter J (2003) The biology of VEGF and its receptors. Nat Med 9:669–676
33. Fukuda R, Zhang H, Kim JW, Shimoda L, Dang CV, Semenza GL (2007) HIF-1 regulates cytochrome oxidase subunits to optimize efficiency of respiration in hypoxic cells. Cell 129:111–122
34. Fukuoka H, Aoyama M, Miyazawa K, Asai K, Goto S (2005) Hypoxic stress enhances osteoclast differentiation via increasing IGF2 production by non-osteoclastic cells. Biochem Biophys Res Commun 328:885–894
35. Gardner LB, Corn PG (2008) Hypoxic regulation of mRNA expression. Cell Cycle 7:1916–1924
36. Gerber H, Malik A, GP Solar, Sherman D, Liang X, Meng G, Hong K, Marsters J, Ferrara N (2002) VEGF regulates haematopoietic stem cell survival by an internal autocrine loop mechanism. Nature 417:954–958
37. Gerber HP, Vu TH, Ryan AM, Kowalski J, Werb Z, Ferrara N (1999) VEGF couples hypertrophic cartilage remodeling, ossification and angiogenesis during endochondral bone formation. Nat Med 5:623–628
38. Giaccia A, Siim B, Johnson R (2003) HIF-1 as a target for drug development. Nat Rev Drug Discov 2:803–811
39. Giaccia AJ, Simon MC, Johnson R (2004) The biology of hypoxia: the role of oxygen sensing in development, normal function, and disease. Genes Dev 18:2183–2194
40. Gibson JS, Milner PI, White R, Fairfax TP, Wilkins RJ (2008) Oxygen and reactive oxygen species in articular cartilage: modulators of ionic homeostasis. Pflugers Arch 455:563–573
41. Goda N, Ryan H, Khadivi B, McNulty W, Rickert R, Johnson R (2003) Hypoxia-inducible factor 1alpha is essential for cell cycle arrest during hypoxia. Mol Cell Biol 23:359–369
42. Gordon J, Simon M (2007) Hypoxia-inducible factors: central regulators of the tumor phenotype. Curr Opin Genet Dev 17:71–77
43. Greijer AE, van der Groep P, Kemming D, Shvarts A, Semenza GL, Meijer GA, van de Wiel MA, Belien JA, van Diest PJ, van der Wall E (2005) Up-regulation of gene expression by hypoxia is mediated predominantly by hypoxia-inducible factor 1 (HIF-1). J Pathol 206:291–304
44. Grimmer C, Balbus N, Lang U, Aigner T, Cramer T, Muller L, Swoboda B, Pfander D (2006) Regulation of type II collagen synthesis during osteoarthritis by prolyl-4-hydroxylases: possible influence of low oxygen tension. Am J Pathol 169:491–502
45. Gu YZ, Hogenesch JB, Bradfield CA (2000) The PAS superfamily: sensors of environmental and developmental signals. Annu Rev Pharmacol Toxicol 40:519–561
46. Guo X, Day T, Jiang X, Garrett-Beal L, Topol L, Yang Y (2004) Wnt/beta-catenin signaling is sufficient and necessary for synovial joint formation. Genes Dev 18:2404–2417
47. Gustafsson M, Zheng X, Pereira T, Gradin K, Jin S, Lundkvist J, Ruas J, Poellinger L, Lendahl U, Bondesson M (2005) Hypoxia requires Notch signaling to maintain the undifferentiated cell state. Dev Cell 9:617–628
48. Haase VH (2005) The VHL tumor suppressor in development and disease: functional studies in mice by conditional gene targeting. Semin Cell Dev Biol 16: 564–574
49. Harper J, Gerstenfeld LC, Klagsbrun M (2001) Neuropilin-1 expression in osteogenic cells: down-regulation during differentiation of osteoblasts into osteocytes. J Cell Biochem 81:82–92
50. Hartmann C, Tabin C (2001) Wnt-14 plays a pivotal role in inducing synovial joint formation in the developing appendicular skeleton. Cell 104:341–351
51. Higgins DF, Kimura K, Iwano M, Haase VH (2008) Hypoxia-inducible factor signaling in the development of tissue fibrosis. Cell Cycle 7:1128–1132
52. Hirsila M, Koivunen P, Gunzler V, Kivirikko K, Myllyharju J (2003) Characterization of the human prolyl 4-hydroxylases that modify the hypoxia-inducible factor. J Biol Chem 278:30772–30780
53. Hofbauer K, Gess B, Lohaus C, Meyer H, Katschinski D, Kurtz A (2003) Oxygen tension regulates the expression of a group of procollagen hydroxylases. Eur J Biochem 270:4515–4522
54. Houck K, Ferrara N, Winer J, Cachianes G, Li B, Leung D (1991) The vascular endothelial growth factor family: identification of a fourth molecular species and characterization of alternative splicing of RNA. Mol Endocrinol 5:1806–1814
55. Hu CJ, Wang LY, Chodosh LA, Keith B, Simon MC (2003) Differential roles of hypoxia-inducible factor 1alpha (HIF-1alpha) and HIF-2alpha in hypoxic gene regulation. Mol Cell Biol 23:9361–9374
56. Huang W, Zhou X, Lefebvre V, de Crombrugghe B (2000) Phosphorylation of SOX9 by cyclic AMP-dependent protein kinase A enhances SOX9's ability to transactivate a Col2a1 chondrocyte-specific enhancer. Mol Cell Biol 20:4149–4158
57. Ilizarov GA (1990) Clinical application of the tension-stress effect for limb lengthening. Clin Orthop Relat Res 8–26
58. Ivan M, Kondo K, Yang H, Kim W, Valiando J, Ohh M, Salic A, Asara J, Lane W, Kaelin W (2001) HIFalpha targeted for VHL-mediated destruction by proline hydroxylation: imlications for O_2 sensing. Science 292:464–468
59. Iyer N, Kotch L, Agani F, Leung S, Laughner E, Wenger R, Gassmann M, Gearhart J, Lawler A, Yu A, Semenza G (1998) Cellular and developmental control of O_2 homeostasis by hypoxia-inducible factor 1alpha. Genes Dev 12:149–162
60. Jaakkola P, Mole D, Tian Y, Wilson M, Gielbert J, Gakell S, Kriegsheim A, Heberstreit H, Mukherji M, Schofield C, Maxwell P, Ratcliffe P (2001) Targeting of HIF-alpha to the von Hippel-Lindau ubiquitylation complex by O_2-regulated prolyl hydroxylation. Science 292:468–472
61. Jacobsen KA, Al-Aql ZS, Wan C, Fitch JL, Stapleton SN, Mason ZD, Cole RM, Gilbert SR, Clemens TL, Morgan EF, Einhorn TA, Gerstenfeld LC (2008) Bone formation during distraction osteogenesis is dependent on both VEGFR1 and VEGFR2 signaling. J Bone Miner Res 23:596–609

62. Jeong C, Lee H, Cha J, Kim J, Kim K, Kim J, Yoon D, Kim K (2007) Hypoxia-inducible factor-1alpha inhibits self-renewal of mouse embryonic stem cells in vitro via negative regulation of the leukemia inhibitory factor-STAT3 pathway. J Biol Chem 282:13672–13679
63. Jin S, White E (2008) Tumor suppression by autophagy through the management of metabolic stress. Autophagy 4:563–566
64. Jogi A, Ora I, Nilsson H, Lindeheim A, Makino Y, Poellinger L, Axelson H, Pahlman S (2002) Hypoxia alters gene expression in human neuroblastoma cells towards an immature and neural crest-like phenotype. Proc Natl Acad Sci 99:7021–7026
65. Kaelin W (2002) How oxygen makes its presence felt. Genes Dev 16:1441–1445
66. Kaelin W, Maher E (1998) The VHL tumor-suppressor gene paradigm. Trends Genet 14:423–426
67. Kallio PJ, Okamoto K, O'Brien S, Carrero P, Makino Y, Tanaka H, Poellinger L (1998) Signal transduction in hypoxic cells: inducible nuclear translocation and recruitment of the CBP/p300 coactivator by the hypoxia-inducible factor-1alpha. EMBO J 17:6573–6586
68. Kallio PJ, Wilson WJ, O'Brien S, Makino Y, Poellinger L (1999) Regulation of the hypoxia-inducible transcription factor 1alpha by the ubiquitin-proteasome pathway. J Biol Chem 274:6519–6525
69. Karsenty G (2003) The complexities of skeletal biology. Nature 423:316–318
70. Keith B, Adelman DM, Simon MC (2001) Targeted mutation of the murine arylhydrocarbon receptor nuclear translocator 2 (Arnt2) gene reveals partial redundancy with Arnt. Proc Natl Acad Sci U S A 98:6692–6697
71. Khan WS, Adesida AB, Hardingham TE (2007) Hypoxic conditions increase hypoxia-inducible transcription factor 2alpha and enhance chondrogenesis in stem cells from the infrapatellar fat pad of osteoarthritis patients. Arthritis Res Ther 9:R55
72. Khatri R, Schipani E (2008) About the importance of being desulfated. Genes Dev 22:2750–2754
73. Kim JW, Tchernyshyov I, Semenza GL, Dang CV (2006) HIF-1-mediated expression of pyruvate dehydrogenase kinase: a metabolic switch required for cellular adaptation to hypoxia. Cell Metab 3:177–185
74. Kingsley D (2001) Genetic control of bone and joint formation. Novartis Found Symp 232:213–222
75. Knowles HJ, Athanasou NA (2008) Hypoxia-inducible factor is expressed in giant cell tumour of bone and mediates paracrine effects of hypoxia on monocyte-osteoclast differentiation via induction of VEGF. J Pathol 215:56–66
76. Kornak U, Mundlos S (2003) Genetic disorders of the skeleton: a developmental approach. Am J Hum Genet 73:447–474
77. Koshiji M, Kageyama Y, Pete E, Horikawa I, Barrett J, Huang L (2004) Hif-1alpha induces cell cycle arrest by functionally counteracting Myc. EMBO J 23:1949–1956
78. Kotch L, Iyer N, Laughner E, Semenza G (1999) Defective vascularization of HIF 1 alpha null embryos is not associated with VEGF deficiency but with mesenchymal cell death. Dev Biol 209:254–267
79. Lafont JE, Talma S, Murphy CL (2007) Hypoxia-inducible factor 2alpha is essential for hypoxic induction of the human articular chondrocyte phenotype. Arthritis Rheum 56:3297–3306
80. Lando D, Peet DJ, Gorman JJ, Whelan DA, Whitelaw ML, Bruick RK (2002) FIH-1 is an asparaginyl hydroxylase enzyme that regulates the transcriptional activity of hypoxia-inducible factor. Genes Dev 16:1466–1471
81. Lee J, Siemann D, Koch C, Lord E (1996) Direct relationship between radiobiological hypoxia in tumors and monoclonal antibody detection of EF5 cellular adducts. Int J Cancer 67:372–378
82. Lee JW, Bae SH, Jeong JW, Kim SH, Kim KW (2004) Hypoxia-inducible factor (HIF-1)alpha: its protein stability and biological functions. Exp Mol Med 36:1–12
83. Lefebvre V, Smits P (2005) Transcriptional control of chondrocyte fate and differentiation. Birth Defects Res Part C Embryo Today 75:200–212
84. Leo C, Giaccia A, Denko N (2004) The hypoxic tumor microenvironment and gene expression. Semin Radiat Oncol 14:207–214
85. Levine B, Klionsky DJ (2004) Development by self-digestion: molecular mechanisms and biological functions of autophagy. Dev Cell 6:463–477
86. Lewis J, Lee J, Underwood J, Harris A, Lewis C (1999) Macrophage responses to hypoxia: relevance to disease mechanisms. J Leukoc Biol 66:889–900
87. Lin Q, Lee Y, Yun Z (2006) Differentiation arrest by hypoxia. J Biol Chem 281:30678–30683
88. Liu L, Simon MC (2004) Regulation of transcription and translation by hypoxia. Cancer Biol Ther 3:492–497
89. Liu XD, Deng LF, Wang J, Qi J, Zhou Q, Wang JS, Wei L, Zhu YP (2007) Regulation of hypoxia inducible factor-1alpha on osteoblast function in osteogenesis. Zhonghua Yi Xue Za Zhi 87:3357–3361
90. Liu XD, Deng LF, Wang J, Qi J, Zhou Q, Wang JS, Wei L, Zhu YP, Clemens T (2007) The regulation of hypoxia inducible factor-1alpha on osteoblast function in postmenopausal osteoporosis. Zhonghua Wai Ke Za Zhi 45:1274–1278
91. Logan M, Martin J, Nagy A, Lobe C, Olsen E, Tabin C (2002) Expression of Cre recombinase in the developing mouse limb bud driven by a Prx1 enhancer. Genesis 33:77–80
92. Lord E, Harwell L, Koch C (1993) Detection of hypoxic cells by monoclonal antibody recognizing 2-nitroimidazole adducts. Cancer Res 53:5721–5726
93. Mack F, Patel J, Biju M, Haase V, Simon M (2005) Decreased growth of Vhl−/− fibrosarcomas is associated with elevated levels of cyclin kinase inhibitors p21 and p27. Mol Cell Biol 25:4565–4578
94. Maes C, Carmeliet P, Moermans K, Stockmans I, Smets N, Collen D, Bouillon R, Carmeliet G (2002) Impaired angiogenesis and endochondral bone formation in mice lacking the vascular endothelial growth factor isoforms VEGF164 and VEGF188. Mech Dev 111:61–73
95. Maes C, Stockmans I, Moermans K, Looveren RV, Smets N, Carmeliet P, Bouillon R, Carmeliet G (2004) Soluble VEGF isoforms are essential for establishing

epiphyseal vascularization and regulating chondrocyte development and survival. J Clin Invest 113:188–199
96. Makino Y, Cao R, Svensson K, Bertilsson G, Asman M, Tanaka H, Cao Y, Berkenstam A, Poellinger L (2001) Inhibitory PAS domain protein is a negative regulator of hypoxia-inducible gene expression. Nature 414: 550–554
97. Maxwell P, Wiesener M, Chang G, Clifford S, Vaux E, Cockman M, Wykoff C, Pugh C, Maher E, Ratcliffe P (1999) The tumour suppressor protein VHL targets hypoxia-inducible factors for oxygen-dependent proteolysis. Nature 399:271–275
98. Maynard MA, Qi H, Chung J, Lee EH, Kondo Y, Hara S, Conaway RC, Conaway JW, Ohh M (2003) Multiple splice variants of the human HIF-3 alpha locus are targets of the von Hippel-Lindau E3 ubiquitin ligase complex. J Biol Chem 278:11032–11040
99. Min J, Yang H, Ivan M, Gertler F, Kaelin WG Jr, Pavletich N (2002) Structure of an HIF-1alpha-pVHL complex: hydroxyproline recognition in signaling. Science 296:1886–1889
100. Mitchell JA, Yochim JM (1968) Intrauterine oxygen tension during the estrous cycle in the rat: its relation to uterine respiration and vascular activity. Endocrinology 83:701–705
101. Morrison SJ, Csete M, Groves AK, Melega W, Wold B, Anderson DJ (2000) Culture in reduced levels of oxygen promotes clonogenic sympathoadrenal differentiation by isolated neural crest stem cells. J Neurosci 20:7370–7376
102. Murphy CL, Polak JM (2004) Control of human articular chondrocyte differentiation by reduced oxygen tension. J Cell Physiol 199:451–459
103. Myllyharju J, Kivirikko K (2004) Collagen, modifying enzymes and their mutations in humans, flies and worms. Trends Genet 20:33–43
104. Niida S, Kaku M, Amano H, Yoshida H, Kataoka H, Nishikawa S, Tanne K, Maeda N, Nishikawa S, Kodama H (1999) Vascular endothelial growth factor can substitute for macrophage colony-stimulating factor in the support of osteoclastic bone resorption. J Exp Med 190:293–298
105. Pacifici M, Jozzo R (1998) Remodeling of the rough endoplasmic reticulum during stimulation of procollagen secretion by ascorbic acid in cultured chondrocytes. A biochemical and morphological study. J Biol Chem 263:2483–2492
106. Papandreou I, Cairns RA, Fontana L, Lim AL, Denko NC (2006) HIF-1 mediates adaptation to hypoxia by actively downregulating mitochondrial oxygen consumption. Cell Metab 3:187–197
107. Papandreou I, Lim AL, Laderoute K, Denko NC (2008) Hypoxia signals autophagy in tumor cells via AMPK activity, independent of HIF-1, BNIP3, and BNIP3L. Cell Death Differ 15:1572–1581
108. Park SK, Dadak AM, Haase VH, Fontana L, Giaccia AJ, Johnson RS (2003) Hypoxia-induced gene expression occurs solely through the action of hypoxia-inducible factor 1alpha (HIF-1alpha): role of cytoplasmic trapping of HIF-2alpha. Mol Cell Biol 23:4959–4971
109. Peng J, Zhang L, Drysdale L, Fong GH (2000) The transcription factor EPAS-1/hypoxia-inducible factor 2alpha plays an important role in vascular remodeling. Proc Natl Acad Sci U S A 97:8386–8391
110. Pfander D, Cramer T, Schipani E, Johnson R (2003) HIF-1alpha controls extracellular matrix synthesis by epiphyseal chondrocytes. J Cell Sci 116:1819–1826
111. Pfander D, Kobayashi T, Knight M, Zelzer E, Chan D, Olsen B, Giaccia A, Johnson R, Haase V, Schipani E (2004) Deletion of Vhlh in chondrocytes reduces cell proliferation and increases matrix deposition during growth plate development. Development 131:2497–2508
112. Pouyssegur J, Dayan F, Mazure NM (2006) Hypoxia signalling in cancer and approaches to enforce tumour regression. Nature 441:437–443
113. Provot S, Zinyk D, Gunes Y, Khatri R, Le Q, Kronenberg H, Johnson R, Longaker M, Giaccia A, Schipani E (2007) Hif-1alpha regulates differentiation of limb bud mesenchyme and joint development. J Cell Biol 177:451–464
114. Rankin EB, Giaccia AJ (2008) The role of hypoxia-inducible factors in tumorigenesis. Cell Death Differ 15:678–685
115. Ratcliffe P, Pugh C, Maxwell P (2000) Targeting tumors through the HIF system. Nat Med 12: 1315–1316
116. Raval RR, Lau KW, Tran MG, Sowter HM, Mandriota SJ, Li JL, Pugh CW, Maxwell PH, Harris AL, Ratcliffe PJ (2005) Contrasting properties of hypoxia-inducible factor 1 (HIF-1) and HIF-2 in von Hippel-Lindau-associated renal cell carcinoma. Mol Cell Biol 25:5675–5686
117. Rios EJ, Fallon M, Wang J, Shimoda LA (2005) Chronic hypoxia elevates intracellular pH and activates Na^+/H^+ exchange in pulmonary arterial smooth muscle cells. Am J Physiol Lung Cell Mol Physiol 289:L867–874
118. Robins JC, Akeno N, Mukherjee A, Dalal RR, Aronow BJ, Koopman P, Clemens TL (2005) Hypoxia induces chondrocyte-specific gene expression in mesenchymal cells in association with transcriptional activation of Sox9. Bone 37:313–322
119. Robinson C, Stringer S (2001) The splice variants of vascular endothelial growth factor (VEGF) and their receptors. J Cell Sci 114:853–865
120. Rodesch F, Simon P, Donner C, Jauniaux E (1992) Oxygen measurements in endometrial and trophoblastic tissues during early pregnancy. Obstet Gynecol 80:283–285
121. Ryan HE, Lo J, Johnson RS (1998) HIF 1 alpha is required for solid tumor formation and embryonic vascularization. EMBO J 17:3005–3015
122. Sacchetti B, Funari A, Michienzi S, DiCesare S, Piersanti S, Saggio I, Tagliafico E, Ferrari S, Robey P, Riminucci M, Bianco P (2007) Self-renewing osteoprogenitors in bone marrow sinusoids can organize a hematopoietic microenvironment. Cell 131:324–326
123. Sainson R, Harris A (2006) Hypoxia-regulated differentiation: let's step it up a Notch. Trends Mol Med 12:141–143
124. Salim A, Nacamuli R, Morgan E, Giaccia A, Longaker M (2004) Transient changes in oxygen tension inhibit osteogenic differentiation and Runx2 expression in osteoblasts. J Biol Chem 279:40007–40016

125. Schipani E, Ryan HE, Didrickson S, Kobayashi T, Knight M, Johnson RS (2001) Hypoxia in cartilage: HIF-1alpha is essential for chondrocyte growth arrest and survival. Genes Dev 15:2865–2876
126. Scortegagna M, Ding K, Oktay Y, Gaur A, Thurmond F, Yan LJ, Marck BT, Matsumoto AM, Shelton JM, Richardson JA, Bennett MJ, Garcia JA (2003) Multiple organ pathology, metabolic abnormalities and impaired homeostasis of reactive oxygen species in Epas1$^{-/-}$ mice. Nat Genet 35:331–340
127. Seagroves T, Johnson R (2002) Two HIFs may be better than one. Cancer Cell 1:211–213
128. Seagroves T, Ryan H, Lu H, Routers B, Knapp M, Thibault P, Laderoute K, Johnson R (2001) Transcription factor HIF-1 is necessary mediator of the Pasteur effect in mammalian cells. Mol Cell Biol 21:3436–3444
129. Semenza G (2008) Mitochondrial autophagy: life and breath of the cell. Autophagy 4:534–536
130. Semenza GL (2003) Targeting HIF-1 for cancer therapy. Nat Rev Cancer 3:721–732
131. Settembre C, Arteaga-Solis E, McKee MD, de Pablo R, Al Awqati Q, Ballabio A, Karsenty G (2008) Proteoglycan desulfation determines the efficiency of chondrocyte autophagy and the extent of FGF signaling during endochondral ossification. Genes Dev 22:2645–2650
132. Shapiro I, Mansfield K, Evans S, Lord E, Koch C (1997) Chondrocytes in the endochondral growth cartilage are not hypoxic. Am J Physiol 272:C1134–C1143
133. Shibuya M (2006) Differential roles of vascular endothelial growth factor receptor-1 and receptor-2 in angiogenesis. J Biochem Mol Biol 39:469–478
134. Shintani T, Klionsky DJ (2004) Autophagy in health and disease: a double-edged sword. Science 306:990–995
135. Simon MC, Keith B (2008) The role of oxygen availability in embryonic development and stem cell function. Nat Rev Mol Cell Biol 9:285–296
136. Smits P, Li P, Mandel J, Zhang Z, Deng JM, Behringer RR, de Crombrugghe B, Lefebvre V (2001) The transcription factors L-Sox5 and Sox6 are essential for cartilage formation. Dev Cell 1:277–290
137. Sowter HM, Ratcliffe PJ, Watson P, Greenberg AH, Harris AL (2001) HIF-1-dependent regulation of hypoxic induction of the cell death factors BNIP3 and NIX in human tumors. Cancer Res 61:6669–6673
138. Srinivasan S, Avadhani NG (2007) Hypoxia-mediated mitochondrial stress in RAW264.7 cells induces osteoclast-like TRAP-positive cells. Ann N Y Acad Sci 1117: 51–61
139. Steinbrech DS, Mehrara BJ, Saadeh PB, Chin G, Dudziak ME, Gerrets RP, Gittes GK, Longaker MT (1999) Hypoxia regulates VEGF expression and cellular proliferation by osteoblasts in vitro. Plast Reconstr Surg 104:738–747
140. Stewart A, Houston B, Farquharson C (2006) Elevated expression of hypoxia inducible factor-2alpha in terminally differentiating growth plate chondrocytes. J Cell Physiol 206:435–440
141. Storm E, Kingsley D (1999) GDF5 coordinates bone and joint formation during digit development. Dev Biol 209:11–27
142. Street J, Bao M, deGuzman L, Bunting S, Peale FV Jr, Ferrara N, Steinmetz H, Hoeffel J, Cleland JL, Daugherty A, van Bruggen N, Redmond HP, Carano RA, Filvaroff EH (2002) Vascular endothelial growth factor stimulates bone repair by promoting angiogenesis and bone turnover. Proc Natl Acad Sci U S A 99:9656–9661
143. Studer L, Csete M, Lee SH, Kabbani N, Walikonis J, Wold B, McKay R (2000) Enhanced proliferation, survival, and dopaminergic differentiation of CNS precursors in lowered oxygen. J Neurosci 20: 7377–7383
144. Svodoba K (1998) Chondrocyte-matrix attachment complexes mediate survival and differentiation. Microsc Res Tech 43:111–122
145. Takahashi Y, Takahashi S, Shiga Y, Yoshimi T, Miura T (2000) Hypoxic induction of prolyl 4-hydroxylase alpha (I) in cultured cells. J Biol Chem 275: 14139–14146
146. Tanaka Y, Abe M, Hiasa M, Oda A, Amou H, Nakano A, Takeuchi K, Kitazoe K, Kido S, Inoue D, Moriyama K, Hashimoto T, Ozaki S, Matsumoto T (2007) Myeloma cell-osteoclast interaction enhances angiogenesis together with bone resorption: a role for vascular endothelial cell growth factor and osteopontin. Clin Cancer Res 13:816–823
147. ten Berge D, Brouwer A, Korving J, Martin JF, Meijlink F (1998) Prx1 and Prx2 in skeletogenesis: roles in the craniofacial region, inner ear and limbs. Development 125:3831–3842
148. Tian H, Hammer RE, Matsumoto AM, Russell DW, McKnight SL (1998) The hypoxia-responsive transcription factor EPAS1 is essential for catecholamine homeostasis and protection against heart failure during embryonic development. Genes Dev 12:3320–3324
149. Tischer E, Mitchell R, Hartman T, Silva M, Gospodarowicz D, Fiddes J, Abraham J (1991) The human gene for vascular endothelial growth factor. Multiple protein forms are encoded through alternative exon splicing. J Biol Chem 266:11947–11954
150. Tracy K, Dibling BC, Spike BT, Knabb JR, Schumacker P, Macleod KF (2007) BNIP3 is an RB/E2F target gene required for hypoxia-induced autophagy. Mol Cell Biol 27:6229–6242
151. Tsang K, Chan D, Cheslett D, Chan W, So C, Melhado I, Chan T, Kwan K, Hunziker E, Yamada Y, Bateman J, Cheung K, Cheah K (2007) Surviving endoplasmic reticulum stress is coupled to altered chondrocyte differentiation and function. PLoS Biol 5:e44
152. Ullah MS, Davies AJ, Halestrap AP (2006) The plasma membrane lactate transporter MCT4, but not MCT1, is up-regulated by hypoxia through a HIF-1alpha-dependent mechanism. J Biol Chem 281:9030–9037
153. Vu T, Shipley J, Bergers G, Berger J, Helms J, Hanahan D, Shapiro S, Senior R, Werb Z (1998) MMP-9/gelatinase B is a key regulator of growth plate angiogenesis and apoptosis of hypertrophic chondrocytes. Cell 93:411–422
154. Wan C, Gilbert SR, Wang Y, Cao X, Shen X, Ramaswamy G, Jacobsen KA, Alaql ZS, Eberhardt AW, Gerstenfeld LC, Einhorn TA, Deng L, Clemens TL (2008) Activation of the hypoxia-inducible factor-1alpha pathway accelerates bone regeneration. Proc Natl Acad Sci U S A 105:686–691

155. Wang GL, Jiang BH, Rue EA, Semenza GL (1995) Hypoxia-inducible factor 1 is a basic-helix-loop-helix-PAS heterodimer regulated by cellular O_2 tension. Proc Natl Acad Sci U S A 92:5510–5514
156. Wang GL, Semenza GL (1993) General involvement of hypoxia-inducible factor 1 in transcriptional response to hypoxia. Proc Natl Acad Sci U S A 90:4304–4308
157. Wang V, Davis DA, Haque M, Huang LE, Yarchoan R (2005) Differential gene up-regulation by hypoxia-inducible factor-1alpha and hypoxia-inducible factor-2alpha in HEK293T cells. Cancer Res 65:3299–3306
158. Wang Y, Wan C, Deng L, Liu X, Cao X, Gilbert S, Bouxsein M, Faugere M, Guldberg R, Gerstenfeld L, Haase V, Johnson R, Schipani E, Clemens T (2007) The hypoxia-inducible factor alpha pathway couples angiogenesis to osteogenesis during skeletal development. J Clin Invest 117:1616–1626
159. Weidemann A, Johnson RS (2008) Biology of HIF-1alpha. Cell Death Differ 15:621–627
160. Wenger RH, Rolfs A, Kvietikova I, Spielmann P, Zimmermann DR, Gassmann M (1997) The mouse gene for hypoxia-inducible factor-1alpha - genomic organization, expression and characterization of an alternative first exon and 5′ flanking sequence. Eur J Biochem 246:155–165
161. Wiesener MS, Jurgensen JS, Rosenberger C, Scholze CK, Horstrup JH, Warnecke C, Mandriota S, Bechmann I, Frei UA, Pugh CW, Ratcliffe PJ, Bachmann S, Maxwell PH, Eckardt KU (2003) Widespread hypoxia-inducible expression of HIF-2alpha in distinct cell populations of different organs. FASEB J 17:271–273
162. Wykoff C, Pugh C, Maxwell P, Harris A, Ratcliffe P (2000) Identification of novel hypoxia dependent and independent target genes of the von Hippel-Lindau (VHL) tumor suppressor by mRNA differential expression profiling. Oncogene 19: 6297–6305
163. Xu Y, Malladi P, Chiou M, Bekerman E, Giaccia AJ, Longaker MT (2007) In vitro expansion of adipose-derived adult stromal cells in hypoxia enhances early chondrogenesis. Tissue Eng 13:2981–2993
164. Yorimitsu T, Klionsky D (2007) Eating the endoplasmic reticulum: quality control by autophagy. Trends Cell Biol 17:279–285
165. Yun Z, Lin Q, Giaccia A (2005) Adaptive myogenesis under hypoxia. Mol Cell Biol 25:3040–3055
166. Yun Z, Maecker H, Johnson R, Giaccia A (2002) Inhibition of PPAR gamma 2 gene expression by the HIF-1-regulated gene DEC-1/Stra13 a mechanism for regulation of adipogenesis by hypoxia. Dev Cell 2:331–341
167. Zelzer E, Glotzer D, Hartmann C, Thomas D, Fukai N, Soker S, Olsen B (2001) Tissue specific regulation of VEGF expression during bone development requires Cbfa1/Runx2. Mech Dev 106:97–106
168. Zelzer E, Levy Y, Kahana C, Shilo B, Rubinstein M, Cohen B (1998) Insulin induces transcription of target genes through the hypoxia-inducible factor 1 alpha. EMBO J 17:5085–5094
169. Zelzer E, Mamluk R, Ferrara N, Johnson R, Schipani E, Olsen B (2004) VEGFA is necessary for chondrocyte survival during bone development. Development 131:2161–2171
170. Zelzer E, McLean W, Ng YS, Fukai N, Reginato AM, Lovejoy S, D'Amore PA, Olsen BR (2002) Skeletal defects in VEGF(120/120) mice reveal multiple roles for VEGF in skeletogenesis. Development 129:1893–1904
171. Zelzer E, Olsen B (2005) Multiple roles of vascular endothelial growth factor (VEGF) in skeletal development, growth and repair. Curr Top Dev Biol 65:169–187
172. Zhang H, Bosch-Marce M, Shimoda LA, Tan YS, Baek JH, Wesley JB, Gonzalez FJ, Semenza GL (2008) Mitochondrial autophagy is an HIF-1-dependent adaptive metabolic response to hypoxia. J Biol Chem 283:10892–10903
173. Zhang K, Kaufman R (2006) Protein folding in the endoplasmic reticulum and the unfolded protein response. Handb Exp Pharmacol 172:69–91

8. BMP Signaling in Skeletogenesis

Kristine D. Estrada and Karen M. Lyons

8.1 Introduction

Bone is a dynamic tissue that provides skeletal support to the body and is essential in the maintenance of hematopoiesis and calcium homeostasis. Bone development and remodeling are tightly regulated by local paracrine factors and systemic hormones. Bone morphogenic proteins (BMPs) were first identified in the 1960s as proteins with the ability to induce ectopic cartilage and bone formation in vivo [87]. The proteins, however, were not identified until the late 1980s, when several polypeptides with BMP activity were cloned and purified [94]. To date, more than 20 BMP-related proteins have been identified and characterized. These molecules constitute the BMP family of secreted factors and form a subgroup of the transforming growth factor β (TGFβ) superfamily. Extensive studies have shown that BMPs are also essential for nonosteogenic developmental processes. For example, BMPs play roles in dorsal-ventral patterning, specification of the epidermis, development of neuronal phenotypes, tooth development, and regulation of apoptosis [10, 16, 21, 26, 61, 105]. The mechanisms by which BMPs regulate these processes will not be discussed here. This chapter will focus on how BMP signaling and crosstalk between other signaling pathways controls chondrogenic, osteogenic, and adipogenic processes.

8.2 The BMP Signaling pathway

The regulation of cellular responses by BMPs is mediated by at least two distinct pathways: the canonical Smad pathway and the noncanonical mitogen-activated protein kinase (MAPK) pathways [11, 53, 89]. BMP signaling is transduced through type I and type II transmembrane serine/threonine kinase receptors. So far, three type II receptors that bind to the BMP ligands have been identified: type II BMP receptor (BMPRII), and type IIA and IIB activin receptors (ActRIIA and ActRIIB) [38, 64, 74, 96]. Three type I receptors have also been identified: activin receptor-like kinase (ALK) 2, ALK3/BMPRIA, and ALK6/BMPRIB [42, 51, 85]. The pattern of oligomerization of the type I and type II BMP receptors is flexible and susceptible to modulation by ligand binding. Specifically, prior to ligand binding, a low level of preformed type I and II BMP heteromeric complexes is present on the cell surface. However, the major fraction of BMP receptors is recruited into the heteromeric complexes only after ligand binding [19]. Binding of BMP-2 to preformed heteromeric BMP receptor complexes triggers the canonical Smad pathway, whereas binding of BMP-2 with the consequent formation of heteromeric receptor complexes triggers the MAPK pathway [63].

F. Bronner et al. (eds.), *Bone and Development*, Topics in Bone Biology 6,
DOI 10.1007/978-1-84882-822-3_8, © Springer-Verlag London Limited 2010

In the canonical Smad pathway, the type II receptors phosphorylate serine and threonine residues of the type I receptors upon ligand binding. In turn, activated type I receptors phosphorylate and thereby activate a subgroup of the Smad family of proteins, called receptor-regulated Smads (R-Smads: Smad1, 5, and 8). Activation is at serines present in their conserved C-terminal SSXS motif. Subsequently, the activated R-Smads form a trimeric complex with a common-partner Smad, Smad4, a component of both the TGFβ and BMP signaling pathways. The R-Smad/Smad4 complex translocates into the nucleus and regulates the transcription of genes by interacting with the DNA-binding proteins or by binding directly to the DNA containing Smad-binding elements. In the noncanonical Smad signaling pathway, BMPs signal via the MAPK pathway by activating TGFβ activated kinase 1 (TAK1). TAK1 leads to the activation of several MAPKs, including JNK, p38, and extracellular signal-regulated kinases (ERKs) [57, 89].

Several mechanisms regulate the duration and intensity of BMP signaling. BMP-mediated responses are regulated extracellularly by antagonists, such as decorin, noggin, and chordin, while BMP responses are regulated intracellularly through attenuation of R-Smad activity by scaffolding proteins that can sequester R-Smad proteins, by inhibitory phosphorylation of R-Smads by MAPK that blocks their nuclear entry, and by the actions of the inhibitory Smads (I-Smads), Smads6 and 7.

I-Smads are structurally related to R-Smads, but lack the C-terminal phosphorylation site present on R-Smads. I-Smads can act as intracellular antagonists of BMP signaling by forming stable associations with activated type I receptors, thereby preventing the phosphorylation of R-Smads [28, 59]. I-Smads can also compete with activated R-Smads for interaction with Smad4 [24]. I-Smads inhibit BMP signaling by recruiting the Smad ubiquitin regulatory factor (Smurf) family of E3 ubiquitin ligases to their respective type I receptors, causing the ubiquitination and degradation of activated type I receptors [37, 58, 83, 84].

8.3 BMP Signaling in Mesenchymal Cell Condensation and Commitment to Chondrogenic Lineage

The process of bone formation begins with aggregation and condensation of mesenchymal cells. This process is associated with an increase in cell–cell and cell–matrix contacts and interactions, which are the result of increased expression and activity of cell adhesion molecules (CAMs), such as neural cadherin (N-cadherin) and neural cell adhesion molecule (N-CAM). N-cadherin interacts with the actin cytoskeleton through the formation of a functional complex with cytoplasmic catenins, such as α- and β-catenin [25, 60]. The spatiotemporal expression pattern of N-cadherin in the developing limb bud suggests that it is required in chondrogenesis. In turn, when N-cadherin activity is disrupted in vitro by NCD-2, an antibody directed against the functional region of N-cadherin, cell condensation and chondrogenesis are inhibited in the micromass cultures of the limb-bud mesenchymal cells. Inhibiting N-cadherin activity in vivo interferes with the development of the embryonic limb bud [65].

BMP signaling is essential in prechondrogenic condensations, with inhibition of BMP signaling by overexpression of either Smad7 [30] or noggin [6, 71] blocking condensation. BMPs promote mesenchymal cell condensation partly by upregulating N-cadherin expression and function [22]. This may involve crosstalk with the Wnt signaling pathway, because BMP-2 modulates the expression of β-catenin and Wnt family members, including Wnt-3a and Wnt-7a, in high-density micromass cultures of the C3H10T1/2 mesenchymal progenitor cell line [15]. Specifically, BMP-2 upregulates Wnt-3a expression and overexpression of Wnt-3a enhances BMP-2-mediated chondrogenesis of C3H10T1/2 cells through the stabilization of β-catenin and regulation of N-cadherin-mediated adhesion [14]. In contrast, BMP-2 downregulates Wnt-7a expression [15] and retroviral expression of Wnt-7a blocks the progression of condensation of limb-bud micromass cultures through alterations in the expression of CAMs [82]. It can be inferred from these studies that crosstalk between BMP and Wnt signaling pathways regulates the initial events in mesenchymal condensation and promotes the commitment of these cells to the chondrogenic lineage.

8.4 BMP Signaling in Chondrogenesis

Bone is formed by intramembranous or endochondral ossification [44, 72, 102]. Intramembranous ossification leads to the formation of flat bones, especially those found in the skull, where mesenchymal cells condense and directly differentiate into osteoblasts. Endochondral ossification is the process by which most other bones are formed. Subsequently, mesenchymal cells condense and then differentiate into chondrocytes that form a matrix template, the growth plate, which is invaded by blood vessels and osteoblasts to initiate ossification.

The chondrocytes in the growth plate undergo a complicated differentiation program of proliferation, maturation, and apoptosis [44, 72, 104]. At the center of condensation, mesenchymal cells differentiate into round, slowly proliferating chondrocytes that express various extracellular matrix and CAMs, such as type II collagen, aggrecan, N-cadherin, and N-CAM, as well as the transcription factor, Sox9. The cells at the border of condensation form the perichondrium. The chondrocytes then align to form a columnar layer of flattened cells that proliferate rapidly and express low levels of the transcription factors, Runx2 and Osterix. Chondrocytes then exit the cell cycle to undergo hypertrophic differentiation and to express the signaling factor, Indian hedgehog (Ihh), as well as type-X collagen. The enlarged, hypertrophic chondrocytes terminally differentiate, mineralize, and undergo apoptosis. Expression of type-X collagen, Runx2, and growth factors that control chondrocyte proliferation and differentiation is enhanced in these cells. Following chondrocyte apoptosis, the residual cartilage matrix serves as a scaffold for trabecular bone.

During embryonic development, BMP signaling is essential for chondrogenesis. Mutations of individual BMPs, as well as compound deletions of either type-I BMP receptors or R-Smads, result in skeletal defects [40, 49, 73, 81, 98]. Moreover, individual BMPs and type-I BMP receptors are expressed in distinct and overlapping regions of the growth plate; this suggests that BMP molecules act in synergy to mediate chondrogenic events [13, 27, 50, 52, 62, 103].

8.4.1 Effect of BMP Signaling on Sox9 Expression

One of the earliest events in chondrogenesis is the commitment of mesenchymal cells to the chondrogenic lineage. Sox9, a member of the Sry-related high-mobility superfamily of transcription factors, is essential in this process. Sox9 is expressed in all cartilage primordia [3], specifically in prechondrogenic condensations during embryogenesis [95]. In mouse chimeras, *Sox9* null cells do not participate in mesenchymal condensations and fail to express chondrocyte-specific markers, such as type-II collagen and aggrecan [3]. Sox9 also plays a role in chondrocyte differentiation and maturation. *Sox9* haploinsufficiency in vivo results in defective cartilage primordia and premature mineralization [4]. In vitro, both $Sox9^{+/-}$ and $Sox9^{-/-}$ mouse embryonic stem cells show reduced type-II collagen expression and Alcian blue staining, exhibiting defects in maturation [23]. Several studies indicate that BMP signaling directly regulates *Sox9* expression. In particular, *Sox9* expression is upregulated in vitro in BMP-2-induced chondrogenesis of C3H10T1/2 cells and in mouse embryonic fibroblasts. In both cell types, *Sox9* expression is required for BMP-2-mediated chondrogenesis. When antisense *Sox9* nucleotides downregulate *Sox9* expression and when Sox9 expression is downregulated by *Sox9*-targeted siRNA, type-II collagen expression and Alcian blue staining are reduced [69, 101]. The regulation of *Sox9* expression by BMP is direct; a

CCAAT box on the *Sox9* promoter is the regulatory sequence responsible for BMP-2-induced *Sox9* expression [69]. The mechanism by which BMP-2 activates *Sox9* expression is attributed to BMP-2-induced association of NF-Y transcription factors with p300, which may contribute to chromatin remodeling at the *Sox9* proximal promoter region [68, 69].

8.4.2 Crosstalk Between BMP Signaling and Other Signaling Pathways: Ihh/PTHrP and FGF

One of the other signal pathways besides BMP that regulates chondrocyte proliferation and differentiation involves the secreted signaling factors, Ihh and parathyroid hormone-related protein (PTHrP). Loss of *Ihh* leads to reduced proliferation and premature maturation of chondrocytes [80]. Similarly, loss of PTHrP results in increased chondrocyte differentiation and accelerated bone growth [35]. *Ihh* is initially expressed in early mesenchymal condensations and, with the initiation of hypertrophic differentiation, it becomes restricted to prehypertrophic chondrocytes. Ihh stimulates the production of PTHrP in the periarticular region of the developing bone. Ihh expression is suppressed when PTHrP signals its receptor, PP-R, which is expressed at high levels in the transitional region between the proliferating and hypertrophic chondrocytes [45, 90]. The interaction between Ihh and PTHrP constitutes a negative feedback loop that regulates hypertrophic differentiation by keeping the chondrocytes in the proliferative state and thereby controlling bone growth (Fig. 8.1d, f).

BMP signaling interacts with the Ihh/PTHrP pathway (see Chap. 4) by increasing the Ihh expression in prehypertrophic chondrocytes (Fig. 8.1h) [54, 55]. Consequently, Ihh upregulates the BMP expression in the adjacent perichondrium and proliferating chondrocytes (Fig. 8.1g). This creates in a positive feedback loop between the two pathways to maintain the rate of chondrocyte proliferation [55, 70]. Evidence that the *Ihh* promoter contains BMP-responsive elements and is activated by treatment with BMP indicates direct regulation of *Ihh* expression by BMPs [73, 77]. Additional evidence of direct

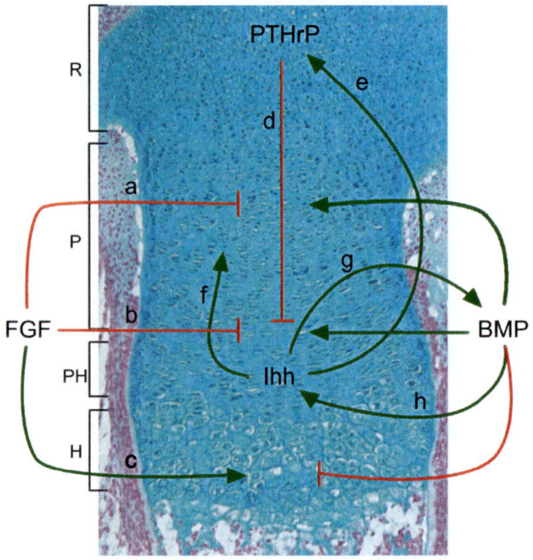

Figure 8.1. Crosstalk between BMP signaling and the Ihh/PTHrP and FGF signaling pathways. FGF signaling has the opposite effect of BMP signaling on chondrogenesis. FGFs inhibit proliferation (*a*), hypertrophic differentiation (*b*), and promote terminal differentiation (*c*). BMP signaling interacts with the Ihh/PTHrP feedback loop to maintain the rate of chondrocyte proliferation and to regulate hypertrophic differentiation. PTHrP inhibits hypertrophic differentiation by maintaining chondrocytes in the proliferative state (*d*). Ihh stimulates the expression of PTHrP in the periarticular region (*e*). Ihh is expressed in the prehypertrophic region and promotes chondrocyte proliferation (*f*). Ihh and BMPs promote the expression of each other (*g*, *h*). *R* resting zone; *P* proliferative zone; *PH* prehypertrophic zone; *H* hypertrophic zone.

regulation comes from Gli transcription factors that upregulate the promoter activity of *Bmp*-4 and -7, as key effectors of hedgehog signaling [39]. Even though both the BMP and Ihh/PTHrP pathways regulate chondrocyte proliferation, neither pathway acts downstream of the other. In particular, double treatment with BMP-2 and cyclopamine, which blocks Ihh signaling, also blocks chondrocyte proliferation. Similarly, overexpression of Ihh does not overcome the block to chondrocyte proliferation, induced by treatment with the BMP antagonist, noggin [55]. Regulation of PTHrP expression by Ihh is also independent of BMP signaling [55, 73].

BMP signaling also interacts with the fibroblast growth factor (FGF) signaling pathways, which plays an important role in chondrogenesis (see Chap. 6 of this volume). This is suggested by the expression patterns of FGFs and their receptors in distinct regions of the growth plate and at various stages of endochondral bone formation [67, 97]. The role of FGF receptors as negative regulators of chondrocyte proliferation has been demonstrated in humans with missense activating mutations in *Fgfr3* [75, 79]. In addition, *Fgf18* deficiency in mice leads to increased zones of proliferative and hypertrophic chondrocytes [48, 66]. These studies indicate that the effect of FGF signaling on chondrocyte proliferation is the opposite of BMP signaling (Fig. 8.1a–c): FGF signaling inhibits chondrocyte proliferation, whereas BMP signaling promotes it. Similarly, FGF signaling inhibits *Ihh* expression, while BMP signaling induces it [48]. Antagonism between FGF and BMP signaling in regulating chondrocyte proliferation and *Ihh* expression has been confirmed in limb explant cultures treated with FGF-2. The molecular mechanism by which these two signaling pathways antagonize each other is unclear. Inactivation by the suppression of ligand expression is not involved, because FGF-2 upregulates the expression of *Bmp*-4 *and Bmp*-7, whereas BMP-2 upregulates the expression of *Fgf18* [54]. Defects in BMP signaling resulting from targeted deletion of type-I BMP receptors [99] or R-Smads [73] in mouse cartilage suggest that the inhibition of FGF signaling by BMP signaling is due to the inactivation of ERK1/2 and STAT1, partly, as the result of inhibiting *Fgfr1* expression in the growth plate.

The mechanism by which the effectors of FGF signaling, ERK1/2 and STAT1, are involved in BMP/FGF antagonism has been examined in vitro. In particular, FGF signaling inhibits BMP signaling through ERK2-mediated phosphorylation of the linker region of Smad1, thereby inactivating Smad1 via Smurf1-mediated ubiquitination and subsequent degradation. In addition, binding of Smurf1 to linker-phosphorylated Smad1 limits the nuclear accumulation of Smad1 by inhibiting its association with nucleoporin [76]. As these studies were conducted with immortalized cell lines and neuroectodermal explants from *Xenopus* embryos, it is uncertain whether linker phosphorylation of R-Smads by ERKs or ERK/STAT inactivation is the general model for BMP/FGF antagonism. Inhibition of BMP signaling by FGFs in the growth plate may involve inactivation of R-Smads by inhibition of C-terminal Smad phosphorylation, rather than via Smad linker phosphorylation. In fact, stimulation or antagonism of FGF pathways leads to respective decreases or increases in C-terminal phosphorylated (activated) Smad1/5, but causes no change in the levels of linker-phosphorylated Smad1/5. Interestingly, Smad1/5 linker phosphorylation was detected primarily in proliferating, but not in resting and hypertrophic chondrocytes [73]. Conceivably, the regulation of linker and C-terminal phosphorylation of R-Smads by BMP and FGF signaling is required to tightly control the duration and intensity of BMP signaling in distinct zones at the growth plate.

8.5 BMP Signaling in Osteogenesis

Progression from chondrocyte proliferation to endochondral ossification requires the upregulation of genes for matrix proteins, transcription factors, and growth factors that coordinate the initiation of mineralization and induction of vascular invasion. BMPs can stimulate ectopic bone formation through increased expression of genes associated with osteoblast differentiation, such as alkaline phosphatase, osteocalcin, osteopontin, and the bone-specific transcription factor, Runx2 [7, 46]. The function of BMPs in osteoblasts has been extensively examined in vitro [9]. More recently, the Cre-*lox*P system, in conjunction with a promoter of an osteoblast-specific *Cre* transgene, such as *Col1a1-Cre* or *Osteocalcin2-Cre*, has been used to investigate the role of BMP signaling in vivo. This system has made the essential role of BMP signaling apparent not only in osteoblast, but also in osteoclast differentiation. Targeted deletion of BMPR1A in osteoblasts, obtained by mating conditional BMPR1A knockout mice with transgenic mice expressing Cre under the control of the *Osteocalcin2* promoter, led to reduced osteoblast activity and bone mass in 3-month-old mice. In 10-month-old mutant mice, on the other hand, bone mass was increased because of a decrease in osteoclast activity [56]. This indicates that BMP signaling plays an essential role in bone cell metabolism. The age-dependent function of BMP signaling in bone formation was further investigated with the aid of a tamoxifen-inducible

Cre-*loxP* system, where the administration of tamoxifen was observed to disrupt BMP signaling in osteoblasts. Targeted deletion of BMPR1A in osteoblasts of mice, either 2 days or 2 months old, caused the bone mass to increase after 3 weeks of tamoxifen administration because bone resorption had decreased [33]. The difference in the bone phenotypes of the conditional BMPR1A knockout mice, in which Cre expression was controlled by either the *Osteocalcin2* or the *Col1a1* promoter, may involve the differences in recombination efficiencies or the timing of recombination. These findings indicate that loss of BMP signaling leads to reduced osteoclast activity, because osteoblast-mediated osteoclast differentiation has been diminished.

8.5.1 Mechanistic Role of BMP Signaling in Osteoclastogenesis

The decrease in osteoclast function that leads to decreased bone resorption may involve interactions between the receptor activator of NF-κB ligand (RANKL) and its receptor, RANK. Osteoblasts express RANKL, while osteoclast precursors express RANK. Thus, cell–cell interactions between RANKL-expressing osteoblasts and RANK-expressing cells promote osteoclast differentiation [36]. Osteoblasts also produce osteoprotegerin (OPG), a decoy receptor for RANKL that can prevent RANKL–RANK interactions [41]. BMP signaling modulates the RANKL–OPG pathway in vitro, as BMP-2 treatment stimulates *Rankl* expression [29,88]. In vivo studies have also shown that BMP signaling regulates the RANKL–OPG pathway by BMP-induced *Opg* expression via Hoxc-8-binding sites located on the *Opg* promoter [33, 34]. Smad1 competes with Hoxc-8, which inhibits *Opg* promoter activity, by binding to the *Opg* Hox sites [91]. BMP signaling may also mediate the RANKL–OPG pathway via secondary mediators such as Wnts, which regulate *Rankl* and *Opg* expression [20]. *Bmpr1a*-deficient calvaria showed upregulation of canonical Wnt signaling via downregulation of the expression of sclerostin, the Wnt pathway inhibitor. In these calvaria, reduction of *Rankl* expression is accompanied by an increase in *Opg*. Treatment of *Bmpr1a*-deficient calvaria with sclerostin reverses the expression patterns of *Rankl* and *Opg* [34]. Similarly, secreted Wnt inhibitors from the Dickkopf (Dkk) family facilitate osteoclastogenesis by enhancing *Rankl* expression and reducing *Opg* expression [17]. It is thus apparent that BMP signaling controls the extent of bone formation by regulating osteoblast-induced osteoclastogenesis by its mediation of the RANKL–OPG pathway, and/or indirectly by its downregulation of Wnt signaling.

8.5.2 Effects of BMP Signaling on Runx2 Activity

Matrix protein expression by osteoblasts during intramembranous and endochondral bone formation is regulated by the transcription factor, Runx2/Cbfa1/Osf2 (hereafter referred to as Runx2), which binds to responsive elements on osteoblast-specific genes to regulate their transcription. The essential role of Runx2 in osteoblast differentiation has been brought out by studies with mice that have a homozygous mutation in *Runx2*. These mice die perinatally and completely lack bone owing to defects in osteoblast maturation [43]. Interestingly, overexpression of either Runx2 or dominant-negative Runx2 causes osteopenia attributed to diminished matrix production and mineralization. In either case, overexpression of Runx2 resulted in diminished function of fully differentiated osteoblasts, as indicated by reduced expression of *osteocalcin*, a marker for terminally differentiated osteoblasts [12,47]. Thus, transcriptional regulation of *Runx2* is crucial in controlling its function during both early and late stages of osteoblast differentiation.

The canonical BMP signaling pathway has been implicated in the regulation of Runx2 transcription and activity [46]. The nuclear matrix targeting signal (NMTS) on the C-terminal region of *Runx2* directs Runx2 to specific sites within the nuclear matrix, thus promoting the expression of osteoblast-specific genes [100]. Deletion mutant studies have identified a R-Smad/Runx2 interaction domain on *Runx2* that overlaps the NMTS [1], where HTY residues on the R-Smad/Runx2 interaction domain initiate BMP-induced osteoblast differentiation [31]. Therefore, R-Smads may facilitate subnuclear targeting of Runx2 to promote the expression of osteoblast-specific genes.

Degradation of Runx2 modulates its transcriptional activity. BMP signaling regulates Runx2

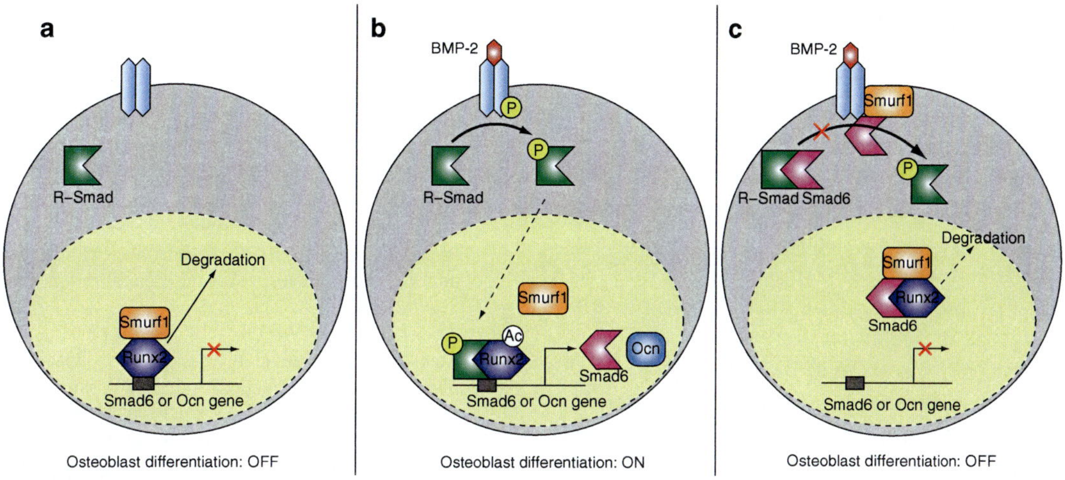

Figure 8.2. Proposed model for BMP-mediated Smad6/Runx2 feedback loop to control osteogenesis. (**a**) Osteoblast differentiation is inhibited in the absence of BMP signaling. In the absence of BMP-2, Smurf1 binds to Runx2 on the Smad6 promoter and induces Runx2 degradation, thus inhibiting *Smad6* transcription. Degradation of Runx2 can also inhibit transcription of genes associated with osteoblast differentiation, such as *osteocalcin* (*Ocn*). (**b**) BMP signaling promotes osteoblast differentiation. In the presence of BMP-2, Runx2 is acetylated, which inhibits Smurf1-mediated degradation. Also, phosphorylated R-Smads replace Smurf1 to promote Runx2-mediated *Smad6* and/or *Ocn* transcription. (**c**) Expression of *Smad6* results in the attenuation of BMP signaling. Smad6 of Smad interacts with Smurf1 to induce Runx2 degradation. Smad6 can also interact with R-Smads and/or BMP receptors to prevent activation (phosphorylation) of R-Smads.

activity by acting on Runx2 stability (Fig. 8.2). Treatment of the pluripotent mesenchymal cell line, C2C12, with BMP-2 causes R-Smads to interact with Runx2 and precludes Smurfl binding on the *Smad6* promoter, thus promoting *Smad6* gene transcription (Fig. 8.2b) [93]. In turn, Smad6 interacts with Smurfl to induce Runx2 degradation (Fig. 8.2c) [78]. Treatment of C2C12 cells with BMP-2 has shown that BMP signaling also protects Runx2 from degradation. BMP-2 stimulates Runx2 acetylation, which inhibits Smurfl-mediated degradation and promotes BMP-induced osteoblast differentiation and bone formation (Fig. 8.2b) [32]. It is unclear, however, whether the tight regulation of Runx2 stability by BMP signaling occurs in vivo.

8.6 BMP Signaling in Adipogenesis and Energy Metabolism

Adipocytes, crucial for the maintenance of proper energy balance, store energy in the form of lipids and expend energy in response to hormonal stimulation. Obesity develops when energy intake exceeds energy expenditure. Understanding the development and regulation of adipogenesis is important in managing the health implications of obesity. Like cartilage and bone, adipose tissue arises from a multipotent stem cell population of mesodermal origin. BMP signaling commits mesenchymal stem cells to the adipocyte lineage, and thus represents the initial stage of adipocyte differentiation [5, 92]. Interestingly, adipocyte and osteoblast commitment can be altered by selective blockage or activation of type-I BMP receptors [8]. Also, BMP-induced commitment of the mesenchymal to the adipocyte lineage is dose-dependent [92].

Once committed, preadipocytes differentiate into adipocytes. Adipose tissue exists as either white (WAT) or brown adipose tissue (BAT). WAT is the primary site of energy storage and is dispersed throughout the body of mammals and birds. Most WAT is subcutaneous and intra-abdominal. BAT provides basal and inducible energy expenditure in the form of thermogenesis. This in turn involves increased expression of uncoupling protein 1 (UCP-1). In humans and rodents, BAT, localized in the intrascapular and paraspinal regions, is abundant during the prenatal and neonatal periods. After birth, only small amounts of BAT remain and its function in adults has been considered negligible [18]. However, recent reports have shown that high energy expenditure in obesity-resistant mice correlates with high expression of UCP-1 in BAT, interspersed between muscle bundles, and that UCP-1 expression is inducible [2]. The regulation of UCP-1 in BAT, as well as brown adipogenesis, may protect against obesity. Moreover, treatment with BMP-7, but not with BMP-2, -4, or -6, induces differentiation of brown preadipocytes, as indicated by increased *UCP-1* expression. Overexpression of BMP-7 in mice has also led to increased brown fat mass, increased energy expenditure, and reduced weight gain [86]. Thus, BMP-7 may prove to be a therapeutic option for treating human obesity.

8.7 Perspectives

Studies using cell-specific Cre-mediated recombination in mice, coupled with in vitro molecular and biochemical assays, have revealed that BMP signaling plays an essential role in all aspects of skeletogenesis. BMP signaling induces the commitment of mesenchymal progenitor cells into the chondrogenic, osteogenic, and adipogenic lineages, and regulates the progression of these cell types through their complex differentiation program. A major challenge is whether the mechanisms by which BMP signaling regulates the expression of target genes in vitro are the general mode for regulation of skeletogenesis in vivo. How BMP signaling interacts with other signaling pathways, such as the Ihh/PTHrP, FGF, and Wnt, is essential to understand how imbalance in signaling affects bone development and homeostasis. Such understanding may lead to the development of new therapies for the treatment of skeletal diseases.

References

1. Afzal F, Pratap J, Ito K, Ito Y, Stein JL, van Wijnen AJ, Stein GS, Lian JB, Javed A (2005) Smad function and intranuclear targeting share a Runx2 motif required for osteogenic lineage induction and BMP2 responsive transcription. J Cell Physiol 204:63–72
2. Almind K, Manieri M, Sivitz WI, Cinti S, Kahn CR (2007) Ectopic brown adipose tissue in muscle provides a mechanism for differences in risk of metabolic syndrome in mice. Proc Natl Acad Sci U S A 104:2366–2371
3. Bi W, Deng JM, Zhang Z, Behringer RR, de Crombrugghe B (1999) Sox9 is required for cartilage formation. Nat Genet 22:85–89
4. Bi W, Huang W, Whitworth DJ, Deng JM, Zhang Z, Behringer RR, de Crombrugghe B (2001) Haploinsufficiency of Sox9 results in defective cartilage primordia and premature skeletal mineralization. Proc Natl Acad Sci U S A 98:6698–6703
5. Bowers RR, Kim JW, Otto TC, Lane MD (2006) Stable stem cell commitment to the adipocyte lineage by inhibition of DNA methylation: role of the BMP-4 gene. Proc Natl Acad Sci U S A 103:13022–13027
6. Capdevila J, Johnson RL (1998) Endogenous and ectopic expression of noggin suggests a conserved mechanism for regulation of BMP function during limb and somite patterning. Dev Biol 197:205–217
7. Chen D, Harris MA, Rossini G, Dunstan CR, Dallas SL, Feng JQ, Mundy GR, Harris SE (1997) Bone morphogenetic protein 2 (BMP-2) enhances BMP-3, BMP-4, and bone cell differentiation marker gene expression during the induction of mineralized bone matrix formation in cultures of fetal rat calvarial osteoblasts. Calcif Tissue Int 60:283–290
8. Chen D, Ji X, Harris MA, Feng JQ, Karsenty G, Celeste AJ, Rosen V, Mundy GR, Harris SE (1998) Differential roles for bone morphogenetic protein (BMP) receptor type IB and IA in differentiation and specification of mesenchymal precursor cells to osteoblast and adipocyte lineages. J Cell Biol 142:295–305
9. Chen D, Zhao M, Mundy GR (2004) Bone morphogenetic proteins. Growth Factors 22:233–241
10. De Robertis EM, Kuroda H (2004) Dorsal-ventral patterning and neural induction in Xenopus embryos. Annu Rev Cell Dev Biol 20:285–308
11. Derynck R, Zhang YE (2003) Smad-dependent and Smad-independent pathways in TGF-beta family signalling. Nature 425:577–584
12. Ducy P, Starbuck M, Priemel M, Shen J, Pinero G, Geoffroy V, Amling M, Karsenty G (1999) A Cbfa1-dependent genetic pathway controls bone formation beyond embryonic development. Genes Dev 13:1025–1036
13. Duprez D, Bell EJ, Richardson MK, Archer CW, Wolpert L, Brickell PM, Francis-West PH (1996) Overexpression of BMP-2 and BMP-4 alters the size and shape of developing skeletal elements in the chick limb. Mech Dev 57:145–157
14. Fischer L, Boland G, Tuan RS (2002) Wnt-3A enhances bone morphogenetic protein-2-mediated chondrogenesis of murine C3H10T1/2 mesenchymal cells. J Biol Chem 277:30870–30878
15. Fischer L, Boland G, Tuan RS (2002) Wnt signaling during BMP-2 stimulation of mesenchymal chondrogenesis. J Cell Biochem 84:816–831
16. Fromigue O, Modrowski D, Marie PJ (2005) Apoptosis in membranous bone formation: role of fibroblast growth factor and bone morphogenetic protein signaling. Crit Rev Eukaryot Gene Expr 15:75–92

17. Fujita K, Janz S (2007) Attenuation of WNT signaling by DKK-1 and -2 regulates BMP2-induced osteoblast differentiation and expression of OPG, RANKL and M-CSF. Mol Cancer 6:71
18. Gesta S, Tseng YH, Kahn CR (2007) Developmental origin of fat: tracking obesity to its source. Cell 131:242–256
19. Gilboa L, Nohe A, Geissendorfer T, Sebald W, Henis YI, Knaus P (2000) Bone morphogenetic protein receptor complexes on the surface of live cells: a new oligomerization mode for serine/threonine kinase receptors. Mol Biol Cell 11:1023–1035
20. Glass DA II, Bialek P, Ahn JD, Starbuck M, Patel MS, Clevers H, Taketo MM, Long F, McMahon AP, Lang RA, Karsenty G (2005) Canonical Wnt signaling in differentiated osteoblasts controls osteoclast differentiation. Dev Cell 8:751–764
21. Graham A, Lumsden A (1996) Patterning the cranial neural crest. Biochem Soc Symp 62:77–83
22. Haas AR, Tuan RS (1999) Chondrogenic differentiation of murine C3H10T1/2 multipotential mesenchymal cells: II. Stimulation by bone morphogenetic protein-2 requires modulation of N-cadherin expression and function. Differentiation 64:77–89
23. Hargus G, Kist R, Kramer J, Gerstel D, Neitz A, Scherer G, Rohwedel J (2008) Loss of Sox9 function results in defective chondrocyte differentiation of mouse embryonic stem cells in vitro. Int J Dev Biol 52:323–332
24. Hata A, Lagna G, Massague J, Hemmati-Brivanlou A (1998) Smad6 inhibits BMP/Smad1 signaling by specifically competing with the Smad4 tumor suppressor. Genes Dev 12:186–197
25. Hinck L, Nathke IS, Papkoff J, Nelson WJ (1994) Dynamics of cadherin/catenin complex formation: novel protein interactions and pathways of complex assembly. J Cell Biol 125:1327–1340
26. Hosoya A, Kim JY, Cho SW, Jung HS (2008) BMP4 signaling regulates formation of Hertwig's epithelial root sheath during tooth root development. Cell Tissue Res 333:503–509
27. Houston B, Thorp BH, Burt DW (1994) Molecular cloning and expression of bone morphogenetic protein-7 in the chick epiphyseal growth plate. J Mol Endocrinol 13:289–301
28. Imamura T, Takase M, Nishihara A, Oeda E, Hanai J, Kawabata M, Miyazono K (1997) Smad6 inhibits signalling by the TGF-beta superfamily. Nature 389:622–626
29. Itoh K, Udagawa N, Katagiri T, Iemura S, Ueno N, Yasuda H, Higashio K, Quinn JM, Gillespie MT, Martin TJ, Suda T, Takahashi N (2001) Bone morphogenetic protein 2 stimulates osteoclast differentiation and survival supported by receptor activator of nuclear factor-kappaB ligand. Endocrinology 142:3656–3662
30. Iwai T, Murai J, Yoshikawa H, Tsumaki N (2008) Smad7 Inhibits chondrocyte differentiation at multiple steps during endochondral bone formation and downregulates p38 MAPK pathways. J Biol Chem 283: 27154–27164
31. Javed A, Afzal F, Bae JS, Gutierrez S, Zaidi K, Pratap J, van Wijnen AJ, Stein JL, Stein GS, Lian JB (2009) Specific residues of RUNX2 are obligatory for formation of BMP2-induced RUNX2-SMAD complex to promote osteoblast differentiation. Cells Tissues Organs 189:133–137
32. Jeon EJ, Lee KY, Choi NS, Lee MH, Kim HN, Jin YH, Ryoo HM, Choi JY, Yoshida M, Nishino N, Oh BC, Lee KS, Lee YH, Bae SC (2006) Bone morphogenetic protein-2 stimulates Runx2 acetylation. J Biol Chem 281:16502–16511
33. Kamiya N, Ye L, Kobayashi T, Lucas DJ, Mochida Y, Yamauchi M, Kronenberg HM, Feng JQ, Mishina Y (2008) Disruption of BMP signaling in osteoblasts through type IA receptor (BMPRIA) increases bone mass. J Bone Miner Res 23:2007–2017
34. Kamiya N, Ye L, Kobayashi T, Mochida Y, Yamauchi M, Kronenberg HM, Feng JQ, Mishina Y (2008) BMP signaling negatively regulates bone mass through sclerostin by inhibiting the canonical Wnt pathway. Development 135:3801–3811
35. Karaplis AC, Luz A, Glowacki J, Bronson RT, Tybulewicz VL, Kronenberg HM, Mulligan RC (1994) Lethal skeletal dysplasia from targeted disruption of the parathyroid hormone-related peptide gene. Genes Dev 8:277–289
36. Katagiri T, Takahashi N (2002) Regulatory mechanisms of osteoblast and osteoclast differentiation. Oral Dis 8:147–159
37. Kavsak P, Rasmussen RK, Causing CG, Bonni S, Zhu H, Thomsen GH, Wrana JL (2000) Smad7 binds to Smurf2 to form an E3 ubiquitin ligase that targets the TGF beta receptor for degradation. Mol Cell 6:1365–1375
38. Kawabata M, Chytil A, Moses HL (1995) Cloning of a novel type II serine/threonine kinase receptor through interaction with the type I transforming growth factor-beta receptor. J Biol Chem 270:5625–5630
39. Kawai S, Sugiura T (2001) Characterization of human bone morphogenetic protein (BMP)-4 and -7 gene promoters: activation of BMP promoters by Gli, a sonic hedgehog mediator. Bone 29:54–61
40. Kingsley DM, Bland AE, Grubber JM, Marker PC, Russell LB, Copeland NG, Jenkins NA (1992) The mouse short ear skeletal morphogenesis locus is associated with defects in a bone morphogenetic member of the TGF beta superfamily. Cell 71:399–410
41. Kobayashi Y, Udagawa N, Takahashi N (2009) Action of RANKL and OPG for osteoclastogenesis. Crit Rev Eukaryot Gene Expr 19:61–72
42. Koenig BB, Cook JS, Wolsing DH, Ting J, Tiesman JP, Correa PE, Olson CA, Pecquet AL, Ventura F, Grant RA et al (1994) Characterization and cloning of a receptor for BMP-2 and BMP-4 from NIH 3T3 cells. Mol Cell Biol 14:5961–5974
43. Komori T, Yagi H, Nomura S, Yamaguchi A, Sasaki K, Deguchi K, Shimizu Y, Bronson RT, Gao YH, Inada M, Sato M, Okamoto R, Kitamura Y, Yoshiki S, Kishimoto T (1997) Targeted disruption of Cbfa1 results in a complete lack of bone formation owing to maturational arrest of osteoblasts. Cell 89:755–764
44. Kronenberg HM (2003) Developmental regulation of the growth plate. Nature 423:332–336
45. Lanske B, Karaplis AC, Lee K, Luz A, Vortkamp A, Pirro A, Karperien M, Defize LH, Ho C, Mulligan RC, Abou-Samra AB, Juppner H, Segre GV, Kronenberg HM

(1996) PTH/PTHrP receptor in early development and Indian hedgehog-regulated bone growth. Science 273:663–666
46. Lee KS, Kim HJ, Li QL, Chi XZ, Ueta C, Komori T, Wozney JM, Kim EG, Choi JY, Ryoo HM, Bae SC (2000) Runx2 is a common target of transforming growth factor beta1 and bone morphogenetic protein 2, and cooperation between Runx2 and Smad5 induces osteoblast-specific gene expression in the pluripotent mesenchymal precursor cell line C2C12. Mol Cell Biol 20:8783–8792
47. Liu W, Toyosawa S, Furuichi T, Kanatani N, Yoshida C, Liu Y, Himeno M, Narai S, Yamaguchi A, Komori T (2001) Overexpression of Cbfa1 in osteoblasts inhibits osteoblast maturation and causes osteopenia with multiple fractures. J Cell Biol 155:157–166
48. Liu Z, Xu J, Colvin JS, Ornitz DM (2002) Coordination of chondrogenesis and osteogenesis by fibroblast growth factor 18. Genes Dev 16:859–869
49. Luo G, Hofmann C, Bronckers AL, Sohocki M, Bradley A, Karsenty G (1995) BMP-7 is an inducer of nephrogenesis, and is also required for eye development and skeletal patterning. Genes Dev 9:2808–2820
50. Lyons KM, Hogan BL, Robertson EJ (1995) Colocalization of BMP 7 and BMP 2 RNAs suggests that these factors cooperatively mediate tissue interactions during murine development. Mech Dev 50:71–83
51. Macias-Silva M, Hoodless PA, Tang SJ, Buchwald M, Wrana JL (1998) Specific activation of Smad1 signaling pathways by the BMP7 type I receptor, ALK2. J Biol Chem 273:25628–25636
52. Mailhot G, Yang M, Mason-Savas A, Mackay CA, Leav I, Odgren PR (2008) BMP-5 expression increases during chondrocyte differentiation in vivo and in vitro and promotes proliferation and cartilage matrix synthesis in primary chondrocyte cultures. J Cell Physiol 214:56–64
53. Massague J (1998) TGF-beta signal transduction. Annu Rev Biochem 67:753–791
54. Minina E, Kreschel C, Naski MC, Ornitz DM, Vortkamp A (2002) Interaction of FGF, Ihh/Pthlh, and BMP signaling integrates chondrocyte proliferation and hypertrophic differentiation. Dev Cell 3:439–449
55. Minina E, Wenzel HM, Kreschel C, Karp S, Gaffield W, McMahon AP, Vortkamp A (2001) BMP and Ihh/PTHrP signaling interact to coordinate chondrocyte proliferation and differentiation. Development 128:4523–4534
56. Mishina Y, Starbuck MW, Gentile MA, Fukuda T, Kasparcova V, Seedor JG, Hanks MC, Amling M, Pinero GJ, Harada S, Behringer RR (2004) Bone morphogenetic protein type IA receptor signaling regulates postnatal osteoblast function and bone remodeling. J Biol Chem 279:27560–27566
57. Moriguchi T, Kuroyanagi N, Yamaguchi K, Gotoh Y, Irie K, Kano T, Shirakabe K, Muro Y, Shibuya H, Matsumoto K, Nishida E, Hagiwara M (1996) A novel kinase cascade mediated by mitogen-activated protein kinase kinase 6 and MKK3. J Biol Chem 271:13675–13679
58. Murakami G, Watabe T, Takaoka K, Miyazono K, Imamura T (2003) Cooperative inhibition of bone morphogenetic protein signaling by Smurf1 and inhibitory Smads. Mol Biol Cell 14:2809–2817
59. Nakao A, Afrakhte M, Moren A, Nakayama T, Christian JL, Heuchel R, Itoh S, Kawabata M, Heldin NE, Heldin CH, ten Dijke P (1997) Identification of Smad7, a TGFbeta-inducible antagonist of TGF-beta signalling. Nature 389:631–635
60. Nelson WJ (2008) Regulation of cell-cell adhesion by the cadherin-catenin complex. Biochem Soc Trans 36:149–155
61. Nie X, Luukko K, Kettunen P (2006) BMP signalling in craniofacial development. Int J Dev Biol 50:511–521
62. Nilsson O, Parker EA, Hegde A, Chau M, Barnes KM, Baron J (2007) Gradients in bone morphogenetic protein-related gene expression across the growth plate. J Endocrinol 193:75–84
63. Nohe A, Hassel S, Ehrlich M, Neubauer F, Sebald W, Henis YI, Knaus P (2002) The mode of bone morphogenetic protein (BMP) receptor oligomerization determines different BMP-2 signaling pathways. J Biol Chem 277:5330–5338
64. Nohno T, Ishikawa T, Saito T, Hosokawa K, Noji S, Wolsing DH, Rosenbaum JS (1995) Identification of a human type II receptor for bone morphogenetic protein-4 that forms differential heteromeric complexes with bone morphogenetic protein type I receptors. J Biol Chem 270:22522–22526
65. Oberlender SA, Tuan RS (1994) Spatiotemporal profile of N-cadherin expression in the developing limb mesenchyme. Cell Adhes Commun 2:521–537
66. Ohbayashi N, Shibayama M, Kurotaki Y, Imanishi M, Fujimori T, Itoh N, Takada S (2002) FGF18 is required for normal cell proliferation and differentiation during osteogenesis and chondrogenesis. Genes Dev 16:870–879
67. Ornitz DM, Marie PJ (2002) FGF signaling pathways in endochondral and intramembranous bone development and human genetic disease. Genes Dev 16:1446–1465
68. Pan Q, Wu Y, Lin T, Yao H, Yang Z, Gao G, Song E, Shen H (2009) Bone morphogenetic protein-2 induces chromatin remodeling and modification at the proximal promoter of Sox9 gene. Biochem Biophys Res Commun 379:356–361
69. Pan Q, Yu Y, Chen Q, Li C, Wu H, Wan Y, Ma J, Sun F (2008) Sox9, a key transcription factor of bone morphogenetic protein-2-induced chondrogenesis, is activated through BMP pathway and a CCAAT box in the proximal promoter. J Cell Physiol 217:228–241
70. Pathi S, Rutenberg JB, Johnson RL, Vortkamp A (1999) Interaction of Ihh and BMP/Noggin signaling during cartilage differentiation. Dev Biol 209:239–253
71. Pizette S, Niswander L (2000) BMPs are required at two steps of limb chondrogenesis: formation of prechondrogenic condensations and their differentiation into chondrocytes. Dev Biol 219:237–249
72. Provot S, Schipani E (2005) Molecular mechanisms of endochondral bone development. Biochem Biophys Res Commun 328:658–665

73. Retting KN, Song B, Yoon BS, Lyons KM (2009) BMP canonical Smad signaling through Smad1 and Smad5 is required for endochondral bone formation. Development 136:1093–1104
74. Rosenzweig BL, Imamura T, Okadome T, Cox GN, Yamashita H, ten Dijke P, Heldin CH, Miyazono K (1995) Cloning and characterization of a human type II receptor for bone morphogenetic proteins. Proc Natl Acad Sci U S A 92:7632–7636
75. Rousseau F, Bonaventure J, Legeai-Mallet L, Pelet A, Rozet JM, Maroteaux P, Le Merrer M, Munnich A (1994) Mutations in the gene encoding fibroblast growth factor receptor-3 in achondroplasia. Nature 371:252–254
76. Sapkota G, Alarcon C, Spagnoli FM, Brivanlou AH, Massague J (2007) Balancing BMP signaling through integrated inputs into the Smad1 linker. Mol Cell 25:441–454
77. Seki K, Hata A (2004) Indian hedgehog gene is a target of the bone morphogenetic protein signaling pathway. J Biol Chem 279:18544–18549
78. Shen R, Chen M, Wang YJ, Kaneki H, Xing L, O'Keefe RJ, Chen D (2006) Smad6 interacts with Runx2 and mediates Smad ubiquitin regulatory factor 1-induced Runx2 degradation. J Biol Chem 281:3569–3576
79. Shiang R, Thompson LM, Zhu YZ, Church DM, Fielder TJ, Bocian M, Winokur ST, Wasmuth JJ (1994) Mutations in the transmembrane domain of FGFR3 cause the most common genetic form of dwarfism, achondroplasia. Cell 78:335–342
80. St-Jacques B, Hammerschmidt M, McMahon AP (1999) Indian hedgehog signaling regulates proliferation and differentiation of chondrocytes and is essential for bone formation. Genes Dev 13:2072–2086
81. Storm EE, Huynh TV, Copeland NG, Jenkins NA, Kingsley DM, Lee SJ (1994) Limb alterations in brachypodism mice due to mutations in a new member of the TGF beta-superfamily. Nature 368:639–643
82. Stott NS, Jiang TX, Chuong CM (1999) Successive formative stages of precartilaginous mesenchymal condensations in vitro: modulation of cell adhesion by Wnt-7A and BMP-2. J Cell Physiol 180:314–324
83. Suzuki C, Murakami G, Fukuchi M, Shimanuki T, Shikauchi Y, Imamura T, Miyazono K (2002) Smurf1 regulates the inhibitory activity of Smad7 by targeting Smad7 to the plasma membrane. J Biol Chem 277:39919–39925
84. Tajima Y, Goto K, Yoshida M, Shinomiya K, Sekimoto T, Yoneda Y, Miyazono K, Imamura T (2003) Chromosomal region maintenance 1 (CRM1)-dependent nuclear export of Smad ubiquitin regulatory factor 1 (Smurf1) is essential for negative regulation of transforming growth factor-beta signaling by Smad7. J Biol Chem 278:10716–10721
85. ten Dijke P, Yamashita H, Ichijo H, Franzen P, Laiho M, Miyazono K, Heldin CH (1994) Characterization of type I receptors for transforming growth factor-beta and activin. Science 264:101–104
86. Tseng YH, Kokkotou E, Schulz TJ, Huang TL, Winnay JN, Taniguchi CM, Tran TT, Suzuki R, Espinoza DO, Yamamoto Y, Ahrens MJ, Dudley AT, Norris AW, Kulkarni RN, Kahn CR (2008) New role of bone morphogenetic protein 7 in brown adipogenesis and energy expenditure. Nature 454:1000–1004
87. Urist MR (1965) Bone: formation by autoinduction. Science 150:893–899
88. Usui M, Xing L, Drissi H, Zuscik M, O'Keefe R, Chen D, Boyce BF (2008) Murine and chicken chondrocytes regulate osteoclastogenesis by producing RANKL in response to BMP2. J Bone Miner Res 23:314–325
89. von Bubnoff A, Cho KW (2001) Intracellular BMP signaling regulation in vertebrates: pathway or network? Dev Biol 239:1–14
90. Vortkamp A, Lee K, Lanske B, Segre GV, Kronenberg HM, Tabin CJ (1996) Regulation of rate of cartilage differentiation by Indian hedgehog and PTH-related protein. Science 273:613–622
91. Wan M, Shi X, Feng X, Cao X (2001) Transcriptional mechanisms of bone morphogenetic protein-induced osteoprotegrin gene expression. J Biol Chem 276:10119–10125
92. Wang EA, Israel DI, Kelly S, Luxenberg DP (1993) Bone morphogenetic protein-2 causes commitment and differentiation in C3H10T1/2 and 3T3 cells. Growth Factors 9:57–71
93. Wang Q, Wei X, Zhu T, Zhang M, Shen R, Xing L, O'Keefe RJ, Chen D (2007) Bone morphogenetic protein 2 activates Smad6 gene transcription through bone-specific transcription factor Runx2. J Biol Chem 282:10742–10748
94. Wozney JM (1989) Bone morphogenetic proteins. Prog Growth Factor Res 1:267–280
95. Wright E, Hargrave MR, Christiansen J, Cooper L, Kun J, Evans T, Gangadharan U, Greenfield A, Koopman P (1995) The Sry-related gene Sox9 is expressed during chondrogenesis in mouse embryos. Nat Genet 9:15–20
96. Yamashita H, ten Dijke P, Huylebroeck D, Sampath TK, Andries M, Smith JC, Heldin CH, Miyazono K (1995) Osteogenic protein-1 binds to activin type II receptors and induces certain activin-like effects. J Cell Biol 130:217–226
97. Yoon BS, Lyons KM (2004) Multiple functions of BMPs in chondrogenesis. J Cell Biochem 93:93–103
98. Yoon BS, Ovchinnikov DA, Yoshii I, Mishina Y, Behringer RR, Lyons KM (2005) Bmpr1a and Bmpr1b have overlapping functions and are essential for chondrogenesis in vivo. Proc Natl Acad Sci U S A 102:5062–5067
99. Yoon BS, Pogue R, Ovchinnikov DA, Yoshii I, Mishina Y, Behringer RR, Lyons KM (2006) BMPs regulate multiple aspects of growth-plate chondrogenesis through opposing actions on FGF pathways. Development 133:4667–4678
100. Zaidi SK, Javed A, Pratap J, Schroeder TM, JW J, Lian JB, van Wijnen AJ, Stein GS, Stein JL (2006) Alterations in intranuclear localization of Runx2 affect biological activity. J Cell Physiol 209:935–942
101. Zehentner BK, Dony C, Burtscher H (1999) The transcription factor Sox9 is involved in BMP-2 signaling. J Bone Miner Res 14:1734–1741

102. Zelzer E, Olsen BR (2003) The genetic basis for skeletal diseases. Nature 423:343–348
103. Zou H, Choe KM, Lu Y, Massague J, Niswander L (1997) BMP signaling and vertebrate limb development. Cold Spring Harb Symp Quant Biol 62: 269–272
104. Zuscik MJ, Hilton MJ, Zhang X, Chen D, O'Keefe RJ (2008) Regulation of chondrogenesis and chondrocyte differentiation by stress. J Clin Invest 118:429–438
105. Zuzarte-Luis V, Hurle JM (2005) Programmed cell death in the embryonic vertebrate limb. Semin Cell Dev Biol 16:261–269

9. Wnt Signaling in Bone Development

Peter V. N. Bodine

9.1 Introduction

This chapter will focus on the role of Wnt signaling in postnatal bone formation and development. Wnts are a large family of 19 secreted carbohydrate- and lipid-modified polypeptides that mediate important biological processes like embryogenesis, organogenesis, and morphogenesis [61, 70, 71, 99]. The proteins bind to a membrane receptor complex composed of a Frizzled (FZD) G-protein coupled receptor and a low-density lipoprotein (LDL) receptor-related protein (LRP) [61, 70, 71]. There are ten different FZDs (1–10) as well as two LRPs (5 and 6), and the binding of Wnt to these receptors activates one of the several intracellular signaling pathways depending on the Wnt, FZD receptor, and the cell type involved [61, 70, 71, 99].

The best-characterized Wnt pathway is termed as canonical or Wnt/β-catenin pathway, and signals through LRP5 or LRP6. The regulatory protein of this pathway is found in a cytoplasmic complex that comprises other proteins like Axin, the adenomatous polyposis coli gene product (APC), glycogen synthase kinase (GSK)-3β, casein kinase 1 (CK1), protein phosphatase 1 (PP1), and the E3 ubiquitin ligase subunit β-Trcp [39]. This cytoplasmic complex facilitates phosphorylation of β-catenin. The phosphorylated β-catenin can be subsequently degraded by the proteosome. When Wnt binds to FZD/LRP, the cytoplasmic protein, disheveled (Dsh), is recruited to the membrane and binds to the receptor complex. In turn, this initiates the recruitment of Axin, GSK-3β, and CK1, which phosphorylates LRP by GSK-3β and CK1. When Axin and GSK-3β are recruited to FZD/LRP, phosphorylation of β-catenin is prevented. As a result, β-catenin accumulates in the cytoplasm, diffuses to the nucleus, and binds to and activates the lymphoid-enhancer binding factor (LEF)/T-cell-specific transcription factors (TCFs), which are members of the high-mobility-group (HMG)-box transcription factor family [61, 70, 71, 86, 99].

Other less well-characterized (noncanonical) pathways are also activated by the Wnts [70, 95]. These include the G-protein-mediated Wnt/calcium pathway [54] and the c-Jun NH_2-terminal kinase (JNK) pathway [97], both of which are also controlled by Dsh [95]. Wnts also stimulate adenylyl cyclase and increase cyclic-adenosine monophosphate (cAMP) levels via a G-protein-coupled mechanism [16, 80]. The functional importance of the canonical pathway as a part of the regulation of the fundamental mammalian processes is well established. The significance of the noncanonical pathways is less well understood, even though they may play a role in cardiogenesis, myogenesis, gastrulation, neuronal morphogenesis, and tumorigenesis.

F. Bronner et al. (eds.), *Bone and Development*, Topics in Bone Biology 6,
DOI 10.1007/978-1-84882-822-3_9,

As Wnt signaling is important in regulating key biological processes, the existence of many extracellular and intracellular regulators of the pathways is not surprising [61,70,99]. Extracelluar regulators include a variety of secreted proteins like Wnt inhibitory factors (WIFs), secreted frizzled-related proteins (sFRPs), dickkopfs (Dkks), and SOST/sclerostin [13, 46, 49, 88, 103]. WIFs and sFRPs bind to Wnts. sFRPs bind to FZD receptors, and Dkks and sclerostin interact with LRPs.

Numerous knockout and transgenic mouse models have been constructed to understand the various mechanisms by which Wnt pathway components act on biological processes. Animal models that offer insights into the mechanisms by which Wnt pathways function in the skeleton will be highlighted in this chapter. Applicable human studies will also be discussed. For recent reviews regarding the role of Wnts in prenatal skeletal development and in other developmental pathways, the reader can refer to [19, 31, 33, 67]. For reviews of the role that Wnt pathways play in the regulation of bone mass, one can refer to [7, 11, 28, 32, 45, 53, 96].

9.2 Effects of LRP5 and LRP6 on Bone Formation and Development

Evidence for the involvement of canonical Wnt signaling in bone formation and development came from human genetic studies of the osteoporosis pseudoglioma (OPPG) syndrome and high bone mass (HBM) phenotypes [6, 22, 51]. Gone et al. [29] reported that numerous nonsense and frame-shift mutations throughout the coding region of the human Wnt coreceptor LRP5 cause OPPG syndrome. These loss-of-function mutations lead to dramatic reductions in trabecular bone volume (TBV), premature fractures, and skeletal deformities that resulted from diminished bone accrual. In addition, loss of LRP5 function was found to lead to developmental eye defects [29].

On the other hand, a gain-of-function mutation in LRP5 has the opposite effect and causes a HBM trait in humans [6, 43, 45, 77]. Two groups, Little et al. [59] and Boyden et al. [14], found the same G171V mutation in two families that had HBM. This mutation resides in the first β-propeller motif of the extracellular domain of LRP5 and leads to a 30–60% increase in hip and spine aerial bone mineral density (aBMD), as evaluated by dual-energy X-ray absorptiometry (DEXA). Radiographs have shown that HBM individuals have bones whose trabecular BMD and cortical thickness are increased, but whose shape is normal [44].

Other gain-of-function mutations of human LRP5 (R154M, G171R, N198S, A214T, A214V, A242T, T253I, M282V, and D111Y) lead to HBM phenotypes like endosteal hyperostosis, Van Buchem disease, autosomal dominate osteosclerosis, and osteopetrosis type I [6, 94]. An interesting observation is that all of the gain-of-function mutations identified to date that cause HBM phenotypes are found in the first β-propeller domain of LRP5 [34]. The mutations are scattered throughout the six blades of this motif, with relief from Dkk1 and sclerostin antagonism [1, 5, 6, 14, 58, 85]. Dkk1 binds to the 3rd and 4th β-propeller motifs of LRP5 and LRP6 and disrupts the canonical signaling by targeting LRP internalization and degradation through kremen [34, 49]. On the other hand, sclerostin binds to and antagonizes LRP5 and LRP6 by interacting with first and second β-propeller domains of the receptors [58].

Knockout and transgenic mouse models of these LRP5 mutations have led to the understanding of the mechanisms by which canonical Wnt signaling regulates bone formation [2, 4, 17, 23, 36, 40, 48, 81, 84]. As first reported by Kato et al. [48], germline deletion of murine LRP5 reduced vertebral TBV by 40% at 8 weeks of age when peak bone mass occurred in the $LRP5^{+/+}$ mice, as determined by histomorphometry. The authors, who disrupted exon 6 of the gene, also noted that $LRP5^{-/-}$ mice had tibial fractures when 2 months of age. This was the result of low bone mass. Moreover, TBV was found to be significantly reduced when the $LRP5^{-/-}$ mice were only 2 weeks old. Even loss of one allele of LRP5 led to a decrease in TBV intermediate between that of wild-type and knockout 24-week-old-animals. Deletion of LRP5 decreased the mineral apposition rate (MAR) in LRP5$^{-/-}$ mice by 50%. This indicates that gene loss led to inhibition of osteoblast function. LRP5 deletion also reduced osteoblast number and calvarial osteoblast proliferation by 50%. However, loss of LRP5 did not alter osteoblast apoptosis and differentiation, osteoclastogenesis or bone resorption. Thus, deletion of LRP5, by reducing osteoblast proliferation and activity, leads to decreased bone accrual in early postnatal mice. There was no difference in the skeletal phenotypes of female and male LRP5$^{-/-}$ mice, and their eye defects were like those of humans with OPPG [48].

Germline deletion of LRP6 also causes a decreased TBV. Total loss of murine LRP6 leads to embryonic lethality [78], but heterozygous mice are viable and can be studied postnatally [50]. In LRP5 and LRP6 double-knockout mice, both distal femur TBV and mid-femur cortical thickness were found reduced in 3-month-old females [36]. These effects appear to be dose-dependent, inasmuch as deletion of two or three alleles has a greater effect than loss of a single allele. Moreover, loss of one LRP6 allele produce a greater decrease in TBV than loss of one LRP5 allele. The spontaneous point mutation of LRP6 known as ringelschwanz (R886W in the Dkk1 binding region) leads to decreased canonical Wnt signaling and to a reduction of the metaphyseal volumetric BMD (vBMD) and of cortical thickness at 14 months of age [52]. Therefore, four alleles of LRP5 and LRP6 seem necessary for normal trabecular and cortical bone formation.

As with the loss-of-function mutation, the LRP5 gain-of-function mice have a phenotype that parallels the human syndrome. The transgenic mice that harbor the G171V mutation of human LRP5 are referred to as the HBM mice [4]. This model was developed by targeting the expression of hLRP5^{G171V} to bone with the aid of the 3.6 kb rat type I collagen promoter. These mice have increased bone formation, but the mechanisms differ from those that lead to decreased bone formation owing to loss of LRP5. Heterozygous HBM mice (LRP5$^{G171V/+}$) have a 100% increase in distal femur trabecular vBMD that can be detected as early as when the mice are 5 weeks of age, and persists until they are at least 1 year old. As in HBM humans, cortical bone thickness in the mouse model is increased by 30%, with the total bone area increased fourfold and the mineralizing surface by 40%. Interestingly, MAR, is not significantly elevated in the HBM mice; this indicates that osteoblast activity is not affected. Alkaline phosphatase (ALP) staining of calvaria is also increased in the LRP5$^{G171V/+}$ mice, while osteoblast apoptosis is decreased by 70% as shown by TUNEL (terminal dNTP transferase-mediated dUTP nick end-labeled) staining. As in LRP5$^{-/-}$ mice, osteoclast number and bone resorption are unchanged by the G171V mutation and the phenotype is similar in both sexes. As true for humans with this gain-of-function mutation, the LRP5$^{G171V/+}$ mice exhibit increased femoral and vertebral bone strength [2], but bone shape and size are normal. Therefore, the principal mechanism that accounts for the increase in bone formation in the HBM mice is the result of an increase in the number of osteoblasts and osteocytes, in turn, due to a decrease in cell death.

Mice with the G171V LRP5 gain-of-function mutation also have a heightened response to the anabolic action of mechanical loading [81], whereas LRP5$^{-/-}$ animals exhibit a diminished response to physical stimuli [84]. These findings point to the important role of LRP5 and Wnt signaling, not only in relation to bone development and accrual, but also for bone modeling and remodeling in response to environmental stimuli.

9.3 Effects of Dkks on Bone Formation and Development

9.3.1 Dkk1

The total loss of murine Dkk1 leads to death of the embryo, because the head does not develop. Limb and digit formation is also affected, with both proliferation and apoptosis altered [73]. Heterozygous mice, however, survive beyond birth and have been studied in detail. The tibias from Dkk1$^{+/-}$ animals exhibit increases in TBV and trabecular bone formation [72]. In comparison with calvarial-derived osteoblasts from wild-type controls, those from heterozygous mice exhibit a reduction in Dkk1 mRNA levels, an increase in canonical Wnt signaling, an elevation of DNA synthesis, and enhanced ALP activity. Thus, partial loss of Dkk1 stimulates osteoblast proliferation, differentiation, and activity. These conclusions have been confirmed by studies of transgenic mice that expressed murine Dkk1 in bone using the 2.3 kb rat type 1A1 collagen promoter [55]. In these mice, TBV is reduced, as are the cortical bone area and the rate of bone formation, because osteoblast differentiation and activity have been suppressed.

An interesting naturally occurring mouse mutant is the doubleridge ($Dkk1^d$), which harbors a hypomorphic allele of Dkk1 and leads to defective skeletal development [65]. Dkk1 expression is reduced by 65–99% of that in the wild type, resulting in hemivertebral fusions and other spinal defects. Interestingly, the skeletal defects are partially corrected in the offspring if the doubleridge mice are mated with LRP5 and LRP6 knockout animals. This finding demonstrates the importance of balancing activating and inhibitory Wnt signals. MacDonald et al. have evaluated the dose-dependent effects of Dkk1 expression on bone formation by generating an allelic series from matings of $Dkk1^{+/-}$ and $Dkk1^{+/d}$ mice [66]. Micro-CT analysis of distal femurs from 8-week-old offspring of these crosses demonstrated an inverse correlation between Dkk1 expression in calvaria and trabecular and cortical bone parameters. Strikingly, a 25% reduction in Dkk1 mRNA levels was sufficient to elevate TBV by 20–30%; this indicates the potent effect of this gene on bone formation and development.

9.3.2 Dkk2

Li et al. examined the role of Dkk2 in osteoblast function and bone formation by deleting the gene in mice [56]. Because Dkk2 is an extracellular antagonist of LRP5 and −6 [61, 70, 99], the authors anticipated that loss of Dkk2 would lead to increased bone formation, but instead found osteopenia, with trabecular and cortical bone mineral content (BMC) and TBV and trabecular number reduced. In addition, Dkk2 deletion led to an increase in osteoid surface without a corresponding elevation in osteoblast number or surface. Moreover, the $Dkk2^{-/-}$ mice exhibited reduced MAR as determined by dynamic histomorphometry. Loss of Dkk2, therefore, seems to cause deficiency in terminal osteoblast differentiation and matrix mineralization. These in vivo analyses were confirmed by in vitro studies of bone marrow-derived and neonatal calvarial-derived osteoblast cultures, which demonstrated that deletion of Dkk2 results in delayed cellular differentiation and matrix mineralization, even though canonical Wnt signaling is elevated. When the expression of Dkk2 mRNA was analyzed as a function of osteogenic differentiation, the levels of this secreted Wnt antagonist were found to increase with advancing osteoblast development. Furthermore, when Dkk2 was overexpressed in bone marrow-derived and neonatal calvarial-derived osteoblast cultures obtained from wild-type mice, matrix mineralization was found to be enhanced. From the viewpoint of development, canonical Wnt signaling may have to be enhanced to induce pre-osteoblast proliferation and for the osteoblast to subsequently progress through cellular differentiation. Terminal differentiation and matrix mineralization thus seem to require suppression of this pathway by antagonists like Dkk2.

9.3.3 Dkk3

Dkk3 is also an osteoblast antagonist, but the mechanism does not involve suppression of Wnt signaling. Aslan et al. used murine C3H10T1/2 mesenchymal stem cells (MSCs) that were engineered to express human bone morphogenetic protein-2 (BMP-2) in a tetracycline-regulated system and identified transcripts involved in bone formation by microarray analysis [3]. The cells were implanted into mice and allowed to form bone in vivo. Histological analysis demonstrated that the cells recapitulated endochondral bone formation as regulated by BMP-2. Among the differentially expressed genes was Dkk3, which peaked at the matrix deposition phase of cartilage and bone formation, but did not appear to block Wnt signaling [68]. When, with use of the tetracycline-regulated system, Dkk3 was engineered into C3H10T1/2 mesenchymal cells that expressed BMP-2, cell division and osteogenesis were inhibited. Micro-CT analysis of bone formed in vivo demonstrated that bone volume was reduced in MSCs that expressed Dkk3 relative to the BMP-2 controls. Thus, as with Dkk1, Dkk3 also diminishes osteoblast proliferation and differentiation.

9.4 Effects of Kremens on Bone Formation and Development

Kremen (Krm) 1 and 2 are single-pass transmembrane coreceptors for Dkk proteins [74]. Deletion of Krm1 and 2, as of Dkk1, affects skeletal development and bone formation, albeit with different and unexpected mechanisms [21]. Germline deletion of either murine Krm1 or 2 alone did not affect bone accrual. On the other hand, complete loss of both genes resulted in extra forelimb digits, a situation that was exacerbated by deletion of one allele of Dkk1. Total ablation of Krm1 and 2 increased TBV up to 200% in 12–23-week-old mice, male or female. This increase was comparable to the gains achieved by the loss of one allele of Dkk1. However, in contrast to digit formation, mice lacking Krm1 and 2 along with one allele of Dkk1 did not exhibit greater increases in TBV. Histomorphometric evaluation of tibias from the animals indicated that the gains in TBV that resulted from deletion of Krm1 and Krm 2 were largely due to a fourfold increase in osteoblast number, with a smaller (38%) elevation of osteoblast activity as measured by MAR. As with other knockout and transgenic models of extracelluar Wnt pathway modulators, loss of murine Krm 1 and Krm 2 did not affect osteoclast numbers or bone resorption.

In vitro analysis of Axin2 mRNA expression by fibroblasts cultured from Krm1,$2^{-/-}$ mouse embryos (MEFs) showed that the levels of this canonical Wnt pathway marker were three to fourfold higher when compared with the wild-type cells [21]. Surprisingly, treatment of the MEFs with *Xenopus* Dkk1 protein-conditioned medium resulted in a dose-dependent decrease in Axin2 expression in both wild-type and Krm1, $2^{-/-}$ cells. Thus, Dkk1 appears to be capable of antagonizing canonical Wnt signaling in the absence of kremens.

9.5 Effects of SOST/sclerostin on Bone Formation and Development

SOST/sclerostin is a member of the DAN cysteine knot-containing family of secreted proteins and blocks both BMP and Wnt signaling [93]. Other members of the DAN family also modulate these pathways [20, 93]. SOST was identified as the gene that is inactivated in sclerosteosis, a bone dysplasia, which is a HBM disease that predominantly affects the Afrikaner population of South Africa [15]. While complete loss of SOST/sclerostin results in an abnormal skeletal phenotype, heterozygote carriers of sclerosteosis have elevated BMD without any of the other pathologies associated with this disease [24]. Another sclerosing bone dysplasia, Van Buchem disease, is also caused by a reduction in sclerostin expression [63]. Patients with Van Buchem disease do not have mutations in the coding region of the SOST gene, but instead harbor a 52-kilobase (kb) noncoding deletion in the downstream region of the gene. This noncoding deletion removes an enhancer that enables expression of SOST/sclerostin in bone. An interesting observation regarding sclerostin is that it is highly expressed in osteocytes [79, 98].

When compared with nontransgenic controls, mice that express human SOST driven by the mouse osteocalcin gene 2 (OG2) promoter/enhancer exhibit reduced BMC of the lumbar vertebrae and femur as measured by PIXImus, as well as reduced TBV, osteoblast surface, and bone formation rate, as determined histologically [98]. These results indicate that SOST/sclerostin inhibits osteoblast proliferation, differentiation, and activity, all of which are also blunted by Dkk1.

In contrast to humans who fail to express sclerostin, $SOST^{-/-}$ mice [57] appear grossly normal with proper digit development, no evidence of facial muscle paralysis, and a lifespan that is comparable with the wild-type controls. However, whole body radiography of 4-month-old male and female SOST knockout mice revealed the characteristic skeletal HBM phenotype of sclerostin deficiency. At 5–6.5 months of age, micro-CT analysis of distal femurs from SOST$^{-/-}$ mice demonstrated a 146–224% increase in trabecular vBMD, compared with wild-type controls. Analysis of the mid-shaft femoral region indicated a 15–22% elevation in periosteal perimeter, and a 93–117% enhancement of cortical bone area in the knockout animals. Histological analysis showed that osteoblast surface was increased by 189–1,007%, whereas MAR was elevated by 20–231% in mice without sclerostin; on the other hand, osteoclast surface was not affected by loss of the gene. Serum levels of the osteoblastic marker, osteocalcin (OC), were elevated by 37–42%, but the levels of the osteoclastic marker TRACP-5b were unaffected by SOST deletion. Bone strength of vertebrae and femurs from SOST$^{-/-}$ mice, in terms of maximum load (N), stiffness (N/mm), and energy to failure (mJ), was increased by 27–56%, when compared with wild-type controls. Thus, loss of SOST/sclerostin leads to robust increases in trabecular and cortical bone formation and strength owing to an elevation of osteoblast number and activity, without an effect on the parameters of osteoclastic function.

Although sclerostin was initially described as a BMP-6-binding protein that suppressed osteoblast proliferation and differentiation by antagonizing BMP signaling [98], more recent work demonstrated that it probably inhibits bone formation by blunting the canonical Wnt pathway through interaction with LRP5 and –6 [58, 85, 88, 92]. More specifically, van Bezooijen et al. [92] have shown that in mouse KS483 MSCs treated with human BMP-4 in the presence and absence of human sclerostin, the transcription profiles were inconsistent with simple BMP antagonism. By employing reporter gene assays to measure BMP and Wnt signaling in osteoblastic cell lines, the authors observed [92] that sclerostin does not antagonize BMP activity, but blocks Wnt activity. Moreover, both sclerostin and Dkk1 inhibited the ability of BMP-4 to activate the canonical Wnt pathway. van Bezooijen et al. [92], thus, concluded that sclerostin suppresses bone formation by antagonizing Wnt signaling that is activated by BMPs and Wnts. As with Dkk1, the HBM mutations of LRP5 also prevent sclerostin from binding and blocking the canonical pathway [20, 58, 85].

9.6 Effects of Wnts on Bone Formation and Development

9.6.1 Wnt-3a, -5a, and -5b

Germline deletion of murine Wnt-5a results in abnormal development of the skeleton, and both endochondral and intramembranous bone formation are affected by loss of this gene [100, 101]. When compared with wild-type controls, long bone length is shortened in the Wnt-5a$^{-/-}$ mice along the proximal-distal axis, culminating in the loss of phalanges [100]. Deficiencies in the function of the apical ectodermal ridge (AER) are not the cause for these skeletal abnormalities, because gene expression analysis failed to show alterations consistent with the changes in AER activity. In contrast, evaluation of progenitor cells within the progress zone of limbs from knockout mice indicated [100] a decrease in progenitor cell DNA synthesis and proliferation, when compared with samples from wild-type controls.

Histological analysis of long bones from Wnt-5a$^{-/-}$ mice showed that chondrocyte hypertrophy and skeletal ossification were delayed relative to Wnt-5a $^{+/+}$ animals [101]. In situ gene expression analysis of long bones from wild-type and knockout mice demonstrated that Wnt-5a is expressed at the boundary of proliferative and pre-hypertrophic chondrocytes, and is required both for chondrocyte proliferation, and the transition of proliferating to pre-hypertrophic cells. Wnt-5a is also produced by cells of the perichondrium/periosteum. Moreover, the expression of Runx2 (runt-related transcription factor 2) and OC was reduced in chondrocytes and osteoblasts of the long bones of Wnt-5a$^{-/-}$ mice. In other words, both cartilage and bone cell differentiation were suppressed.

Surprisingly, and in contrast to the results with the knockout mice, transgenic expression of Wnt-5a in chondrocytes using the type 2a1 collagen promoter also led to suppression of chondrocyte proliferation and differentiation [101]. As Wnt-5b is synthesized by chondrocytes at the boundary of pre-hypertrophic and hypertrophic cells, the authors examined the effects of transgenic expression for this close relative of Wnt-5a, using the type 2a1 collagen promoter. They found that chondrocyte differentiation prior to hypertrophic development was delayed, whereas chondrocyte proliferation was increased. Further evaluation of these transgenic mouse lines revealed that overexpression of Wnt-5a in chondrocytes prevents articular/resting epiphyseal cells (Zone I) from entering the proliferative phase (Zone II), but promotes differentiation to pre-hypertrophic cells. Overexpression of Wnt-5b stimulates the entrance of cells into Zone II, but prevents cell-cycle withdrawal and subsequent hypertrophy. Thus, Wnt-5a and -5b are both required to modulate the transition, proliferation, and differentiation of chondrocytes from the epiphysis to the growth plate.

Takada et al. have evaluated the skeletal phenotypes of the Wnt-3a$^{+/-}$ and Wnt-5a$^{+/-}$ mice [87]. Wnt-3a signals through the canonical β-catenin pathway and perhaps other pathways [16, 80, 91], whereas Wnt-5a has consistently been shown to activate noncanonical pathways [61, 70, 71, 99]. Deletion of one allele of either Wnt-3a or Wnt-5a results in decreased femoral distal BMD and TBV, when compared with the wild-type controls. However, these two knockout mouse lines also differ in the fact that loss of Wnt-5a led to a three to fourfold increase in the number of bone marrow adipocytes, whereas removal of Wnt-3a had no effect on adipogenesis. Treatment of murine bone marrow mesenchymal stem cells (BMSCs) in vitro with Wnt-5a protein blocked the induction of adipogenesis by troglitazone and enhanced osteogenesis; moreover, this trans-differentiation effect occurred in the absence of β-catenin [87]. The authors determined that the intracellular signaling pathway for Wnt-5a action on adipogenesis/osteogenesis of BMSCs involved the activation of calmodulin-dependent protein kinase II (CamKII). This leads to suppression of peroxisome proliferator activated receptor (PPAR)-γ trans-activation (adipogenic pathway) and enhancement of Runx2 trans-activation (osteogenic pathway).

9.6.2 Wnt-7b

Although considered to be a canonical Wnt [61, 70, 71, 99], Wnt-7b has also been reported to signal through a noncanonical pathway to regulate bone formation and development [91]. Using Cre-loxP technology to create a null allele by deleting the essential exon 3 of Wnt-7b from early mesenchymal progenitor cells, Tu et al. [91] used the Dermo1 (twist2) promoter to express Cre recombinase (Dermo1-Cre; Wnt7b$^{n/c3}$). The Wnt-7b mutant mice were viable at birth and exhibited no obvious phenotype. However, histological examination of long bones from embryonic animals indicated that Wnt-7b had lost its ability to suppress bone formation and the bones thus exhibited delayed chondrocyte maturation [91]. Osteogenesis was suppressed because of reduced expression of the osteoblast transcription factor, Osterix. Also, Wnt-7b did not appear to signal through β-catenin, but instead activated a G-protein-coupled receptor pathway that involved $G\alpha_{q/11}$ and protein kinase C (PKC) δμ [91].

9.6.3 Wnt-10b

Wnt-10b signals through the β-catenin pathway and is expressed by normal human osteoblasts [30, 89]. In addition, mechanical stimulation of mouse MC-3T3-E1 osteoblasts in vitro increases Wnt-10b mRNA levels [81]. Wnt-10b is also expressed in murine pre-adipocytes and marrow vascular cells [10, 83]. Transgenic expression of Wnt-10b in mice using the FABP4 promoter that targets the gene to marrow decreases both white and brown fat formation, provides resistance to diet-induced obesity, and increases glucose tolerance [47, 62]. In addition, mice with transgenic expression of Wnt10b exhibit increased bone formation [8]. In both male and female FABP4-Wnt10b mice, the TBV of the distal femur is increased fourfold, with the increase seen from 8 weeks to 23 months of age. However, the properties of cortical bone are largely unaffected by the transgene. Female FABP4-Wnt10b mice are also resistant to ovariectomy-induced trabecular bone loss at 3 months of age. Consistent with these results, female Wnt-10b$^{-/-}$ mice had 30% reduction in serum OC and in TBV of the distal femur at 8 weeks of age [8]. Concentrations of TRACP-5b did not change in the mutants, and similar to the loss-of-function and gain-of-function mutations of LRP5, bone formation, but not resorption, was altered by germline deletion.

To further characterize the role that Wnt-10b plays in bone formation, Bennett et al. [9] developed a transgenic mouse line that, with the aid of the human OC promoter (Oc-Wnt10b), expresses murine Wnt-10b in osteoblasts. Oc-Wnt10b mice require water-softened or ground chow to thrive when weaned. Incisor eruption is delayed in mandibles of the transgenic animals, with normal values attained at postnatal day 16. At 3 months of age, Oc-Wnt10b mice have a threefold elevation of femoral TBV, when compared with the nontransgenic controls, but with no other effects on cortical bone parameters. The osteoblast surface in these mice is increased 1.4-fold, with a slight increase in MAR, a measure of osteoblast activity. Compared with nontransgenic controls, the Oc-Wnt10b transgenic mice display an increase in trabecular bone formation, essentially owing to an increase in osteoblast number. As osteoblast proliferation and apoptosis are unaltered by transgenic expression of Wnt-10b, it is apparent that osteoblast differentiation was enhanced. As true for the Wnt-10b$^{-/-}$ mice, the Oc-Wnt10b animals do not exhibit changes in osteoclast number.

9.7 Effects of sFRPs on Bone Formation and Development

9.7.1 sFRP-1

Germline deletion of murine sFRP-1 leads to increased bone formation and accelerated chondrocyte differentiation in the absence of aberrant effects on nonskeletal tissues [12, 26, 90]. Robust sFRP-1 promoter activity is found in many embryonic tissues of the sFRP-1$^{-/-}$ mice (brain, skeleton, kidney, eye, spleen, and heart), but inactivation of this gene does not appear to compromise normal embryonic development [90]. Loss of this Wnt antagonist does, however, increase distal femur TBV by 80% in adult 35-week-old female mice [12]. In addition, other trabecular bone parameters like connectivity density, trabecular number, trabecular thickness, and trabecular spacing are improved by loss of the gene. However, loss of sFRP-1 has no effect on parameters of cortical bone. Interestingly, trabecular vBMD of the distal femur in sFRP-1$^{-/-}$ mice did not begin to differ until the animals were 13 weeks of age. However, as the mice aged, the sFRP-1$^{+/+}$ animals lost trabecular bone, while the sFRP-1$^{-/-}$ mice gained trabecular bone, so that, by 38 weeks of age, BMD had increased 100%. This increase was maintained until the animals were at least 52 weeks of age. Thus, deletion of sFRP-1 delays and enhances the onset of peak bone mass and suppresses senile bone loss. Although sFRP-1$^{-/-}$ males also have a HBM phenotype, it is not as pronounced as in females [12]. Dynamic histomorphometric analysis of proximal femurs from 35-week-old sFRP-1$^{+/+}$ and sFRP-1$^{-/-}$ female mice showed that deletion of sFRP-1 increased MAR by 30%. Histology and TUNEL staining of calvaria from 33-week-old female mice demonstrated that loss of sFRP-1 also led to a 15–20% increase in calvarial thickness and to a 50% decrease in osteoblast and osteocyte apoptosis. When bone marrow from 27-week-old sFRP-1$^{+/+}$ and sFRP-1$^{-/-}$ female mice was cultured in the presence of ascorbic acid, β-glycerolphosphate, and dexamethasone, deletion of sFRP-1 caused the number of ALP + cells to increase three to fourfold. Analysis of the differentiating cultures for LacZ expression showed that osteoblast development and matrix mineralization increased as sFRP-1 promoter activity became elevated. This suggests that control of Wnt signaling by sFRP-1 modulates osteoblast differentiation and function. In addition, evaluation of bone marrow cultures from knockout mice by TUNEL staining showed that cellular apoptosis was suppressed by 70%, when compared with cultures from wild-type controls. Measurement of DNA synthesis in cultures derived from newborn sFRP-1$^{+/+}$ and sFRP-1$^{-/-}$ mice calvaria showed that osteoblast proliferation also increased twofold in the knockout cells during the proliferative phase. However, when the sFRP-1$^{-/-}$ cultures reached confluence and proliferation ceased, the rate of DNA synthesis returned to normal. This indicates that the transition from proliferation to differentiation was not altered by loss of sFRP-1. Deletion of sFRP-1 thus can be seen to enhance osteoblast proliferation, differentiation, and function, at the same time suppressing osteoblast and osteocyte apoptosis.

One mechanism to explain the increase in osteoblast differentiation seen in sFRP-1$^{-/-}$ mice bone marrow cultures is elevated Runx2 expression. When RNA was isolated from the long bones of the sFRP-1$^{-/-}$ mice, Runx2 message levels increased four to eightfold over those in the controls [25]. Analysis of the Runx2 promoter identified a putative LEF/TCF response element about 100 bp upstream from the transcription start site, which in turn is adjacent to a Runx2-binding site. Cotransfection of MC-3T3-E1 mouse osteoblastic cells with a 0.6 kb Runx2 promoter-luciferase construct, TCF-1, and various Wnts showed that the Wnts upregulated Runx2 promoter activity. Moreover, this effect was suppressed by cotransfection with sFRP-1. Thus, the increase in Runx2 expression owing to Wnts is blocked by sFRP-1.

In addition to being a negative regulator of osteoblast physiology and bone formation, sFRP-1 also suppresses chondrocyte differentiation and cartilage formation [26]. Promoter activity for LacZ gene expression in embryonic cartilaginous tissues from the sFRP-1$^{-/-}$ mice is abundant in chondrocytes of developing epiphyses of limbs and joints of growing digits. Deletion of sFRP-1 leads to shortening of the hypertrophic zone and growth plate, decreased chondrocyte proliferation, and increased hypertrophic zone calcification; this suggests an acceleration of chondrocyte maturation in the knockout animals. Consistent with these observations is that expression of Runx2 and collagen type 10a1 protein is enhanced in pre-hypertrophic and hypertrophic chondrocytes of sFRP-1$^{-/-}$ mice. Transcription profiling of MEFs from the knockout mice that had differentiated into chondrocytes in vitro demonstrated an increase in Runx2 and collagen type 2a1 mRNA levels, a suppression of Indian Hedgehog mRNA levels, a delay of Sox9 mRNA expression, and an acceleration of collagen type 10a1 mRNA expression. In addition, loss of sFRP-1 led to a reduction in the message levels of other Wnt pathway antagonists and a subsequent elevation of Wnt/β-catenin pathway activity.

9.7.2 sFRP-3

Another secreted Wnt antagonist, sFRP-3, also plays a role in bone and cartilage physiology. Using Cre-lox technology to delete murine sFRP-3 (also known as FrzB for Frizzled motif in bone development [46]) in the germline, Lories et al. [64] described the skeletal phenotype of these knockout animals. As in the sFRP-1$^{-/-}$ mice [90], loss of sFRP-3 did not result in an overt developmental phenotype [64]. However, postnatally, the sFRP-3$^{-/-}$ mice displayed alterations in their joints and in the biomechanical properties of cortical bone. Although unchallenged adult (10–12-week-old) knockout mice appeared to have normal articular cartilage, the sFRP-3$^{-/-}$ animals exhibited enhanced cartilage damage after treatment with papain, collagenase, or methylated bovine serum albumin. Treatments also led to an enhancement of canonical Wnt signaling and matrix metalloproteinase (MMP)-3 expression and activity in articular cartilage. The subchondral bone area, mineral content, and density were normal in the sFRP-3$^{-/-}$ mice. pQCT and micro-CT analysis of femurs from 10- to 20-week-old knockout animals showed elevated cortical BMC and thickness. Biomechanical evaluation of long bones from the knockout mice suggested that they were stiffer than bones from wild-type controls, consistent with the increase in cortical thickness seen in the knockouts. As murine sFRP-3 is expressed in the periosteum [64], in vivo mechanical loading of the ulnae resulted in an enhanced elevation of periosteal bone volume. Moreover, the cortical bone of sFRP-3$^{-/-}$ mice responded to a lower peak strain rate than did that of sFRP-3$^{+/+}$ animals. Thus, while sFRP-1 is a negative regulator of chondrocyte maturation and trabecular bone formation, sFRP-3 suppresses cartilage degradation in models of osteoarthritis and inhibits cortical bone formation and response to mechanical stimulation.

9.7.3 sFRP-4

The senescence-accelerated mouse strain, SAMP6, has a naturally occurring mutation that causes low peak bone mass and an enhanced age-related bone loss that results from impaired osteoblastogenesis [42, 69]. By generating congenic strains and doing segregation analysis of chromosome 13, Nakanishi et al. [76] identified sFRP-4 as the gene that is responsible for the low bone mass, that was confirmed by the finding [75] that in transgenic mouse that overexpressed sFRP-4 in osteoblasts, the use of the murine 2.3-kb collagen 1a1 promoter also had lower TBV at 8 weeks of age. This drop had resulted from a reduction in osteoblast proliferation.

Thus, three of the five sFRPs appear to play a role in modulating bone formation in mice. This provides further support for the role played by Wnt signaling in bone formation.

9.8 Effects of Downstream Wnt Pathway Components on Bone Formation and Development

9.8.1 Axin2

Axin inhibits Wnt signaling intracellularly [61, 70, 99]. The skull structures of Axin2$^{-/-}$ mice have malformations owing to premature cranial suture fusion [102]. These malformations resemble craniosynostosis in humans. Deletion of Axin2 led to enhanced cellular proliferation as measured by BrdU labeling, and enhanced osteoblast differentiation, as measured by ALP in cultures of neonatal calvarial-derived osteoblasts. Osteopontin and OC expression were stimulated and matrix mineralization was increased, but osteoblast apoptosis was not affected. Levels of activated β-catenin in whole calvaria were elevated, but osteoblast apoptosis was unaffected. Thus, loss of Axin2 leads to an increase in Wnt signaling in osteoblasts that, in turn, brings about an increase in cellular proliferation and differentiation.

In a subsequent study, Yu et al. [60] found that in the calvaria of Axin2$^{-/-}$ mice, osteoprogenitor cells had higher nuclear β-catenin levels, and that this correlated with an increase in the levels of cyclin D1 and its target, CDK4. This increase, in turn, stimulated osteoprogenitor proliferation. Loss of Axin2 expression also enhanced osteoblastic BMP-2 and -6 production, and increased phospho-Smad1/5/8 levels. It also promoted the interaction between cytoplasmic β-catenin and osteoblast-cadherin at the membranes of mature osteoblasts. Thus, Axin2 plays a role in suppressing both nuclear and membrane functions of β-catenin in calvarial osteoblasts, an action that is partly mediated by inducing BMP expression and canonical signaling.

9.8.2 β-Catenin, APC, and TCF-1

Additional support for the importance of the β-catenin pathway in osteogenesis has come from the report by Hu et al. [38], who found that 18.5-day embryos of conditional knockout mice (β-cat$^{c/c}$) have skeletons that lack bone, but not cartilage. Osteoblast differentiation was arrested at the early progenitor stages, and only type I collagen and ALP were expressed. This means that β-catenin signaling is required for osteoblasts to complete differentiation and synthesize properly formed bone. Hill et al. [35] and Day et al. [18] described similar findings. To study the effects of β-catenin in limb and head mesenchyme, Hill et al. [35] used β-cat$^{\Delta Prx1/-}$ mice and showed that β-catenin activity is required for an early step of osteoblast differentiation. On the other hand, stabilization of the β-catenin function in the mesenchyme of β-catΔex3$^{Prx/+}$ animals suppresses chondrogenesis rather than stimulate osteoblastogenesis. Day et al. [18] used Catnby$^{c/c}$;Dermo1 (twist-2)-Cre mice to inactivate β-catenin in early mesenchymal progenitor cells. They also utilized Catnby$^{c/-}$/Col2a1-Cre mice to remove functional β-catenin from late mesenchymal cells that were committed to the chondrocyte lineage. They concluded that β-catenin signaling is necessary to inhibit chondrocyte differentiation while allowing formation of osteoblasts.

Holmen et al. [37] studied the role of osteoblastic β-catenin signaling during postnatal murine bone acquisition by conditionally deleting either β-catenin or APC, using the OC promoter to drive Cre expression. Both trabecular and cortical bone volume were reduced in the Δβ-catenin mice and this correlated with diminished osteoblast differentiation and matrix mineralization, as well as with an increase in osteoclast differentiation and activity. The latter resulted from downregulation of osteoblastic osteoprotegerin (OPG) expression and upregulation of a receptor that was activated by nuclear factor-κB ligand (RANKL) expression. On the other hand, the Δ-APC mice that had elevated osteoblastic β-catenin levels exhibited an osteopetrotic phenotype that resulted primarily from reduced osteoclast differentiation and activity, because osteoblastic OPG expression had been upregulated and RANKL expression had been downregulated. Using targeted Cre-lox technology to delete portions of the β-catenin gene in murine osteoblasts, Glass et al. [27] reported that creation of a constitutively active form of β-catenin produced an osteopetrotic phenotype that resulted from a decrease in osteoclastogenesis and bone resorption, because OPG expression had increased. Conversely, targeted deletion of functional β-catenin had the opposite effect and produced osteopenia that resulted from an increase in osteoclastogenesis and bone resorption because of a decrease in OPG expression by the osteoblast. Interestingly, germline deletion of TCF-1 in mice produced a similar, low bone mass phenotype, also because of diminished OPG expression. Surprisingly, no significant changes in osteoblastogenesis or bone formation were seen in any of these transgenic or knockout mouse models. In a study to characterize the molecular events associated with Wnt-3a action on mouse C3H10T1/2 pluripotent mesenchymal stem cells, Jackson et al. [41] also found that OPG expression was upregulated following activation of the β-catenin pathway. Thus, the canonical Wnt pathway seems to regulate both bone formation and coupled bone resorption via cells of the osteoblast lineage. Alterations of LRP5 and LRP6 activity appear to result in bone-formation changes, whereas regulation of downstream pathway components like β-catenin and TCF-1 primarily changes bone resorption. The reason for this is not clear, but modulation of downstream components is likely to be refractory to feedback control and may therefore represent extreme phenotypes.

Rodda and McMahon [82] evaluated the role of β-catenin in skeletogenesis. By using the collagen 2α1 promoter to drive Cre expression (*Col2α1-cre3; β-catenin*$^{c/c}$), they created mice that lack this signaling protein in the progenitors of chondrocytes and osteoblasts. The tibias from these animals lack a mineralized bone matrix; instead, hypertrophic chondrocytes are associated with mineralization. This phenotype confirms a role for β-catenin in osteoblastogenesis. In situ hybridization of tibias from the β-catenin knockout mice for the expression of osteoblast marker genes showed that collagen 1a1, Runx2, and Osterix mRNAs were present, while the message for OC was absent. On the other hand, markers of proliferating chondrocytes and postmitotic hypertrophic chondrocytes, collagen 2α1 and collagen 10α1, respectively, were expressed. Thus, loss of β-catenin did not affect early osteoblast formation, but delayed terminal differentiation of the cells; this suggests that Wnt signaling acts downstream of Osterix. Moreover, in the absence of β-catenin, the early osteoblasts reverted to chondrocytes.

9.9 Summary and Conclusions

Figure 9.1 summarizes the effects of Wnt pathway components on chondrogenesis and osteogenesis at the cellular level. Canonical signaling needs to be suppressed to allow entry of MSCs into the chondrocyte (Chond) lineage. However, after commitment, both canonical and noncanonical pathways are stimulated to enable progression of chondroprogenitors (CPs) to the pre-hypertrophic (Pre-HC) stage. At this point, antagonists like sFRP-1 are required to lower canonical signaling for maturation of these cells to hypertrophic chondrocytes (HCs). In contrast to chondrogenesis, canonical and noncanonical pathways need to be activated for the entry of skeletal progenitor cells (SPCs) into the osteoblast lineage. Beyond the osteoprogenitor (OP) stage, β-catenin (β-Cat) signaling is required for

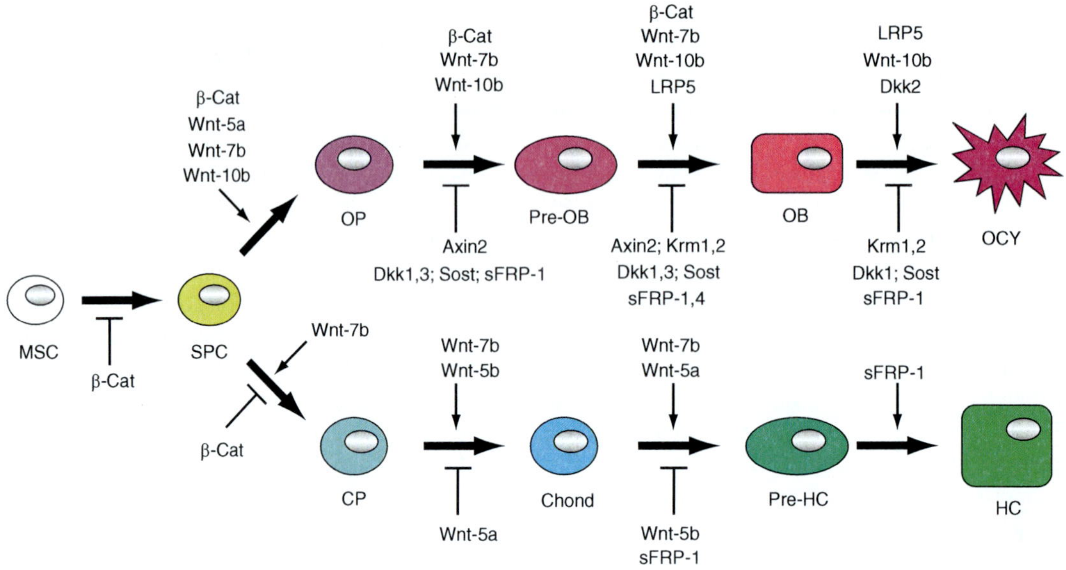

Figure 9.1. Wnt pathway regulation of chondrogenesis and osteogenesis. Please refer to the text for discussion of the model and for definition of the abbreviations.

the differentiation of these cells to pre-osteoblasts (Pre-OBs), mature osteoblasts (OBs), and perhaps, to osteocytes (OCYs) as well.

Over the past decade, it has become clear that Wnt signaling plays a vital role in embryonic and postnatal bone formation and development. Much evidence associates the canonical pathway with these skeletal processes, but recent findings indicate that noncanonical signaling is also involved. Modulation of extracellular and transmembrane components of the Wnt pathway largely affects bone formation, but interference with the intracellular machinery of bone formation also controls bone resorption via RANKL signaling. The reasons for these mechanistic differences may reside in the refractory nature of downstream pathway components to feedback regulation. Endochondral and intramembranous bone formation are both controlled by Wnts, which are important in inducing progenitor cell commitment and differentiation along the chondrocyte and osteoblast lineages. A key area for future research in this field is to better understand how these pathways intersect with other fundamental skeletal modulatory proteins like BMPs, hedgehogs, and fibroblast growth factors.

References

1. Ai M, Holmen SL, Van Hul W, Williams BO, Warman ML (2005) Reduced affinity to and inhibition by DKK1 form a common mechanism by which high bone mass-associated missense mutations in LRP5 affect canonical Wnt signaling. Mol Cell Biol 25:4946–4955
2. Akhter MP, Wells DJ, Short SJ, Cullen DM, Johnson ML, Haynatzki GR, Babij P, Allen KM, Yaworsky PJ, Bex F, Recker RR (2004) Bone biomechanical properties in LRP5 mutant mice. Bone 35:162–169
3. Aslan H, Ravid-Amir O, Clancy BM, Rezvankhah S, Pittman D, Pelled G, Turgeman G, Zilberman Y, Gazit Z, Hoffmann A, Gross G, Domany E, Gazit D (2006) Advance molecular profiling in vitro detects novel function of dickkopf-3 in regulation of bone formation. J Bone Miner Res 21:1935–1945
4. Babij P, Zhao W, Small C, Kharode Y, Yaworsky PJ, Bouxsein ML, Reddy PS, Bodine PVN, Robinson JA, Bhat B, Moran RA, Bex F (2003) High bone mass in mice expressing a mutant LRP5 gene. J Bone Miner Res 18:960–974
5. Balemans W, Devogelaer J-P, Cleiren E, Piters E, Caussin E, Van Hul W (2007) Novel LRP5 missense mutation in a patient with high bone mass phenotype results in decreased DKK1-mediated inhibition of Wnt signaling. J Bone Miner Res 22:708–716
6. Balemans W, van Hul W (2007) The genetics of low-density lipoprotein receptor-related protein 5 in bone: a story of extremes. Endocrinology 148:2622–2629
7. Baron R, Rawadi G (2007) Wnt signaling and the regulation of bone mass. Curr Osteoporos Rep 5:73–80

8. Bennett CN, Longo KA, Wright WS, Suva LJ, Lane TF, Hankenson KD, MacDougald OA (2005) Regulation of osteoblastogenesis and bone mass by Wnt10b. Proc Natl Acad Sci U S A 102 3324–3329
9. Bennett CN, Ouyang H, Ma YL, Zeng Q, Gerin I, Sousa KM, Lane TF, Krishnan V, Hankenson KD, MacDougald OA (2007) Wnt-10b increases postnatal bone formation by enhancing osteoblast differentiation. J Bone Miner Res 22:1924–1932
10. Bennett CN, Ross SE, Longo KA, Bajnok L, Hemati N, Johnson KW, Harrison SD, MacDougald OA (2002) Regulation of Wnt signaling during adipogenesis. J Biol Chem 277:30998–31004
11. Bodine PVN, Komm BS (2006) Wnt signaling and osteobla stogenesis. Rev Endocrine Metab Disord 7:33–39
12. Bodine PVN, Zhao W, Kharode YP, Bex FJ, Lambert A-J, Goad MB, Gaur T, Stein GS, Lian JB, Komm BS (2004) The Wnt antagonist secreted frizzled-related protein-1 is a negative regulator of trabecular bone formation in adult mice. Mol Endocrinol 18:1222–1237
13. Bovolenta P, Esteve P, Ruiz JM, Cisneros E, Lopez-Rios J (2008) Beyond Wnt inhibition: new functions of secreted Frizzled-related proteins in development and disease. J Cell Sci 121:737–746
14. Boyden LM, Mao J, Belsky J, Mitzner L, Farhi A, Mitnick MA, Wu D, Insogna K, Lifton RP (2002) High bone density due to a mutation in LDL-receptor-related protein 5. N Engl J Med 346:1513–1521
15. Brunkow ME, Gardner JC, Van Ness J, Paeper BW, Kovacevich BR, Proll S, Skonier JE, Zhao L, Sabo PJ, Fu Y-H, Alisch RS, Gillett L, Colbert T, Tacconi P, Galas D, Hamersma H, Beighton P, Mulligan JT (2001) Bone dysplasia sclerosteosis results from loss of the SOST gene product, a novel cysteine knot-containing protein. Am J Hum Genet 68:577–589
16. Chen AE, Ginty DD, Fan C-M (2005) Protein kinase A signaling via CREB control myogenesis induced by Wnt proteins. Nature 433:317–322
17. Clement-Lacroix P, Ai M, Morvan F, Roman-Roman S, Vayssiere B, Belleville C, Estrera K, Warman ML, Baron R, Rawadi G (2005) Lrp5-independent activation of Wnt signaling by lithium chloride increases bone formation and bone mass in mice. Proc Natl Acad Sci U S A 102 17406–17411
18. Day TF, Guo X, Garrett-Beal L, Yang Y (2005) Wnt/beta-Catenin signaling in mesenchymal progenitors controls osteoblast and chondrocyte differentiation during vertebrate skeletogenesis. Dev Cell 8:739–750
19. Day TF, Yang Y (2008) Wnt and hedgehog signaling pathways in bone development. J Bone Joint Surg 90:19–24
20. Ellies DL, Viviano B, McCarthy J, Rey J-P, Itasaki N, Saunders S, Krumlauf R (2006) Bone density ligand, sclerostin, directly interacts with LRP5 but not LRP5G171V to modulate Wnt activity. J Bone Miner Res 21:1738–1749
21. Ellwanger K, Saito H, Clement-Lacroix P, Maltry N, Niedermeyer J, Lee WK, Baron R, Rawadi G, Westphal H, Niehrs C (2008) Targeted disruption of the Wnt regulator Kremen induces limb defects and high bone density. Mol Cell Biol 28:4875–4882
22. Ferrari SL, Deutsch S, Antonarakis SE (2005) Pathogenic mutations and polymorphisms in the lipoprotein receptor-related protein 5 reveal a new biological pathway for the control of bone mass. Curr Opin Lipidol 16:207–214
23. Fujino T, Asaba H, Kang MJ, Ikeda Y, Sone H, Takada S, Kim DH, Ioka RX, Ono M, Tomoyori H, Okubo M, Murase T, Kamataki A, Yamamoto J, Magoori K, Takahashi S, Miyamoto Y, Oishi H, Nose M, Okazaki M, Usui S, Imaizumi K, Yanagisawa M, Sakai J, Yamamoto TT (2003) Low-density lipoprotein receptor-related protein 5 (LRP5) is essential for normal cholesterol metabolism and glucose-induced insulin secretion. Proc Natl Acad Sci U S A 100:229–324
24. Gardner JC, van Bezooijen RL, Mervis B, Hamdy NAT, Lowik CWGM, Hamersma H, Beighton P, Papapoulos SE (2005) Bone mineral density in Sclerosteosis; affected individuals and gene carriers. J Clin Endocrinol Metab 90:6392–6395
25. Gaur T, Lengner CJ, Hovhannisyan H, Bhat RA, Bodine PV, Komm BS, Javed A, van Wijnen AJ, Stein JL, Stein GS, Lian JB (2005) Canonical WNT signaling promotes osteogenesis by directly stimulating Runx2 gene expression. J Biol Chem 280:33132–33140
26. Gaur T, Rich L, Lengner CJ, Hussain S, Trevant B, Ayers A, Stein JL, Bodine PVN, Komm BS, Stein GS, Lian JB (2006) Secreted frizzled-related protein-1 regulates Wnt Signaling for BMP2 induced chondrocyte differentiation. J Cell Physiol 208:87–96
27. Glass DA II, Bialek P, Ahn JD, Starbuck M, Patel MS, Clevers H, Taketo MM, Lang RA, Karsenty G (2005) Canonical Wnt signaling in differentiated osteoblasts controls osteoclast differentiation. Dev Cell 8:751–764
28. Glass DA II, Karsenty G (2006) Molecular bases of the regulation of bone remodeling by the canonical Wnt signaling pathway. Curr Top Dev Biol 73:43–84
29. Gong Y, Slee RB, Fukai N, Rawadi G, Roman-Roman S, Reginato AM, Wang H, Cundy T, Glorieux FH, Lev D, Zacharin M, Oexle K, Marcelino J, Suwairi W, Heeger S, Sabatakos G, Apte S, Adkins WN, Allgrove J, Arslan-Kirchner M, Batch JA, Beighton P, Black GC, Boles RG, Boon LM, Borrone C, Brunner HG, Carle GF, Dallapiccola B, De Paepe A, Floege B, Halfhide ML, Hall B, Hennekam RC, Hirose T, Jans A, Juppner H, Kim CA, Keppler-Noreuil K, Kohlschuetter A, LaCombe D, Lambert M, Lemyre E, Letteboer T, Peltonen L, Ramesar RS, Romanengo M, Somer H, Steichen-Gersdorf E, Steinmann B, Sullivan B, Superti-Furga A, Swoboda W, van den Boogaard MJ, Van Hul W, Vikkula M, Votruba M, Zabel B, Garcia T, Baron R, Olsen BR, Warman ML; The Osteoporosis-Pseudoglioma Syndrome Collaborative G (2001) LDL receptor-related protein 5 (LRP5) affects bone accrual and eye development. Cell 107:513–523
30. Hale LV, Halladay DL, Galvin RJS, Onyia JE, Frolik CA (2004) The Wnt pathway in human bone cells and bone-related cells: Taqman gene expression analysis. J Bone Miner Res 19:S275
31. Hartmann C (2007) Skeletal development - Wnts are in control. Mol Cells 24:177–184

32. Hartmann C (2006) A Wnt canon orchestrating osteoblastogenesis. Trends Cell Biol 16:151–158
33. Hayward P, Kalmar T, Arias AM (2008) Wnt/Notch signaling and information processing during development. Development 135:411–424
34. He X, Semenov M, Tamai K, Zeng X (2004) LDL receptor-related proteins 5 and 6 in Wnt/beta-catenin signaling: arrow points the way. Development 131:1663–1677
35. Hill TP, Spater D, Taketo MM, Birchmeier W, Hartmann C (2005) Canonical Wnt/beta-catenin signaling prevents osteoblasts from differentiating into chondrocytes. Dev Cell 8:727–738
36. Holmen SL, Giambernardi TA, Zylstra CR, Buckner-Berghuis BD, Resau JH, Hess JF, Glatt V, Bouxsein ML, Ai M, Warman ML, Williams BO (2004) Decreased BMD and limb deformities in mice carrying mutations in both LRP5 and LRP6. J Bone Miner Res 19:2033–2040
37. Holmen SL, Zylstra CR, Mukherjee A, Sigler RE, Faugere MC, Bouxsein ML, Deng L, Clemens TL, Williams BO (2005) Essential role of beta-catenin in postnatal bone acquisition. J Biol Chem 280: 21162–21168
38. Hu H, Hilton MJ, Tu X, Yu K, Ornitz DM, Long F (2005) Sequential roles of Hedgehog and Wnt signaling in osteoblast development. Development 132:49–60
39. Huang H, He X (2008) Wnt/beta-catenin signaling: new (and old) players and new insights. Curr Opin Cell Biol 20:119–125
40. Iwaniec UT, Wronski TJ, Liu J, Rivera MF, Arzaga RR, Hansen G, Brommage R (2007) Parathyroid hormone stimulates bone formation in mice deficient in Lrp5. J Bone Miner Res 22:394–402
41. Jackson A, Vayssiere B, Garcia T, Newell W, Baron R, Roman-Roman S, Rawadi G (2005) Gene array analysis of Wnt-regulated genes in C3H10T1/2 cells. Bone 36:585–598
42. Jilka RL, Weinstein RS, Takahashi K, Parfitt AM, Manolagas SC (1996) Linkage of decreased bone mass with impaired osteoblastogenesis in a murine model of accelerated senescence. J Clin Invest 97:1732–1740
43. Johnson ML (2004) The high bone mass family–the role of Wnt/LRP5 signaling in the regulation of bone mass. J Musculoskelet Neuronal Interact 4:135–138
44. Johnson ML, Gong G, Kimberling W, Recker SM, Kimmel DB, Recker RR (1997) Linkage of a gene causing high bone mass to human chromosome 11 (11q12–13). Am J Hum Genet 60:1326–1332
45. Johnson ML, Harnish K, Nusse R, Van Hul W (2004) LRP5 and Wnt signaling: a union made for bone. J Bone Miner Res 19:1749–1757
46. Jones SE, Jomary C (2002) Secreted Frizzled-related proteins: searching for relationships and patterns. Bioessays 24:811–820
47. Kang S, Bajnok L, Longo KA, Petersen RK, Hansen JB, Kristiansen K, MacDougald OA (2004) Effects of Wnt signaling on brown adipocyte differentiation and metabolism mediated by PGC-1alpha. Mol Cell Biol 25:1272–1282
48. Kato M, Patel MS, Levasseur R, Lobov I, Chang BH, Glass DA II, Hartmann C, Li L, Hwang TH, Brayton CF, Lang RA, Karsenty G, Chan L (2002) Cbfa1-independent decrease in osteoblast proliferation, osteopenia, and persistent embryonic eye vascularization in mice deficient in Lrp5, a Wnt coreceptor. J Cell Biol 157:303–314
49. Kawano Y, Kypta R (2003) Secreted antagonists of the Wnt signaling pathway. J Cell Sci 116:2627–2634
50. Kelly OG, Pinison KI, Skarnes WC (2004) The Wnt co-receptors Lrp5 and Lrp6 are essential for gastrulation in mice. Development 131:2803–2815
51. Koay MA, Brown MA (2005) Genetic disorders of the LRP5-Wnt signalling pathway affecting the skeleton. Trends Mol Med 11:129–137
52. Kokubu C, Heinzmann U, Kokubu T, Sakai N, Kubota T, Kawai M, Wahl MB, Galceran J, Grosschedl R, Ozono K, Imai K (2004) Skeletal defects in ringelschwanz mutant mice reveal that Lrp6 is required for proper somitogenesis and osteogenesis. Development 131:5469–5480
53. Krishnan V, Bryant HU, MacDougald OA (2006) Regulation of bone mass by Wnt signaling. J Clin Invest 116:1202–1209
54. Kuhl M, Sheldahl LC, Park M, Miller JR, Moon RT (2000) The Wnt/Ca2 + pathway: a new vertebrate Wnt signaling pathway takes shape. Trends Genet 16:279–283
55. Li J, Sarosi I, Cattley RC, Pretorious J, Asuncion F, Grisanti M, Morony S, Adamu S, Geng Z, Qiu W, Kostenuik P, Lacey DL, Simonet WS, Bolon B, Qian X, Shalhoub V, Orminsky MS, Ke HZ, Li X, Richards WG (2006) Dkk1-mediated inhibition of Wnt signaling in bone results in osteopenia. Bone 39:754–766
56. Li X, Liu P, Liu W, Maye P, Zhang J, Zhang Y, Hurley M, Guo C, Boskey A, Sun L, Harris SE, Rowe DW, Ke HZ, Wu D (2005) Dkk2 has a role in terminal osteoblast differentiation and mineralized matrix formation. Nat Genet 37:945–952
57. Li X, Ominsky MS, Niu Q-T, Sun N, Daugherty B, D'Agostin D, Kurahara C, Gao Y, Cao J, Gong J, Asuncion F, Barrero M, Warmington K, Dwyer D, Stolina M, Morony S, Sarosi I, Kostenuik PJ, Lacey DL, Simonet WS, Ke HZ, Paszty C (2008) Targeted deletion of the sclerostin gene in mice results in increased bone formation and bone strength. J Bone Miner Res 23: 860–869
58. Li X, Zhang Y, Kang H, Liu W, Liu P, Zhang J, Harris SE, Wu D (2005) Sclerostin binds to LRP5/6 and antagonizes canonical Wnt signaling. J Biol Chem 280:19883–19887
59. Little RD, Carulli JP, Del Mastro RG, Dupuis J, Osborne M, Folz C, Manning SP, Swain PM, Zhao SC, Eustace B, Lappe MM, Spitzer L, Zweier S, Braunschweiger K, Benchekroun Y, Hu X, Adair R, Chee L, FitzGerald MG, Tulig C, Caruso A, Tzellas N, Bawa A, Franklin B, McGuire S, Nogues X, Gong G, Allen KM, Anisowicz A, Morales AJ, Lomedico PT, Recker SM, Van Eerdewegh P, Recker RR, Johnson ML (2002) A mutation in the LDL receptor-related protein 5 gene results in the autosomal dominant high-bone-mass trait. Am J Hum Genet 70:11–19
60. Liu B, Yu HMI, Hsu W (2007) Craniosynostosis caused by Axin2 deficiency is mediated through distinct functions of beta-catenin in proliferation and differentiation. Dev Biol 301:298–308

61. Logan CY, Nusse R (2004) The Wnt signaling pathway in development and disease. Annu Rev Cell Dev Biol 20:781–810
62. Longo KA, Wright WS, Kang S, Gerin I, Chiang SH, Lucas PC, Opp MR, MacDougald OA (2004) Wnt10b inhibits development of white and brown adipose tissues. J Biol Chem 279:35503–35509
63. Loots GG, Kneissel M, Keller H, Baptist M, Chang J, Collette NM, Ovcharenko D, Plajzer-Frick I, Rubin EM (2005) Genomic deletion of a long-range bone enhancer misregulates sclerostin in Van Buchem disease. Genome Res 15:928–935
64. Lories RJU, Peeters J, Bakker A, Tylzanowski P, Derese I, Schrooten J, Thomas JT, Luyten FP (2007) Articular cartilage and biomechanical properties of the long bones in Frzb-knockout mice. Arthritis Rheum 56: 4095–4103
65. MacDonald BT, Adamska M, Meisler MH (2004) Hypomorphic expression of Dkk1 in the doubleridge mouse: dose dependence and compensatory interactions with Lrp6. Development 131:2543–2552
66. MacDonald BT, Joiner DM, Oyserman SM, Sharma P, Goldstein SA, He X, Hauschka PV (2007) Bone mass is inversely proportional to Dkk1 levels in mice. Bone 41:331–339
67. Macsai CE, Foster BK, Xian CJ (2008) Roles of Wnt signaling in bone growth, remodeling, skeletal repair disorders and fracture repair. J Cell Physiol 215:578–587
68. Mao B, Niehrs C (2003) Kremen2 modulates Dickkopf2 activity during Wnt/LRP6 signaling. Gene 302:179–183
69. Matsushita M, Tsuboyama T, Kasai R, Okumura H, Yamamuro T, Higuchi K, Higuchi K, Kohno A, Yonezu T, Utani A (1986) Age-related changes in bone mass in the senescence-accelerated mouse (SAM): SAM-R/3 and SAM-P/6 as new murine models for senile osteoporosis. Am J Pathol 125:276–283
70. Miller JR (2002) The Wnts. Genome Biol 3:REVIEWS3001
71. Moon RT, Kohn AD, De Ferrari GV, Kaykas A (2004) WNT and beta-catenin signalling: diseases and therapies. Nat Rev Genet 5:691–701
72. Morvan F, Boulukos K, Clement-Lacroix P, Roman-Roman S, Suc-Royer I, Vayssiere B, Ammann P, Martin P, Pinho S, Pognonec P, Mollat P, Niehrs C, Baron R, Rawadi G (2006) Deletion of a single allele of the Dkk1 gene leads to an increase in bone formation and bone mass. J Bone Miner Res 21:934–945
73. Mukhopadhyay M, Shtrom S, Rodriguez-Esteban C, Chen L, Tsukui T, Gomer L, Dorward DW, Glinka A, Grinberg A, Huang SP, Niehrs C, Belmonte JC, Westphal H (2001) Dickkopf1 is required for embryonic head induction and limb morphogenesis in the mouse. Dev Cell 1:423–434
74. Nakamura T, Nakamura T, Matsumoto K (2008) The functions and possible significance of Kremen as a gatekeeper of Wnt signaling in development and pathology. J Cell Mol Med 12:391–408
75. Nakanishi R, Akiyama H, Kimura H, Otsuki B, Shimizu M, Tsuboyama T, Nakamura T (2008) Osteoblast-targeted expression of Sfrp4 in mice results in low bone mass. J Bone Miner Res 23:271–277
76. Nakanishi R, Shimizu M, Mori M, Akiyama H, Okudaira S, Otsuki B, Hashimoto M, Higuchi K, Hosokawa M, Tsuboyama T, Nakamura T (2006) Secreted frizzled-related protein 4 is a negative regulator of peak BMD in SAMP6 mice. J Bone Miner Res 21:1713–1721
77. Patel MS, Karsenty G (2002) Regulation of bone formation and vision by LRP5. N Engl J Med 346:1572–1574
78. Pinison KI, Brennan J, Monkley S, Avery BJ, Skarnes WC (2000) An LDL-receptor-related protein mediates Wnt signaling in mice. Nature 407:535–538
79. Poole KES, van Bezooijen RL, Loveridge N, Hamersma H, Papapoulos SE, Lowik CW, Reeve J (2005) Sclerostin is a delayed secreted product of osteocytes that inhibits bone formation. FASEB J 19:1842–1844
80. Pourquie O (2005) A new canon. Nature 433:208–209
81. Robinson JA, Chatterjee-Kishore M, Yaworsky PJ, Cullen DM, Zhao W, Li C, Kharode Y, Sauter L, Babij P, Brown EL, Hill AA, Akhter MP, Johnson ML, Recker RR, Komm BS, Bex FJ (2006) Wnt/beta-catenin signaling is a normal physiological response to mechanical loading in bone. J Biol Chem 281:31720–31728
82. Rodda SJ, McMahon AP (2006) Distinct roles for hedgehog and canonical Wnt signaling in specification, differentiation and maintenance of osteoblast progenitors. Development 133:3231–3244
83. Ross SE, Hemati N, Longo KA, Bennett CN, Lucas PC, Erickson RL, MacDougald OA (2000) Inhibition of adipogenesis by Wnt signaling. Science 289:950–953
84. Sawakami K, Robling AG, Ai M, Pitner ND, Liu D, Warden SJ, Li J, Rowe DW, Duncan RL, Warman ML, Turner CH (2006) The Wnt co-receptor is essential for skeletal mechanotransduction but not for the anabolic bone response to parathyroid hormone treatment. J Biol Chem 281:23698–23711
85. Semenov MV, He X (2006) LRP5 mutations linked to high bone mass diseases cause reduced LRP5 binding and inhibition by SOST. J Biol Chem 281:38276–38284
86. Sharpe C, Lawrence N, Martinez Arias A (2001) Wnt signalling: a theme with nuclear variations. Bioessays 23:311–318
87. Takada I, Mihara M, Suzawa M, Ohtake F, Kobayashi S, Igarashi M, Youn MY, Takeyama K, Nakamura T, Mezaki Y, Takezawa S, Yogiashi Y, Kitagawa H, Yamada G, Takada S, Minami Y, Shibuya H, Matsumoto K, Kato S (2007) A histone lysine methyltransferase activated by non-canonical Wnt signalling suppresses PPAR-gamma transactivation.[see comment]. Nat Cell Biol 9:1273–1285
88. ten Dijke P, Krause C, de Gorter DJJ, Lowik CWGM, van Bezooijen RL (2008) Osteocyte-derived sclerostin inhibits bone formation: its role in bone morphogenetic protein and Wnt signaling. J Bone Joint Surg 90(suppl 1):31–35
89. Trendelenburg V, Schaeublin M, Halleux C, Gasser JA, Guth S, Porter J, Curtis D, Seuwen K, John MR (2004) Expression of extracellular WNT pathway components in adult human trabecular bone cells. J Bone Miner Res 19:S144
90. Trevant B, Gaur T, Hussain S, Symons J, Komm BS, Bodine PVN, Stein GS, Lian JB (2008) Expression of

secreted frizzled-related protein 1, a Wnt antagonist, in brain, kidney and skeleton is dispensable for normal embryonic development. J Cell Physiol 217:113–126

91. Tu X, Joeng KS, Nakayama KI, Nakayama K, Rajagopal J, Carroll TJ, McMahon AP, Long F (2007) Noncanonical Wnt signaling through G protein-linked PKCdelta activation promotes bone formation. Dev Cell 12:113–127
92. van Bezooijen RL, Svensson JP, Eefting D, Visser A, van der Horst G, Karperien M, Quax PHA, Vrieling H, Papapoulos SE, ten Dijke P, Lowik CWGM (2007) Wnt but not BMP signaling is involved in the inhibitory action of sclerostin on BMP-stimulated bone formation. J Bone Miner Res 22:19–28
93. van Bezooijen RL, ten Dijke P, Papapoulos SE, Lowick CWGM (2005) SOST/sclerostin, an osteocyte-derived negative regulator of bone formation. Cytokine Growth Factor Rev 16:319–327
94. Van Wesenbeeck L, Cleiren E, Gram J, Beals RK, Benichou O, Scopelliti D, Key L, Renton T, Bartels C, Gong Y, Warman ML, De Vernejoul MC, Bollerslev J, Van Hul W (2003) Six novel missense mutations in the LDL receptor-related protein 5 (LRP5) gene in different conditions with an increased bone density. Am J Hum Genet 72: 763–771
95. Veeman MT, Axelrod JD, Moon RT (2003) A second canon: functions and mechanisms of beta-catenin-independent Wnt signaling. Dev Cell 5:367–377
96. Westendorf JJ, Kahler RA, Schroeder TM (2004) Wnt signaling in osteoblasts and bone diseases. Gene 341:19–39
97. Weston CR, Davis RJ (2002) The JNK signal transduction pathway. Curr Opin Genet Dev 12:14–21
98. Winkler DG, Sutherland MK, Geoghegan JC, Yu C, Hayes T, Skonier JE, Shpektor D, Jonas M, Kovacevich BR, Staehling-Hampton K, Appleby M, Brunkow ME, Latham JA (2003) Osteocyte control of bone formation via sclerostin, a novel BMP antagonist. EMBO J 22:6267–6276
99. Wodarz A, Nusse R (1998) Mechanisms of Wnt signaling in development. Annu Rev Cell Dev Biol 14:59–88
100. Yamaguchi TP, Bradley A, McMahon AP, Jones S (1999) A Wnt5a pathway underlies outgrowth of multiple structures in the vertebrate embryo. Development 126:1211–1223
101. Yang Y, Topol L, Lee H, Wu J (2003) Wnt5a and Wnt5b exhibit distinct activities in coordinating chondrocyte proliferation and differentiation. Development 130:1003–1015
102. Yu HMI, Jerchow B, Sheu TJ, Liu B, Costantini F, Puzas JE, Birchmeier W, Hsu W (2005) The role of Axin2 in calvarial morphogenesis and craniosynostosis. Development 132:1995–2005
103. Zorn AM (2001) Wnt signaling: antagonistic dickkopfs. Curr Biol 11:R592–R5R5

10. Development of the Craniofacial Complex

Rena N. D'Souza, L-Bruno Ruest, Robert J. Hinton, and Kathy K. H. Svoboda

10.1 Introduction

The craniofacial complex comprises the head, face, and oral cavity and is the most distinguishing of all the structures in the human body, imparting unique identities to individuals. Structures of the craniofacial complex, such as the mandible, palate, temporomandibular joint (TMJ), and dentition, each offer valuable paradigms for studying development, structure, and functions. This chapter will provide a background for the succeeding chapter that will compare, in detail, the differences in bone and tooth development. The chapter's goals are to review the classical and current knowledge of branchial arch development, mandibular and temporomandibular joint (TMJ) formation, palatogenesis, and tooth development. Information on defects or disorders that arise from perturbations in genes, their protein products, and relevant signaling pathways is integrated into each section. The overarching goal is to emphasize how the knowledge of fundamental developmental processes can be translated to regenerative approaches targeted at restoring the integrity and function of craniofacial tissues.

10.2 Development of the Craniofacial Skeleton

Ossification of the skeleton of the head utilizes both endochondral and intramembranous processes (Fig. 10.1). The neurocranium that comprises the cranial base that underlies the brain is formed by endochondral ossification of cartilages that originate from the mesoderm (chondrocranium). In contrast, the neurocranium creating the cranial vault develops from the cells from the paraxial mesoderm or neural crest that undergo intramembranous ossification (Fig. 10.1) [31, 35, 76, 150]. The cranial sutures between the mesodermal bones involve cells originating from the neural crest. The skeleton of the face, i.e., the viscerocranium, develops from the neural crest cells that undergo both intramembranous and endochondral ossification (Fig. 10.1). After delaminating from the neural crest, these cells undergo an epithelial-to-mesenchymal transition and eventually migrate anterior to the developing brain and into the pharyngeal arches, which are structures located on the ventral aspect of the embryos. Each arch produces a specific cartilage. Two bilateral cartilaginous rods known as

F. Bronner et al. (eds.), *Bone and Development*, Topics in Bone Biology 6,
DOI 10.1007/978-1-84882-822-3_10, © Springer-Verlag London Limited 2010

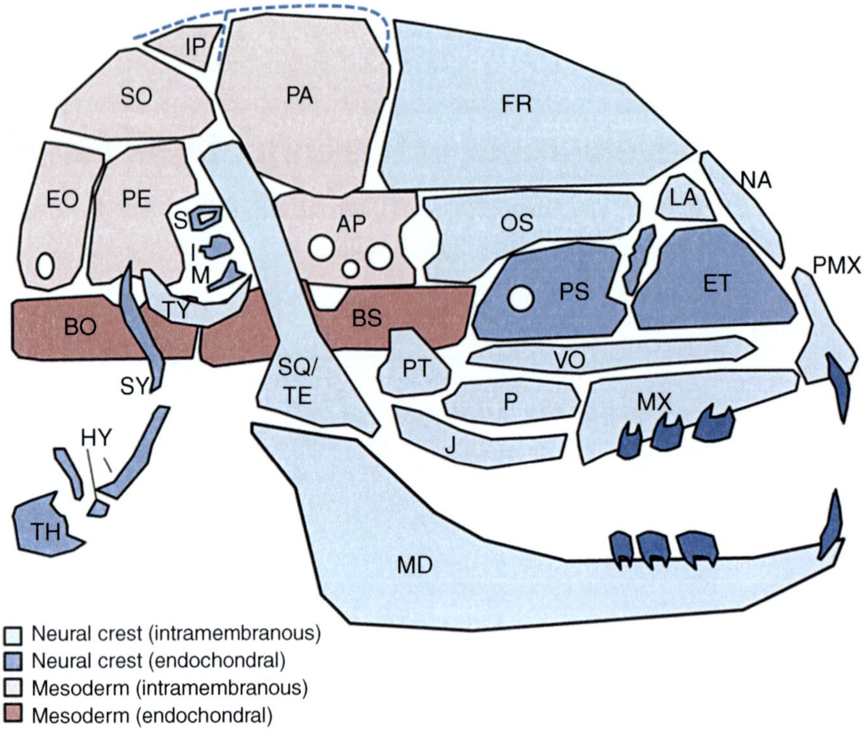

Figure 10.1. Mouse skull showing the contributions of neural crest and mesodermal mesenchyme to the cranial skeleton. Darker colors indicate skeletal structures that undergo endochondral ossification, and lighter colors indicate structures that are formed by intramembranous ossification. As teeth do not form by endochondral or intramembranous ossification, they are shown in another hue of blue to indicate neural crest cell contributions during their formation. *AP* alisphenoid; *BO* basoccipital; *BS* basisphenoid; *EO* exoccipital; *ET* ethmoid; *FR* frontal; *HY* hyoid components; *I* incus; *IP* interparietal; *J* jugal (zygoma); *LA* lacrimal; *M* malleus; *MD* mandible; *MX* maxilla, *NA* nasal; *OS* orbitosphenoid; *P* palatine; *PA* parietal; *PE* petrosal (including mastoid process); *PMX* premaxilla; *PS* presphenoid; *PT* pterygoid; *S* stapes; *SO* supraoccipital; *SQ/TE* squamosal/temporal; *SY* styloid process; *TH* thyroid; *TY* tympanic ring; and *VO* vomer. (Adapted from Noden and Trainor [150], with permission from Wiley-Blackwell, and from Chai and Maxson [35], copyright 2006, reprinted with permission from Wiley).

"Meckel's cartilages" are associated with the first arch and give rise to the lower jaw (mandible) and the malleus and incus. The second arch produces a part of the body and the lesser horns of the hyoid (Reitchert's cartilage), styloid process, and stapes; the third arch gives rise to the body and greater horns of the hyoid. The thyroid cartilage and the cricoid cartilage are created from the fourth and the sixth arches, respectively. The first pharyngeal arch has typically been subdivided into the mandibular and maxillary (upper jaw) prominences. Mapping data indicate that the maxillary prominences contribute to the formation of structures that are associated with the lower jaw [34, 116, 172], with the maxilla, palatine, and jugal (zygomatic arch) originating from the neural crest cells that migrate toward the postoptic region above the maxillo-mandibular cleft.

The development of the facial skeleton above the mandible involves the orderly and integrated growth and movement of different prominences that eventually fuse and expand to form the face [31, 35, 76, 150]. Fusion failure results in orofacial clefts. The five different facial prominences are the frontonasal, medionasal (2), nasolateral (2), maxillary (2), and mandibular (2). The mandibular prominences, constituting the first pharyngeal arch, fuse at the midline days before the other prominences fuse. The development of the first pharyngeal arch is discussed subsequently. The frontonasal prominence grows downward and forms the forehead, middle of the nose, philtrum of the upper lip, premaxilla, and primary palate. The medial and lateral nasal prominences develop on each side of the nasal pit, which becomes the nostrils.

These prominences eventually migrate medially and fuse with the frontonasal prominence to form the nose. The maxillary prominences also move forward toward the midline and fuse with the frontonasal prominence to complete the upper lip and, with the lateronasal prominences, form the nasolacrimal grooves. The maxillary prominences form the sides of the face and the associated bones of the zygomatic arches, maxilla, and secondary palate.

During the process of bone formation, the endochondral and intramembranous bones use the same mechanisms of osteoblast differentiation, similar to the axial and appendicular skeletons [101, 110]. As *Runx2*-null mice [109, 155] are born without endochondral and intramembranous bones, it is evident that the transcriptional factor, Runx2, is essential for bone differentiation. The activation of *Sox9* is also required for the formation of the osteo-chondro-progenitor that will differentiate into the chondrocytes [78, 125]. The differentiation of the chondrocytes into hypertrophic chondrocytes and the subsequent differentiation steps, including ossification, are mediated by *Runx2*; Sox9 activity is not essential for intramembranous bone formation.

10.3 Development of the Mandible

The mandible is a unique mammalian structure that allows mastication during feeding. Its development involves cells that, originating from the neural crest, populate the first pharyngeal arch. These cells are influenced by signals from the ectoderm, core paraxial mesoderm, and pharyngeal pouch endoderm that induce the endochondral differentiation of the neural crest cells to create the two bilateral cartilaginous rods known as "Meckel's cartilages" and differentiate into the osteoblasts forming the intramembranous bone.

Mandibular development begins with the condensation of the neural crest mesenchymal cells that form the mandibular blastema and continues as a subpopulation of these cells differentiates into chondrocytes that then form Meckel's cartilage. The two rods of the proximal Meckel's cartilage differentiate into the malleus. The distal ends of the Meckel's cartilage project inward toward the embryo midline, where they meet at the site of the eventual symphysis of the lower jaw.

Meckel's cartilage serves as a scaffold for the ensuing ossification [168, 169, 220]. Unlike long bones that undergo endochondral ossification, the mandible ossifies mostly through an intramembranous process. During embryogenesis, the ossification of the mandible starts on the external side along the first distal third of the Meckel's cartilage and proceeds rapidly toward the oral side [168, 169]. Ossification then ensues along the cartilage, proximally and distally. The ossification of the condylar and coronoid processes represents a continuous addition of intramembranous bone and occurs independently of the scaffold provided by the Meckel's cartilage.

Interestingly, part of the neural crest-derived mesenchyme does not differentiate into bone, but provides the alveolar spacing essential for tooth development. Skeletal muscles develop along the ossification front, initiating the jaw-opening reflex [106]. This initial jaw opening articulates with the developing incus via the Meckel's and malleus cartilages and is reminiscent of the articulation between the articular of the lower jaw and the quadrate (ancestral incus) seen in early gnathostomes [35, 48, 77]. The evolutionary process that has modified the lower jaw articulation is intimately related to the development of the mammalian hearing system. The jaw-opening reflex is essential for the development of the secondary cartilage capping the condyle; this condylar cartilage forms the articulation with the squamosal bone to create the definitive articulation of the lower jaw with the skull.

10.3.1 Molecular Regulation of Mandibular Development

Of the genes involved in neural crest cell formation, migration and differentiation, most modulate mandible development. Mutation or alteration of their expression can result in mandibular defects. This is also true for the genes expressed by the surrounding tissues, which influence the neural crest cell development in the mandibular pharyngeal arch.

Other factors influencing bone development and mandible patterning are Sonic hedgehog (Shh), Fgf8, Bmp4, and endothelin-1 signaling. These factors, expressed by the mandibular arch ectoderm or pharyngeal pouch endoderm on the underlying neural crest cells, predominantly act in the course of early mandible development.

Shh signaling is essential for the survival of the neural crest cell population that forms the mandible [90]. The absence of Shh signaling by targeted deletion in the mouse results in several craniofacial defects, including holoprosencephaly. Most Shh-negative embryos die early during embryonic development. It is difficult to establish the function of *Shh* in neural crest cells and mandible development [37]. McMahon et al. conditionally inactivated *Smo*, thus blocking the transcription of Shh-dependent genes [131]. This allowed Shh signaling to proceed normally in other mouse tissues [90]. The neural crest cell-derived craniofacial skeleton and the mandible were greatly reduced in size because of excessive death by the neural crest cells. These results demonstrate that Shh plays an essential role in neural crest cell survival.

Bone morphogenetic protein 4 (Bmp4) and fibroblast growth factor 8 (Fgf8) are both expressed by the mandibular arch ectoderm. *Bmp4* is expressed more distally and induces the ectodermal expression of the homeobox transcription factor, *Dlx2* (Fig. 10.2) [209, 224, 225]. *Fgf8* is expressed more proximally, inducing the mesenchymal expression of *Dlx2*, along with *Lhx6* and *Lhx7*. It appears that each factor represses the other, creating a proximo-distal boundary in the pharyngeal arch ectoderm that can be defined by the mutually exclusive domains of *Dlx2* expression. The absence of Bmp4 signaling

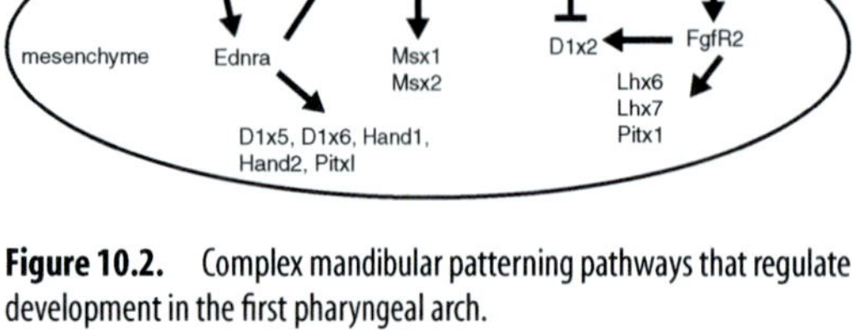

Figure 10.2. Complex mandibular patterning pathways that regulate development in the first pharyngeal arch.

is lethal during early embryonic development [235]. When Bmp4 was conditionally inactivated in the pharyngeal arch ectoderm and pharyngeal pouch endoderm [120], severe mandibular defects resulted, and the level of expression correlated with that of the remaining *Bmp4* expression. In embryos with minimal *Bmp4* expression, only the distal mandible development is affected, as evidenced by the absence of incisors. Embryos with near or total loss of *Bmp4* expression in the mandibular arch have no mandibular structure except for small, indeterminate intramembranous bones proximal to the squamosal bone. These findings indicate that mandibular development depends on different Bmp4 thresholds, as reflected during the expression of the genes *Msx1* and *Msx2* in the underlying crest cells and the expression of *Fgf8* in the ectoderm [120]. With less *Bmp4* expression, more *Fgf8* is expressed in the ectoderm, with the expression expanding distally. Bmp4 may therefore play a role in neural crest cell patterning and survival [87, 187, 188]. *Msx1*-null mice are born with mild distal mandibular defects: the incisors and molars are missing, and the alveolae normally encasing the teeth are filled by membranous bone [187]. In the *Msx2* knockout mice, the distal mandible is severely malformed, and teeth may be absent [188]. In the compound *Msx1/Msx2* double-mutant embryos, the mandible is much shorter and the proximal mandible and TMJ formation are affected. In addition, distal mandibular defects are present; these may be due to additive gene effects [87]. Bmp4 signaling, through the activation of the *Msx* genes, is therefore essential for mandibular patterning and tooth formation. This indicates that Bmp4 also has a role in distal mandibular development.

Of interest are the increased rates of apoptosis in the *Bmp4* conditional knockout embryos, resulting from an upregulation of *Fgf8* expression [120]. Conditional inactivation of the *Fgf8* gene in the pharyngeal arch ectoderm leads to a massive loss of neural crest cells by apoptosis [223]. However, Fgf8 is also a patterning factor that regulates the expression of mesenchymal genes, such as *Dlx2*, *Lhx6*, and *Lhx7* as well as the oral-aboral polarity [209, 224, 225]. An *Fgf8* hypomorphic allele has been used to circumvent the problem of neural crest cell loss; the expression of this hypomorphic allele is lower than that of the wild-type allele, but is sufficient to prevent early embryonic death [60]. Embryos with one null and one hypomorphic *Fgf8* allele exhibit micrognathia, but the shape of the mandible is fairly normal [60]. However, the development of more proximal structures is affected when the TMJ fails to form and the mandible fuses with the squamosal bone and maxilla. This proximal transformation suggests that Fgf8 is also a factor patterning the lower jaw. Fgf8 patterning function is probably mediated by *Pitx1*, another gene regulated by the growth factor [209]. The distal mandible of *Pitx1* mutant mouse embryos is normal. However, the proximal mandibular structures are severely malformed, with most of the ramus missing. This is consistent with the role of Ffg8 in proximal mandible patterning [114].

Endothelin signaling also plays an important role in the patterning of the lower jaw bone. Endothelin-1 (Edn1) is secreted by the mandibular arch ectoderm, core paraxial mesoderm, and pharyngeal pouch endoderm, and binds to the endothelin-A receptor (Ednra) expressed in the neural crest cells (Fig. 10.2) [39, 179, 180]. Initially thought to be a signaling mechanism that guides the neural crest cell migration to the pharyngeal arch, the inactivation of either gene revealed that endothelin signaling is instead essential for inducing a mandibular identity in the neural crest cells [179]. In the absence of endothelin signaling in the mouse, the lower jaw undergoes transformation into upper jaw-like structures, including duplication of the maxilla, palatine, and zygomatic arch bones [179, 180]. This homeotic transformation may be an atavism, because the lower jaw is a mirror image of the upper jaw, as observed in more primitive animals (e.g., sharks) or in evolutionary ancestors of mammals [47, 48]. This transformation is caused by the downregulation of the expression of the mandibular genes (i.e., *Dlx5*, *Dlx6*, *Hand1*, and *Hand2*) in the first pharyngeal arch and the gain of maxillary gene expression (i.e., *Wnt5a*, *Dlx1*, and *Dlx2*) in the same arch [179]. A similar phenotype was observed in *Dlx5/Dlx6* knockout mouse embryos; therefore, the regulation of homeobox genes is essential for lower jaw patterning [17, 47]. Recent data suggest that endothelin signaling is the earliest patterning mechanism for the lower jaw, probably upstream of Bmp4 and Fgf8, inasmuch as the expression of the *Bmp4* and Fgf8-dependent gene *Pitx1* is affected in the absence of endothelin signaling [179, 180, 185, 186].

10.3.2 Patterning of the Mandibular Neural Crest Cells

Structural patterning of the body is associated with the regulation of the homeobox genes, and the mandible is no exception. The neural crest cells populating the mandibular arch are also referred to as the "Hox-less crest cells," as they are not influenced by *Hox* genes prior to their migration [43, 115]. This absence of *Hox* gene influence is essential for their patterning. As revealed by the inactivation of the *Hoxa2* gene in the mouse, abrogating the gene expression characterizing the second pharyngeal arch results in the duplication of the first arch structures (malleus and incus), instead of the formation of second arch structures [66, 173]. As the expression of the Hox genes is linked to retinoic acid signaling, it is not surprising that similar phenotypes were observed in different retinoic acid receptor mutant mice [121, 122, 129, 134]. Thus, in the absence of Hox signaling, second arch neural crest cells behave like first arch crest cells; this suggests that the expression of *Hox* genes in the first arch represses a mandibular phenotype. To determine whether the *Hox* genes inhibit lower jaw patterning, ectopic expression of the *Hoxa2* genes in the mandibular arch was studied in chicken and Xenopus embryos [68, 156], in which the mandibular structures were transformed into second arch-like structures. This mandible-to-hyoid homeotic transformation indicates that the neural crest cells carry prepatterning information; therefore, the absence of Hox signaling is essential to maintain mandibular identity. On the other hand, neural crest cells have absolute plasticity, based on neural crest transplant experiments [184, 221]. The findings indicate that neural crest cells do carry some prepatterning information. Interspecies transplantation of similar axial neural crests between duck and quail embryos [190] demonstrates the presence of prepatterning information. In these chimeric birds, the quails develop a duck bill, whereas the ducks develop a quail beak. This not only shows that the crest cells carry prepatterning information, but that this prepatterning cannot be changed by the surrounding environment. Structural patterning is, however, associated with the expression of the homeobox genes. As no *Hox* gene is expressed early in the mandibular arch crest cell, other homeobox genes must compensate to establish mandible patterning, a function that is due to the *Dlx* genes.

Dlx genes (like *Hox* genes) are duplicated and found in tandem in the genome. They are expressed along a proximo-distal gradient, with *Dlx1* and *Dlx2* more proximal, *Dlx5* and *Dlx6* more distal, and *Dlx3* and *Dlx4* in between [47, 48]. On the basis of the gradient, it seems likely that Dlx1 and Dlx2 regulate the patterning of the more proximal structures, with Dlx5 and Dlx6 patterning the more distal structures. Inactivation of the gene encoding *Dlx2*, or the genes encoding *Dlx1* and *Dlx2*, has shown that the two genes are essential for the patterning of the upper jaw; their absence leads to palatine, maxillary, and zygomatic defects [164, 165]. The duplication of the proximal structures (e.g., incus) of the mandibular arch led surprisingly to the malformation of the middle-ear ossicles. This duplication implies that other genes are involved in the patterning of the middle-ear structures and the mandible.

The mandibular patterning of the first arch neural crest cells is absent when both *Dlx5* and *Dlx6* are inactivated, with the lower jaw replaced by upper jaw-like structures [17, 47]. This homeotic transformation is caused by the downregulation of genes that are normally expressed in the mandibular arch, such as *Hand2*, and the upregulation of genes associated with maxillary development, including *Dlx1* and *Dlx2*. This transformation is also an atavism, as described earlier. Axial patterning requires retinoic acid signaling, and the *Hox* genes are involved; in the mandibular neural crest cells, this interaction is provided by the endothelin/Dlx pathway [179, 180], a pathway also essential for the expression of transcriptional factors like *Hand1* and *Hand2*. Dlx6 directly activates the expression of *Hand2* by binding to the enhancer that drives the expression in the mandibular pharyngeal arch [36]. The two bHLH factors, Hand1 and Hand2, are essential for early embryonic development, as *Hand1*-null and *Hand2*-null embryos die at embryonic ages 8.5 or 10.5 days, respectively [56, 208].

In mice whose *Hand 2's* endothelin-dependent pharyngeal arch enhancer was removed by targeted deletion, the mandible is hypoplastic and porotic, and malformations are observed in the distal segment and in the angular process [62, 239]. These defects are consistent with the expression pattern of the Hand2 gene in the mandibular arch [178]. When the expression of both *Hand2* and *Hand1* genes is reduced, more severe distal defects are observed [12]. Both branches of the mandible are fused at the symphysis, and only one incisor forms; in other words, Hand1 can partially compensate for the loss of Hand2 function. The most interesting phenotype in the pharyngeal arch-specific *Hand2* mutant embryos is the porotic bone. This phenotype is caused by premature ossification of the mandible, with the depletion of the pool of crest-derived mesenchymal cells that differentiate into osteoblasts [62]. This premature ossification is caused by the loss of the Hand2 physical repression on the transcriptional activity of Runx2, a master regulator of bone differentiation. However, according to Ruest and Clouthier [180], the later expression of Hand2 in the mandibular arch is independent of endothelin signaling. This raises the question of what regulates Hand2 expression after activation by the endothelin/Dlx pathway and what regulates the onset of ossification in the mandibular arch. Conceivably, this is Bmp signaling. Endothelin signaling is intermingled with Bmp4 signaling [179]. Possibly, an unknown factor(s), released by the neural crest cells, influences ectodermal gene expression. This uncertainty reflects the complexity of the signaling mechanisms that regulate mandibular patterning and development.

Endothelin signaling appears to be one of the earliest patterning mechanisms to establish a mandibular identity in the neural crest that populates the first arch, and does so by regulating *Dlx5*, *Dlx6*, *Bmp4*, *Pitx1*, *Hand1*, and *Hand2* expression [179, 180, 185, 186]. What is more, without endothelin signaling, the mandibular identity is lost and upper jaw-like structures develop in place of the mandibular arch. These findings indicate that endothelin signaling may repress upper jaw development and induce mandibular development ectopically. The restricted expression of Edn1 may explain why this situation does not occur, inasmuch as Ednra is expressed in all head neural crest cells [179, 186]. Kurihara's group in Japan produced transgenic mice that ectopically expressed the edn1 ligand. This caused activation of the Ednra receptor signaling in all head neural crest cells, and not only in those in the pharyngeal arches [185]. In the transgenic embryos, the maxilla is transformed into lower jaw-like structures, including Meckel's cartilage and a mandible-like formation. This homeotic transformation is accompanied by expression in the maxillary prominence of the lower jaw markers, *Dlx5*, *Dlx6*, *Pitx1*, and *Hand2*, a transformation that is mostly visible in the Hox-less-derived neural crest cells, with no effect on the development of the lower pharyngeal arch structures. As mentioned earlier, *Hox* genes are essential for the development of neural-crest-derived structures in the lower pharyngeal arches with the absence of *Hoxa2* expression causing an anterior-to-posterior transformation. The ectopic expression of *Hoxa2* in the Hox-less mandibular arch causes a posterior-to-anterior transformation [66, 68, 156,173]. The ectopic activation of endothelin signaling is reminiscent of the posterior-to-anterior transformation with *Hoxa2*. Retinoic acid regulates the expression of Hox homeobox genes in the posterior arch structures; this regulatory function in anterior structures is probably assumed by edn1 functions.

10.4 Temporomandibular Joint

10.4.1 Initiation as a Secondary Cartilage

All movements of the mandible take place at the articulation of the mandible with the cranium, the temporomandibular joint (TMJ). These bilateral synovial joints have an interesting developmental history that makes them different from the joints of the limbs. The general structure of the TMJ resembles that of most synovial joints, but the cartilage capping the mandibular condyle (mandibular condylar cartilage or MCC) is a *secondary cartilage* [16], a term indicating that the morphogenesis of the TMJ and its components begins after the bone of the mandible is present and after analogous joints in the limbs are formed. For the most part, the secondary cartilages are transient, occurring in numerous locations in the developing craniofacial complex [231]. They persist postnatally in the mandibular condyle, in the angular process of the mandible and the intermaxillary suture [82, 160]. The primary cartilages of the limbs typically arise via interaction between the mesenchyme and epithelium [75], while secondary cartilages typically develop in response to local biomechanical stimuli [16, 74]. The first sign of the future MCC, adjacent to the intramembranous bone of the mandible, is a condensation of the alkaline phosphatase-positive cells that are continuous anteriorly with the periosteum of the mandible [199]. Even though these cells are osteoblastic in nature [200], they seem to be bipotent, becoming chondrogenic when mobility and loading are normal and osteogenic, when motion is limited or loads are low or absent [82, 161]. This is reflected in the fact that cells in the MCC anlage express not only mRNA for osteogenic lineage markers (e.g., *collagen*, *Runx2*, and *Osterix*), but also mRNA for *Sox 9*, a marker for chondrogenic differentiation [201]. Secondary cartilages such as the MCC are also characterized by very rapid differentiation of chondrocytes to hypertrophic chondrocytes, with extensive overlap between collagen types II and X. This differs from the stratification in different zones of the growth plate of limb cartilages [28, 61, 198].

10.4.2 Stages of TMJ Morphogenesis

Human TMJ morphogenesis does not commence until the embryo is 7 or 8 weeks old. By that time, which is called the *blastematic stage* [135], the major joints of the limbs are fully formed, and their structure resembles that of the adult joint [65, 139]. During this stage, the mesenchymal cells condense, such that the mandibular condyle and the temporal bone becomes recognizable [13, 117, 135, 226]. The condylar blastema grows dorsally and cranially, eventually to approximate the separate temporal blastema [14, 109]; this process is not completed until around 12 weeks [14, 242]. The mesenchyme located between the condylar and temporal blastemata comprises a third blastema that is thought to give rise to the articular disc [135, 226]. It is important to emphasize that the condylar condensation has no connection to primary cartilages, such as Meckel's cartilage or the cartilage anlage of the malleus (a middle ear ossicle). Premyoblasts that form the lateral pterygoid muscle appear around 6–7 weeks, and by 7 weeks, muscle fibers appear to attach to the condylar mesenchymal condensation [114, 117, 151].

During weeks 9–11 in utero, known as the *cavitation stage*, cells in the center of the condylar blastema differentiate into chondrocytes [14, 117]. At the same time, the mesenchyme separating the condylar and temporal components becomes denser; this signals a more definitive anlage of the future articular disc. Coincident with this, small clefts between the disc anlage and the condyle can be observed [151, 159, 226]. These events reflect the initial formation of the inferior joint cavity, which is typically completed through the coalescence of the clefts by week 10. Interestingly, the upper joint space does not become evident until week 11 or 11.5 [226]. By week 12, two parts of the lateral pterygoid muscle appear: an upper part, in contact with the medial aspect of the disc, and a lower part, in contact with the condyle [151].

The *maturation stage* of TMJ development [135, 226] begins in week 12. All the major components of the TMJ, present in a form that approximates their eventual postnatal structure, commence a period of continued growth and consolidation. The disc is comprised of densely

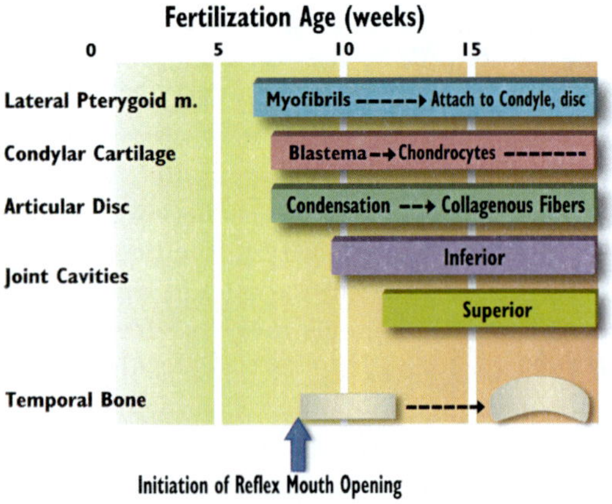

Figure 10.3. Timeline of human TMJ development showing changes in different joint components.

packed fibroblasts and exhibits a thinned area centrally, with thickening laterally and medially [63]. The joint capsule which, at 9–11 weeks, is a stained zone near the periphery of the mesenchymal block [135, 226], becomes clearly evident by week 14 [151]. The temporal component that has been described as convex or flat during the cavitation stage [135, 167, 226] now assumes a slightly concave shape that is reminiscent of what is seen postnatally, although no true eminence is present. The development of the human TMJ is schematized in Fig. 10.3.

Human fetuses can open their mouth beginning at the age of 8.5 weeks; this is a component of total contralateral head, trunk, and rump flexion [84]. After 11 weeks, mouth-opening reflexes are accompanied by progressively fewer trunk and extremity movements; by 15 weeks, mouth opening occurs without head or other movements [84]. As the superior and inferior joint cavities arise between 10 and 11.5 weeks, cavitation in the TMJ may be stimulated by these early jaw movements. However, the reflex mouth opening reported at 8.5 weeks is independent of the TMJ, which is only in the process of formation at this time. Some investigators [11, 135] have suggested that these early movements take place at the malleus/incus joint at the rostral end of the Meckel's cartilage. If this is the case, it is intriguing to speculate whether initiation of chondrogenesis in the condylar cartilage at 9 weeks is engendered by these early reflex movements. This may be true because the ex utero limitation of jaw movements in mouse fetuses are observed to reduce growth at the condylar cartilage [73]. Similarly, the absence of fetal swallowing in human newborns is strongly associated with micrognathia [195].

10.4.3 Postnatal Growth and Maturation

Unlike the limbs, in which growth and articulation are carried out by separate growth and articulation cartilages, the MCC incorporates both the functions in a single tissue. The MCC is an active site of endochondral growth during prenatal and early postnatal life (Fig. 10.4), yet its thickness decreases to two-thirds by 6 months of age in humans [32]. The MCC continues to grow at an ever-attenuating rate until the mid to late teens [237]; notwithstanding that, during puberty, it is subject to increasing loads owing to muscle hypertrophy. In the rat, the percent of cells undergoing mitosis in the MCC declines with age to 47% of the value at weaning at puberty, and to 7% by full adulthood [230]. A solid subchondral plate of bone seals off the cartilage from the medullary spaces by 20 years of age [86, 215], effectively preventing further endochondral ossification by denying blood vessels from the marrow access to the deeper layers of the cartilage. Over the ensuing years, the near- or complete loss of the prechondroblastic (mitotic) cells and reductions in overall cellularity, including chondrocytes, transform the MCC into a relatively homogeneous fibrocartilage [123, 124]. This completes a cycle in which the MCC, initially a site of rapid growth with minimal loading, takes on both growth and articular functions, and is ultimately transformed into a purely articular (fibro) cartilage. It has only recently become apparent that the unusual developmental history of the MCC and the resultant differences in its histological structure and composition from limb cartilages give rise to material properties and growth characteristics that must be taken into account in attempts to develop constructs that mimic native TMJ tissues [8, 232] or to stimulate the overall length of the mandible beyond its normal growth potential [166].

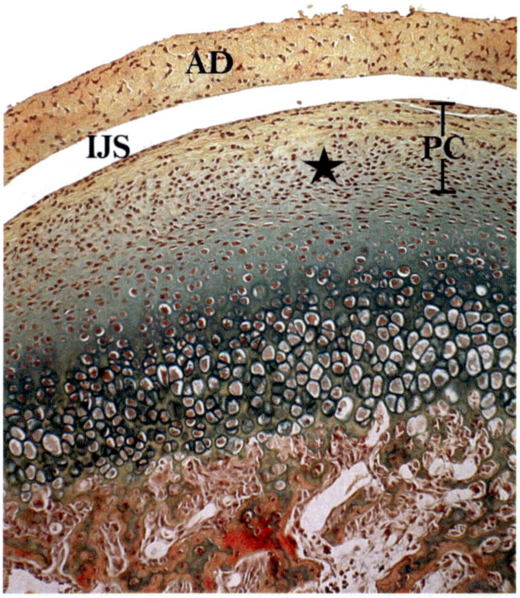

Figure 10.4. Mandibular condylar cartilage (MCC) in a rapidly growing rat. AD, articular disc; IJS, inferior joint space; PC, perichondrium. The star designates the inner layer of the perichondrium where cells in the MCC undergo division, when compared with the deeper-lying chondrocytes in a growth plate. Attwood stain.

10.5 Palate Development

10.5.1 Classic Theories of Palatal Morphogenesis

The palatal structures are composed of the cranial neural crest-derived mesenchyme and pharyngeal ectoderm [79, 99, 147]. The epithelia that cover the palatal shelves can be divided into oral, nasal, and medial edge epithelia (MEE). The nasal and oral epithelia differentiate into pseudostratified and squamous epithelia, whereas the MEE is removed from the fusion line (Fig. 10.5).

The secondary palate originates as an outgrowth of the maxillary prominences on or about embryonic day 11.5 in the mouse (E11.5-m) and 6 weeks post-conception (p.c.) in humans (6 week-h). The palate shelves initially grow vertically along the sides of the tongue (E13.5-m; p.c. 7 week-h), and then rise above the tongue as

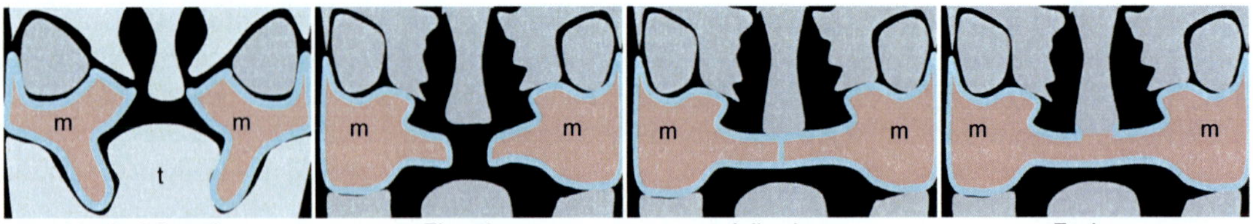

Figure 10.5. Coronal view of a normal palate shelf and the key stages of mouse palatal development. At days E12-E13 in the gestation of the mouse, the palatal shelves grow downward along the tongue (t). At E13-E13.5 days, the palatal shelves become elevated above the tongue. At E14.5, the palatal shelves adhere to each other in the midline. After E15.5 days, the MES completely degrades and the palate fuses. (Reprinted with permission from Yu et al. [241]).

the latter drops in the oral cavity, owing to the forward and downward growth of the mandible (E14.0-m; p.c. 8 weeks-h). With continued growth, the shelves appose at the midline (E14.5-m; p.c. 10 weeks-h) and eventually fuse (E15.5-m; p.c. 13 week-h) [144]. Numerous genes that are similar in mice [241] and humans [26, 144, 196] are expressed (Table 10.1) during palatal development.

During fusion, the epithelium covering the tip of opposing palatal shelves adheres, intercalates, and thins into a single-layer midline epithelial seam (MES) [147]. The disintegration of this seam results in the confluence of the palatal mesenchyme. Tremendous interest has arisen in the cellular mechanisms underlying MES degradation. The epithelial-mesenchymal transition (EMT) is one of the proposed models that regulate the MEE cell fate [79, 96, 99, 147, 202]. However, other mechanisms have been proposed, such as apoptosis [44, 141, 217], in which all the MEE cells are thought to die during fusion. Alternatively, the MES cells may disappear by migrating from the midline toward the nasal and oral epithelia [29, 94]. Conceivably, apoptosis, migration, and EMT may all occur [133, 141, 147]. The fusion of the external surface of the bilateral maxillary processes with the nasofrontal prominence in the chick is similar to palatal fusion (Fig. 10.6) [211]. The outer periderm layer dies through apoptosis, and the lateral edge epithelium of the intermaxillary segment of the nasofrontal process fuses with the medial edge epithelium of the external maxillary process to form a seam that transitions to a confluent mesenchyme (Fig. 10.6) [211].

10.5.2 Molecular Mechanisms in Embryonic Palatal Development

The genes that are expressed to induce the different stages of palatal development have been examined through observations of human and animal oral facial clefts. Cleft lip with or without cleft palate (CL/P) is a complex trait caused by many genes and environmental factors [143].

The failure of the palatal shelf formation is a rare, but severe defect. Signaling networks between the epithelium and mesenchyme involve signaling molecules and growth factors such as Shh, members of the transforming growth factor β (TGFβ) super family including BMPs and TGFβs, FGFs, and their receptors (FgfR), as well as other effectors and targets [144]. FGF signaling during early palatal development alters cell proliferation within both mesenchyme and epithelium in the palatal shelves, and induces an increase in apoptosis within the epithelium. In Fgf10 and FgfR2b mouse mutants, the initial development of the palatal shelves was altered and the pups had a fully developed cleft palate (CP) [170]. By signaling via its receptor [170] in the palatal shelf epithelium, the mesenchymally derived Fgf10 supports epithelial proliferation and survival and induces the expression of Shh within the epithelium. Shh, in turn, signals to the mesenchyme and stimulates cell proliferation. Signaling activities are generally subject to tight spatiotemporal control and, in many instances, too much or too little signal is detrimental to the developing organ. This situation is well illustrated in anomalies caused by deregulated hedgehog (Hh) and FGF signaling [149, 171]. Fgf10/FgfR2b activity plays a crucial role during

Table 10.1. Syndromic genes associated with cleft and palate

Syndrome	Clinical features	Genes	Reference
Apert syndrome	AD; high arched palate, bifid uvula, and cleft palate	FGFR2	[72, 130]
Bamforth–Lazarus syndrome	AR; hypothyroidism, athyroidal, CPO, choanal atresia, spiky hair	FOXE1	[33, 72]
Branchio-oculo facial syndrome	AD; pseudocleft of the upper lip resembling a poorly repaired cleft lip	TFAP2A	[72, 137]
Down syndrome	Macroglossia, microstomia, atlantoaxial subluxation	Duplication of portion of chromosome 21	[98]
Ectrodactyly-ectodermal dysplasia-cleft syndrome	AD; triad of ectrodactyly, ectodermal dysplasia, and facial clefting	P63	[72]
Fetal alcohol syndrome	Disorder characterized by a pattern of minor facial anomalies, prenatal, and postnatal growth retardation	Alcohol dehydrogenase 1B	[1, 69]
Goldenhar syndrome	Oculo auricular vertebral dysplasia; AD; incomplete development of the ear, nose, soft palate, lip, mandible	Pericentric inversion of chromosome 9	[108, 230]
Hereditary lymphedema-distichiasis syndrome	AD; lymphedema of the limbs, double rows of eyelashes, cardiac defects, and cleft palate	FOXC mutations	[52]
Kallmann syndrome	AR disorder; Hypogonadotropic hypogonadism and anosmia	FGFR1 mutations	[50, 72]
Margarita Island ectodermal dysplasia [71]	AR; unusual facies, dental anomalies, syndactyly, and cleft lip/cleft palate	PVRL1 (nectin-1) mutation	[72, 212]
Pierre Robin sequence	AD; triad of micrognathia, glossoptosis, and cleft palate	Loci 2q24.1–33.3, 4q32qter, 11q2123.1, and17q2124.325.1	[40, 162]
Smith–Lemli-Opitz syndrome	AR; defects in cholesterol biosynthesis, growth retardation, dysmorphic facial features including CLP/CPO, postaxial polydactyly	DHCR	[72, 142]
Stickler syndrome	AD; midface hypoplasia, micrognathia, Pierre robin sequence, retinal detachment and early cataracts, deafness, hypermobility of joints	Col11A1, Col11A2, Col2A1	[206, 234]
Treacher-Collins syndrome	AD; craniofacial deformities such as: downward slanting eyes, micrognathia, conductive hearing loss, underdeveloped zygoma	Mutation in TCOF1 gene at chromosome 5q32-q33.1	[49]
van der Woude syndrome	AD; cleft lip palate, distinctive pits of the lower lips, or both	IRF 6 (interferon regulatory factor 6) mutations	[72, 111]
Velocardiofacial syndrome	AD; cleft palate, heart defects, abnormal facial structure, and learning problems	Chromosome 22q11 microdeletion	[45, 140]
Unnamed syndrome	CL/P and hereditary diffuse gastric cancer	CDH1	[245]
Unnamed syndrome	Chromodomain helicase DNA-binding proteins; CL/P in Charge syndrome	CHD7	[182]
Unnamed syndrome	Bilateral CL/P, colobomas of the optic nerve and retina, agenesis of the corpos callosum. Dysphagia, reduced esophageal peristalsis	PAX 9	[72] #5801
Unnamed syndrome	X-linked mental retardation and CL/P	PH8	[2]
Unnamed syndrome	Holoprosencephaly 7, a spectrum of forebrain and midline anomalies and midline CL	PTCH	[72]
Unnamed syndrome	CPO, craniofacial anomalies, osteoporosis, and cognitive defects	SATB2	[72]
Unnamed syndrome	Holoprosencephaly, a spectrum of anomalies ranging from severe (cyclopia) to subtle midline assymetries CL/P part of the spectrum	SHH	[86, 180]
Unnamed syndrome	Anomalies with most features of DiGeorge/velocardiofacial syndromes: CPO, thymus, and parathyroid gland hypoplasia, vertebra, facial, and cardiac outflow anomalies	TBX1	[86, 305]

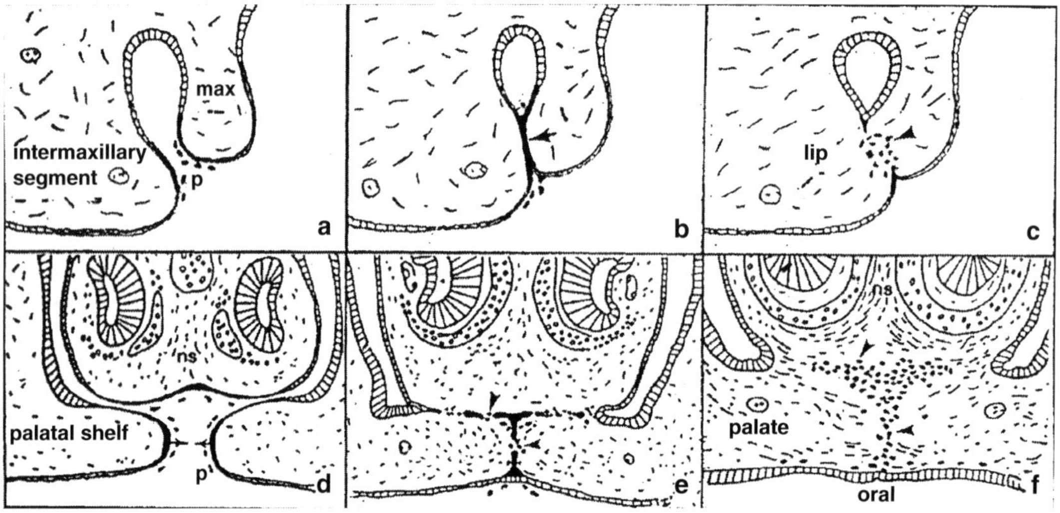

Figure 10.6. Comparison of the morphogenesis of the upper lip (**a**–**c**) with that of the palate (**d**–**f**). After the bilateral maxillary processes (max) fuse externally with the intermaxillary segment, the resulting epithelial seam (*arrow*, **b**) gives rise to mesenchyme (*arrowhead*, **c**) to produce a confluent lip. At a later time, the palatal shelves arising internally from the maxillary processes fuse with each other (*arrows*, **d**) and with the nasal septum (ns) above them, creating an epithelial seam that transforms to mesenchyme (*arrowheads*, **e**) to produce the confluent palate (*arrowheads*, **f**). *p* sloughed periderm cells. Reprinted with permission from Griffith and Hay [70], at www.dev.biologists.org, and Sun et al. [211] copyright 2000, with permission from Elsevier).

palatogenenesis, but appears subject to the tight spatiotemporal regulation prevailing in mice lacking *Shox2*. *Shox2*-mutant mice develop a very rare type of CP, where the soft palate is intact, but the hard palate has a cleft [80]. This condition is also found in humans. Abnormal proliferation and apoptosis may cause the cleft. Yet, many factors that play a role in palatogenesis including *Msx1, Bmp4, Pax9, Lhx8, Osr2, Tgfβ3*, and *Jag 2* are normally expressed [80]. In contrast, Fgf10 and Fgfr2b are expressed at ectopic sites within the mesenchyme of Shox2-mutant mice [240]. These studies emphasize the importance of the precise timing and sites of signaling activities that are necessary for normal development.

The mutation of activin-βA causes a severe facial primordial development defect, which may be responsible for the retardation of palatal shelf development and complete CP. In addition, other genes, including *Msx1, Lhx8, Shox2*, and *Osr2*, assume important roles in the palatal shelf growth. The targeted mutation of these genes in mice generates CP; this indicates that these factors are essential for palatogenesis [240].

Under normal conditions, the palatal shelves do not fuse with other oral structures. However, in mice that do not express Fgf10, the palatal shelf epithelium fuses with the tongue and mandible [170]. The loss-of-function mutations of Fgf10 result in anterior palatal shelf fusion with the tongue. At the same time, the middle and posterior palatal shelf regions adhere to the mandible, thus preventing the elevation of the palatal shelf [6]. There is a severe reduction in the *Jagged 2* expression, encoding a ligand for the Notch family receptors and the ectopic production of Tgfβ3 in the nasal epithelia of mutant mice. On the basis of the analysis of *Jag2* mutant embryos, it is apparent that Jag2-Notch signaling prevents inappropriate palatal shelf adhesion to other oral epithelia through its control of the oral epithelial differentiation. Mutations in TBX22 have been reported in families with X-linked CP and ankiloglossia [24, 128, 236]. *Tbx22* is expressed in the developing palate and tongue in mice; this suggests an important role in regulating tongue and palate development.

The role of Tgfβ3 during palatal fusion has been studied extensively [58, 158]. For fusion to occur, the MEE must adhere to the palatal shelf. TGfβ3 is expressed in the MEE before and during fusion, and mediates MEE adhesion of the opposing palatal shelves through filopodia. E-cadherin is required for fusion, whereas the filopodia seem to be crucial for the proper alignment and guidance of cell sheets that are fated to fuse, but not for the fusion itself [191]. Tgfβ3 is implicated in controlling the remodeling of the extracellular matrix through regulation of the expression of matrix metalloproteinases (MMPs), MMP13, MMP2, and the tissue inhibitor of metalloproteinase (TIMP)-2 [19]. TGFβ3 signaling functions in the MEE to mediate epithelial–mesenchymal interactions leading to changes that regulate palatal fusion. For example, EMT of the MES may constitute the major mechanism that underlies the disappearance of the MES, which generates mesenchyme continuity and prevents palatal clefts [146]. The establishment of the concept of EMT as the prevailing mechanism of MES disappearance has led to studies attributing roles to various molecules including Tgfβ3, Lef1, Smad, RhoA, phosphatidylinositol 3-kinase (PI-3 kinase), MMPs, Twist, and Snail [97, 99, 145]. In *Tgfβ*- or *Egfr*-mutant mice, the fate of MEE cells is altered [95, 136], and the MEE cells fail to undergo apoptosis and persist along the midline, thereby preventing normal fusion.

10.5.3 Ossification of the Palate

Palatal fusion indicates the ossification process that forms the hard palatal tissues in the anterior two-thirds of the palate. This entails the successful fusion of three embryonic structures, namely, the lateral edges of the primary palate with the two anterior edges of the secondary palate. This process requires the synchronization of shelf movements, together with the growth and withdrawal of the tongue and the growth of the mandible and head [31]. Any form of disruption during the formative stages results in a pathological cleft.

A wide range of studies on craniofacial skeletal maturation has shown that the fusion of the palatal shelves along their length to form the midpalatal (MP) suture occurs in the course of the ossification of the maxillae and palatine bones before the development of mandibular condyle [80, 105, 152, 157]. Ossification is observed where mesenchymal cells condense, the surrounding tissue vascularizes, and cells differentiate into osteoblasts. A number of growth and differentiation factors are involved in this process, e.g., BMPs, core-binding proteins, FGFs, and Hh proteins. These interact with various signaling pathways to regulate the patterning of undifferentiated mesenchyme. Bmp-6 and the transcription factor Gli1 are also expressed during intramembranous bone formation [89, 103]. As in the craniofacial sutures, the MP and TP suture osteoblasts express Tgfβ1,2, and 3, while the suture cells primarily express Tgfβ3 [3, 4].

Cranial sutures are the growth sites for the neurocranium, with the dura mater providing the signaling molecules to regulate suture patency [153]. The MP and TP sutures have different structures and are not in contact with the dura mater. Opperman's group has proposed that these facial sutures are growth centers [6, 7] and that the nasal capsular cartilage produces signaling molecules that regulate the fusion of the MP and TP sutures (Fig. 10.7) [4]. The nasal cartilage maintains the TP sutures as growth sites with or without nasal cartilage. Conceivably, the nasal cartilage regulates mid-facial growth [4].

Cyclic forces constitute an effective mechanical stimulus for the regulation of osteogenesis and osteoclastogenesis in the growth of sutures in neonatal rats [229]. At the early stage of sutural expansion, when osteoblasts and fibroblasts have proliferated, application of tensile forces has led to a cyst-like zone at the conjuncture of the bony front and the sutural connective tissue. New bone is deposited along the nasal septum and at the front of the cyst until the new bone front is formed, with the original structure restored by the suture [119].

Utilizing the MP suture expansion in mice has provided insight into how mechanical stress modulates remodeling of bones and cartilage. The expansive force across the MP suture promotes bone resorption through the activation of osteoclasts and bone formation through the increased proliferation and differentiation of periosteal cells [83]. Similarly, when expansion by orthodontic wire was done in growing rats, the secondary cartilage underwent chondrogenic and osteogenic differentiation in the maxillary arch. These induced changes have been attributed to progenitor cells differentiating from chondroblast to osteoblast. When this occurs, many sutures

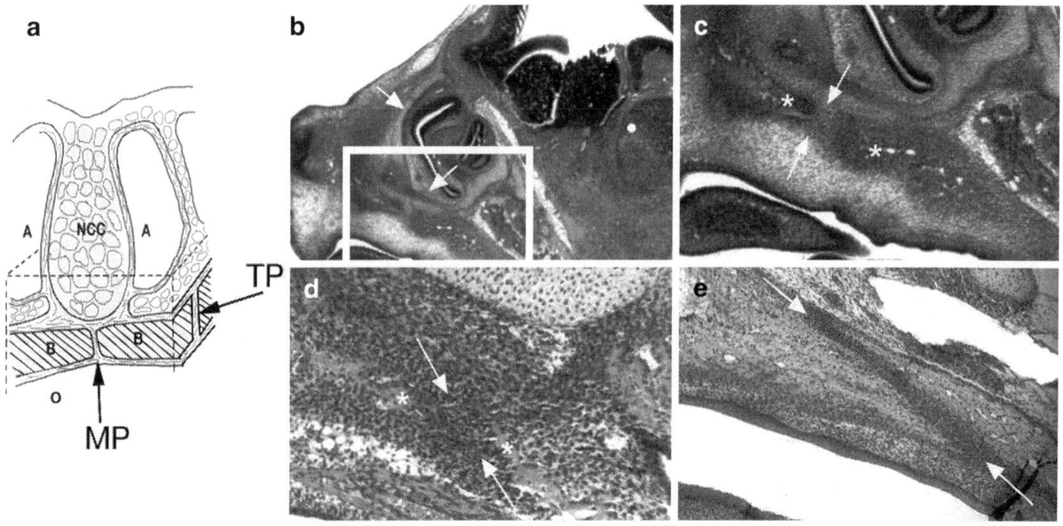

Figure 10.7. (**a**) Relationship between the nasal capsular (NC) cartilages and the transpalatal suture. *Dotted lines* indicate cut lines for removing the palate from the embryo and the NC cartilage from above the sutures. (**b**–**e**) Micrographs of parasagittal sections through fetal rat heads, showing the prenatal development of transpalatal (TP) sutures. (**b**) At E16, NC cartilages (*arrows*) can be seen directly above the presumptive TP suture region (in *box*). (**c**) High-power micrograph of the region in the box, showing the advancing palatal plate of the maxilla and horizontal plate of the palatal bone (*asterisks*) on either side of the presumptive TP suture (between *arrows*). (**d**) At E18, the advancing bone fronts (*asterisks*) overlap, creating a highly cellular suture blastema (between *arrows*). (**e**) By E20, an elongated TP suture (between *arrows*) continues to form as the bone fronts proceed to overlap. *A* airway; *B* shelves of maxillary bones; *MP* mid-palatal suture; *NCC* nasal capsular cartilage; *O* oral cavity; *TP* transpalatal suture. (Reprinted with permission from Adab et al. [3]).

temporarily form secondary cartilage. Histological observations at days 7, 10, and 14 have shown that intramembranous bone formation occurred at the boundary between the precartilaginous and cartilaginous cell layers, with osteocalcin detected in the calcified matrix [214]. The cellular events that take place at the MP suture cartilage expansion force are similar to what occurs when endochondral bone is formed at the boundary between the maxillary bone and cartilage. On the other hand, intramembranous osteogenesis appears at the internal aspect of the cartilaginous layer [107].

To stimulate new bone formation, rat organ cultures with distracted palatal sutures were treated with Bmp-7 and Nell-1 for 8 days in vitro. Nell-1 increased chondrocyte hypertrophy and endochondral bone formation, whereas Bmp-7 enhanced chondrocyte proliferation and differentiation in the distracted palates of the 4-week-old male rats. This study indicates that Nell-1 is involved in the rapid osteoblast differentiation in palate sutures [42]. When TGF-β1 was applied during the early stages of rat MP expansion, bone formed, presumably at the suture site [189].

10.5.4 Oral and Palatal Musculature and Related Deformities

Defects encompassed in overt cleft lip and palate range from the so-called microform clefts to complete unilateral or bilateral clefts of the lip and palate. The orbicularis oris (OO) muscle consists of many muscular fiber strata that are differently oriented and surround the mouth opening. At approximately 7 weeks p.c. in humans, the two maxillary prominences fuse with the medial nasal prominence; however, lip fusion is not complete until the epithelial seam disappears through EMT and/or apoptosis [31]. By 8 weeks p.c., there appears a dense, continuous band of mesenchymal cells that give rise to the OO muscle; discernible OO muscle fibers are present by 12 weeks and the complete OO muscle architecture is formed by 16 weeks [93]. Any delay in fusion may result in a subepithelial OO defect, such as the altered migration of the mesenchymal cells. Subepithelial (nonvisible) defects of the OO muscle represent the mildest form of cleft lip, constituting a part of the phenotypic spectrum of CL/P. This defect is a ridge of tissue, resembling a scar on the upper lip along the philtrum [5].

Histological studies have shown that the above-described defects extend to the muscle fibers of the superior OO muscle. A method using high-resolution ultrasonography was developed to visualize the OO muscle noninvasively [148]. OO defects differ significantly between first-degree relatives of the CL/P individuals and controls, with the differences detected by ultrasound, consistent with the information from autopsies [127, 148]. Interestingly, in the Bmp4 knockout mouse, bilateral cleft lips can be seen at E14.5, even though this condition occurs only in 22% of newborns [93]. This suggests that the initial cleft lip is rescued or healed in utero, leaving only the subepithelial OO defect. Two individuals with OO defects were found to have mutations in BMP4, whereas none was found in the controls [150]. The strong evidence that OO discontinuities are part of the phenotypic spectrum of CL/P is important for estimating the clinical recurrence risk for families with members affected with CL/P.

The mildest form of CP is termed as a "submucosal CP." This is made up of a bifid uvula, palatal muscle diastasis, and a notch in the posterior surface of the hard palate [67]. Defects in the nasopharyngeal structure and/or function may lead to velopharyngeal incompetence (VPI). Although most VPI is caused by CP, the population prevalence of VPI owing to other causes is approximately 2.5% [20]. VPI may be caused by submucosal muscular defects of the levator veli palatini or musculus uvulae. Most of the soft-palate muscles are derived from myotome cells, which invade pharyngeal arch 4 and then migrate to the palate, with innervation from the vagus nerve. One muscle (tensor veli palatini) is derived from myotome cells that invade arch 1 and are innervated by the trigeminal nerve [213]. In the mouse, the tensor veli palatini, levator veli palatini, medial pterygoid, and lateral pterygoid muscles are myogenic fields, beginning with gestational day 15. The palatoglossus, palatopharyngeus, and musculus uvulae, however, are not yet in evidence [222]. The presence of these anatomical features in unaffected individuals may constitute an elevated risk for producing clefts in offspring [233].

10.5.5 Small Ubiquitin-Like Modifier (SUMO) Modification of Signaling Pathways in Palatogenesis

The molecular understanding of nonsyndromic (NS) CL/P is further complicated because penetrance may differ significantly when a given mutation is placed on different strains. This reflects the fact that CL/P pathogenesis is subject to both genetic and environmental modifiers. One posttranslational mechanism is due to the SUMO [157]. SUMO proteins are ubiquitously expressed throughout the eukaryotic kingdom [243]. SUMO1 shows strong expression in the medial edge epithelial of the secondary palate [7]. A translocation breakpoint interrupting SUMO1 was found in a patient with CLP [7]. This translocation defect is the cause of CL/P and has been confirmed in SUMO1-deficient mice [7]. Moreover, mutations in TBX22 profoundly affect sumoylation, with changes in this process at least partially responsible for loss of function [10]. Other SUMO targets include Smad4, Msx1, p63, Pax9, Eya1, and FGF signaling [157], a change in some of which may affect the SUMO pathway. Destabilizing the normal balance of expression and activity for genes such as TBX22, Msx1, SATB2, and p63 during early pregnancy is likely to constitute a risk for the occurrence of CL/P. On elucidating the relationship of environmental factors, the SUMO pathway and the networks of craniofacial genes influenced by posttranscriptional modification may be crucial to understanding the idiopathic forms of orofacial clefts.

10.5.6 Overview of the Genetic Etiology of Cleft Palate

Disturbances at any stage during palate development, e.g., defective palatal shelf growth, failed or delayed elevation, and blocked fusion, can result in CP [38, 54]. As one of the most common congenital craniofacial defects, CP occurs in approximately 1 per 750 live births in the United States [38, 59]. Clefts occur more frequently among Asians (about 1:400) and certain American Indians than in Europeans. Clefts are relatively less common among Africans and African Americans (about 1:1,500) [204].

The etiology of CL/P is due to a combination of genetic and environmental factors [72, 143]. Characterization of the genomic sequences will pinpoint variations in the stages of craniofacial morphogenesis. Classification of CL/P into syndromic (Table 10.1) and NS genes (Table 10.2) helps to understand the molecular and genetic mechanisms that affect these types of craniofacial defects [30, 35, 71]. In addition, there is strong evidence that environmental factors such as alcohol consumption, tobacco, and anticonvulsants increase the risk of CL/P [192, 238]. On the other hand, folic acid may have a protective effect on CL/P and neural tube defects [21, 25, 55, 88, 112]. Recent data from the National Birth Defect Prevention Network have shown that neural tube defects have decreased from 5/10,000 to less than 2/10,000 after the food supply was fortified with folic acid. This vitamin and the proteins that facilitate its uptake and metabolism may be candidate genes in craniofacial development [55, 113, 193, 216, 244].

10.6 Tooth Development

From an evolutionary perspective, mammalian dentition is considered as a segmental or sequentially arranged organ system, in which specific numbers of teeth are spatially organized along the linear axes of the jaws. Biochemical and developmental pathways that control the initiation of tooth development in different vertebrate species are remarkably conserved. For developmental biologists, the developing tooth model is useful for studying the modes of patterning and morphogenesis that determine the position, size, shape, and number during organogenesis. For stem cell biologists and tissue engineering experts, the forming and fully developed tooth is an attractive model that offers both challenges and opportunities. Adult teeth house reservoirs of postnatal or "niche" stem cells that differentiate into bone and dentin and other tissues. These cells have been utilized in tissue engineering to regenerate mineralized tissues [64, 197]. As the implantation of a bioengineered "test tube tooth" would not result in life-threatening consequences, there is burgeoning interest in the field of bioengineering to utilize the wealth of genetic knowledge about tooth development to regenerate whole tooth organs for replacement therapies. Understanding the basic principles that guide the development of teeth, one of the most complex mammalian organ systems, is critical for regenerative medicine.

Teeth develop in distinct stages that are easily recognizable under the microscope (Fig. 10.8). They are the lamina, bud, cap, and bell (early and late) stages of tooth development [218]. As the molecular events that transform the tooth bud into a fully formed mineralized tooth have become known, the following functional terms can be used to describe the developing tooth organ: initiation, morphogenesis, cell or cytodifferentiation, and matrix apposition. The first visible sign of tooth development, becoming evident around 5 weeks of human development and at embryonic day 11 (E11) in mouse gestation, is a thickening of the oral epithelium that lines the frontonasal, maxillary, and mandibular arches. At this stage, the *dental lamina* is inductive and can direct the mesenchyme to a tooth-forming mesenchyme. As development progresses, the dental lamina grows into a *bud* that is distinguished by a well-demarcated zone of condensed ectomesenchyme called the *dental papilla*. At this stage, the inductive or tooth-forming potential is transferred from the dental epithelium to the dental papilla. At the cap stage, further elongation occurs, and the ectodermal component is referred to as the *dental* or *enamel* organ. The enamel organ and dental papilla become encapsulated by the *dental follicle*, a thin layer of mesenchymal cells that separate the dental papilla from the other connective tissues of the jaws.

The transition from the bud to the cap stage marks the onset of crown formation. Similar to the signaling centers found in other tissues, the tooth organ utilizes the *enamel knot* as an important organizing center that initiates cuspal patterning [91]. In this region, a unique set of signaling molecules is expressed. They modulate the shape of the crown and the underlying dental papilla. The enamel knot undergoes programmed cell death or apoptosis after cuspal patterning is completed at the onset of the early bell stage. The dental organ then assumes the shape of a bell as cells continue to divide

Table 10.2. Nonsyndromic genes: interaction effects of genes and environmental risk factors on oral clefts

Gene	Functional role	Risk factor	References
Cytochrome P450 proteins (CYP) CYPIA1, CYPIA2, CYPIB1 CYP2E1	Highly polymorphic, having multiple functional alleles; role in detoxification; metabolism of endogenous morphogens in the developing fetus	Negative gene–smoking interaction effect	[81]
Epoxide hydrolase (EPHX)	Class of proteins that catalyze the hydration of chemically reactive epoxides into their corresponding dihydrodiol products		
EPHX	Plays an important role in both the bioactivation and detoxification of exogenous chemicals, such as PAHs, which are present in cigarette smoke	Negative gene–smoking interaction effect	[9,81]
EPHX1 Y113H	Variant of EPHX 1 found in the fetus and maternal smoking	Positive gene–smoking interaction effect	[196]
Glutathione transferase gene family (GST)	Families of dimeric phase II enzymes that catalyze the conjugation of reduced glutathione with electrophilic groups of a wide variety of environmental agents		
GSTM1	Major gene detoxifying PAHs and widely studied in many disorders and cancers	Negative gene–smoking interaction effect	[196]
GSTT1	Expressed in a variety of tissues/organs, such as erythrocytes, lung, kidney, brain, skeletal muscles, heart, and small intestine; elevated expression profile at the craniofacial regions during embryonic development	Positive gene–smoking interaction effect	[196]
GSTP1	Major gene detoxifying PAHS; involvement in a variety of disorders and cancers. Major enzyme involved in the inactivation of cigarette smoker's metabolites; most important isoform at the embryonic and early fetal developmental stages	Positive gene–smoking interaction effect	[196]
GST A4/GSTM3	Two other types of GST gene family members	Positive gene–smoking interaction effect	[196]
Hypoxia-induced factor-1	Mechanism by which maternal smoking may affect embryonic development owing to the production of carbon monoxide that interferes with oxygen transfer to the placenta, or nicotine that constricts the uterine wall resulting in hypoxia	Positive gene–smoking interaction effects	[196]
Arylamine *N*-acetyltransferase gene family	N-conjugation of arylamine by the action of *N*-acetyltransferases (NAT), UDP glucoronosyltransferases (UGTs), or sulfotransfereases (SULTSO) produces nontoxic compounds		
NAT 1	Expressed in many tissues, such as erythrocytes, bladder, lymphocytes, neural tissues, liver, and intestines	Negative gene–smoking interaction effects	[113,203,205]
NAT pseudogene (NATP1)	Pseudogenes identified, which are located at chromosome 8p23.1–8p21.3		[113,203,205]
NAT 2	Expressed in the liver and epithelial cells of the intestine	Positive gene–smoking interaction effects	[196]
Methylenetetrahydrofolate reductase (MTHFR) MTHFRC677T	Metabolism of folate by reducing methylenetetrahydrofolate, primary donor for methionin synthesis. Variant of methylenetetrahydrofolate reductase	Positive gene–vitamin interaction effect Negative gene-smoking interaction effect	[18,132]
Other metabolic genes			
NAD(P)H quinine oxidoreductase (NQO1)	Flavoenzyme that catalyzes two electron reduction of quinine compounds to hydroquinone and is inducible by oxidative stress, dioxin, and PAHS found in cigarette smoke	Negative gene–smoking interaction effect	[196]
SULT1A1	Catalyzes transfer of the sulfonate group from the active sulfate to a substrate to form the respective sulfate or sulfamate ester	Negative gene–smoking interaction effects	[196]

(*continued*)

Table 10.2. (continued)

Gene	Functional role	Risk factor	References
UDP glycosyltransferases (UGTs) UGT1A7 variant	Catalyzes conjugation reactions where hydrophobic chemicals are transformed into water-soluble compounds. Potential maternal effects on embryonic development	Positive gene–smoking interaction effects	[41, 194, 196]
Developmental genes for oral clefts			
Transforming growth factor A (TGF α)	Transmembrane protein expressed at the medial edge of the epithelium (MEE) of fusing palatal shelves. Its receptor epidermal growth factor is expressed in the degenerating MEE	Positive gene–interaction effects (smoking, alcohol drinking, vitamins)	[85, 126]
Transforming growth factor β-3 (TGF β3)	Regulator of many biological processes such as proliferation, differentiation, epithelial-mesenchymal transformation, and apoptosis	Positive–gene interaction effects (smoking, alcohol drinking)	[126]
Muscle segment homeobox1 (MSX1)	Transcriptional repressor important in craniofacial, limb, and nervous system development	Positive–gene interaction effects (smoking and alcohol drinking)	[126, 138, 176]
MSX2	Similar to MSX1; rare cause of isolated cleft lip with or without cleft palate		[138, 176]
Acyl-CoA desaturase ACOD4	Pericentric inversion disrupts a gene (ACOD4) on chromosome 4q21 that codes for a novel acyl-CoA desaturase enzyme occurs in a single two generation family with CL		[15]
Retinoic acid receptor	Odds ratios for transmission of alleles at THRA1 were significant when ethnic group was included	Negative gene–smoking interaction effects	[126]
CHD7	Chromodomain helicase DNA-binding proteins		[53]
ESR1	Ligand-activated TF estrogen receptor		[154]
FGF/FGFR families FGF8 FGF3 FGF10 FGF18 FGFR1 FGFR2 FGFR3	Expressed during craniofacial development and can rarely harbor mutations that result in human clefting syndromes		[174]
SPRY1/SPRY2	Loss-of-function mutations in FGFR1 cause a syndromic form of clefting		[228]
TBX10	Ectopically expressed in dancer cleft lip and palate-mutant mice		[228]
GABRB3	β3 subunit of GABA receptor CL/P		[72]
GLI2	Mutations in GLi2 cause holoprosencephaly-like features with cleft lip and palate		[228]
ISGF3G	Similar to IRF6		[228]
Other candidate genes			
SKI, FOXE1, JAG2, LHX8	Rare causes of isolated cleft lip with or without cleft palate		[228]

at differential rates. The outermost layer of cuboidal cells is called the *external dental epithelium*, whereas the cells that encase the dental papilla are the *internal dental epithelium*. The latter gives rise to the ameloblasts, cells responsible for enamel formation. Functional layers develop within the enamel organ, which allow it to expand and change the fate of the dental papilla. The star-shaped cells of the stellate reticulum are rich in glycosaminoglycans that are thought to sequester fluids, as well as growth factors that lead to its expansion. The narrow layer of flattened cells termed the *stratum intermedium*, which expresses high levels of alkaline phosphatase, develops adjacent to the inner dental epithelium and influences differentiation into ameloblasts, as well as the process of enamel biomineralization.

Shortly after the shape of the crown is determined, the cells of the internal dental epithelium at the sites of the future cusp tips stop dividing and signal the underlying dental papilla cells to organize themselves along the epithelial–mesenchymal interface. These newly differentiated cells are called *odontoblasts*, cells that are responsible for the synthesis and secretion of

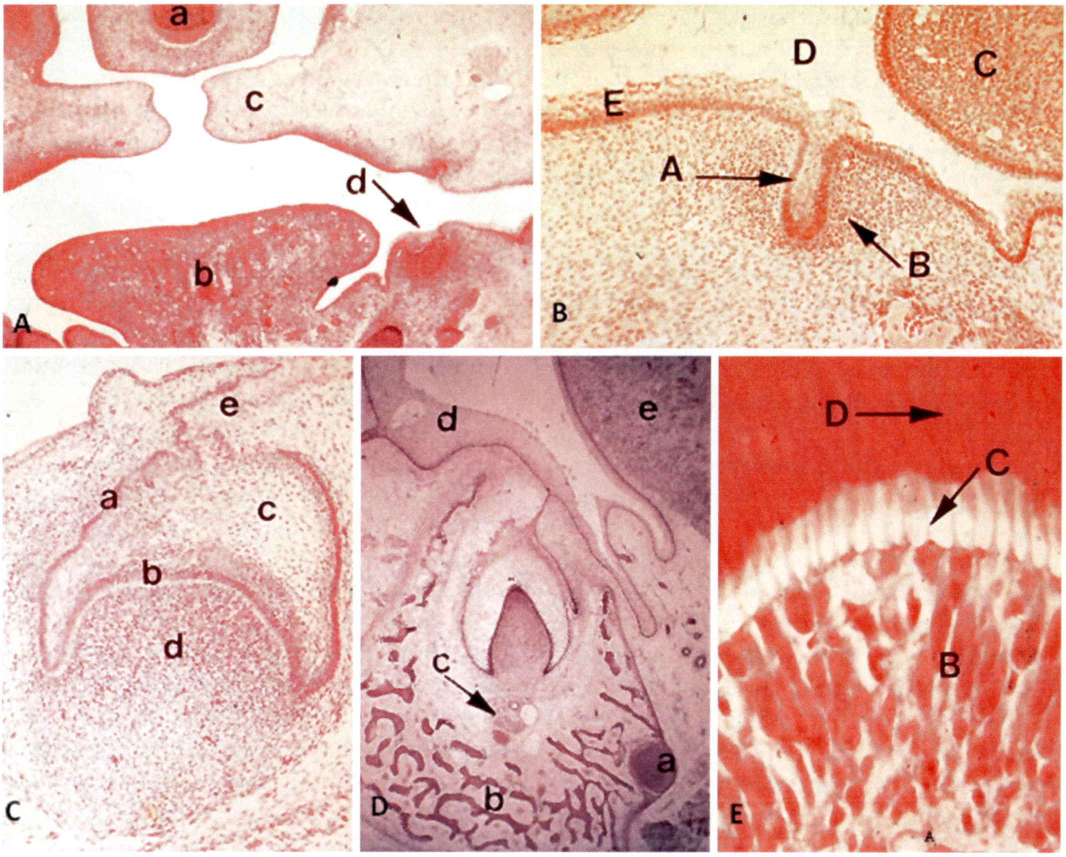

Figure 10.8. Histologic depiction of tooth development. (**a**) lamina phase (a = nasal septum; b = tongue; c = palatal shelves; d = dental lamina). (**b**) bud stage (a = ectodermal outgrowth; b = dental mesenchyme; c = tongue; d = oral cavity space; e = oral ectoderm). (**c**) cap or transition to early bell stage (a = outer dental epithelium; b = internal dental epithelium; c = stellate reticulum; d = dental papilla ectomesenchyme; e = dental lamina). (**d**) late bell stage (a = nerve bundle; b = alveolar bone; c = vasculature; d = oral ectoderm; e = tongue). Note the extension of the dental lamina on the right aspect of the dental organ that will form the succeeding incisor. (**e**) onset of dentinogenesis (a = dental pulp; b = cluster of odontoblasts that appear crowded at the tip; c = odontoblastic process; d = dentin).

the dentin matrix that shares the biochemical properties with bone. The dental papilla is now termed the dental *pulp*. After the odontoblasts deposit the first layer of predentin, inner dental epithelium cells develop into ameloblasts or enamel-producing cells. As enamel is deposited over the dentin matrix, the ameloblasts retreat to the outside and undergo apoptosis. In contrast, the odontoblasts line the inner surface of the dentin and remain metabolically active throughout the life of the tooth. The inner and outer dental epithelia combine in the area of the cervical loop to form Hertwig's epithelial root sheath. This structure influences the differentiation of the odontoblasts from the dental papilla, as well as the cementoblasts from the follicle mesenchyme, thus forming root dentin and cementum, respectively. The dental follicle that gives rise to the components of the periodontium (the periodontal ligament fibroblasts, alveolar bone of the tooth socket, and the cementum) also plays a role during tooth eruption, the last phase of odontogenesis.

10.6.1 Signaling Interactions During Tooth Development

Epithelial–mesenchymal interactions that involve an exchange of molecular information between the ectoderm and mesenchyme drive critical events in tooth morphogenesis. As is true for the limb bud, no single transcription factor or growth factor is responsible for odontogenesis; rather, a series of interactions involving several molecules leads to the development of the complex tooth form [92]. Signaling is reciprocal in nature. In other words, information is exchanged to and from the dental epithelium to the mesenchyme, and to and from the dental mesenchyme to the epithelium. For example, when the dental epithelium is separated from the mesenchyme, cusp patterning does not occur. Similarly, in the absence of the dental epithelium, the dental mesenchyme does not differentiate into odontoblasts [177].

The website (http://honeybee.helsinki.fi/toothexp) lists all molecules expressed in tooth organs. The two principal groups of molecules involved in the information exchange between the tooth epithelium and mesenchyme are the transcription factors and growth factors. The key mediators are the BMPs, FGFs, and WNT families: *Shh*, transcriptional molecules like the *Msx-1,-2* homeobox genes, *l*ymphoid *e*nhancer-binding *f*actor *1* (Lef-1) and Pax9, a member of the paired-box-containing transcription factor gene family. For a description of the actions and interactions of these molecules, see [46, 100].

10.6.2 The Role of the Extracellular Matrix (ECM) in Tooth Morphogenesis and Cytodifferentiation

The basement membrane ECM directs the budding and folding of dental epithelium during morphogenesis [219]. Molecules like collagens type I, III, and IV, along with laminin and various proteoglycans, are expressed in the basement membrane at the tooth epithelial–mesenchymal interface [177]. The MMPs, such as gelatinase, cleave type-IV collagen and contribute to the overall degradation of the basement membrane [181]. The expression of the protease inhibitors, TIMPs 1, 2, and 3, also correlates with tooth morphogenesis. Earlier in vitro studies have shown that the integrity of the basement membrane influences the budding and folding of the dental epithelium during morphogenesis and the spatial ordering of the cells that undergo terminal differentiation [219].

10.6.3 Dentin Biomineralization

The formation of dentin follows the same principles that guide the formation of other mesenchymal-derived mineralized tissues, e.g., cementum or bone. The odontoblasts are terminally differentiated cells that synthesize and secrete a type-I collagen-rich organic matrix called *predentin*. As the odontoblasts retreat toward the center of the tooth, cellular processes that subsequently mineralize remain in the matrix. Apatite crystals are deposited in an orderly manner, with disruptions resulting in a defective matrix, as seen in several dentinogeneses imperfectae and dysplasias.

For several decades, researchers have sought answers to these fundamental questions:

What is the exact composition of the dentin matrix and what biochemical features distinguish dentin from bone and cementum? Are there dentin-specific markers and can they be used to characterize the nature of the replacement cells responsible for forming reparative dentin? How do the physical features and conformational structures of the ECM molecules facilitate the calcification of dentin? Do these macromolecules interact with each other during the mineralization of dentin, and do they form supramolecular complexes that promote the deposition of hydroxyapatite crystals? What is the nature of the ECM molecules that modulate the initiation, rate, and extent of dentin deposition? What is the nature of the genes that encode the ECM molecules for dentin? Are defects in these genes responsible for inherited dentin disorders, namely dentinogenesis imperfecta (DGI) and dentin dysplasia? What genes regulate the expression of key dentin ECM molecules?

The noncollagenous proteins (NCPs) of the dentin matrix are thought to play a unique role in modulating the mineralization of dentin. Experimental evidence for this role is provided by the discovery that mutations in the dentin sialophosphoprotein (DSPP) gene are responsible for the defects seen in DGI types II and III [51]. As 90% of the organic matrix is type-I collagen, it is not surprising that patients with DGI type I caused by mutations in the type-I collagen gene have severe dentinal defects [104].

In recent years, a family of dentin and bone NCPs that have attracted attention are the small integrin-binding ligand, N-linked glycoprotein (SIBLING) proteins. This group comprises DSPP, dentin matrix protein 1 (DMP1), bone sialoprotein (BSP), and osteopontin (OPN) [57]. As they are polyanionic molecules, SIBLING proteins are active in the mineralization of a collagen-containing matrix and are also thought to promote crystal growth within predentin.

10.6.4 Dentin Sialophosphoprotein (DSPP)

DSPP is a member of the SIBLING family that makes dentin matrix distinguishable from the bone. It is transcribed from a single mRNA that encodes DSP at the 5′ end and DPP at the 3′ end of a large precursor molecule [175]. Because of the abundance of at least two proteins in dentin ECM, DSPP is likely to be cleaved posttranslationally by a proteinase. The expression profiles of DSP and DPP show tooth-specific colocalization in the preameloblasts, the newly differentiated odontoblasts in predentin and dentin matrix. DSPP does occur in bone, but with far fewer osteoblasts expressed than in dentin and odontoblasts [163].

DSP, discovered by Butler et al. [27], has no specific function to date; it does not promote mineralization in vitro [22]. In contrast, DPP, discovered by Veis and Perry [227], may modulate mineralization. It contains unusually large amounts of acidic residues, such as aspartic acid and phosphoserine, and can initiate and modulate the formation and growth of hydroxyapatite crystals [23]. Expressed in odontoblasts, DPP binds to collagen at the mineralization front and may modulate binding of other NCPs to the growing hydroxyapatite crystals in a specific conformation [118].

More recently, a proteoglycan form of DSP (DSP-PG) has been isolated and characterized, but its precise role is still unknown [210].

Each of the three DSPP-derived variants, DSP, DPP, and DSP-PG, may play a unique role in the mineralization of dentin. Conversion of DSPP to DSP and DPP in dentin may require activation and the activating molecule(s), once identified, may have therapeutic value. As the precursor of DSPP is a large molecule, it is likely that structural changes are needed to enable the DPP to bind calcium to the collagen fibers. In other words, the rate and extent of biomineralization may be controlled by the activation and structural changes involving DSPP.

Mutations in the human DSPP gene give rise to DGI-II and DGI-III, causing the dentin to be severely affected. Studies with DSPP-null mice have provided evidence for defects in the mineralization of dentin. The SIBLING protein, therefore, is critical for normal dentinogenesis [207].

10.7 Future Perspectives

Many medical and dental scientists envision the day when diagnostic tools will be available to establish a personalized genetic and molecular profile of a patient's condition. Such a "molecular fingerprint" can also provide clues about gene changes and their effects on encoded proteins and the signaling pathways that are altered in the development and progression of the disease. In coming decades, identification and analysis of molecules that regulate the development of the craniofacial complex will provide insights that can be translated into clinical therapies to treat the spectrum of disorders and diseases that affect this part of the body. Knowledge of the mechanisms that drive the formation of mandible, palate, TMJ, and the teeth will provide a basis for developing new regenerative strategies aimed at restoring normal structure and function.

Acknowledgment

The authors acknowledge the excellent editorial assistance provided by Ms. Jeanne Santa Cruz in the preparation of the original manuscript for this chapter. Data described in this chapter were gathered during the course of the following funded research grants: March of Dimes 6-FY06-321 (KKHS), Cleft Palate Foundation (LBR), NIH/NIDCR U24 DE16472 (LBR, KKHS, RDS), NIH/NIDCR T32 DE108380 (RDS), NIH/NIDCR R01 DE013368 and R01 DE019471(RDS), and NIH/NIDCR R01 DE015401 (RH).

References

1. Abel EL (2006) Fetal alcohol syndrome: a cautionary note. Curr Pharm Des 12:1521–1529
2. Abidi FE, Miano MG, Murray JC, Schwartz CE (2007) A novel mutation in the PHF8 gene is associated with X-linked mental retardation with cleft lip/cleft palate. Clin Genet 72:19–22
3. Adab K, Sayne JR, Carlson DS, Opperman LA (2002) Elevated TGF-b1, TGF-b2, TGF-b3 and Msx2 expression are associated with morphogenesis of facial sutures and active bone growth from these sites. J Dent Res 81:A221
4. Adab K, Sayne JR, Carlson DS, Opperman LA (2003) Nasal capsular cartilage is required for rat transpalatal suture morphogenesis. Differentiation 71:496–505
5. Akita S, Hirano A (2005) Surgical modifications for microform cleft lip repairs. J Craniofac Surg 16: 1106–1110
6. Alappat SR, Zhang Z, Suzuki K, Zhang X, Liu H, Jiang R, Yamada G, Chen Y (2005) The cellular and molecular etiology of the cleft secondary palate in Fgf10 mutant mice. Dev Biol 277:102–113
7. Alkuraya FS, Saadi I, Lund JJ, Turbe-Doan A, Morton CC, Maas RL (2006) SUMO1 haploinsufficiency leads to cleft lip and palate. Science 313:1751
8. Almarza AJ, Athanasiou KA (2004) Design characteristics for the tissue engineering of cartilaginous tissues. Ann Biomed Eng 32:2–17
9. An S, Dickens MA, Bleu T, Hallmark OG, Goetzl EJ (1997) Molecular cloning of the human Edg2 protein and its identification as a functional cellular receptor for lysophosphatidic acid. Biochem Biophys Res Commun 231:619–622
10. Andreou AM, Pauws E, Jones MC, Singh MK, Bussen M, Doudney K, Moore GE, Kispert A, Brosens JJ, Stanier P (2007) TBX22 missense mutations found in patients with X-linked cleft palate affect DNA binding, sumoylation, and transcriptional repression. Am J Hum Genet 81:700–712
11. Avery JK (1987) Development, structure and function of temporomandibular joint, oral development and histology. Williams & Williams, Baltimore, pp 348–364
12. Barbosa AC, Funato N, Chapman S, McKee MD, Richardson JA, Olson EN, Yanagisawa H (2007) Hand transcription factors cooperatively regulate development of the distal midline mesenchyme. Dev Biol 310:154–168
13. Baume LJ (1962) Ontogenesis of the human temporomandibular joint 1. Development of the condyles. J Dent Res 41:1327–1338
14. Baume LJ, Holz J (1970) Ontogenesis of the human temporomandibular joint: 2. Development of the temporal components. J Dent Res 49:864–875
15. Beiraghi S, Zhou M, Talmadge CB, Went-Sumegi N, Davis JR, Huang D, Saal H, Seemayer TA, Sumegi J (2003) Identification and characterization of a novel gene disrupted by a pericentric inversion inv(4) (p13.1q21.1) in a family with cleft lip. Gene 309:11–21
16. Beresford WA (1981) Chondroid bone, secondary cartilage, and metaplasia. Urban and Schwartzenberg, Baltimore
17. Beverdam A, Merlo GR, Paleari L, Mantero S, Genova F, Barbieri O, Janvier P, Levi G (2002) Jaw transformation with gain of symmetry after Dlx5/Dlx6 inactivation: mirror of the past? Genesis 34: 221–227
18. Blanton SH, Kolle BS, Hecht JT, Mulliken JB, Martin ER (2000) No evidence supporting MTHFR as a risk factor in the development of familial NSCLP. Am J Med Genet 92:370–371
19. Blavier L, Lazaryev A, Groffen J, Heisterkamp N, DeClerck YA, Kaartinen V (2001) Tgf-beta3-induced palatogenesis requires matrix metalloproteinases. Mol Biol Cell 12:1457–1466
20. Boorman JG, Varma S, Ogilvie CM (2001) Velopharyngeal incompetence and chromosome 22q11 deletion. Lancet 357:774
21. Boot MJ, Steegers-Theunissen RP, Poelmann RE, Van Iperen L, Lindemans J, Gittenberger-de Groot AC (2003) Folic acid and homocysteine affect neural crest and neuroepithelial cell outgrowth and differentiation in vitro. Dev Dyn 227:301–308
22. Boskey A, Spevak L, Tan M, Doty SB, Butler WT (2000) Dentin sialoprotein (DSP) has limited effects on in vitro apatite formation and growth. Calcif Tissue Int 67:472–478
23. Boskey AL, Maresca M, Doty S, Sabsay B, Veis A (1990) Concentration-dependent effects of dentin phosphophoryn in the regulation of in vitro hydroxyapatite formation and growth. Bone Miner 11:55–65
24. Braybrook C, Doudney K, Marcano AC, Arnason A, Bjornsson A, Patton MA, Goodfellow PJ, Moore GE, Stanier P (2001) The T-box transcription factor gene TBX22 is mutated in X-linked cleft palate and ankyloglossia. Nat Genet 29:179–183
25. Briggs RM (1976) Vitamin supplementation as a possible factor in the incidence of cleft lip/palate deformities in humans. Clin Plast Surg 3:647–652
26. Britto JA, Evans RD, Hayward RD, Jones BM (2002) Toward pathogenesis of Apert cleft palate: FGF, FGFR, and TGF beta genes are differentially expressed in sequential stages of human palatal shelf fusion. Cleft Pal Craniofac J 39:332–340
27. Butler WT, Bhown M, Dimuzio MT, Linde A (1981) Nonocollagenous proteins of dentin. Isolation and partial characterization of rat dentin proteins and proteoglycans using a three-step preparative method. Coll Relat Res 1:187–199
28. Buxton PG, Hall B, Archer CW, Francis-West P (2003) Secondary chondrocyte-derived Ihh stimulates proliferation of periosteal cells during chick development. Development 130:4729–4739
29. Carette MJ, Ferguson MW (1992) The fate of medial edge epithelial cells during palatal fusion in vitro: an analysis by DiI labelling and confocal microscopy. Development 114:379–388
30. Carinci F, Pezzetti F, Scapoli L, Martinelli M, Carinci P, Tognon M (2000) Genetics of nonsyndromic cleft lip and palate: a review of international studies and data

regarding the Italian population. Cleft Pal Craniofac J 37:33–40
31. Carlson BM (2004) Human embryology and developmental biology, 3rd edn. Mosby, Philadelphia, vol xv, p 527
32. Carlson DS (1994) Growth of the temporomandibular joint. In: Zarb GA, Carlsson GE, Sessle BJ, Mohl ND (eds) Temporomandibular joint and masticatory muscle disorders. Munksgaard, Copenhagen 128–153
33. Castanet M, Park SM, Smith A, Bost M, Leger J, Lyonnet S, Pelet A, Czernichow P, Chatterjee K, Polak M (2002) A novel loss-of-function mutation in TTF-2 is associated with congenital hypothyroidism, thyroid agenesis and cleft palate. Hum Mol Genet 11:2051–2059
34. Cerny R, Lwigale P, Ericsson R, Meulemans D, Epperlein HH, Bronner-Fraser M (2004) Developmental origins and evolution of jaws: new interpretation of "maxillary" and "mandibular". Dev Biol 276:225–236
35. Chai Y, Maxson RE Jr (2006) Recent advances in craniofacial morphogenesis. Dev Dyn 235:2353–2375
36. Charite J, McFadden DG, Merlo G, Levi G, Clouthier DE, Yanagisawa M, Richardson JA, Olson EN (2001) Role of Dlx6 in regulation of an endothelin-1-dependent, dHAND branchial arch enhancer. Genes Dev 15: 3039–3049
37. Chiang C, Litingtung Y, Lee E, Young KE, Corden JL, Westphal H, Beachy PA (1996) Cyclopia and defective axial patterning in mice lacking Sonic hedgehog gene function. Nature 383:407–413
38. Christensen K, Juel K, Herskind AM, Murray JC (2004) Long term follow up study of survival associated with cleft lip and palate at birth. Br Med J 328:12
39. Clouthier DE, Hosoda K, Richardson JA, Williams SC, Yanagisawa H, Kuwaki T, Kumada M, Hammer RE, Yanagisawa M (1998) Cranial and cardiac neural crest defects in endothelin-A receptor-deficient mice. Development 125:813–824
40. Cole A, Lynch P, Slator R (2008) A new grading of Pierre Robin sequence. Cleft Pal Craniofac J 45:603–606
41. Collier AC, Tingle MD, Paxton JW, Mitchell MD, Keelan JA (2002) Metabolizing enzyme localization and activities in the first trimester human placenta: the effect of maternal and gestational age, smoking and alcohol consumption. Hum Reprod 17:2564–2572
42. Cowan CM, Cheng S, Ting K, Soo C, Walder B, Wu B, Kuroda S, Zhang X (2006) Nell-1 induced bone formation within the distracted intermaxillary suture. Bone 38:48–58
43. Creuzet S, Couly G, Le Douarin NM (2005) Patterning the neural crest derivatives during development of the vertebrate head: insights from avian studies. J Anat 207:447–459
44. Cuervo R, Covarrubias L (2004) Death is the major fate of medial edge epithelial cells and the cause of basal lamina degradation during palatogenesis. Development 131:15–24
45. Cuneo BF (2001) 22q11.2 deletion syndrome: DiGeorge, velocardiofacial, and conotruncal anomaly face syndromes. Curr Opin Pediatr 13:465–472
46. D'Souza RN, Klein OD (2007) Unraveling the molecular mechanisms that lead to supernumerary teeth in mice and men: current concepts and novel approaches. Cells Tissues Organs 186:60–69
47. Depew MJ, Lufkin T, Rubenstein JL (2002) Specification of jaw subdivisions by Dlx genes. Science 298:381–385
48. Depew MJ, Simpson CA, Morasso M, Rubenstein JL (2005) Reassessing the Dlx code: the genetic regulation of branchial arch skeletal pattern and development. J Anat 207:501–561
49. Dixon J, Jones NC, Sandell LL, Jayasinghe SM, Crane J, Rey JP, Dixon MJ, Trainor PA (2006) Tcof1/Treacle is required for neural crest cell formation and proliferation deficiencies that cause craniofacial abnormalities. Proc Natl Acad Sci U S A 103:13403–13408
50. Dode C, Fouveaut C, Mortier G, Janssens S, Bertherat J, Mahoudeau J, Kottler ML, Chabrolle C, Gancel A, Francois I, Devriendt K, Wolczynski S, Pugeat M, Pineiro-Garcia A, Murat A, Bouchard P, Young J, Delpech M, Hardelin JP (2007) Novel FGFR1 sequence variants in Kallmann syndrome, and genetic evidence that the FGFR1c isoform is required in olfactory bulb and palate morphogenesis. Hum Mutat 28:97–98
51. Dong J, Amor D, Aldred MJ, Gu T, Escamilla M, MacDougall M (2005) DLX3 mutation associated with autosomal dominant amelogenesis imperfecta with taurodontism. Am J Med Genet A 133A:138–141
52. Fang J, Dagenais SL, Erickson RP, Arlt MF, Glynn MW, Gorski JL, Seaver LH, Glover TW (2000) Mutations in FOXC2 (MFH-1), a forkhead family transcription factor, are responsible for the hereditary lymphedema-distichiasis syndrome. Am J Hum Genet 67:1382–1388
53. Felix TM, Hanshaw BC, Mueller R, Bitoun P, Murray JC (2006) CHD7 gene and non-syndromic cleft lip and palate. Am J Med Genet A 140:2110–2114
54. Ferguson MW (1988) Palate development. Development 103:41–60
55. Finnell RH, Shaw GM, Lammer EJ, Brandl KL, Carmichael SL, Rosenquist TH (2004) Gene-nutrient interactions: importance of folates and retinoids during early embryogenesis. [Review] [132 refs]. Toxicol Appl Pharmacol 198:75–85
56. Firulli AB, McFadden DG, Lin Q, Srivastava D, Olson EN (1998) Heart and extra-embryonic mesodermal defects in mouse embryos lacking the bHLH transcription factor Hand1. Nat Genet 18:266–270
57. Fisher LW, Torchia DA, Fohr B, Young MF, Fedarko NS (2001) Flexible structures of SIBLING proteins, bone sialoprotein, and osteopontin. Biochem Biophys Res Commun 280:460–465
58. Fitzpatrick DR, Denhez F, Kondaiah P, Akhurst RJ (1990) Differential expression of TGF beta isoforms in murine palatogenesis. Development 109:585–595
59. Fogh-Andersen P (1971) Epidemiology and etiology of clefts. In: Bergsma D (ed) Birth defects: original article series. Williams and Wilkins, Baltimore
60. Frank DU, Fotheringham LK, Brewer JA, Muglia LJ, Tristani-Firouzi M, Capecchi MR, Moon AM (2002) An

Fgf8 mouse mutant phenocopies human 22q11 deletion syndrome. Development 129:4591–4603
61. Fukada K, Shibata S, Ohya K, Kuroda T (1999) In situ hybridisation study of type I, II, X collagens and aggregan mRNSa in the developing condylar cartilage of fetal mouse mandible. J Anat 195:321–329
62. Funato N, Chapman SL, McKee MD, Funato H, Morris JA, Shelton JM, Richardson JA, Yanagisawa H (2009) Hand2 controls osteoblast differentiation in the branchial arch by inhibiting DNA binding of Runx2. Development 136:615–625
63. Furstman L (1963) The early development of the human temporomandibular joint. Am J Orthod 49:672–682
64. Galler KM, Cavender A, Yuwono V, Dong H, Shi S, Schmalz G, Hartgerink JD, D'Souza RN (2008) Self-assembling peptide amphiphile nanofibers as a scaffold for dental stem cells. Tissue Eng A 14:2051–2058
65. Gardner E, O'Rahilly R (1968) The early development of the knee joint in staged human embryos. J Anat 102:289–299
66. Gendron-Maguire M, Mallo M, Zhang M, Gridley T (1993) Hoxa-2 mutant mice exhibit homeotic transformation of skeletal elements derived from cranial neural crest. Cell 75:1317–1331
67. Gosain AK, Conley SF, Marks S, Larson DL (1996) Submucous cleft palate: diagnostic methods and outcomes of surgical treatment. Plast Reconstr Surg 97: 1497–1509
68. Grammatopoulos GA, Bell E, Toole L, Lumsden A, Tucker AS (2000) Homeotic transformation of branchial arch identity after Hoxa2 overexpression. Development 127:5355–5365
69. Green ML, Singh AV, Zhang Y, Nemeth KA, Sulik KK, Knudsen TB (2007) Reprogramming of genetic networks during initiation of the fetal alcohol syndrome. Dev Dyn 236:613–631
70. Griffith CM, Hay ED (1992) Epithelial-mesenchymal transformation during palatal fusion: carboxyfluorescein traces cells at light and electron microscopic levels. Development 116:1087–1099
71. Gritli-Linde A (2007) Molecular control of secondary palate development. Dev Biol 301:309–326
72. Gritli-Linde A (2008) The etiopathogenesis of cleft lip and cleft palate usefulness and caveats of mouse models. Curr Top Dev Biol 84:37–138
73. Habib H, Hatta T, Udagawa J, Zhang L, Yoshimura Y, Otani H (2005) Fetal jaw movement affects condylar cartilage development. J Dent Res 84:474–479
74. Hall BK (1968) The fate of adventitious and embryonic articular cartilage in the skull of the common fowl, Gallus Domesticus (Aves: Phasianidae). Aust J Zool 16:795–805
75. Hall BK (2005) Bones and cartilage: developmental and evolutionary skeletal biology. Elsevier, Amsterdam
76. Hanken J, Hall BK (eds) (1993) The skull, vol 1. Development, University of Chicago Press, Chicago, XIV, p 587 S
77. Hanken J, Hall BK (eds) (1993) The skull, volume 3: Functional and evolutionary mechanisms. University of Chicago Press, Chicago, X, p 460 S
78. Hardingham TE, Oldershaw RA, Tew SR (2006) Cartilage, SOX9 and Notch signals in chondrogenesis. J Anat 209:469–480
79. Hay ED (1995) An overview of epithelio-mesenchymal transformation. Acta Anat 154:8–20
80. Hilliard SA, Yu L, Gu S, Zhang Z, Chen YP (2005) Regional regulation of palatal growth and patterning along the anterior-posterior axis in mice. J Anat 207:655–667
81. Hines RN, McCarver DG (2002) The ontogeny of human drug-metabolizing enzymes: phase I oxidative enzymes. J Pharmacol Exp Ther 300:355–360
82. Hinton RJ (1988) Response of the intermaxillary suture cartilage to alterations in masticatory function. Anat Rec 220:376–387
83. Hou B, Fukai N, Olsen BR (2007) Mechanical force-induced midpalatal suture remodeling in mice. Bone 40:1483–1493
84. Humphrey T (1968) The development of mouth opening and related rflexes involving the oral area of human fetuses. Ala J Med Sci 5:126–157
85. Hwang SJ, Beaty TH, Panny SR, Street NA, Joseph JM, Gordon S, McIntosh I, Francomano CA (1995) Association study of transforming growth factor alpha (TGF alpha) TaqI polymorphism and oral clefts: indication of gene-environment interaction in a population-based sample of infants with birth defects. Am J Epidemiol 141:629–636
86. Ingervall B, Carlsson GE, Thilander B (1976) Postnatal development of the human temporomandibular joint. I. A microradiographic study. Acta Odontol Scand 34:133–139
87. Ishii M, Han J, Yen HY, Sucov HM, Chai Y, Maxson RE Jr (2005) Combined deficiencies of Msx1 and Msx2 cause impaired patterning and survival of the cranial neural crest. Development 132:4937–4950
88. Itikala PR, Watkins ML, Mulinare J, Moore CA, Liu Y (2001) Maternal multivitamin use and orofacial clefts in offspring. Teratology 63:79–86
89. Iwasaki M, Le AX, Helms JA (1997) Expression of indian hedgehog, bone morphogenetic protein 6 and gli during skeletal morphogenesis. Mech Dev 69:197–202
90. Jeong J, Mao J, Tenzen T, Kottmann AH, McMahon AP (2004) Hedgehog signaling in the neural crest cells regulates the patterning and growth of facial primordia. Genes Dev 18:937–951
91. Jernvall J, Kettunen P, Karavanova I, Martin LB, Thesleff I (1994) Evidence for the role of the enamel knot as a control center in mammalian tooth cusp formation: non-dividing cells express growth stimulating Fgf-4 gene. Int J Dev Biol 38:463–469
92. Jernvall J, Thesleff I (2000) Reiterative signaling and patterning during mammalian tooth morphogenesis. Mech Dev 92:19–29
93. Jiang R, Bush JO, Lidral AC (2006) Development of the upper lip: morphogenetic and molecular mechanisms. Dev Dyn 235:spc1
94. Jin J-Z, Ding J (2006) Analysis of cell migration, transdifferentiation and apoptosis during mouse secondary palate fusion. Development 133:3341–3347

95. Kaartinen V, Voncken JW, Shuler C, Warburton D, Bu D, Heisterkamp N, Groffen J (1995) Abnormal lung development and cleft palate in mice lacking TGF-beta 3 indicates defects of epithelial-mesenchymal interaction. Nat Genet 11:415–421
96. Kaartinen V, Cui XM, Heisterkamp N, Groffen J, Shuler CF (1997) Transforming growth factor-beta3 regulates transdifferentiation of medial edge epithelium during palatal fusion and associated degradation of the basement membrane. Dev Dyn 209:255–260
97. Kaartinen V, Haataja L, Nagy A, Heisterkamp N, Groffen J (2002) TGFbeta3-induced activation of RhoA/Rho-kinase pathway is necessary but not sufficient for epithelio-mesenchymal transdifferentiation: implications for palatogenesis. Int J Mol Med 9:563–570
98. Kallen B, Mastroiacovo P, Robert E (1996) Major congenital malformations in Down syndrome. Am J Med Genet 65:160–166
99. Kang P, Svoboda KK (2005) Epithelial-mesenchymal transformation during craniofacial development. J Dent Res 84:678–690
100. Kapadia H, Mues G, D'Souza R (2007) Genes affecting tooth morphogenesis. Orthod Craniofac Res 10:237–244
101. Karsenty G (2008) Transcriptional control of skeletogenesis. Annu Rev Genomics Hum Genet 9:183–196
102. Keith DA (1982) Development of the human temporomandibular joint. Br J Oral Surg 20:217–224
103. Kerrigan JJ, Mansell JP, Sengupta A, Brown N, Sandy JR (2000) Palatogenesis and potential mechanisms for clefting. J R Coll Surg Edinb 45:351–358
104. Kim JW, Simmer JP (2007) Hereditary dentin defects. J Dent Res 86:392–399
105. Kjaer I (1992) Human prenatal palatal shelf elevation related to craniofacial skeletal maturation. Eur J Orthod 14:26–30
106. Kjaer I (1997) Mandibular movements during elevation and fusion of palatal shelves evaluated from the course of Meckel's cartilage. J Craniofac Genet Dev Biol 17:80–85
107. Kobayashi ET, Hashimoto F, Kobayashi Y, Sakai E, Miyazaki Y, Kamiya T, Kobayashi K, Kato Y, Sakai H (1999) Force-induced rapid changes in cell fate at midpalatal suture cartilage of growing rats. J Dent Res 78:1495–1504
108. Kokavec R (2006) Goldenhar syndrome with various clinical manifestations. Cleft Palate Craniofac J 43: 628–634
109. Komori T, Yagi H, Nomura S, Yamaguchi A, Sasaki K, Deguchi K, Shimizu Y, Bronson RT, Gao YH, Inada M, Sato M, Okamoto R, Kitamura Y, Yoshiki S, Kishimoto T (1997) Targeted disruption of Cbfa1 results in a complete lack of bone formation owing to maturational arrest of osteoblasts. Cell 89:755–764
110. Komori T (2006) Regulation of osteoblast differentiation by transcription factors. J Cell Biochem 99:1233–1239
111. Kondo S, Schutte BC, Richardson RJ, Bjork BC, Knight AS, Watanabe Y, Howard E, de Lima RL, Daack-Hirsch S, Sander A, McDonald-McGinn DM, Zackai EH, Lammer EJ, Aylsworth AS, Ardinger HH, Lidral AC, Pober BR, Moreno L, Arcos-Burgos M, Valencia C, Houdayer C, Bahuau M, Moretti-Ferreira D, Richieri-Costa A, Dixon MJ, Murray JC (2002) Mutations in IRF6 cause Van der Woude and popliteal pterygium syndromes. Nat Genet 32: 285–289
112. Lammer EJ, Shaw GM, Iovannisci DM, Finnell RH (2004) Periconceptional multivitamin intake during early pregnancy, genetic variation of acetyl-N-transferase 1 (NAT1), and risk for orofacial clefts. Birth Defects Res A Clin Mol Teratol 70:846–852
113. Lammer EJ, Shaw GM, Iovannisci DM, Van Waes J, Finnell RH (2004) Maternal smoking and the risk of orofacial clefts: Susceptibility with NAT1 and NAT2 polymorphisms. Epidemiology 15:150–156
114. Lanctot C, Moreau A, Chamberland M, Tremblay ML, Drouin J (1999) Hindlimb patterning and mandible development require the Ptx1 gene. Development 126:1805–1810
115. Le Douarin NM, Brito JM, Creuzet S (2007) Role of the neural crest in face and brain development. Brain Res Rev 55:237–247
116. Lee SH, Bedard O, Buchtova M, Fu K, Richman JM (2004) A new origin for the maxillary jaw. Dev Biol 276:207–224
117. Lee SK, Kim YS, Oh HS, Yang KH, Kim EC, Chi JG (2001) Prenatal development of the human mandible. Anat Rec 263:314–325
118. Linde A, Goldberg M (1993) Dentinogenesis. Crit Rev Oral Biol Med 4:679–728
119. Liu C, Song R, Song Y (2000) Sutural expansion osteogenesis for management of the bony-tissue defect in cleft palate repair: experimental studies in dogs. Plast Reconstr Surg 105:2012–2025; discussion 26–27
120. Liu W, Selever J, Murali D, Sun X, Brugger SM, Ma L, Schwartz RJ, Maxson R, Furuta Y, Martin JF (2005) Threshold-specific requirements for Bmp4 in mandibular development. Dev Biol 283:282–293
121. Lohnes D, Mark M, Mendelsohn C, Dolle P, Dierich A, Gorry P, Gansmuller A, Chambon P (1994) Function of the retinoic acid receptors (RARs) during development (I). Craniofacial and skeletal abnormalities in RAR double mutants. Development 120: 2723–2748
122. Lohnes D, Mark M, Mendelsohn C, Dolle P, Decimo D, LeMeur M, Dierich A, Gorry P, Chambon P (1995) Developmental roles of the retinoic acid receptors. J Steroid Biochem Mol Biol 53:475–486
123. Luder HU (1997) Frequency and distribution of articular tissue features in adult human mandibular condyles: a semiquantitative light microscopic study. Anat Rec 248:18–28
124. Luder HU (1998) Age changes in the articular tissue of human mandibular condyles from adolescence to old age: a semiquantitative light microscopic study. Anat Rec 251:439–447
125. Mackie EJ, Ahmed YA, Tatarczuch L, Chen KS, Mirams M (2008) Endochondral ossification: how cartilage is converted into bone in the developing skeleton. Int J Biochem Cell Biol 40:46–62
126. Maestri NE, Beaty TH, Hetmanski J, Smith EA, McIntosh I, Wyszynski DF, Liang KY, Duffy DL, VanderKolk C (1997) Application of transmission disequilibrium tests to nonsyndromic oral clefts: including candidate

genes and environmental exposures in the models. Am J Med Genet 73:337–344
127. Marazita ML (2007) Subclinical features in non-syndromic cleft lip with or without cleft palate (CL/P): review of the evidence that subepithelial orbicularis oris muscle defects are part of an expanded phenotype for CL/P. Orthod Craniofac Res 10:82–87
128. Marcano AC, Doudney K, Braybrook C, Squires R, Patton MA, Lees MM, Richieri-Costa A, Lidral AC, Murray JC, Moore GE, Stanier P (2004) TBX22 mutations are a frequent cause of cleft palate. J Med Gen 41:68–74
129. Mark M, Lohnes D, Mendelsohn C, Dupe V, Vonesch JL, Kastner P, Rijli F, Bloch-Zupan A, Chambon P (1995) Roles of retinoic acid receptors and of Hox genes in the patterning of the teeth and of the jaw skeleton. Int J Dev Biol 39:111–121
130. Martelli H Jr, Paranaiba LM, de Miranda RT, Orsi J Jr, Coletta RD (2008) Apert syndrome: report of a case with emphasis on craniofacial and genetic features. Pediatr Dent 30:464–468
131. Marti E, Bovolenta P (2002) Sonic hedgehog in CNS development: one signal, multiple outputs. Trends Neurosci 25:89–96
132. Martinelli M, Scapoli L, Pezzetti F, Carinci F, Carinci P, Stabellini G, Bisceglia L, Gombos F, Tognon M (2001) C677T variant form at the MTHFR gene and CL/P: a risk factor for mothers? Am J Med Genet 98:357–360
133. Martinez-Alvarez C, Blanco MJ, Perez R, Rabadan MA, Aparicio M, Resel E, Martinez T, Nieto MA (2004) Snail family members and cell survival in physiological and pathological cleft palates. Dev Biol 265:207–218
134. Mendelsohn C, Lohnes D, Decimo D, Lufkin T, LeMeur M, Chambon P, Mark M (1994) Function of the retinoic acid receptors (RARs) during development (II). Multiple abnormalities at various stages of organogenesis in RAR double mutants. Development 120:2749–2771
135. Merida-Velasco JR, Rodriguez-Vasquez JF, Merida-Velasco JA, Sanchez-Montesinos I, Espin-Ferra J, Jimenez-Collado J (1999) Development of the human temporomandibular joint. Anat Rec 255:20–33
136. Miettinen PJ, Chin JR, Shum L, Slavkin HC, Shuler CF, Derynck R, Werb Z (1999) Epidermal growth factor receptor function is necessary for normal craniofacial development and palate closure. Nat Genet 22:69–73
137. Milunsky JM, Maher TA, Zhao G, Roberts AE, Stalker HJ, Zori RT, Burch MN, Clemens M, Mulliken JB, Smith R, Lin AE (2008) TFAP2A mutations result in branchio-oculo-facial syndrome. Am J Hum Genet 82:1171–1177
138. Mitchell LE, Murray JC, O'Brien S, Christensen K (2001) Evaluation of two putative susceptibility loci for oral clefts in the Danish population. Am J Epidemiol 153:1007–1015
139. Moffett BC, DeHaan RL, Ursprung H (1965) The morphogenesis of joints, organogenesis. Holt, Rinehart, and Winston, New York, pp 301–313
140. Moreno F, Zuazo E, Gonzalez S, Bereciartu P (2009) 22q11 deletion syndrome: an expanding phenotype. Neurologia 24:69–71
141. Mori C, Nakamura N, Okamoto Y, Osawa M, Shiota K (1994) Cytochemical identification of programmed cell death in the fusing fetal mouse palate by specific labelling of DNA fragmentation. Anat Embryol (Berl) 190:21–28
142. Muenke M (2002) The pit, the cleft and the web. Nat Genet 32:219–220
143. Murray JC (2002) Gene/environment causes of cleft lip and/or palate. Clin Genet 61:248–256
144. Murray JC, Schutte BC (2004) Cleft palate: players, pathways, and pursuits. J Clin Invest 113: 1676–1678
145. Nawshad A, Hay ED (2003) TGFbeta3 signaling activates transcription of the LEF1 gene to induce epithelial mesenchymal transformation during mouse palate development. J Cell Biol 163:1291–1301
146. Nawshad A, LaGamba D, Hay ED (2004) Transforming growth factor beta (TGFbeta) signalling in palatal growth, apoptosis and epithelial mesenchymal transformation (EMT). Arch Oral Biol 49: 675–689
147. Nawshad A (2008) Palatal seam disintegration: To die or not to die? that is no longer the question. Dev Dyn 237:2643–2656
148. Neiswanger K, Weinberg SM, Rogers CR, Brandon CA, Cooper ME, Bardi KM, Deleyiannis FW, Resick JM, Bowen A, Mooney MP, de Salamanca JE, Gonzalez B, Maher BS, Martin RA, Marazita ML (2007) Orbicularis oris muscle defects as an expanded phenotypic feature in nonsyndromic cleft lip with or without cleft palate. Am J Med Genet A 143: 1143–1149
149. Nie X, Luukko K, Kettunen P (2006) FGF signalling in craniofacial development and developmental disorders. Oral Dis 12:102–111
150. Noden DM, Trainor PA (2005) Relations and interactions between cranial mesoderm and neural crest populations. J Anat 207:575–601
151. Ogutcen-Toller M, Juniper RP (1993) The embryonic development of the human lateral pterygoid muscle and its relationships with the temporomandibular joint disc and Meckel's cartilage. J Oral Maxillofac Surg 51:772–778
152. Okano J, Suzuki S, Shiota K (2006) Regional heterogeneity in the developing palate: morphological and molecular evidence for normal and abnormal palatogenesis. Congenit Anom (Kyoto) 46:49–54
153. Opperman LA (2000) Cranial sutures as intramembranous bone growth sites. Dev Dyn 219:472–485
154. Osoegawa K, Vessere GM, Utami KH, Mansilla MA, Johnson MK, Riley BM, L'Heureux J, Pfundt R, Staaf J, van der Vliet WA, Lidral AC, Schoenmakers EF, Borg A, Schutte BC, Lammer EJ, Murray JC, de Jong PJ (2008) Identification of novel candidate genes associated with cleft lip and palate using array comparative genomic hybridisation. J Med Genet 45:81–86
155. Otto F, Thornell AP, Crompton T, Denzel A, Gilmour KC, Rosewell IR, Stamp GW, Beddington RS, Mundlos S, Olsen BR, Selby PB, Owen MJ (1997) Cbfa1, a candidate gene for cleidocranial dysplasia syndrome, is essential for osteoblast differentiation and bone development. Cell 89:765–771

156. Pasqualetti M, Ori M, Nardi I, Rijli FM (2000) Ectopic Hoxa2 induction after neural crest migration results in homeosis of jaw elements in Xenopus. Development 127:5367–5378
157. Pauws E, Stanier P (2007) FGF signalling and SUMO modification: new players in the aetiology of cleft lip and/or palate. Trends Genet 23:631–640
158. Pelton RW, Hogan BL, Miller DA, Moses HL (1990) Differential expression of genes encoding TGFs beta 1, beta 2, and beta 3 during murine palate formation. Dev Biol 141:456–460
159. Perry HT, Xu Y, Forbes DP (1985) The embryology of the temporomandibular joint. J Craniomand Prac 3:125–132
160. Petrovic A (1972) Mechanisms and regulation of mandibular condylar growth. Acta Morphol Neerl Scand 10:25–34
161. Petrovic AG, Stutzmann JJ, Oudet CL, McNamara JA Jr (1975) Control processes in the postnatal growth of the condylar cartilage of the mandible, determinants of mandibular form and growth. Center for Human Growth and Development, University of Michigan, Ann Arbor, pp 101–154
162. Prows CA, Bender PL (1999) Beyond Pierre Robin sequence. Neonatal Netw 18:13–19
163. Qin C, Brunn JC, Cadena E, Ridall A, Tsujigiwa H, Nagatsuka H, Nagai N, Butler WT (2002) The expression of dentin sialophosphoprotein gene in bone. J Dent Res 81:392–394
164. Qiu M, Bulfone A, Martinez S, Meneses JJ, Shimamura K, Pedersen RA, Rubenstein JL (1995) Null mutation of Dlx-2 results in abnormal morphogenesis of proximal first and second branchial arch derivatives and abnormal differentiation in the forebrain. Genes Dev 9:2523–2538
165. Qiu M, Bulfone A, Ghattas I, Meneses JJ, Christensen L, Sharpe PT, Presley R, Pedersen RA, Rubenstein JL (1997) Role of the Dlx homeobox genes in proximodistal patterning of the branchial arches: mutations of Dlx-1, Dlx-2, and Dlx-1 and -2 alter morphogenesis of proximal skeletal and soft tissue structures derived from the first and second arches. Dev Biol 185:165–184
166. Rabie ABM, She TT, Hagg U (2003) Functional appliance therapy accelerates and enhances condylar growth. Am J Orthod Dentofac Orthop 123:40–48
167. Radlanski RJ, Lieck S, Bontschev NE (1999) Development of the human temporomandibular joint. Computer-aided 3D-reconstructions. Eur J Oral Sci 107:25–34
168. Radlanski RJ, Renz H, Klarkowski MC (2003) Prenatal development of the human mandible. 3D reconstructions, morphometry and bone remodelling pattern, sizes 12–117 mm CRL. Anat Embryol (Berl) 207:221–232
169. Radlanski RJ, Renz H (2006) Genes, forces, and forms: mechanical aspects of prenatal craniofacial development. Dev Dyn 235:1219–1229
170. Rice R, Spencer-Dene B, Connor EC, Gritli-Linde A, McMahon AP, Dickson C, Thesleff I, Rice DP (2004) Disruption of Fgf10/Fgfr2b-coordinated epithelial-mesenchymal interactions causes cleft palate. J Clin Invest 113:1692–1700
171. Rice R, Thesleff I, Rice DPC (2005) Regulation of Twist, Snail, and Id1 is conserved between the developing murine palate and tooth. Dev Dyn 234:28–35
172. Richman JM, Buchtova M, Boughner JC (2006) Comparative ontogeny and phylogeny of the upper jaw skeleton in amniotes. Dev Dyn 235:1230–1243
173. Rijli FM, Mark M, Lakkaraju S, Dierich A, Dolle P, Chambon P (1993) A homeotic transformation is generated in the rostral branchial region of the head by disruption of Hoxa-2, which acts as a selector gene. Cell 75:1333–1349
174. Riley BM, Mansilla MA, Ma J, Daack-Hirsch S, Maher BS, Raffensperger LM, Russo ET, Vieira AR, Dode C, Mohammadi M, Marazita ML, Murray JC (2007) Impaired FGF signaling contributes to cleft lip and palate. Proc Natl Acad Sci U S A 104:4512–4517
175. Ritchie HH, Li X (2001) A novel rat dentin mRNA coding only for dentin sialoprotein. Eur J Oral Sci 109:342–347
176. Romitti PA, Lidral AC, Munger RG, Daack-Hirsch S, Burns TL, Murray JC (1999) Candidate genes for nonsyndromic cleft lip and palate and maternal cigarette smoking and alcohol consumption: evaluation of genotype-environment interactions from a population-based case-control study of orofacial clefts. Teratology 59:39–50
177. Ruch JV (1987) Determinisms of odontogenesis. Revis Biol Celular 14:1–99
178. Ruest LB, Dager M, Yanagisawa H, Charite J, Hammer RE, Olson EN, Yanagisawa M, Clouthier DE (2003) dHAND-Cre transgenic mice reveal specific potential functions of dHAND during craniofacial development. Dev Biol 257:263–277
179. Ruest LB, Xiang X, Lim KC, Levi G, Clouthier DE (2004) Endothelin-A receptor-dependent and -independent signaling pathways in establishing mandibular identity. Development 131:4413–4423
180. Ruest LB, Clouthier DE (2009) Elucidating timing and function of endothelin-A receptor signaling during craniofacial development using neural crest cell-specific gene deletion and receptor antagonism. Dev Biol 328:94–108
181. Sahlberg C, Reponen P, Tryggvason K, Thesleff I (1992) Association between the expression of murine 72 kDa type IV collagenase by odontoblasts and basement membrane degradation during mouse tooth development. Arch Oral Biol 37:1021–1030
182. Sanlaville D, Etchevers HC, Gonzales M, Martinovic J, Clement-Ziza M, Delezoide AL, Aubry MC, Pelet A, Chemouny S, Cruaud C, Audollent S, Esculpavit C, Goudefroye G, Ozilou C, Fredouille C, Joye N, Morichon-Delvallez N, Dumez Y, Weissenbach J, Munnich A, Amiel J, Encha-Razavi F, Lyonnet S, Vekemans M, Attie-Bitach T (2006) Phenotypic spectrum of CHARGE syndrome in fetuses with CHD7 truncating mutations correlates with expression during human development. J Med Genet 43:211–217
183. Sano K, Sekine J, Pe MB, Inokuchi T (1992) Bromodeoxyuridine Immunohistochemistry for Evaluating Age-Related Changes in the Rat Mandibular Condyle Decalcified by Intravenous Infusion. Biotech Histochem 67(5):297–302

184. Santagati F, Rijli FM (2003) Cranial neural crest and the building of the vertebrate head. Nat Rev Neurosci 4:806–818
185. Sato T, Kawamura Y, Asai R, Amano T, Uchijima Y, Dettlaff-Swiercz DA, Offermanns S, Kurihara Y, Kurihara H (2008) Recombinase-mediated cassette exchange reveals the selective use of Gq/G11-dependent and -independent endothelin 1/endothelin type A receptor signaling in pharyngeal arch development. Development 135:755–765
186. Sato T, Kurihara Y, Asai R, Kawamura Y, Tonami K, Uchijima Y, Heude E, Ekker M, Levi G, Kurihara H (2008) An endothelin-1 switch specifies maxillomandibular identity. Proc Natl Acad Sci U S A 105:18806–18811
187. Satokata I, Maas R (1994) Msx1 deficient mice exhibit cleft palate and abnormalities of craniofacial and tooth development. Nat Genet 6:348–356
188. Satokata I, Ma L, Ohshima H, Bei M, Woo I, Nishizawa K, Maeda T, Takano Y, Uchiyama M, Heaney S, Peters H, Tang Z, Maxson R, Maas R (2000) Msx2 deficiency in mice causes pleiotropic defects in bone growth and ectodermal organ formation. Nat Genet 24:391–395
189. Sawada M, Shimizu N (1996) Stimulation of bone formation in the expanding mid-palatal suture by transforming growth factor-beta 1 in the rat. Eur J Orthod 18:169–179
190. Schneider RA, Helms JA (2003) The cellular and molecular origins of beak morphology. Science 299:565–568
191. Schock F, Perrimon N (2002) Molecular mechanisms of epithelial morphogenesis. Annu Rev Cell Dev Biol 18:463–493
192. Shaw GM, Lammer EJ, Zhu H, Baker MW, Neri E, Finnell RH (2002) Maternal periconceptional vitamin use, genetic variation of infant reduced folate carrier (A80G), and risk of spina bifida.. Am J Med Genet 108:1–6. Erratum (2002) 113(4):392
193. Shaw GM, Zhu H, Lammer EJ, Yang W, Finnell RH (2003) Genetic variation of infant reduced folate carrier (A80G) and risk of orofacial and conotruncal heart defects. Am J Epidemiol 158:747–752
194. Shaw WC, Brattstrom V, Molsted K, Prahl-Andersen B, Roberts CT, Semb G (2005) The Eurocleft study: intercenter study of treatment outcome in patients with complete cleft lip and palate. Part 5: discussion and conclusions. Cleft Pal Craniofac J 42:93–98
195. Sherer DM, Metlay LA, Woods JR Jr (1995) Lack of mandibular movement manifested by absent fetal swallowing: a possible factor in the pathogenesis of micrognathia. Am J Perinat 12:30–33
196. Shi M, Wehby GL, Murray JC (2008) Review on genetic variants and maternal smoking in the etiology of oral clefts and other birth defects. Birth Defects Res C Embryo Today 84:16–29
197. Shi S, Gronthos S (2003) Perivascular niche of postnatal mesenchymal stem cells in human bone marrow and dental pulp. J Bone Miner Res 18:696–704
198. Shibata S, Suzuki S, Tengan T, Ishi M, Kuroda T (1996) A histological study of the developing condylar cartilage of the fetal mouse mandible using coronal sections. Arch Oral Biol 41:47–54
199. Shibata S, Fukada K, Suzuki S, Yamashita Y (1997) Immunohistochemistry of collagen types II and X, and enzyme-histochemistry of alkaline phosphatase in developing condylar cartilage of the fetal mouse mandible. J Anat 191:561–570
200. Shibata S, Suda N, Yoda S, Fukuoka H, Ohyama K, Yamashita Y, Komori T (2004) Runx2-deficient mice lack manmdibular condylar cartilage and have deformed Meckel's cartilage. Anat Embryol 208:273–280
201. Shibata S, Suda N, Suzuki S, Fukuoka H, Yamashita Y (2006) An in situ hybridization study of Runx2, Osterix, and Sox9 at the onset of condylar cartilage formation in fetal mouse mandible. J Anat 208: 169–177
202. Shuler CF, Halpern DE, Guo Y, Sank AC (1992) Medial edge epithelium fate traced by cell lineage analysis during epithelial-mesenchymal transformation in vivo. Dev Biol 154:318–330
203. Sim E, Payton M, Noble M, Minchin R (2000) An update on genetic, structural and functional studies of arylamine N-acetyltransferases in eucaryotes and procaryotes. Hum Mol Genet 9:2435–2441
204. Slavkin HC (1992) Incidence of cleft lips, palates rising. J Am Dent Assoc 123:61–65
205. Smelt VA, Upton A, Adjaye J, Payton MA, Boukouvala S, Johnson N, Mardon HJ, Sim E (2000) Expression of arylamine N-acetyltransferases in pre-term placentas and in human pre-implantation embryos. Hum Mol Genet 9:1101–1107
206. Snead MP, Yates JR (1999) Clinical and Molecular genetics of Stickler syndrome. J Med Genet 36:353–359
207. Sreenath T, Thyagarajan T, Hall B, Longenecker G, D'Souza R, Hong S, Wright JT, MacDougall M, Sauk J, Kulkarni AB (2003) Dentin sialophosphoprotein knockout mouse teeth display widened predentin zone and develop defective dentin mineralization similar to human dentinogenesis imperfecta type III. J Biol Chem 278:24874–24880
208. Srivastava D, Thomas T, Lin Q, Kirby ML, Brown D, Olson EN (1997) Regulation of cardiac mesodermal and neural crest development by the bHLH transcription factor, dHAND. Nat Genet 16:154–160
209. St Amand TR, Zhang Y, Semina EV, Zhao X, Hu Y, Nguyen L, Murray JC, Chen Y (2000) Antagonistic signals between BMP4 and FGF8 define the expression of Pitx1 and Pitx2 in mouse tooth-forming anlage. Dev Biol 217:323–332
210. Sugars RV, Olsson ML, Waddington R, Wendel M (2006) Substitution of bovine dentine sialoprotein with chondroitin sulfate glycosaminoglycan chains. Eur J Oral Sci 114:89–92
211. Sun D, Baur S, Hay ED (2000) Epithelial-mesenchymal transformation is the mechanism for fusion of the craniofacial primordia involved in morphogenesis of the chicken lip. Dev Biol 228: 337–349
212. Suzuki K, Hu D, Bustos T, Zlotogora J, Richieri-Costa A, Helms JA, Spritz RA (2000) Mutations of PVRL1, encoding a cell-cell adhesion molecule/herpesvirus receptor, in cleft lip/palate-ectodermal dysplasia. Nat Genet 25:427–430
213. Sweeney L (1998) Basic concepts in embryology: a student's survival guide. McGraw-Hill, New Jersy, p 443

214. Takahashi I, Mizoguchi I, Nakamura M, Sasano Y, Saitoh S, Kagayama M, Mitani H (1996) Effects of expansive force on the differentiation of midpalatal suture cartilage in rats. Bone 18:341–348
215. Takenoshita Y (1982) Development with age of the human mandibular condyle: part II. Assessment of mineral content and microradiographic study. Dentomaxillofac Radiol 11:17–24
216. Tang LS, Santillano DR, Wlodarczyk BJ, Miranda RC, Finnell RH (2005) Role of Folbp1 in the regional regulation of apoptosis and cell proliferation in the developing neural tube and craniofacies. Am J Med Genet C Semin Med Genet 135:48–58
217. Taniguchi K, Sato N, Uchiyama Y (1995) Apoptosis and heterophagy of medial edge epithelial cells of the secondary palatine shelves during fusion. Arch Histol Cytol 58:191–203
218. Ten Cate A (1998) Oral histology: development, structure, and function, 5th edn, Mosby, St. Louis.
219. Thesleff I, Pratt RM (1980) Tunicamycin inhibits mouse tooth morphogenesis and odontoblast differentiation in vitro. J Embryol Exp Morphol 58:195–208
220. Tomo S, Ogita M, Tomo I (1997) Development of mandibular cartilages in the rat. Anat Rec 249: 233–239
221. Trainor P, Krumlauf R (2000) Plasticity in mouse neural crest cells reveals a new patterning role for cranial mesoderm. Nat Cell Biol 2:96–102
222. Trotman CA, Hou D, Burdi AR, Cohen SR, Carlson DS (1995) Histomorphologic analysis of the soft palate musculature in prenatal cleft and noncleft A/Jax mice. Cleft Pal Craniofac J 32:455–462
223. Trumpp A, Depew MJ, Rubenstein JL, Bishop JM, Martin GR (1999) Cre-mediated gene inactivation demonstrates that FGF8 is required for cell survival and patterning of the first branchial arch. Genes Dev 13:3136–3148
224. Tucker AS, Al Khamis A, Ferguson CA, Bach I, Rosenfeld MG, Sharpe PT (1999) Conserved regulation of mesenchymal gene expression by Fgf-8 in face and limb development. Development 126: 221–228
225. Tucker AS, Yamada G, Grigoriou M, Pachnis V, Sharpe PT (1999) Fgf-8 determines rostral-caudal polarity in the first branchial arch. Development 126:51–61
226. van der Linden EJ, Burdi AR, de Jongh HJ (1987) Critical periods in the prenatal morphogenesis of the human lateral pterygoid muscle, the mandibular condyle, the articular disc, and medial articular capsule. Am J Orthod 91:22–28
227. Veis A, Perry A (1967) The phosphoprotein of the dentin matrix. Biochem 6:2409–2416
228. Vieira AR, Avila JR, Daack-Hirsch S, Dragan E, Felix TM, Rahimov F, Harrington J, Schultz RR, Watanabe Y, Johnson M, Fang J, O'Brien SE, Orioli IM, Castilla EE, Fitzpatrick DR, Jiang R, Marazita ML, Murray JC (2005) Medical sequencing of candidate genes for nonsyndromic cleft lip and palate. PLoS Genet 1:e64
229. Vij K, Mao JJ (2006) Geometry and cell density of rat craniofacial sutures during early postnatal development and upon in vivo cyclic loading. Bone 38:722–730
230. Vilkki SK, Hukki J, Nietosvaara Y, Hurmerinta K, Suominen E (2002) Microvascular temporomandibular joint and mandibular ramus reconstruction in hemifacial microsomia. J Craniofac Surg 13: 809–815
231. Vinkka H (1982) Secondary cartilages in the facial skeleton of the rat. Proc Finn Dent Soc 78(suppl 7): 1–137
232. Wang L, Detamore MS (2007) Tissue engineering the mandibular condyle. Tissue Eng 13:1955–1971
233. Weinberg SM, Neiswanger K, Martin RA, Mooney MP, Kane AA, Wenger SL, Losee J, Deleyiannis F, Ma L, De Salamanca JE, Czeizel AE, Marazita ML (2006) The Pittsburgh Oral-Facial Cleft study: expanding the cleft phenotype. Background and justification. Cleft Pal Craniofac J 43:7–20
234. Wilkin DJ, Mortier GR, Johnson CL, Jones MC, de Paepe A, Shohat M, Wildin RS, Falk RE, Cohn DH (1998) Correlation of linkage data with phenotype in eight families with Stickler syndrome. Am J Med Genet 80:121–127
235. Winnier G, Blessing M, Labosky PA, Hogan BL (1995) Bone morphogenetic protein-4 is required for mesoderm formation and patterning in the mouse. Genes Dev 9:2105–2116
236. Wong FK, Hagg U (2004) An update on the aetiology of orofacial clefts. Hong Kong Med J 10:331–336
237. Wright DM, Moffett B (1974) The postnatal development of the human temporomandibular joint. Am J Anat 141:235–249
238. Wyszynski DF, Duffy DL, Beaty TH (1997) Maternal cigarette smoking and oral clefts: a meta-analysis. Cleft Pal Craniofac J 34:206–210
239. Yanagisawa H, Clouthier DE, Richardson JA, Charite J, Olson EN (2003) Targeted deletion of a branchial arch-specific enhancer reveals a role of dHAND in craniofacial development. Development 130:1069–1078
240. Yu L, Gu S, Alappat S, Song Y, Yan M, Zhang X, Zhang G, Jiang Y, Zhang Z, Zhang Y, Chen Y (2005) Shox2-deficient mice exhibit a rare type of incomplete clefting of the secondary palate. Development 132:4397–4406
241. Yu W, Ruest L, Svoboda K (2009) Regulation of epithelial-mesenchymal transition in palatal fusion. Exp Biol Med 234(5):483–491
242. Yuodelis RA (1966) Ossification of the human temporomandibular joint. J Dent Res 45:192198
243. Zhang FP, Mikkonen L, Toppari J, Palvimo JJ, Thesleff I, Janne OA (2008) Sumo-1 function is dispensable in normal mouse development. Mol Cell Biol 28:5381–5390
244. Zhu H, Curry S, Wen S, Wicker NJ, Shaw GM, Lammer EJ, Yang W, Jafarov T, Finnell RH (2005) Are the betaine-homocysteine methyltransferase (BHMT and BHMT2) genes risk factors for spina bifida and orofacial clefts? Am J Med Genet A 135:274–277
245. Frebourg T, Oliveira C, Hochain P, Karam R, Manouvrier S, Graziadio C, Vekemans M, Hartmann A, Baert-Desurmont S, Alexandre C, Lejeune Dumoulin S, Marroni C, Martin C, Castedo S, Lovett M, Winston J, Machado JC, Attie T, Jabs EW, Cai J, Pellerin P, Triboulet JP, Scotte M, Le Pessot F, Hedouin A, Carneiro F, Blayau M, Seruca R (2006) Cleft lip/palate and cdh1/e-cadherin mutations in families with hereditary diffuse gastric cancer. J Med Genet 43(2):138-142.

11. Dentin and Bone: Similar Collagenous Mineralized Tissues

Mary J. MacDougall and Amjad Javed

Teeth are individual organs that consist of an exposed crown structure and an internally embedded root structure. Each tooth is an individual organ that, through location and function, is coordinated to form a highly ordered and symmetrical patterned unit known as the dentition. Humans have two successive sets of teeth, the primary dentition or baby teeth, which are replaced by the permanent dentition. The tooth forms three distinct mineralized extracellular matrices, enamel, dentin, and cementum, which are temporally and spatially integrated to form the hardest structure in the human body. The tooth crown is covered by an outer layer of enamel with an inner, more resilient mineralized dentin layer in juxtaposition, followed by an unmineralized predentin matrix adjacent to the dental pulp chamber. The root is covered by a thin outer layer of cementum over the inner layers of dentin and predentin. Therefore, the most abundant matrix of the tooth is dentin that covers both the crown and root structures. This chapter will discuss dentin, the mineralized connective tissue of the teeth, and compare and contrast its formation and structure with that of bone.

11.1 Odontogenesis

Tooth formation is the result of complex reciprocal interactions that are mediated through ligands and receptors between the oral epithelium and cranial neural crest-derived ectomesenchyme [125, 130]. Tooth development proceeds in distinct and characteristic structural and differentiation stages: dental lamina, bud, cap, bell, crown, and root. The first indication of tooth formation is a thickening of the oral epithelium, which occurs at approximately 7 weeks of gestation in humans and embryonic day 11 in mice. The epithelial thickening invaginates into the underlying ectomesenchyme that is derived from the cranial neural crest; this in turn leads to mesenchymal condensation during the bud stage. At the cap stage, the epithelium further wraps around the condensed mesenchyme. During the transition from cap to bell stage, the ectomesenchyme cells in contact with the basement membrane begin to undergo cytodifferentiation and produce the dentin extracellular matrix (DECM) in a process known as dentinogenesis. This occurs at about 18 weeks in human

F. Bronner et al. (eds.), *Bone and Development*, Topics in Bone Biology 6,
DOI 10.1007/978-1-84882-822-3_11, © Springer-Verlag London Limited 2010

embryonic development, with deciduous teeth as the result.

11.1.1 Primary Dentinogenesis

The process of dentinogenesis follows a specific temporal-spatial pattern that comprises the cytodifferentiation of the odontoblasts, highly specialized polarized cells from the dental pulp mesenchyme, and leads to the formation of the DECM bilayer [35, 72, 111]. Cytodifferentiation begins at the principal cusp tips and proceeds in both directions toward the cervical aspects of the tooth. The cusp tip regions are initially associated with the special inductive organization centers of the tooth, known as enamel knots.

Undifferentiated mesenchymal cells within the dental papilla come into contact with the basement membrane at the undersurface of the inner enamel epithelium. The dental papilla cells divide, with the mitotic spindle forming in a direction that is perpendicular to the basement membrane. Only the daughter cells in direct contact with the basement member will continue to differentiate into odontoblasts. Initially, these cells have large nuclei with little cytoplasm or organelles. As cytodifferentiation progresses, the cells enlarge their cytoplasm by increasing the number of Golgi complexes and the rough endoplasmic reticulum. The cells become more cylindrical in shape and polarize, with the nucleus shifting toward the dental papilla. These cells are then referred to as preodontoblasts (Fig. 11.1).

The preodontoblasts differentiate further into odontoblasts, cells that are tall and columnar (50–60 μm in length) and form a single layer with the configuration of an epithelial column. Functional secretory odontoblasts are polarized and no longer undergo mitosis. Odontoblasts have a highly developed rough endoplasmic reticulum, Golgi apparatus, mitochondria, and secretory granules that produce the DECM. Once terminally differentiated, the odontoblasts form tight junctions. They also form a unique

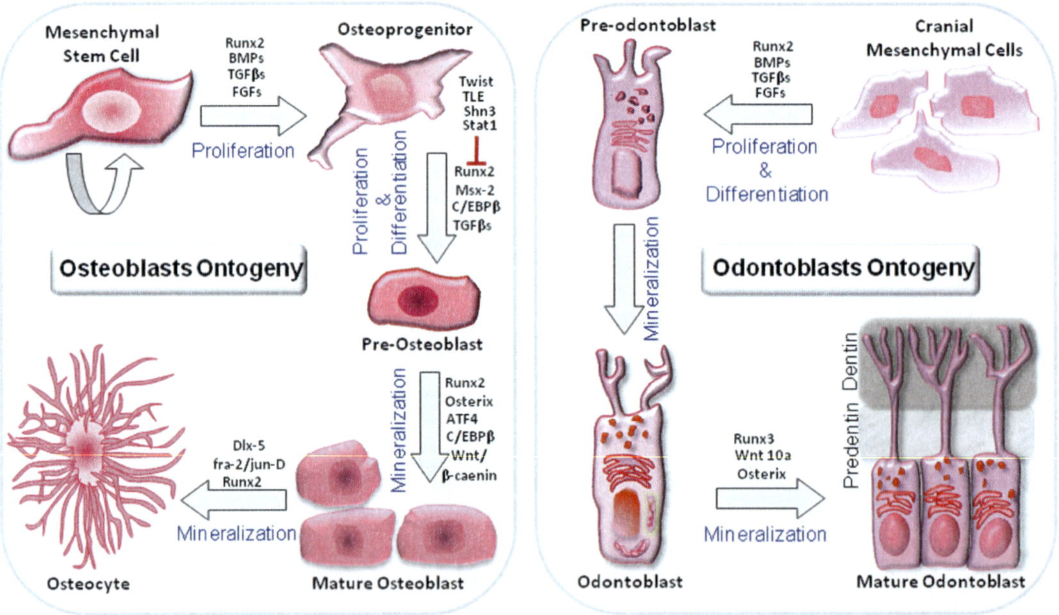

Figure 11.1. Osteoblast and odontoblast lineage progression and phenotypic features. Sequence and stages of the osteoblast and odontoblast lineage from a self-renewing, pluripotent mesenchymal stem cell are illustrated. Several mediators that influence odontoblast and osteoblast development are indicated. These include transforming growth factor β (TGFβ), the bone morphogenetic proteins (BMPs), and fibroblast growth factors (FGFs). Also listed are the key transcription factors involved in genetic control of osteoblast and odontoblast maturation, and/or expression of osteoblast/odontoblast-specific genes. Factors that negatively regulate Runx2 activity at earlier stages are also listed. The diagram shows the morphological features of odontoblast lineage cells at each stage, from stem cells to polarized functional odontoblast, and the osteoblast lineage cells at each stage, from stem cell to osteocytes.

unidirectional, long branched process, termed the odontoblastic cell process, which is separated from the cell body by a terminal web and cell junctions and is devoid of cytoplasmic organelles, but contains coated vesicles. The odontoblastic cell process traverses the developing DECM, forming numerous branches distally from the cell body, and becomes encased in the DECM as the odontoblasts retreat toward the pulp chamber, causing elongation of the cellular processes. The dentin that forms around these processes is termed *dentinal tubules*. These give the structure its unique "Swiss cheese" appearance. The diameter and density of the dentin tubules vary, being larger (3 µm) and more abundant near the pulp. Human dentin contains about 65,000 tubules per mm^2 near the pulp and about 15,000 tubules per mm^2 at the periphery, near the enamel.

The initial matrix produced by the odontoblasts is termed the mantle dentin. This layer contains coarser collagen fibrils and small, spherical, membrane-enriched vesicles, termed matrix vesicles that are 50–150 nm in diameter. These vesicles are formed by buds from the cell membrane and are associated with calcifying epiphyseal cartilage, bone, and dentin [5]. They are rich in alkaline phosphatase, accumulate calcium, and contain the first formed mineral crystals of the DECM which act as initiation sites. The mantle dentin becomes localized distally to the odontoblasts, adjacent to the later forming enamel matrix of the crown.

The mature odontoblasts synthesize and secrete the DECM that forms the bulk of the tooth's matrix and consists of two distinct layers: the mineralized predentin and the mineralized dentin [8]. Predentin is an unmineralized layer about 15 µm wide, which lines the entire surface of the dentin next to the odontoblast cell layer. Predentin prevents the internal resorption of dentin and the cells from becoming engulfed within the mineralized matrix. The latter contains coarse collagen fibrils and, except in pathological conditions, is always found adjacent to the cells. The dentin is located distally from the odontoblasts in contact with the overlaying mantle dentin. In these layers, the collagen fibrils are thinner and more densely packed, many running around the dentinal tubules.

The peritubular dentin is the mineralized dentin matrix that surrounds the dentinal tubules in the form of a ring. It is more highly mineralized than the dentin between the peritubular dentin. This inter-dispersed dentin, known as the intertubular dentin, makes up most of the mineralized dentin. As already pointed out, the peritubular dentin houses the odontoblastic cell processes and tissue fluid, as well as the nerves within 200 µm of the pulp chamber. Peritubular dentin is rich in glutamic acid containing protein, but contains no collagen [37, 138]. The structures are thought to be mineralized by a noncollagenous proteolipid–phospholipid complex by the way of small crystals similar to those found in intertubular dentin [37].

After the initial secretion of dentin by odontoblasts, the epithelial-derived ameloblasts secrete the components of the enamel extracellular matrix; this is known as amelogenesis. The matrix interface of the dentin and enamel is called the *dentin enamel junction*; its components originate from odontoblasts and ameloblasts. In the course of amelogenesis, the inner enamel epithelium-derived cells differentiate into ameloblasts and produce the extracellular matrix for the enamel. These cells differentiate only after dentin formation has been initiated. Enamel matrix differs from dentin and bone in that it is not rich in collagen. Its major components are the structural proteins amelogenin, enamelin, ameloblastin, amelotin, proteinase kallikrein 4, and matrix metalloproteinase 20.

11.1.2 Radicular Dentin Formation

After the crown has been completed, epithelial cells of the inner and outer dental epithelium form Hertwig's epithelial root sheath at the most distal margins of the enamel organ. Hertwig's epithelial root sheath sets the pattern for the shape of the root, its size and length and may determine the differentiation of root odontoblasts and cementoblasts. The root dentin matrix contains a small interglobular, hypomineralized region, known as the *Tomes' granular layer*. The odontoblasts that form the root or radicular dentin differ slightly from those located within the crown, in that they have fine cell branches that give it a brush-like appearance. On the basis of what is seen in human radicular dentin dysplasia, root odontoblast and dentin formation is independent of crown dentin formation. Mantle dentin is also formed in the root peripheral to the granular layer of Tomes, but is not continuous.

11.1.3 Secondary Dentin

Secondary dentin is formed after the tooth crown and root dentin have been completed. Secondary dentin forms on the entire pulpal surface, with slightly more on the ceiling and floor of the pulp chamber. In the course of development, secondary dentin induces a reduction in the size and shape of the pulp chamber and pulp horns at the cusp tips. This process is known as pulpal recession and is thought to reduce the general permeability of the dentin and protect the viable pulp. The continuous growth of peritubular dentin results in partial or complete blocking of the tubules with age. In general, as dentin ages, it becomes more brittle, harder, and translucent; it is then termed as sclerotic dentin. Interestingly, secondary dentin is formed throughout the lifespan of a tooth by the same postmitotic odontoblasts that were formed during late embryonic development–early childhood, and become the permanent teeth.

11.2 Osteogenesis

Bone is a specialized connective tissue that, together with cartilage, makes up the skeletal system. Bone and cartilage serve three essential functions: (1) mechanical; (2) protective; and (3) metabolic. In bone, as in all connective tissues, the fundamental constituents are the osteoblasts, osteocytes, osteoclasts, and the abundant extracellular matrix composed of collagen fibers and noncollagenous protein [103].

In mammals, osteogenesis or bone development is the last embryonic event in the development of the skeleton. Once the mesenchymal condensation for each future skeletal element has formed, between embryonic days 10.5 and 12.5 in mouse, each can evolve along two paths. Cells in the condensed mesenchyme differentiate directly into osteoblasts to form the skull and clavicle bones by intramembranous ossification [40]. For the other skeletal elements, the condensed mesenchyme cells differentiate into chondrocytes that form the cartilage anlagen of the future bone. Terminally differentiated chondrocytes undergo hypertrophy and form a calcified matrix. Apoptosis of the chondrocyte in the calcified cartilage results in blood vessel invasion and recruitment of osteoblast [23, 47]. Osteoblasts deposit the bone matrix and, as the bone marrow forms, multi-nucleated osteoclasts arise [46]. Endochondral ossification consists of the sequential appearance of cartilage anlagen, calcified cartilage and mineralized bone.

11.2.1 Cytodifferentiation of Osteoblasts

Developmentally, osteoblasts originate from local mesenchymal cells, bone marrow stromal stem cells, or connective tissue mesenchymal stem cells. These precursor cells, upon appropriate stimuli, undergo proliferation and differentiate into preosteoblasts and then into mature osteoblasts. Osteoblasts never appear or function individually, but are always found in clusters lining the bone matrix layer that they are producing. Three forms of the osteoblast cell lineage are recognized: the progenitor osteoblasts; mature osteoblasts; and osteocytes (Fig. 11.1).

In the early stages of osteoblast development, progenitor cells proliferate extensively, expressing growth-related genes (histones, c-myc, and c-fos) and a number of matrix genes (type-I collagen, fibronectin, some growth factors such as BMP2/TGFβ). The genes are active for a number of days and their products are joined by gene products associated with a mature matrix, such as ALP and MGP [70]. When the matrix and matrix-maturing proteins are no longer expressed, the gene products associated with mineralization begin to be expressed (e.g., BSP, OPN, and OSC). This leads to hydroxyapatite accumulation and complete mineralization. When the cuboidal- and columnar-shaped osteoblasts have completed forming new bone, the matrix surrounds some cells that then differentiate into osteocytes; other osteoblasts undergo apoptosis and disintegrate. Approximately 15% of osteoblasts become osteocytes, the end-stage phenotype of an osteoblast. Osteocytes are spatially and morphologically distinct from the rest of the osteoblast lineage. They are completely encased in bone and have long branched cellular processes that allow them to contact each other, as well as the cells lining the bone surface.

In contrast, odontoblasts form a continous single layer of cells lining the entire tooth pulp chamber and, under normal conditions, do not become completely embedded in the mineralized matrix as osteocytes. Odontoblasts seem to be a hybrid of osteoblasts and osteocytes, and are polarized with an extensive, unidirectionally formed cellular process.

11.3 Cell Lines and Models of Osteoblast and Odontoblast Cultures

A number of in vitro cell models have been used to investigate the differentiation of osteoprogenitor cells into osteoblasts [122]. Model systems have been developed to analyze how dental pulp progenitor cells differentiate into odontoblasts [93, 128]. In addition, primary cultures from calvarial bone tissue, bone marrow stromal cells, and dental pulp have helped to understand the early phenotypic commitment, cell-specific cytodifferentiation, and matrix-mediated mineralization.

Since the first attempt by Niizima to culture odontogenic cells [95], a variety of culture systems have been reported. Some of these have used outgrowths of isolated pulp-tissue explants [82, 129], or isolated cells from dental pulp plated as a monolayer [81, 128]. Isolated pulp tissue or pulp cells from developing or adult teeth differentiate in vitro into matrix producing cells that mineralize. Pulp cells grown in osteogenic supportive media that contain ascorbic acid and beta-glycerophosphate with or without dexamethasone form multilayer cellular nodules that undergo differentiation with the up-regulation of alkaline phosphatase and production of a mineralized matrix (VonKossa stain). As these cells express bone proteins, e.g., collagen types I and III, osteonectin, osteopontin, and fibronectin, investigators have focused on determining whether they are odontoblasts or osteoblasts. Once DSP and DPP were identified as odontoblastic markers, cells associated with nodules in pulp cultures were characterized as odontoblast-like, because they expressed DSP and DPP very robustly, were polarized, and produced a mineralized matrix [80, 81]. These findings indicate that some dental pulp cells differentiate into the more specialized odontoblast phenotype in vitro [41, 80]. Culture systems using human crowns or thick slices of human or rat teeth have also been used to mimic the natural cellular architecture and environment [24].

Immortalized cell lines derived from stroma, bone, or other mesenchymal/mesodermal tissues have yielded transcription factors and genes involved in osteoblastic differentiation (see Table 11.1). Unlike the supply of primary cell cultures, that of immortalized cells has the advantage of being virtually unlimited. Moreover, cells transformed by T antigen of SV40 can grow in serum concentrations that do not support survival of parental or primary cells. Unlike cell lines such as C3H10T1/2 and NIH 3T3, virus-transformed cells do not require growth factor when grown in serum-free media [118]. The T antigen also disrupts homeostasis by modulating cellular proliferation and apoptosis and, in transgenic mice, induces choroid plexus tumors and intestinal hyperplasia [64]. Established cell lines are often genomically altered, tumorigenic, and display gross chromosomal abnormalities. Indeed, cytogenetic studies have confirmed that most of these cells possess a highly rearranged hyperdiploid karyotype with 10–22% polyploidy. In addition, established cell lines generally reflect a “frozen state of differentiation” that represents the tissue and its developmental stage at the time of isolation.

The establishment of culture conditions conducive for odontoblastic differentiation from pulp cells has led to the production of immortalized odontoblast-like cell lines. The first of these came from mice. MO6-G3 is a mouse cell line with odontoblast-like properties that was established by using stable transfection with a temperature-sensitive SV40 large T antigen [80, 87]. MDPC-23, another mouse line, was established through spontaneous immortalization using a 3T3 protocol [41]. Other immortalized odontoblast-like cell lines have been established from rat, bovine,

Table 11.1. Most-widely used cell line/models for osteoblast differentiation

Cell line	Morphology	Species/age	Tissue	Method	Differentiation potential	References
MC3T3 E1	Adherent fibroblast-like	Mouse C57BL/6 New born	Calvaria	Clonal expansion	Preosteoblast, poor differentiation and mineralization	[66]
C3H10T1/2	Adherent fibroblast-like	Mouse C3H fetal 14–17dpc	Whole embryo	Clonal expansion	Chondrocyte, adipocyte, muscle osteoblast, poor mineralization	[108]
UMR 106	Adherent epithelial	Rat sprague Dawley, adult	Bone	Induced by 32p radiation	Differentiated osteoblast, good mineralization	[84]
Saos-2	Adherent epithelial	Human 11-year old female	Bone	Osteosarcoma	Differentiated osteoblast, poor mineralization, pRb and P53 deficient	[27]
ROS 17/2.8	Adherent epithelial	Rat sprague Dawley, adult	Bone	Osteosarcoma	Differentiated osteoblast, poor mineralization, high OC expression	[110]
MLO-Y4	Adherent dendritic	C57BL/6 transgenic mice 14 day old	Long bone	T-antigen expressed by OC promoter	Osteocyte characteristics, High levels of OC and Connexin 43	[59]
Most-widely used cell line/models for odontoblast differentiation						
M06-G3	Polarized odontoblastic cell process	Mouse Swiss Webster E 18	Pulp molars	SV40 T-antigen	Odontoblast-like, DECM markers, mineralized matrix	[77]
MDPC-23	Multiple cell processes	Mouse CD-1 E-18 & E-19	Pulp molars	Spontaneous immortalized	Odontoblast-like, DECM markers, High ALP	[41]
DPM	Spindle shaped	Mouse E18	Pulp molars	Immorto-mouse	Differentiate to odontoblast-like cells, DECM markers, mineralized matrix	[9]
OCL	Fibroblastic	C57BL/6 EGFP transgenic mice E 18.5	Pulp molars	Spontaneous immortalized	Odontoblast-like, DECM markers mineralized matrix	[1]
RPC-C2	Fibroblastic	Rat Wistar, 7-week-old	Pulp incisor	Spontaneous	Dental pulp, high ALP	[58]
RDP 4–1 KN-1, 2, 3	Fibroblastic	Rat Wistar, 1-week-old	Pulp	Spontaneous	Dental pulp, type I collagen, ALP High ALP, DSPP and Runx2,	[60, 96]
T4–4 T3–2	Polarized, odontoblastic process	Rat sprague Dawley, 3–5 days Postnatal	Molar tooth germ	Human telomerase	Odontoblast-like, DECM markers, mineralized matrix	[42]
tCPC-B, C, D tCPC-12	Fibroblastic spindle-shaped	Bovine, 6-month-old	Molars dental papilla	SV40 T-antigen	Odontoblast like, DPP, OSC, collagen type I	[126]
HPC-T tHPC#V2	Fibroblastic spindle-shaped	Human impacted 3rd molars 16–19 years	Pulp	SV40 T-antigen	High ALP odontoblast-like, DECM markers	[30, 100]
HDP-Htert	Fibroblastic	Human third molar	Pulp	Telomerase hTERT	Odontoblast-like, DECM markers, ALP, mineralized matrix	[65]

and human tissues [30, 42, 126], and have been used in studies of the biocompatibility of dental materials, the regulation of gene expression, and the identification of genes expressed by dental pulp, but not by odontoblasts [77, 78].

11.4 Transcriptional Control of Osteoblast and Odontoblast Differentiation

Development of functional osteoblast or odontoblast lines requires interplay between transcription factors that are primarily expressed in osteoblasts and/or those that are expressed more broadly. Runx2, a member of the Runt domain family of regulatory proteins and Osterix/SP7, a member of the zinc-finger containing SP family, are essential for osteoblast and odontoblast differentiation [15, 18, 67, 92]. Osterix/SP7 is genetically downstream of Runx2, is critical for maintenance of odontoblasts, and is thought to exert its function in later stages of osteoblast differentiation. Runx2 is expressed throughout the osteoblast differentiation period and regulates the transcription of various genes that are markers for different stages of osteoblast differentiation [2, 21, 50, 69]. Runx2-target genes include genes expressed by immature and differentiated osteoblasts, such as TGF-β receptor, collagen type I α1, α2, ALP, Osterix, Vitamin D receptor, galectin-3, BSP, OPN, OSC, and collagenase [69]. In odontoblasts, Runx2 downregulates specific dentin markers such as DSPP [12, 14]. Furthermore, forced expression of Runx2 in odontoblasts causes loss of their columar morphology, a decrease in dentin matrix thickness, downregulation of collagen type I α1 expression, and loss of DSPP expression [89]. Another Runx family member, Runx3, restricts Osterix expression in dental pulp cells, thus allowing odontoblasts to differentiate [149].

Runx2-mediated differential transcriptional control during osteoblast differentiation is regulated by posttranslational modification, and its interactions with other nonbone-specific transcription factors, such as Smads, C/EBPs, Statb2, AP-1, Dlx5, and ATF4 [19, 39, 45, 50, 114, 146]. Runx2 activity is suppressed during early stages of mesenchymal cell commitment toward osteoblast lineage by Groucho/TLE, Stat1, Shn3, Msx1, Bapx1, and Twist [3, 51, 55, 63, 115, 127]. The ability of Runx2 to activate or repress gene transcription is in part achieved through chromatin modification of a gene and a promoter's conformation [52]. Runx2 directly interacts and recruits p300 acetyltransferase and histone deacetylase to regulate target genes [53, 117]. Thus, Runx2 and its associated regulatory protein complex are important to direct mesenchymal precursor cells toward the osteoblast/odontoblast lineage.

11.4.1 Growth Factors and Hormones

The stages of osteoblast differentiation are regulated by a complex series of signaling molecules and associated transcription factors. Furthermore, bone and tooth cells produce growth factors and cytokines that regulate cell proliferation, differentiation, and survival in both auto- and paracrine fashion.

Of the TGFβ superfamily, the most important matrix-inductive molecules are the protein members of the bone morphogenetic protein (BMP) family. BMPs are produced by almost all skeletal cell types and their receptors are present on ectodermal, mesodermal, and endodermal derived cells, including osoteoblasts and odontoblasts. Stimulation of mesenchymal cells by BMP2 dramatically induces the expression of both Runx2 and Osterix, in turn leading to osteoblast and odontoblast differentiation [11, 145]. Induction of Runx2 and Osterix by BMP2 and subsequent upregulation of osteoblast-specific genes involves Dlx5, Smad transducers, and MAPK pathway. In odontoblasts, regulation of DSPP by BMP2 is mediated by NF-Y signaling [13]. BMP4 and BMP7 induce reparative dentin formation in dogs [93, 131] and ferrets [119]. Rutherford and coworkers have shown that when they applied recombinant human osteogenic protein-1 to exposed molars and premolars of nonhuman primates, there resulted an increase in reparative dentins, with the thickness of the new dentin directly proportional to the amount of BMP7 applied [112, 113].

Indian hedgehog and Wnt/β-catenin signaling pathways exert positive regulatory roles for bone formation at various stages of differentiation. These pathways are indispensable for osteoblast differentiation and bone development, with Ihh acting upstream of the Wnt signaling. The endogenous ligand, Wnt7b, is thought to regulate osteogenesis [48]. Wnt10a is associated with dentinogenesis because it regulates dentin sialophosphoprotein [143].

During bone and tooth formation, there is a distinct spatial and developmental pattern of FGF receptor and ligand molecule expression in epithelial and mesenchymal cells. Most FGFs suppress proliferation and promote skeletal cell differentiation [98]. FGF-3 and FGF-10 have redundant functions in the tooth mesenchyme, downregulating growth factors in postmitotic odontoblasts [62].

Insulin-like growth factors increase osteoprogenitor number, stimulate proliferation, reduce bone marrow stromal cell apoptosis, and encourage recruitment and migration of osteoblasts to the bone surface, while exerting prosurvival effects on osteoblasts. IGFs are produced by osteoblastic cells in response to parathyroid hormone, estrogens, and BMPs. IGFs accumulate in the bone matrix, stimulate proliferation and differentiation of osteoprogenitors and cause increased longitudinal bone growth [54, 75]. In mice with a conditional knockout of the IGF-I receptor in mature osteoblasts, trabecular bone volume is decreased and bone matrix mineralization is impaired. This suggests that IGF-I signaling in mature osteoblasts plays a key role in matrix mineralization [148]. IGF-I also functions as an autocrine/paracrine regulator of tooth development [56]. Exogenous IGF-1 added to mouse pulp cultures stimulates mitotic activity, cell differentiation, promotes odontoblast development, and dentin formation [9, 10].

The activity of vitamin D hormone regulates skeletal metabolism both directly and indirectly. Both the vitamin D receptor and the metabolic enzymes that transform vitamin D into the functionally active metabolite are expressed in the progenitor and mature osteoblasts and odontoblasts. Yet, VDR signaling in early developmental stages inhibits osteoblast differentiation, whereas VDR activation in mature osteoblasts enhances their function and bone synthesis. In addition, vitamin D exerts indirect regulation of bone via its regulatory role in calcium and phosphate homeostasis [121]. In odontoblasts, disruption of VDR results in altered dentin maturation and mineralization, with the resulting teeth exhibiting an increase in pulp chambers, hypoplastic dentin, and increased predentin thickness, with fewer dentin tubules [150].

Estrogens and androgens are each required for optimum skeletal function. This is not the case for teeth. The hormones act directly via osteoblast receptors that give rise to genomic or nongenomic signals. They also act indirectly in response to mechanical loading, modulation of the Wnt/β-catenin signaling, or interaction with the GH/IGF-I axis. Androgens and estrogens also exert antiresorptive effects by inhibiting osteoclast generation, activity, and enhancing osteoclast apoptosis [133].

11.5 Composition of Matrix Synthesized by Osteoblasts and Odontoblasts

Odontoblasts and osteoblasts each synthesize a collagenous extracellular matrix with organic components in common that undergoes mineralization. Eighteen percent of the organic components of dentin and 86% of the organic components of bone are type I collagen. In addition, the organic components include type I trimer, type III, type V, and type VI collagens, and several noncollagenous proteins (NCP) [7, 71, 106]. The latter consist of MGP, OSN, BSP, OPN, OSC, MEPE, Dmp1, DSP, and DPP (see Table 11.2). The major class of NCPs is the small integrin-binding ligand, N-linked glycoproteins (SIBLING) family that consist of OPN, BSP, MEPE, DMP1, DSP, and DPP [26]. These genes have been mapped to human chromosome 4q21

Table 11.2. Noncollagenous matrix proteins

Gene name	Gene symbol/ chromosome	Protein properties	Center for Bone and teeth		References
			Bone	Teeth	
Fibronectin	FN1 2p14–16	Relatively abundant, may help regulate osteoblast differentiation	Embryonic lethal	ND	[31]
Osteonectin	SPARC 5q31–33	"Bone connector" may regulate mineralization	Osteoporosis	ND	[17]
Thrombo-spondin 2	THBS2 6q27	Regulates the proliferation of mesenchymal progenitors	Endocortical bone increased	ND	[68]
Osteocalcin	BGP 1q25-q31	Binds calcium. Influence energy metabolism by regulating insulin	Increased bones	ND	[22]
Matrix-gla-protein	MGP 12p12.3	Inhibits mineralization	Normal bones but calcified cartilage and blood vessels	Inhibits tooth mineralization	[57, 74]
SIBLINGS (small integrin-binding ligand, N-linked glycoprotein family)					
Bone sialoprotein	BSP 4q21.1	Binds to integrins, may assist cancer cells	Reduced bone formation	ND	[83]
Osteopontin	SPP1 4q21.1	Increases angiogenesis and modulate osteoclast differentiation	Normal bones	Normal teeth	[109]
Dentin matrix protein-1	DMP1 4q21.1	Regulates bone and tooth mineralization, cause autosomal recessive hypophosphatemia	Rickets and osteomalacia	Hypomineralized dentin	[25, 147]
Dentin sialophospho-protein	DSPP 4q21.1	Regulation of dentin mineralization and tubular structures, causes DGI types II/III and DD type II	high trabecular bone, effect bone turnover	Hypomineralized dentin, Pulpal calcifications	[120, 135]
Matrix extracellular glycoprotein	MEPE 4q21.1	Inhibits mineralization and may induce osteomalacia	Increased bone mass, osteoblast number, activity	ND	[38]
Noncollagenous matrix proteins with attached sugars					
Biglycan	BGN	Function uncertain, may bind to TGFβ and collagen	Osteopenia	Small female molars crowns, low carbonate content	[6, 142]
Decorin	DCN 12q21.33	Binds to collagen and TGFβ. Inhibits cell attachment to fibronectin	Normal bones, abnormal collagen fibril	Increased carbonate content	[6, 16]
Fibromodulin	FMOD 1q32.1	Binds to collagen, TGFβ, and regulates collagen fibrillogenesis	Normal bones, abnormal collagen fiber in tail tendon	Impaired dentin mineralization, delayed enamel formation	[34, 123]
Aggrecan	ACAN 15q26.1	Major structural macromolecules in cartilage, binds both hyaluronan and link protein	Perinatal lethal, dwarfism, and craniofacial abnormalities	Poor dentin mineralization, twisted porous enamel	[137]
Hyaluronan and proteoglycan link protein 1	HAPLN1 (CRTL1) 5q14.3	Stabilizes aggregates of aggrecan and hyaluronan, giving cartilage its tensile strength and elasticity	Perinatal lethal, chondrodysplasia	Normal	[136]

within a gene cluster. SIBLINGs also share common gene structure features, including a small noncoding first exon, the start codon and first two amino acids encoded by exon 2, and a last exon that contains most of the coding segment. These proteins share features such as the Arg–Gly–Asp (RGD) motif that mediates cell attachment/signaling via its reaction with cell-surface integrins and posttranslational modifications, such as phosphorylation and glycosylation [26, 104]. SIBLINGs proteins are secreted during the formation and mineralization of both dentin and bone, but are also associated with other mineralized tissues such as cartilage and enamel. Furthermore, several reports have shown that SIBLINGs are expressed in nonmineralized tissues such as kidney and salivary glands [97]. The protein levels of the SIBLINGS found in dentin differ quantitatively from those in bone [106]. DSPP, the major protein marker associated with dentin formation, has a much lower expression in bone. The levels of DSP and DPP polypeptide fragments in bone-matrix extracts are only 1:400th of those in dentin [105, 106]. These proteins are encoded by a single gene, DSPP, expressed as a large transcript that is processed posttranslationally [79]. Recently, a third DSPP-derived protein, dentin glycoprotein, has been isolated from porcine dentin [144]. The noncollagenous proteins of dentin and bone are believed to be essential for initiation, inhibition, and regulation of matrix mineralization.

11.5.1 Mechanical Influence

Bone has the remarkable and well-documented capacity to respond to physical forces. In the absence of loading, bone mass is lost. In the presence of loading, bone mass is either maintained or increased. The response of bone to alterations in applied forces depends on how these are perceived by the sensor cells and by the manner in which the forces are transmitted [36]. To withstand or resist loads, bones must constantly undergo adaptive remodeling.

Osteocytes, with their vast interconnected canalicular network, are thought to be the key in sensing mechanical strain and in orchestrating signals that lead to bone resorption or formation. Osteocytes, the descendants of osteoblasts, are the most abundant bone cell type, constituting 90–95% of bone cells in the adult skeleton. Especially in cortical bone, osteocytes play a unique role, serving as mechanosensors [101].

Both osteocytes and osteoblasts, as descendents of the same cell lineage, are highly responsive to circulating hormones and cytokines, but their responses to mechanical loading differ. Primary cilia in osteoblasts do not mediate calcium flux in response to fluid flow. Primary osteoblasts are less sensitive to shear stress than primary osteocytes, and the ion channels that respond to strain are not the same in osteoblasts as in osteocytes. In osteocytes, prostaglandin produced in response to shear stress is inhibited when the cytoskeleton is disrupted. This is not the case in osteoblasts. Under mechanical strain, osteocytes increase glucose uptake, RNA production, and express several genes, including OSC, Dmp1, MEPE, and IGF-1 [32, 33, 43].

Wnt/β-catenin signaling is important in osteoblast differentiation and for the synthesis of bone matrix. Osteocytes, however, utilize the Wnt/β-catenin pathway to transmit signals of mechanical loading to cells on the bone surface. The many different mechanical responses to mechanical stress reflect the highly dynamic nature of osteocytes. Although embedded in bone, they extend and retract their dendritic processes in response to mechanical stimuli, while their cell body undergoes deformation [4]. Targeted deletion of osteocytes causes bone to become fragile, because of intracortical porosity and the incidence of microfractures; it also causes loss of trabecular bone. Yet bones of osteocyte-null animals are resistant to unloading-induced bone loss. Osteocytes are therefore necessary to maintain bone mass in response to normal loads. In the absence of loads, osteocytes send signals to induce resorption [124]. The reduced remodeling of the aging human skeleton and its inability to overcome microdamage efficiently are attributed to the loss of osteocytes.

11.5.2 Remodeling and Repair

Once growth and modeling of the skeleton have been completed, the bones alter their internal structure by remodeling, i.e., the localized removal of previously laid down bone and replacement with newly formed bone. Remodeling is a complex process and requires interactive cellular activity that is regulated by a variety of biochemical and mechanical factors. Remodeling allows bone to retain its strength by repairing microdamage and enabling it to respond to mechanical stress. Remodeling thus is an important aspect of mineral metabolism.

Remodeling is either directed or stochastic. Bone repairs microfractures by directed remodeling at the damaged site. In stochastic remodeling, bone is renewed at random. This prevents accumulation of older, densely mineralized, and brittle bone [102].

Bone remodeling involves a group of cells termed the bone remodeling unit (BMU) [28]. Some ~20% of cancellous bone undergoes remodeling at any time, involving a very large number of BMUs. The lifecycle of a BMU involves the following steps in sequence: origination and organization of the BMU, activation of the osteoclast, old bone resorption, osteoblast recruitment, new bone matrix formation, and mineralization. Mechanical stimuli and a variety of hormones and cytokines, such as vitamin Dhormone, PTH, IL-6, sex steroids, IGF, among the others, initiate a BMU. BMU activation is a continuing process, with new cells actively recruited throughout the life of a BMU. Although the precise signals are unknown, bone lining cells continuously change shape and produce more matrix-degrading enzymes that then expose some of the collagen and mineralized matrix. The increase in RANK ligand production also promotes fusion and maturation of preosteoclasts. The BMU resorption lasts several weeks and proceeds at the rate of 15 μm per day. In the course of resorption, growth factors such as TGFβ, IGF, and FGF, which are in the bone niche, are released, promoting coupling between resorption and formation. Osteoblasts converge at the bottom of cavities created by bone resorption and begin to produce matrix and mineralize until the cavity is filled with new bone. Normally, the rates of bone resorption and formation are essentially the same, but the disturbance of the remodeling balance is associated with a variety of metabolic bone diseases, including osteoporosis.

Dentin resorption is a part of the normal process of deciduous tooth exfoliation, as well as of pathological conditions [29]. Dentin is resorbed from the internal pulp chamber or the outer aspect of the root surface. The cells that remove dentin are termed odontoclasts and are similar in all respects to osteoclasts [20]. A common side effect of orthodontic treatment is dental root resorption.

Tertiary dentin is produced in reaction to an intense insult or injury to the tooth, and takes place rapidly and only at the site of the stimulus. Tertiary dentin is of two types: reactionary, formed by preexisting odontoblasts; and reparative, formed by newly differentiated odontoblasts-like cells [88, 131, 132]. Reactionary dentin results from a mild injury or insult, with the odontoblasts still viable. Reparative dentin is produced when the injury destroys the odontoblasts. This causes progenitor or pluripotent cells to be recruited from within the dental pulp to constitute a replacement of viable odontoblasts. As reparative dentin production is rapid, the cells often become embedded in the matrix, so that no initial tubular dentin structure forms osteodentin.

11.6 Genetic Syndromes and Diseases

Human skeletal disorders arise as a consequence of gain-of-function and loss-of-function mutations in signaling pathways. Disturbances in intramembranous bone formation are associated with craniofacial disorders, whereas defects in endochondral ossifications are associated with dwarfism. Haploinsufficiency of MSX2 is marked by a decrease in parietal ossification (parietal foramina). Gain of function mutation in MSX2 is associated with craniosynostosis [49, 139]. Mutations in MSX1 are associated with autosomal dominant hypodontia [134]. FGF receptors are major players in cranial skeletogenesis and mutations in FGFR2 and FGFR3 cause craniosynostosis [90, 107]. These are dominant mutations that cause increased signaling by the mutant receptor [94]. As most mutations of FGFR3 are associated with dwarfism (see Chap. 6), the primary function of this receptor is endochondral rather than intramembranous ossification. Heterogeneous mutations in Runx2 are associated with the autosomal dominant disease, cleidocranial dysplasia, which affects both bone and tooth phenotypes. Bone CCD defects include short stature, delayed closure of the fontanelles, and hyoplastic or missing clavicles. CCD dental defects include formation of extensive supranumerary teeth, altered cementum formation, and an abnormal cycle of tooth resorption-eruption, with most CCD defects due to inactivating mutations in Runx2 [91, 99].

Heritable dentin diseases affect both primary and permanent dentitions. They mostly exhibit an autosomal-dominant pattern of inheritance and are divided into two groups, dentinogenesis imperfecta (DGI) and dentin dysplasia, each with subclassifications [116]. DGI has been classified into three subgroups: Type I (DGI-I), associated with osteogenesis imperfecta (brittle bone disease), caused by heterogeneous mutations of Type I collagen; Type II (DGI-II), the classically inherited disease; and Type III (DGI-III), found in a southern Maryland tri-racial population [116]. DGI presents with gray to brownish-blue discoloration of the teeth and rapid attrition of the crowns, because the dentin matrix is poorly mineralized [140]. The pulp chamber is obliterated by the abnormal production of the mineralized dentin matrix with its poorly organized dentin tubules. The dentin of DGI teeth has a lower mineral content, with fewer hydroxyapatite crystals [61].

DD is less frequent and has been subclassified into two forms: Type I (DD-I), also known as rootless teeth associated with crescent-shaped pulp; and Type II (DD-II), associated with thistle-tube pulp [116]. Clinically, DD-I presents with teeth of normal shape and size with well-formed coronal enamel and dentin. The teeth tend to be mobile and often are exfoliated prematurely, because the roots are short or missing. The pulp chamber is filled with matrix, resulting in a crescent-shaped appearance. Although the crown dentin is normal, there are large masses of calcified atubular dentin with pulpal remnants near the pulp [85]. DD-II also presents with teeth of normal size and shape; they sometimes are amber or translucent in color. Radiographically, the primary teeth show that the pulp chamber has been completely obliterated. The permanent teeth display a hypertrophic dentin matrix with thistle-tube appearance [86]. The dentin matrix is highly calcified, with an irregular organization that lacks dentinal tubular patterning. DGI types II and III, and DD-II are the result of heterogeneous mutations in DSPP [44, 76]. The first reports of mutations in DGI were of four unrelated Chinese families [141, 151], some of whose members also presented with hearing loss. DMP1 heterogeneous mutations have been associated with autosomal recessive hypophosphatemia, implicating this protein in phosphate homeostasis [25, 73].

11.7 Common Properties of Bone and Dentin

The formation of dentin is closely related to bone in a number of ways, including composition and formation. Both bone and dentin are composed of a collagenous matrix that mostly consists of Type I collagen and a mineral phase with hydroxyapaptite plate-like crystals. As they form, odontoblasts and osteoblasts secrete an unmineralized matrix laid down in close association with the predentin or osteoid of the cells. Mineralization of dentin and bone extracellular matrix is initiated with the aid of matrix vesicles and later involves secretion of families of a specialized matrix protein. Bone and dentin secrete similar extracellular matrix proteins, but the relative proportion of these proteins may differ dramatically. Both odontoblasts and osteoblasts are mesenchymally-derived cells. However, the cells forming dentin originate from neural crest ectomesenchyme, whereas those forming bone are derived from neural crest mesenchyme, paraxial mesoderm, and lateral plate mesoderm. The signaling pathways involved in odontoblast and osteoblast differentiation are similar. Growth factors and hormones common to both regulate their formation. Abnormalities in both dentin and bone formation lead to a number of similar diseases and syndromes. As already discussed critical differences involve the morphology of the cells. Odontoblasts are tall columnar cells that form a continuous single layer with an epitheloid configuration. Cells involved in bone are much more complex and include three distinct phenotypes: osteoblasts, mature osteoblasts, and osteocytes. More importantly, only bone has the ability to remodel.

References

1. Arany S, Nakata A, Kameda T, Koyota S, Ueno Y, Sugiyama T (2006) Phenotype properties of a novel spontaneously immortalized odontoblast lineage cell line. Biochem Biophys Res Commun 342:718–724
2. Banerjee C, McCabe LR, Choi JY, Hiebert SW, Stein JL, Stein GS, Lian JB (1997) Runt homology domain proteins in osteoblast differentiation: AML3/CBFA1 is a major component of a bone-specific complex. J Cell Biochem 66(1):1–8
3. Bialek P, Kern B, Yang X, Schrock M, Sosic D, Hong N, Wu H, Yu K, Ornitz DM, Olson EN, Justice MJ, Karsenty G (2004) A twist code determines the onset of osteoblast differentiation. Dev Cell 6:423–435
4. Bonewald LF, Johnson ML (2008) Osteocytes, mechanosensing and Wnt signaling. Bone 42(4):606–615
5. Bonucci E (1967) Fine structure of early cartilage calcification. J Ultrastruct Res 20:33
6. Boskey AL, Young MF, Kilts T, Verdelis K (2005) Variation in mineral properties in normal and mutant bones and teeth. Cells Tissues Organs 181(3–4):144–153
7. Butler WT (1998) Dentin matrix proteins. Eur J Oral Sci 106(suppl 1): 204–210
8. Butler WT, Brunn JC, Qin C (2003) Dentin extracellular matrix (ECM) proteins: comparison to bone ECM and contribution to dynamics of dentinogenesis. Connect Tissue Res 44(suppl 1):171–178
9. Catón J, Bringas P Jr, Zeichner-David M (2007) Establishment and characterization of an immortomouse-derived odontoblast-like cell line to evaluate the effect of insulin-like growth factors on odontoblast differentiation. J Cellular Biochem 100:450–463
10. Caviedes-Bucheli J, Angel-Londoño P, Díaz-Perez A, Orozco MP, Alvarez JL, Lombana N, Díaz E, Muñoz HR (2007) Variation in the expression of insulin-like growth factor-1 in human pulp tissue according to the root-development stage. J Endod 33(11):1293–1295
11. Celil AB, Campbell PG (2005) BMP-2 and insulin-like growth factor-I mediate Osterix (Osx) expression in human mesenchymal stem cells via the MAPK and protein kinase D signaling pathways. J Biol Chem 280(36):31353–31359
12. Chen S, Chen L, Jahangiri A, Chen B, Wu Y, Chuang HH, Qin C, MacDougall M (2008) Expression and processing of small intergrin-binding ligand N-linked glycoproteins in mouse odontoblastic cells. Arch Oral Biol 53(9):879–889
13. Chen S, Gluhak-Heinrich J, Martinez M, Li T, Wu Y, Chuang HH, Chen L, Dong J, Gay I, MacDougall M (2008) Bone morphogenetic protein 2 mediates dentin sialophosphoprotein expression and odontoblast differentiation via NF-Y signaling. J Biol Chem 283(28):19359–19370
14. Chen S, Gu TT, Sreenath T, Kulkarni AB, Karsenty G, MacDougall M (2002) Spatial expression of Cbfa1/Runx2 isoforms in teeth and characterization of binding sites in the DSPP gene. Connect Tissue Res 43(2–3): 338–344
15. Choi JY, Pratap J, Javed A, Zaidi SK, Xing L, Balint E, Dalamangas S, Boyce B, van Wijnen AJ, Lian JB, Stein JL, Jones SN, Stein GS (2001) Subnuclear targeting of Runx/Cbfa/AML factors is essential for tissue-specific differentiation during embryonic development. Proc Natl Acad Sci U S A 98(15):8650–8655
16. Danielson KG, Baribault H, Holmes DF, Graham H, Kadler KE, Iozzo RV (1997) Targeted disruption of decorin leads to abnormal collagen fibril morphology and skin fragility. J Cell Biol 136:729–743
17. Delany AM, Amling M, Priemel M, Howe C, Baron R, Canalis E (2000) Osteopenia and decreased bone formation in osteonectin-deficient mice. J Clin Invest 105(7): 915–923
18. D'Souza RN, Aberg T, Gaikwad J, Cavender A, Owen M, Karsenty G, Thesleff I (1999) Cbfa1 is required for epithelial-mesenchymal interactions regulating tooth development in mice. Development 126(13):2911–2920
19. Dobreva G, Chahrour M, Dautzenberg M, Chirivella L, Kanzler B, Fariñas I, Karsenty G, Grosschedl R (2006) SATB2 is amultifunctional determinant of craniofacial patterning and osteoblast differentiation. Cell 125: 971–986
20. Domon T, Sugaya k, Yawaka Y, Osanai M, Hanaizumi Y, Takaahashi S, Wakita M (1994) Electron microscopic and histochemical studies of the mononuclear odontoblasts of the human. Ant Rec 240:42–51
21. Ducy P, Zhang R, Geoffroy V, Ridall AL, Karsenty G (1997) Osf2/Cbfa1: a transcriptional activator of osteoblast differentiation. Cell 89:747–754
22. Ducy P, Desbois C, Boyce B, Pinero G, Story B, Dunstan C, Smith E, Bonadio J, Goldstein S, Gundberg C, Bradley A, Karsenty G (1996) Increased bone formation in osteocalcin-deficient mice. Nature 382(6590):448–452
23. Erlebacher A, Filvaroff EH, Gitelman SE, Derynck R (1995) Toward a molecular understanding of skeletal development. Cell 80:371–378
24. Farges JC, Couble ML, Magloire H, Hartmann DJ, Bleicher F (1995) Ultrastructural characterization of mesenchymal and epithelial cells co-cultured from human dental root apical explants. Connect Tissue Res 33(1–3):37–46
25. Feng JQ, Ward LM, Liu S, Lu Y, Xie Y, Yuan B, Yu X, Rauch F, Davis SI, Zhang S, Rios H, Drezner MK, Quarles LD, Bonewald LF, White KE (2006) Loss of DMP1 causes rickets and osteomalacia and identifies a role for osteocytes in mineral metabolism. Nat Genet 38(11):1310–1315
26. Fisher LW, Fedarko NS (2003) Six genes expressed in bones and teeth encode the current members of the SIBLING family of proteins. Connect Tissue Res 44(suppl 1): 33–40
27. Fogh J, Wright WC, Loveless JD (1977) Absence of HeLa cell contamination in 169 cell lines derived from human tumors. J Natl Cancer Inst 58(2):209–214
28. Frost HM (1969) Tetracycline-based histological analysis of bone remodeling. Calcif Tissue Res 3(3):211–237
29. Furseth R (1968) The resorption oprocesses of human deciduous teeth studied by light mcriscopy, microadiography and electron microscopy. Arch Oral Biol 13:417

30. Galler K, Schweikl H, Thonemann B, D'Souza RN, Schmalz G (2006) Human pulp-derived cells immortalized with Simian Virus 40 T-antigen. Eur J Oral Sci 114:138–146
31. George EL, Georges-Labouesse EN, Patel-King RS, Rayburn H, Hynes RO (1993) Defects in mesoderm, neural tube and vascular development in mouse embryos lacking fibronectin. Development 119(4):1079–1091
32. Gluhak-Heinrich J, Pavlin D, Yang W, MacDougall M, Harris SE (2007) MEPE expression in osteocytes during orthodontic tooth movement. Arch Oral Biol 52(7): 684–690
33. Gluhak-Heinrich J, Ye L, Bonewald LF, Feng JQ, MacDougall M, Harris SE, Pavlin D (2003) Mechanical loading stimulates dentin matrix protein 1 (DMP1) expression in osteocytes in vivo. J Bone Miner Res 18(5):807–817
34. Goldberg M, Septier D, Oldberg A, Young MF, Ameye LG (2006) Fibromodulin-deficient mice display impaired collagen fibrillogenesis in predentin as well as altered dentin mineralization and enamel formation. J Histochem Cytochem 54(5):525–537
35. Goldberg M, Smith AJ (2004) Cells and extracellular matrices of dentin and pulp: a biological basis for repair and tissue engineering. Crit Rev Oral Biol Med 15(1):13–27
36. Goldstein SA (1987) The mechanical properties of trabecular bone: dependence on anatomic location and function. J Biomech 20(11–12):1055–1061
37. Gotlive B, Veis A (2007) Peritubular dentin, a vertebrate apatitic mineralized tissue without collagen: role of a phospholipid-proteolipid complex. Calcif Tissue Int 81:191–205
38. Gowen LC, Petersen DN, Mansolf AL, Qi H, Stock JL, Tkalcevic GT, Simmons HA, Crawford DT, Chidsey-Frink KL, Ke HZ, McNeish JD, Brown TA (2003) Targeted disruption of the osteoblast/osteocyte factor 45 gene (OF45) results in increased bone formation and bone mass. J Biol Chem 278(3):1998–2007
39. Gutierrez S, Javed A, Tennant DK, van Rees M, Montecino M, Stein GS, Stein JL, Lian JB (2002) CCAAT/enhancer-binding proteins (C/EBP) beta and delta activate osteocalcin gene transcription and synergize with Runx2 at the C/EBP element to regulate bone-specific expression. J Biol Chem 277(2):1316–1323
40. Hall BK, Miyake T (1992) The membranous skeleton: the role of cell condensations in vertebrate skeletogenesis. Anat Embryol 186:107–124
41. Hanks CT, Fang D, Sun Z, Edwards CA, Butler WT (1998) Dentin-specific proteins in MDPC-23 cell line. Eur J Oral Sci 106:260–266
42. Hao J, Narayanan K, Ramachandran A, He G, Almushayt A, Evans C, George A (2002) Odontoblast cells immortalized by telomerase produce mineralized dentin-like tissue both in vitro and in vivo. J Biol Chem 277:19976–19981
43. Harris SE, Gluhak-Heinrich J, Harris MA, Yang W, Bonewald LF, Riha D, Rowe PS, Robling AG, Turner CH, Feng JQ, McKee MD, Nicollela D (2007) DMP1 and MEPE expression are elevated in osteocytes after mechanical loading in vivo: theoretical role in controlling mineral quality in the perilacunar matrix. J Musculoskelet Neuronal Interact 7(4):313–315
44. Hart PS, Hart TC (2007) Disorders of human dentin. Cells Tissues Organs 186(1):70–77
45. Hassan MQ, Javed A, Morasso MI, Karlin J, Montecino M, van Wijnen AJ, Stein GS, Stein JL, Lian JB (2004) Dlx3 transcriptional regulation of osteoblast differentiation: temporal recruitment of Msx2, Dlx3, and Dlx5 homeodomain proteins to chromatin of the osteocalcin gene. Mol Cell Biol. 24(20):9248–9261
46. Hofstetter W, Wetterwald A, Cecchini MG, Mueller C, Felix R (1995) Detection of transcripts and binding sites for colony-stimulating factor-1 during bone development. Bone 17:145–151
47. Horton WA (1993) Morphology of connective tissue: cartilage. In: Connective tissue and its heritable disorders. Wiley, New York, NY, pp 73–84
48. Hu H, Hilton MJ, Tu X, Yu K, Ornitz DM, Long F (2005) Sequential roles of Hedgehog and Wnt signaling in osteoblast development. Development 132:49–60
49. Jabs EW, Müller U, Li X, Ma L, Luo W, Haworth IS, Klisak I, Sparkes R, Warman ML, Mulliken JB, Sneadf ML, Maxson R (1993) A mutation in the homeodomain of the human MSX2 gene in a family affected with autosomal dominant craniosynostosis. Cell 75(3):443–450
50. Javed A, Bae JS, Afzal F, Gutierrez S, Pratap J, Zaidi SK, Lou Y, van Wijnen AJ, Stein JL, Stein GS, Lian JB (2008) Structural coupling of Smad and Runx2 for execution of the BMP2 osteogenic signal. J Biol Chem 283(13): 8412–8422
51. Javed A, Guo B, Hiebert S, Choi JY, Green J, Zhao SC, Osborne MA, Stifani S, Stein JL, Lian JB, van Wijnen AJ, Stein GS (2000) Groucho/TLE/R-esp proteins associate with the nuclear matrix and repress RUNX (CBF(alpha)/AML/PEBP2(alpha)) dependent activation of tissue-specific gene transcription. J Cell Sci 113(pt 12):2221–2231
52. Javed A, Gutierrez S, Montecino M, van Wijnen AJ, Stein JL, Stein GS, Lian JB (1999) Multiple Cbfa/AML sites in the rat osteocalcin promoter are required for basal and vitamin D-responsive transcription and contribute to chromatin organization. Mol Cell Biol 19(11):7491–7500
53. Jensen ED, Schroeder TM, Bailey J, Gopalakrishnan R, Westendorf JJ (2008) Histone deacetylase 7 associates with Runx2 and represses its activity during osteoblast maturation in a deacetylation-independent manner. J Bone Miner Res 23(3):361–372
54. Jilka RL (2007) Molecular and cellular mechanisms of the anabolic effect of intermittent PTH. Bone 40(6): 1434–1446
55. Jones DC, Wein MN, Oukka M, Hofstaetter JG, Glimcher MJ, Glimcher LH (2006) Regulation of adult bone mass by the zinc finger adapter protein Schnurri-3. Science 312:1223–1227
56. Joseph BK, Savage NW, Daley TJ, Young WG (1996) In situ hybridization evidence for a paracrine/autocrine role for insulin-like growth factor-I in tooth development. Growth Factors 13(1–2): 11–17

57. Kaipatur NR, Murshed M, McKee MD (2008) Matrix Gla protein inhibition of tooth mineralization. J Dent Res 87(9):839–844
58. Kasugai S, Adachi M, Ogura H (1988) Establishment and characterization of a clonal cell line (RPC-C2A) from dental pulp of the rat incisor. Arch Oral Biol 33:887–891
59. Kato Y, Windle JJ, Koop BA, Mundy GR, Bonewald LF (1997) Establishment of an osteocyte-like cell line, MLO-Y4. J Bone Miner Res 12(12):2014–2023
60. Kawase T, Orikasa M, Suzuki A (1990) A clonal prostaglandinresponsive cell line (RDP 4–1) derived from rat dental pulp. Bone Miner 11:163–175
61. Kerebel B, Daculsi G, Menenteau J, Kerebel LM (1981) The inorganic phase in dentinogenesis imperfecta. J Dent Res 60(9):1655–1660
62. Kettunen P, Laurikkala J, Itäranta P, Vainio S, Itoh N, Thesleff I (2000) Association of FGF-3 and FGF-10 with signaling networks regulation tooth morphogenesis. Dev Dyn 219(3):322–332
63. Kim S, Koga T, Isobe M, Kern BE, Yokochi T, Chin YE, Karsenty G, Taniguchi T, Takayanagi H (2003) Stat1 functions as a cytoplasmic attenuator of Runx2 in the transcriptional program of osteoblast differentiation. Genes Dev 17:1979–1991
64. Kim SH, Roth KA, Coopersmith CM, Pipas JP, Gordon JI (1994) Expression of wild-type and mutant simian virus 40 large tumor antigens in villus-associated enterocytes of transgenic mice. Proc Natl Acad Sci U S A 91:6914–6918
65. Kitagawa M, Ueda H, Iizuka S, Sakamoto K, Oka H, Kudo Y, Ogawa I, Miyauchi M, Tahara H, Takata T (2007) Immortalization and characterization of human dental pulp cells with odontoblastic differentiation. Arch Oral Biol 52(8):727–731
66. Kodama H, Amagai Y, Sudo H, Kasai S, Yamamoto S (1981) Establishment of a clonal osteogenic cell line from newborn mouse calvaria. Jpn J Oral Biol 23: 899–901
67. Komori T, Yagi H, Nomura S, Yamaguchi A, Sasaki K, Deguchi K, Shimizu Y, Bronson RT, Gao YH, Inada M, Sato M, Okamoto R, Kitamura Y, Yoshiki S, Kishimoto T (1997) Targeted disruption of Cbfa1 results in a complete lack of bone formation owing to maturational arrest of osteoblasts. Cell 89:755–764
68. Kyriakides TR, Zhu YH, Smith LT, Bain SD, Yang Z, Lin MT, Danielson KG, Iozzo RV, LaMarca M, McKinney CE, Ginns EI, Bornstein P (1998) Mice that lack thrombospondin 2display connective tissue abnormalities that are associated with disordered collagen fibrillogenesis, an increased vascular density, and a bleeding diathesis. J Cell Biol 140:419–430
69. Lian JB, Javed A, Zaidi SK, Lengner C, Montecino M, van Wijnen AJ, Stein JL, Stein GS (2004) Regulatory controls for osteoblast growth and differentiation: role of Runx/Cbfa/AML factors. Crit Rev Eukaryot Gene Expr 14(1–2):1–41
70. Lian JB, Stein GS, Stein JL, van Wijnen AJ (1998) Osteocalcin gene promoter: unlocking the secrets for regulation of osteoblast growth and differentiation. J Cell Biochem Suppl 30–31:62–72
71. Linde A, Goldberg M (1993) Dentinogenesis. Crit Rev Oral Biol Med 4(5):679–728
72. Linde A (1984) Dentin and dentinogenesis, vol 1–2. CRC Press, Boca Raton, FL, pp 55–92
73. Lorenz-Depiereux B, Bastepe M, Benet-Pagès A, Amyere M, Wagenstaller J, Müller-Barth U, Badenhoop K, Kaiser SM, Rittmaster RS, Shlossberg AH, Olivares JL, Loris C, Ramos FJ, Glorieux F, Vikkula M, Jüppner H, Strom TM (2006) DMP1 mutations in autosomal recessive hypophosphatemia implicate a bone matrix protein in the regulation of phosphate homeostasis. Nat Genet 38(11):1248–1250
74. Luo G, Ducy P, McKee MD, Pinero GJ, Loyer E, Behringer RR, Karsenty G (1997) Spontaneous calcification of arteries and cartilage in mice lacking matrix GLA protein. Nature 386:78–81
75. Lupu F, Terwilliger JD, Lee K, Segre GV, Efstratiadis A (2001) Roles of growth hormone and insulin-like growth factor 1 in mouse postnatal growth. Dev Biol 229:141–162
76. MacDougall M, Dong J, Acevedo AC (2006) Molecular basis of human dentin disease. Am J Hum Genet 140(23):2536–2546
77. MacDougall M, Unterbrink A, Carnes D, Rani S, Luan X, Chen S (2001) Utilization of MO6-G3 immortalized odontoblast cells in studies regarding dentinogenesis. Adv Dent Res 15:25–29
78. MacDougall M, Selden JK, Nydegger J, Carnes DL (1998) Immortalized mouse odontoblast cell line M06-G3 application for in vitro biocompatibility testing. Am J Dent 11:511–516
79. MacDougall M, Simmons D, Luan X, Nydegger J, Feng J, Gu TT (1997) Dentin phosphoprotein and dentin sialoprotein are cleavage products expressed from a single transcript coded by a gene on human chromosome 4: dentin phosphoprotein DNA sequence determination. J Biol Chem 272:835–842
80. MacDougall M, Thiemann F, Ta H, Hsu P, Chen LS, Snead ML (1995) Temperature sensitive simian Virus 40 large T Antigen immortalization of murine odontoblast cell cultures: establishment of clonal odontoblast cell line. Conn Tiss Res 33:97–103
81. MacDougall M (1992) Dentin excellular matrix protein expression by odontoblastic cell cultures. In Slavkin H, Price P (eds) The fourth international conference on the chemistry and biology of mineralized tissues. Elsevier, New York, pp 117–124
82. Magloire H, Hartmann DJ, Couble ML, Grimaud J, Herage D, Ville G (1984) Tooth morphogenesis and differentiation, vol 125. INSERM, Paris, pp 119–126
83. Malaval L, Wade-Guéye NM, Boudiffa M, Fei J, Zirngibl R, Chen F, Laroche N, Roux JP, Burt-Pichat B, Duboeuf F, Boivin G, Jurdic P, Lafage-Proust MH, Amédée J, Vico L, Rossant J, Aubin JE (2008) Bone sialoprotein plays a functional role in bone formation and osteoclastogenesis. J Exp Med 205(5):1145–1153
84. Martin TJ, Ingleton PM, Underwood JC, Michelangeli VP, Hunt NH, Melick RA (1976) Parathyroid hormone-responsive adenylate cyclase in induced transplantable osteogenic rat sarcoma. Nature 260(5550):436–438

85. Melnick M, Levin LS, Brady J (1980) Dentin dysplasia type I: a scanning electron microscopic analysis of the primary dentition. Oral Surg 50:335–339
86. Melnick M, Eastman JR, Goldblatt LI, Michaud M, Bixler D (1977) Dentin dysplasia, type II: a rare autosomal dominant disorder. Oral Surg 44:592–599
87. Mesgouez C, Oboef M, Mauro N, Colon P, MacDougall M, Machtou P, Sautier JM, Berdal A (2006) Ultrastructural and immunohistochemical characterization of immortalized odontoblasts M06-G3. Intern Endodont J 38:1–11
88. Mitsiadis TA, Rahiotis C (2004) Parallels between tooth development and repair: conserved molecular mechanisms following carious and dental injury. J Dent Res 83(12):896–902
89. Miyazaki T, Kanatani N, Rokutanda S, Yoshida C, Toyosawa S, Nakamura R, Takada S, Komori T (2008) Inhibition of the terminal differentiation of odontoblasts and their transdifferentation into osteoblasts in Runx2 transgenic mice. Arch Histol Cytol 71(2): 131–146
90. Muenke M, Schell U, Hehr A, Robin NH, Losken HW, Schinzel A, Pulleyn LJ, Rutland P, Reardon W, Malcolm S, Winter RM (1994) A common mutation in the fibroblast growth factor receptor 1 gene in Pfeiffer syndrome. Nat Genet 8(3):269–274
91. Mundlos S, Otto F, Mundlos C, Mulliken JB, Aylsworth AS, Albright S, Lindhout D, Cole WG, Henn W, Knoll JH, Owen MJ, Mertelsmann R, Zabel BU, Olsen BR (1997) Mutations involving the transcription factor CBFA1 cause cleidocranial dysplasia. Cell 89:773–779
92. Nakashima K, Zhou X, Kunkel G, Zhang Z, Deng JM, Behringer RR, de Crombrugghe B (2002) The novel zinc finger-containing transcription factor osterix is required for osteoblast differentiation and bone formation. Cell 108:17–29
93. Nakashima M (1990) The induction of reparative dentine in the amputated dental pulp of the dog by bone morphogenetic protein. Archs Oral Biol 35(7):493–497
94. Naski MC, Ornitz DM (1998) FGF signaling in skeletal development. Front Biosci 3 781–794
95. Niizima M (1956) Dental papilla in tissue culture. Am J Anat 99:351–389
96. Nomiyama K, Kitamura C, Tsujisawa T, Nagayoshi M, Morotomi T, Terashita M, Nishihara T (2007) Effects of lipopolysaccharide on newly established dental pulp-derived cell line with odontoblastic properties. J Endod 33:1187–1191
97. Ogbureke KU, Fisher LW (2004) Expression of SIBLINGs and their partner MMPs in salivary glands. J Dent Res 83(9):664–670
98. Ornitz DM, Marie PJ (2002) FGF signaling pathways in endochondral and intramembranous bone development and human genetic disease. Genes Dev 16(12): 1446–1465
99. Otto F, Thornell AP, Crompton T, Denzel A, Gilmour KC, Rosewell IR, Stamp GW, Beddington RS, Mundlos S, Olsen BR, Selby PB, Owen MJ (1997) Cbfa1, a candidate gene for cleidocranial dysplasia syndrome, is essential for osteoblast differentiation and bone development. Cell 89:765–771
100. Panagakos FS (1998) Transformation and preliminary characterization of primary human pulp cells. J Endodon 24:171–175
101. Parfitt AM (1987) Bone remodeling and bone loss: understanding the pathophysiology of osteoporosis. Clin Obstet Gynecol 30(4):789–811
102. Parfitt AM, Mathews CH, Villanueva AR, Kleerekoper M, Frame B, Rao DS (1983) Relationships between surface, volume, and thickness of iliac trabecular bone in aging and in osteoporosis. Implications for the microanatomic and cellular mechanisms of bone loss. J Clin Invest 72(4):1396–1409
103. Puzas JE (1996) Osteoblast cell biology, lineage and functions In: Favus MJ (eds) Primer on the metabolic bone diseases and disorders of mineral metabolism. Lippincott-Raven, Philadelphia, PA, pp 11–16
104. Qin C, Baba O, Butler WT (2004) Post-translational modifications of sibling proteins and their roles in osteogenesis and dentinogenesis. Crit Rev Oral Biol Med 15(3):126–136
105. Qin C, Brunn JC, Cadena E, Ridall A, Butler WT (2003) Dentin sialoprotein in bone and dentin sialophosphoprotein gene expressed by osteoblasts. Connect Tissue Res 44(suppl 1):179–183
106. Qin C, Brunn JC, Jones J, George A, Ramachandran A, Gorski JP, Butler WT (2001) A comparative study of sialic acid-rich proteins in rat bone and dentin. Eur J Oral Sci 109:133–141
107. Reardon W, Winter RM, Rutland P, Pulleyn LJ, Jones BM, Malcolm S (1994) Mutations in the fibroblast growth factor receptor 2 gene cause Crouzon syndrome. Nat Genet 8(1):98–103
108. Reznikoff CA, Brankow DW, Heidelberger C (1973) Establishment and characterization of a cloned line of C3H mouse embryo cells sensitive to postconfluence inhibition of division. Cancer Res 33(12):3231–328
109. Rittling SR, Matsumoto HN, McKee MD, Nanci A, An XR, Novick KE, Kowalski AJ, Noda M, Denhardt DT (1998) Mice lacking osteopontin show normal development and bone structure but display altered osteoclast formation in vitro. J Bone Miner Res 13(7):1101–1111
110. Rodan SB, Fischer MK, Egan JJ, Epstein PM, Rodan GA (1984) The effect of dexamethasone on parathyroid hormone stimulation of adenylate cyclase in ROS 17/2.8 cells. Endocrinology 115(3):951–958
111. Ruch JV, Lesot H, Begue-Kirn C (1995) Odontoblast differentiation. Int J Dev Biol 39:51–68
112. Rutherford RB, Wahle J, Tucker M, Sampath K, Rueger D, Charette M (1993) Induction of reparative dentine formation in monkeys by recombinant humanosteogenic protein-1. Arch Oral Biol 38:571–576
113. Rutherford RB, Wahle J, Tucker M, Rueger D, Charette M (1994) The time-course of the induction of reparative dentine formation in monkeys by recombinant human osteogenic protein-1. Arch Oral Biol 39:833–838
114. Sabatakos G, Sims NA, Chen J, Aoki K, Kelz MB, Amling M, Bouali Y, Mukhopadhyay K, Ford K, Nestler EJ, Baron R (2000) Overexpression of ΔFosB transcription factor(s) increases bone formation and inhibits adipogenesis. Nat Med 6:985–990

115. Satokata I, Ma L, Ohshima H, Bei M, Woo I, Nishizawa K, Maeda T, Takano Y, Uchiyama M, Heaney S, Peters H, Tang Z, Maxson R, Maas R (2000) Msx2 deficiency in mice causes pleiotropic defects in bone growth and ectodermal organ formation. Nat Genet 24:391–395
116. Shields ED, Bixler D, El-Kafrawy AM (1973) A proposed classification for heritable human dentine defect with a description of a new entity. Arch Oral Biol 18:543–553
117. Sierra J, Villagra A, Paredes R, Cruzat F, Gutierrez S, Javed A, Arriagada G, Olate J, Imschenetzky M, Van Wijnen AJ, Lian JB, Stein GS, Stein JL, Montecino M (2003) Regulation of the bone-specific osteocalcin gene by p300 requires Runx2/Cbfa1 and the vitamin D3 receptor but not p300 intrinsic histone acetyltransferase activity. Mol Cell Biol 23:3339–3351
118. Slinskey A, Barnes D, Pipas JM (1999) Simian virus 40 large T antigen J domain and Rb-binding motif are sufficient to block apoptosis induced by growth factor withdrawal in a neural stem cell line. J Virol 73(8):6791–6799
119. Smith AJ, Robias RS, Cassidy N, Plant G, Browne RM, Begue-Kirn C, Ruch JV, Lesot H (1994) Odontoblast stimulation in ferrets by dentine matrix components. Archs Oral Biol 39:13–22
120. Sreenath T; Thyagarajan T; Hall B, Longenecker G, D'Souza R, Hong S, Wright JT, MacDougall M, Sauk J, Kulkarni AB (2003) Dentin sialophosphoprotein knockout mouse teeth display widened predentin zone and develop defective dentin mineralization similar to human dentinogenesis imperfecta type III. J Biol Chem 278:24874–24880
121. St-Arnaud R (2008) The direct role of vitamin D on bone homeostasis. Arch Biochem Biophys 473(2):225–230
122. Stein GS, Lian JB, Owen TA (1990) Relationship of cell growth to the regulation of tissue-specific gene expression during osteoblast differentiation. FASEB J 4:3111–3123
123. Svensson L, Aszódi A, Reinholt FP, Fässler R, Heinegård D, Oldberg A (1999) Fibromodulin-null mice have abnormal collagen fibrils, tissue organization, and altered lumican deposition in tendon. J Biol Chem 274(14):9636
124. Tatsumi S, Ishii K, Amizuka N, Li M, Kobayashi T, Kohno K, Ito M, Takeshita S, Ikeda K (2007) Targeted ablation of osteocytes induces osteoporosis with defective mechanotransduction. Cell Metab 5:464–475
125. Thesleff I (2003) Epithelial-mesenchymal signalling regulating tooth morphogenesis. J Cell Sci 116:1647–1648
126. Thonemann B, Schmalz G (2000) Bovine dental papilla-derived cells immortalized with HPV 18 E6/E7. Eur J Oral Sci 108:432–441
127. Tribioli C, Lufkin T (1999) The murine Bapx1 homeobox gene plays a critical role in embryonic development of the axial skeleton and spleen. Development 126:5699–5711
128. Tsukamoto Y, Fukutani S, Shinike T, Kubota T, Sato S, Suzuki Y, Mori M (1993) Mineralized nodule formation by cultures of human dental pulp-derived fibroblasts. Arch Oral Biol 37:1045–1055
129. Tsukamoto Y, Fukutani S, Takeuchi S, Tanaka Y, Mori M (1988) Cultivation of fibroblast-like cells derived from human dental pulp, demonstrated 1,25(OH)2D3 sensitive alkaline phosphatase. Jpn J of Oral Biol 30:851–854
130. Tucker A, Sharpe P (2004) The cutting-edge of mammalian development; how the embryo makes teeth. Nat Rev 5:499–508
131. Tziafas D (2004) The future role of a molecular approach to pulp-dentinal regeneration. Caries Res 38:314–320
132. Tziafas D, Hurmerinta K (1990) Inductive influences of demineralized dentin and bone matrix on pulp cells: an approach of secondary dentinogenesis. J Dent Res 69:75–81
133. Vanderschueren D, Gaytant J, Boonen S, Venken K (2008) Androgens and bone. Curr Opin Endocrinol Diabetes Obes 15(3):250–254
134. Vastardis H, Karimbus N, Guthua SW, Seidman JG, Seidman CE (1996) A human MSX1 homeodomain missense mutation causes selective tooth agenesis. Nat Genet 13:417–421
135. Verdelis K, Ling Y, Sreenath T, Haruyama N, MacDougall M, van der Meulen MC, Lukashova L, Spevak L, Kulkarni AB, Boskey AL (2008) DSPP effects on in vivo bone mineralization. Bone 43(6): 983–990
136. Watanabe H, Yamada Y (1999) Mice lacking link protein develop dwarfism and craniofacial abnormalities. Nat Genet 21(2):225–229
137. Watanabe H, Kimata K, Line S, Strong D, Gao LY, Kozak CA, Yamada Y (1994) Mouse cartilage matrix deficiency (cmd) caused by a 7 bp deletion in the aggrecan gene. Nat Genet 7(2):154–157
138. Weiner A, Veis A, Beniash Em Arad T, Dillon JW, Sabsay B, Siddiqui F (1999) Peritubular dentin formation: crystal organization and the macromolecular constituents in human teeth. J Struct Biol 126:27–41
139. Wilkie AO, Tang Z, Elanko N, Walsh S, Twigg SR, Hurst JA, Wall SA, Chrzanowska KH, Maxson RE Jr (2000) Functional haploinsufficiency of the human homeobox gene MSX2 causes defects in skull ossification. Nat Genet 24(4):387–390
140. Witkop CJ (1957) Hereditary defects in enamel and dentin. Acta Genet 7:236–239
141. Xiao S, Yu C, Chou X, Yuan W, Wang Y, Bu L, Fu G, Qian M, Yang J, Shi Y, Hu L, Han B, Wang Z, Huang W, Liu J, Chen Z, Zhao G, Kong X (2001) Dentinogenesis imperfecta 1 with or without progressive hearing loss is associated with distinct mutations in DSPP. Nat Genet 27(2):201–204
142. Xu T, Bianco P, Fisher LW, Longenecker G, Smith E, Goldstein S, Bonadio J, Boskey A, Heegaard AM, Sommer B, Satomura K, Dominguez P, Zhao C, Kulkarni AB, Robey PG, Young MF (1998) Targeted disruption of the biglycan gene leads to an osteoporosis-like phenotype in mice. Nat Genet. 20(1):78–82
143. Yamashiro T, Zheng L, Shitaku Y, Saito M, Tsubakimoto T, Takada K, Takano-Yamomoto T, Thesleff I (2007) Wnt10a regulates dentin sialophosphoprotein mRNA expression and possibly links odontoblast differentiation and tooth morphogenesis. Differentiation 75(5): 452–462
144. Yamakoshi Y, Hu JCC, Fukae M, Zhang H, Simmer JP (2006) Dentin glycoprotein: the protein in the middle

of the dentin sialophophoprotien chimera. J Biol Chem 280(17):17472–17479
145. Yamamoto N, Akiyama S, Katagiri T, Namiki M, Kurokawa T, Suda T (1997) Smad1 and smad5 act downstream of intracellular signalings of BMP-2 that inhibits myogenic differentiation and induces osteoblast differentiation in C2C12 myoblasts. Biochem Biophys Res Commun 238:574–580
146. Yang X, Matsuda K, Bialek P, Jacquot S, Masuoka HC, Schinke T, Li L, Brancorsini S, Sassone-Corsi P, Townes TM, Hanauer A, Karsenty G (2004) ATF4 is a substrate of RSK2 and an essential regulator of osteoblast biology; implication for Coffin-Lowry syndrome. Cell 117(3):387–398
147. Ye L, MacDougall M, Zhang S, Xie Y, Zhang J, Li Z, Lu Y, Mishina Y, Feng JQ (2004) Deletion of dentin matrix protein-1 leads to a partial failure of maturation of predentin into dentin, hypomineralization, and expanded cavities of pulp and root canal during postnatal tooth development. J Biol Chem 279(18): 19141–19148
148. Zhang M, Xuan S, Bouxsein ML, von Stechow D, Akeno N, Faugere MC, Malluche H, Zhao G, Rosen CJ, Efstratiadis A, Clemens TL (2002) Osteoblast-specific knockout of the insulin-like growth factor (IGF) receptor gene reveals an essential role of IGF signaling in bone matrix mineralization. J Biol Chem 277(46):44005–44012
149. Zheng L, Iohara K, Ishikawa M, Into T, Takano-Yamamoto T, Matsushita K, Nakashima M (2007) Runx3 negatively regulates osterix expression in dental pulp cells. Biochem J 405(1):69–75
150. Zhang X, Rahemtulla FG, MacDougall MJ, Thomas HF (2007) Vitamin D receptor deficiency affects dentin maturation in mice. Arch Oral Biol 52(12): 1172–1179
151. Zhang X, Zhao J, Li C, Gao S, Qiu C, Liu P, Wu G, Qiang B, Lo WHY, Shen Y (2001) DSPP mutation in dentinogenesis imperfecta Shields type II. Nat Genet 27:151–152

12. Evolution of Bone Proteins

Eddie Wang and Seung-Wuk Lee

12.1 Introduction

The ability to biomineralize has evolved many times in living organisms. In eukaryotes, various organisms have evolved that form elaborate structures composed of calcium carbonate, calcium phosphate (CaP), or silica [61]. In particular, the advent of CaP biomineralization in vertebrates led to the formation of bone, dentin, and enamel/enameloid. These tissues provided critical improvements to defense, predation, and locomotion, ultimately allowing colonization of dry land [19, 88]. Given the importance of mineralized tissues to the vertebrate way of life, it is important to know how and when these tissues first formed and how they evolved.

Theories on the origins and evolution of vertebrate mineralized tissues initially were based on the fossil record. Subsequently, molecular biologists began to isolate and characterize the active proteins that control mineralization. More recently, bolstered by the influx of new genome sequencing data, evolutionary biologists have pieced together the origins of the proteins. This chapter will focus on recent discoveries in the evolution of mineralized tissue proteins (MTPs). In addition, we will highlight how directed evolution is being harnessed to learn more about the mechanisms by which MTPs control mineral growth and to create new molecules for modulating CaP biomineralization.

Over 200 proteins have been identified in bone, most of which originate in the serum [18, 79]. The genes giving rise to these proteins include genes for transcription factors, signaling molecules, their receptors, and their downstream signaling proteins. Many of these genes are orthologous or paralogous to genes that exist throughout metazoans. This chapter will therefore review the genes of extracellular matrix (ECM) proteins, because many are specific to mineralized tissues, with no counterparts in tissues of nonmineralizing animals.

12.2 Gene Duplication

An important concept to review in this chapter is gene duplication, a process that gives rise to new genetic material subject to mutation and selection. The redundancy of the duplicate allows for mutations to accumulate [41, 46, 72, 108]. These mutations may be deleterious, leading to loss of function and pseudogenization [64, 97, 108]. On the other hand, the duplicate may survive, maintaining its original function, taking on part of the function of its parent gene (subfunctionalization), or obtaining a new function (neofunctionalization) [28, 105, 108].

Gene duplication generally occurs in three ways: (1) Unequal crossing over, which generates linked genes on a chromosome (tandem duplication);

F. Bronner et al. (eds.), *Bone and Development*, Topics in Bone Biology 6,
DOI 10.1007/978-1-84882-822-3_12, © Springer-Verlag London Limited 2010

(2) Retroposition, which involves RNA being retrotranscribed to DNA and inserted into the genome; or (3) chromosomal/whole-genome duplication (WGD) [108]. WGD produces many duplicate genes that co-evolve to form new gene networks. The potential effects of WGD are especially pronounced because genes produced by WGD survive better than genes copied in smaller scale duplications [12].

First proposed in a seminal work by Susumu Ohno and now known as the 2R hypothesis, vertebrate genomes are believed to have undergone two rounds of WGD in relatively quick succession [16, 72]. The results of the 2R hypothesis can be seen in the genomes of jawed vertebrates where sets of paralogous genes are located on multiple chromosomes, whereas in urochordates and cephalochordates there is only one set of corresponding linked genes [46, 62, 74]. Importantly, as has been demonstrated for the HOX gene clusters and others, WGD also results in the duplication of the clusters' adjacent regions [46]. The first vertebrate WGD is believed to have occurred before the split between jawless fish (Agnatha) and the jawed vertebrates (Gnathostomata) (Fig. 12.1a), while the second occurred prior to the split between cartilagenous fish (Chondrichthyes) and bony fish (Osteichthyes) (Fig. 12.1b) [71]. In addition, Hufton et al. have proposed that the era prior to the first WGD was

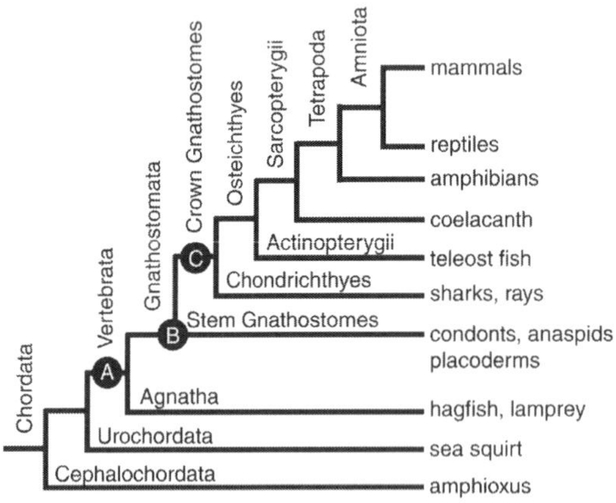

Figure 12.1. Phylogeny of Chordates. (A) First whole-genome duplication, possible emergence of MGP, and pro-α1(II) precursor from fibrillar clade A collagen ancestor. (B) Second whole-genome duplication. Possible emergence of BGP precursor from MGP and SPARCL1 precursor from SPARC. (C) Origin of endochondral bone [52, 55, 71, 77].

characterized by widespread genome rearrangement [41]. The timing of the large-scale gene duplications at the dawn of vertebrates suggests that these duplications were critical to forming the precursors of genes that ultimately gave rise to modern-day vertebrate mineralization.

12.3 Collagens

No discussion of proteins related to mineralized tissue can exclude collagens, inasmuch as they comprise 85–90% of the organic matrix of bone [61]. Other than in enamel, fibrillar collagens act as the scaffolds on which CaP is mineralized. Type I collagen is mineralized in bone, the non-enamel portions of teeth, tendons, and ligaments, whereas mineralized cartilage contains mostly type II collagen [8]. Fibrillar collagens are not limited to mineralized tissues or to organisms with mineralized components. Fibrillar collagens are in fact a conserved feature of almost all multicellular animals from sponges to humans [6]. The pervasiveness of collagens emphasizes their importance in the survival and development of metazoan lineages.

Vertebrate fibrillar collagens can be divided into three clades (A–C). The A clade includes collagen types I–III and the pro-α2(V) chain; the B clade includes the pro-α1(V), pro-α3(V), and type XI chains; and the C clade includes pro-α1(XXIV) and pro-α1(XXVII), which are expressed in mineralized bone and cartilage, respectively [7, 95]. Their sequences have the same general composition. The procollagen fibril is composed of three pro-α chains, with each chain composed of an uninterrupted central triple helical collagenous domain of ~338 Gly-Xaa-Yaa triplets flanked by an N-propeptide and a C-propeptide [1, 24]. The C-propeptide contains the most conserved region and is necessary for α chain recognition [1]. The N-propeptide of clade A collagens contains a von Willebrand factor-type C module, whereas clades B and C contain thrombospondin amino-terminal-like domain modules. Clades A and B collagens contain a minor triple helix in the N-propeptide, which is absent in Clade C collagens. In addition, Clade C collagens have a shorter major triple helix that contains multiple points where the perfect repeats of Gly-Xaa-Yaa are broken. Finally, Clade A and B vertebrate collagens have longer chain recognition sequences in their C-propeptide than Clade C and invertebrate fibrillar collagens [1, 95].

At the DNA level, the central triple-helical domain of collagen is coded by exons that are multiples of 54 base pairs (bp) or multiples of 54–9 bp (e.g., 99 bp). Amazingly, this gene structure is also seen in sponge collagens. This suggests a strong selective pressure to maintain the size and organization of the collagenous sequence [24, 25]. It is postulated that the ancestral fibrillar collagen gene was created by multiple duplications of an ancient 54 bp exon and that unequal crossing-over led to a 54 + 45 bp exon [24, 103]. The identity and role of the 54 bp exon before the appearance of collagen, however, is unknown. Collagen-like domains have been identified in various prokaryotic and viral proteins; however, there is insufficient evidence to suggest that either is related to the ancestor of modern collagens [24, 92].

Several studies have attempted to tackle the questions of how and when orthologs to the vertebrate fibrillar collagen clades arose. Boot-Handford and colleagues have postulated that the three clades emerged in the common ancestor of vertebrates [6]. Their reasoning is based on the absence of the extended C-propeptide chain selection sequence in invertebrates and that insertion of the extended chain selection sequence must have occurred in the vertebrate ancestor by a rare genomic event. This ancestral collagen was then duplicated to form the ancestors of the A and B clades, with further duplications leading to the various members of the clades [6]. In contrast, Aouacheria and collaborators [1] argued that divergence into three clades occurred far earlier. Their hypothesis is based on the fact that certain invertebrate protostome collagens were grouped more closely to one clade than another and that it was unlikely for the lengthened chain selection sequence to be gained and then lost in clade C [14]. They proposed that because the extended chain selection sequence region appeared to be in a highly divergent area of the sequence, the lengthened sequences were not due to a rare genomic event but rather the result of "a long evolutionary process" [1]. In agreement with Aouacheria et al. [1], a study of deuterostome fibrillar collagen genes by Wada et al. [95] linked fibrillar collagens from amphioxus, ascidians, and echinoderms to clades A–C; this suggests that the gene duplications that led to the three clades predated the split between echinoderms and chordates [95]. Results by Wasa et al. [95] point toward independent convergent insertion of longer chain selection sequences in clades A and B. In a recent follow-up study, Exposito et al. [25] analyzed the sequences of sponge and sea anemone fibrillar collagens and concluded that ancestral orthologs to the three vertebrate clades may have formed before the divergence of sponges.

In mammals, the clade A fibrillar collagens are each linked to Hox gene clusters (COL1A2 to HOXA, COL1A1 to HOXB, COL2A1 to HOXC, COL5A2 and COL3A1 to HOXD); this may mean that the fibrillar collagens were duplicated along with the Hox genes in the same WGD events [1, 3]. Analysis of Hox clusters and collagen genes indicated that three events gave rise to collagens type I and II: first, an ancestral collagen duplicated into precursors of pro-α2(V) and a type I and II ancestor. Then, one duplication led to pro-α2(I) and another led to the pro-α1(I) and pro-α1(II) lineage [3, 68]. Although the three-step gene duplication pathway seems inconsistent with two rounds of WGD, it may be an artifact and therefore may not contradict the 2R hypothesis [46]. Experimental results agree with the theory that the modern clade A collagens appeared at the time of WGDs. Specifically, collagen pro-α1(II) was identified in hagfish and lampreys while only an undifferentiated, ancestral clade A like collagen was found in lancelets. This means that the duplication that led to the formation of pro-α1(II) must have occurred in stem vertebrates before the split between agnathans and gnathostomes, a period in time that corresponds to the first vertebrate WGD [107]. Whether or not the collagen type I precursor formed at the same time is not known. The concomitant formation of new fibrillar collagen types with an increase in the number of genes available for evolution by WGD may have been a driving force for the formation of new, specialized vertebrate tissues [107].

The presence of Type I collagen in multiple tissues and the overall ubiquity of fibrillar collagens among metazoans suggests that although collagen is the mineralization substrate, it is not the only determinant of hard tissue mineralization. Accordingly, in vitro systems designed to mineralize collagen fibrils in the absence of additives or serum have often failed to reconstitute the structural characteristics of natural mineralized collagen [73]. This points to the importance of noncollagenous proteins in regulating collagen mineralization.

12.4 BGP and MGP

Members of the Vitamin K-dependent (VKD) protein family are characterized by posttranslational modification of glutamic acid residues to γ-carboxyglutamic acid (Gla) [55]. Amongst the VKD protein family, BGP (Bone Gla protein, aka osteocalcin) and MGP (Matrix Gla protein) play regulatory roles in skeletal and dental mineralization and maintenance, although the exact nature of their role is not known.

MGP is a 10 kDa protein expressed in fetal and adult tissues, but accumulates predominantly in cartilage, bone, and dentin [11, 29, 55], where it inhibits calcification. In chick embryo limb buds, overexpression of MGP inhibits cartilage mineralization and prevents endochondral ossification; MGP knockout or mutant mice exhibit abnormal calcification of cartilage and arteries [63, 102].

BGP is a 5.6 kDa protein secreted by osteoblasts and odontoblasts [55, 78]. Unlike MGP, it is specific to calcified tissues, although a small amount enters the circulation. BGP is one of the most abundant noncollagenous proteins in bone, yet its function is unknown. It may have a role in the regulation of mineral turnover. The bone mass of BGP-deficient mice is greater and the degree of mineral maturation higher than in controls [9, 21]. BGP acts as a chemoattractant for osteoclast-like cells, possibly in combination with osteopontin [13, 82]. On the basis of recent results, non-Gla-modified BGP may act as a hormone that is involved in the regulation of energy metabolism [56]. Structurally, the Gla residues are critical determinants of hydroxyapatite and calcium-binding affinity and protein conformation [20, 38, 70].

Gene sequencing, multiple sequence alignment, and phylogenetic analysis have helped elucidate the evolutionary link between BGP and MGP. In the most comprehensive analysis, Laize et al. [55] examined 28 BGP and 20 MGP sequences and found BGP and MGP genes to be organized into four exons and three introns, with the intron phase conserved among BGP and MGP sequences. In addition, the relative exon lengths are also conserved. The presence of conserved residues (23 in MGP and 20 in BGP), critical for protein structure or function, made it possible to identify several conserved sequence motifs, including a transmembrane signal peptide, a γ-carboxyglutamyl carboxylase targeting site, two invariable cysteine residues involved in disulfide formation, proteolytic cleavage sites, a C-terminal carboxypeptidase processing site, and a C-terminal Gla domain. In the latter, most glutamates are carboxylated and the domain includes a conserved motif involved in γ-carboxyglutamyl carboxylase recognition. In addition, the presence of a conserved MGP phosphorylation motif was established. Further evidence of the relationship between MGP and BGP is that the exons of each gene encode the same domains in each protein. For example, exon 1 always codes for the transmembrane signal peptide and its cleavage site.

The origins of MGP and BGP can also be inferred from phylogenetic analysis. Molecular clock calculations placed the origin of MGP at 480 ± 133 Myr ago and the origin of BGP at 381 ± 102 Myr ago [55]. It is very likely that the similarity of BGP and MGP is due to gene duplication rather than convergence. Laize et al. [55] postulate that the first round of vertebrate WGD led to the formation of the MGP precursor gene and then to the evolution of cartilage, while the second round of WGD led to the formation of the BGP gene precursor by duplication of MGP. The origins of BGP and MGP are consistent with the fact that they have no identified homologs in nonvertebrates including *Ciona intestinalis*, the closest sequenced nonvertebrate ancestor of vertebrates. Further evidence that MGP evolved first is that an MGP-like immunoreactive protein, but no BGP, was identified in lamprey and that, unlike MGP, no BGP has been identified in cartilaginous fish. Finally, these findings indicate that BGP was not involved in the earliest instances of tissue mineralization. This is because the absence of BGP from sharks suggests that the stem group vertebrates, the first group to have mineralized tissues, also lacked BGP [48].

12.5 Secretory Calcium-Binding Phosphoproteins

In a series of studies, Kawasaki et al. [50] have shown that many of the matrix proteins involved in bone and tooth mineralization can be grouped into a family with the same evolutionary origin and named it the secretory calcium-binding phosphoprotein (SCPP) family. The family includes dentin/bone, enamel, salivary, and milk proteins. The SCPPs of dentin/bone form a subfamily including dentin sialophosphoprotein (DSPP), dentin matrix acidic phosphoprotein I (DMPI), integrin-binding sialoprotein, ak a bone sialoprotein (BSP), matrix extracellular phosphoglycoprotein (MEPE) and secreted phosphoprotein 1, aka osteopontin (OPN). Bone and dentin both contain the five proteins (DSPP, DMPI, BSP, MEPE, OPN), but the relative amounts differ in each [47]. Enamel matrix proteins (EMPs) form another SCPP subfamily. They include enamel matrix protein (EMP), amelogenin (AMEL), ameloblastin (AMBN), amelotin (AMTN), odontogenic ameloblast-associated protein (ODAM), and enamelin (ENAM), all secreted by ameloblasts. Table 12.1 lists the SCPPs associated with mineralized tissue. Related to the enamel genes are the milk caseins and salivary proteins, including statherin and histatins 1 and 3.

Table 12.1. List of Mineralized Tissue Associated SCPPs and their precursors SPARC and SPARCL1

Gene symbol	Protein name	Mineralized tissue distribution
SPARC	Secreted protein, acidic, cysteine-rich (osteonectin)	Dentin/bone
SPARCL1	Secreted protein, acidic, cysteine-rich like 1 protein	–
DSPP[a]	Dentin sialophosphoprotein	Dentin/bone
DMP1[a]	Dentin matrix acidic phosphoprotein 1	Dentin/bone
IBSP (BSP)[a]	Integrin-binding sialoprotein (bone sialoprotein)	Dentin/bone
MEPE[a]	Matrix extracellular phosphoglycoprotein	Dentin/bone
SPP1 (OPN)[a]	Secreted phosphoprotein 1 (Osteopontin)	Dentin/bone
AMEL	Amelogenin	Enamel
ENAM[a]	Enamelin	Enamel
AMBN	Ameloblastin	Enamel
AMTN	Amelotin	Enamel
ODAM	Odontogenic, ameloblast-associated protein	Enamel, milk, saliva

[a]SIBLING Family Proteins [26].
Source: From Kawasaki and Weiss [52].

The protein sequences of the SCPP family show very limited sequence homology and therefore their evolutionary relationships were determined by similarities in biochemical characteristics and gene structure. Biochemically, the proteins are all secreted, as indicated by the presence of a signal peptide; most are enriched with negatively charged acidic amino acids (Asp and Glu). Almost all have one or more Ser-Xaa-Glu (SXE) motifs, where the serine residues are often phosphorylated and all have sequences rich in Pro, Gln, Arg, Lys, and Ser residues and poor in Cys residues [43]. The concentration of negatively charged acidic amino acids including phosphoserine allows these proteins to interact strongly with calcium ions or calcium-bearing mineral surfaces [47, 50]. However, their amino acid distributions indicate instrinsically disordered structures [43]. In terms of gene structure, the SCPP genes have a 5′ untranslated region spanning all of exon 1 and the 5′ end of exon 2. They have their entire signal peptide and mature protein N-terminus coded by exon 2, and their introns are all phase 0 (intron–exon boundaries between codons) [47,50]. Finally, except for amelogenin, which was translocated to the X-chromosome, all SCPP genes are clustered into two regions on chromosome 4 [50]. One cluster contains the dentin/bone proteins, while the other contains the EMPs, saliva, and milk proteins. The split between the genes is probably the result of intrachromosomal rearrangement that took place before the split of ray-finned and lobe-finned fish [47]. The close arrangement of SCPPs on a single chromosome suggests that they were formed by tandem duplication and may have been subject to common spatial and temporal regulation gene regulation [50].

Within the SCPP family, the dentin/bone proteins form a subgroup known as the small integrin-binding ligand N-linked glycoproteins (SIBLING) [26, 27]. ENAM is also considered to be a distantly related member [26, 43]. Based on their gene structure and biochemical similarities, SIBLING proteins are believed to have arisen from a common ancestor, although the exact order and timing of th eir evolution remains unknown. The SIBLING proteins have similar gene structures. Exon 3 contains a casein kinase II phosphorylation site (SSEE); exon 4 has a proline-rich region, whereas exon 5 often contains a second casein kinase II site. Exons 4 and 5 contain the integrin-binding RGD sequence. The phosphorylation sites are often within acidic serine–aspartate-rich MEPE-associated motifs (ASARM) [8, 84]. The SIBLING proteins are typically rich in acidic amino acid residues and are extensively modified posttranslationally by phosphorylation, sulfation, and glycosylation [27]. Based on their primary sequence, the SIBLING proteins seem intrinsically disordered. This was confirmed for BSP and OPN, both are unstructured [27]. Structural flexibility is common for protein domains that have multiple binding partners, even though, on binding, the proteins may take on a single conformation [26]. Known binding partners of members of the SIBLING family include bone/tooth mineral, integrins, collagen, complement Factor H, and CD44 [8, 26, 27]. Importantly, many of the SIBLING proteins can be fragmented proteolytically into active segments. Segments for DSPP are dentin sialoprotein, dentin phosphophoryn, and dentin glycoprotein [52, 104]. SIBLING proteins and their active fragments inhibit and nucleate hydroxyapatite in vitro, the degree and end result depending on concentration, degree of posttranslational modification, and mobility (in solution or adsorbed) [8, 36, 42]. Sibling protein knockout studies have led to normally formed or somewhat altered, but grossly functional, bones and teeth [8, 26].

The EMPs form a second subfamily among SCPPs and are also believed to have been formed from a common ancestor by tandem gene duplication [88]. They are expressed by ameloblasts, have conserved features in their N-terminal regions, but are highly divergent in the other molecular regions and are considered more proline/glutamine (P/Q) rich than the acidic dentin/bone proteins [47, 88]. The phylogeny of EMPs is controversial, possibly due to the limited number of available non-mammalian sequences [50, 88]. Sire et al. [88], in a recent and extensive study, have shown that an ancestral ENAM was duplicated to form the precursors of ODAM, AMTN, and AMBN. The ancestral AMBN was then duplicated to form the precursors of AMEL and of modern AMBN (Fig. 12.2) [88]. The view that an ancestral ENAM protein is the precursor to all EMPs is in agreement with the classification of ENAM as a more distantly related SIBLING protein.

Casein genes have evolved from a common ancestor, as did the statherin/histatins [50, 86, 106]. They and the salivary SCPPs maintain the solubility of calcium phosphate in the supersaturated environments of milk and saliva [31, 40]. These proteins are absent in nonmammalian tetrapods and have arisen from an EMP in stem group mammals [47].

SPARCL1 (secreted protein, acidic, cysteine-rich like 1 protein) is the ancestor of the SCPP

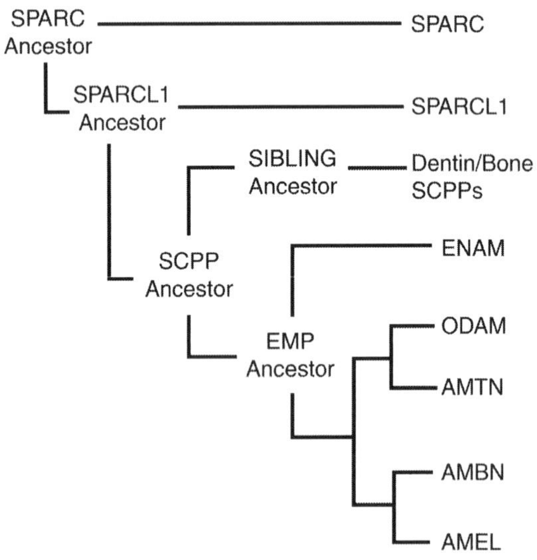

Figure 12.2. Proposed evolutionary origin of SCPPs beginning with SPARC (Osteonectin). Adapted from Sire et al. [88] (with permission from Karger, Basel).

genes. It was formed by duplication of SPARC, also known as osteonectin. SPARC and SPARCL1 are multifunctional, and are associated with proteins, cations, growth factors, and cells [47]. SPARC is an ancient gene present in protostomes and deuterostomes and in humans is one of the most abundant noncollagenous proteins in dentin and bone [51]. SPARCL1 is expressed primarily in the brain [47]. Evidence for SPARC and SPARCL1 being ancestral to the SCPP genes can be derived from their biochemical and gene structures. Both proteins are composed of three domains, where domain I, like SCPPs, is intrinsically disordered [47]. Domain I of SPARCL1 has an amino acid composition similar to SCPPs, is larger (414 amino acids vs. 52 in SPARC), and contains 104 acidic and 55 basic amino acids, compared with the 18 acidic amino acids in SPARC [47]. In addition, it contains multiple SXE motifs (nine in humans, compared with two in SPARC [51]). The concentration of acidic amino acids allows both proteins to bind calcium ions weakly [47]. At the genetic level, SPARC and SPARCL1, like the SCPPs, have a signal peptide coded in exon 2 and all introns are phase-0 in domain I [50]. At the genome level, SPARCL1 is on chromosome 4, adjacent to the dentin/bone SCPP cluster, whereas SPARC is on chromosome 5. SPARCL1 may therefore have arisen from duplication of SPARC and obtained its larger, disordered domain 1 subsequently. The SCPP genes would then have arisen from SPARCL1's domain 1 by tandem duplication [48]. Phylogenetic evidence suggests that the duplication event that led to SPARCL1 occurred in the Paleozoic jawless vertebrates and coincided with the development of mineralized skeletons based on the fossil record. This would have occurred before the divergence of sharks and bony fish and after the origin of the lamprey (Fig. 12.1a). On the basis of the timing and chromosomal locations of SPARC and SPARCL1, their duplication probably occurred during the second WGD [47].

Kawasaki et al. [47] postulate that skeletal mineralization initially relied on SPARC and perhaps non-SCPP proteins. They reason that because many SCPP genes are specialized for mineralization, they may have arisen in the course of modification of mineralized tissues, rather than having arisen before mineralization and then being co-opted. Kawasaki et al. also postulate that because collagen type IV associated SPARC is a conserved feature of basal lamina, it would have been co-opted in the initial formation of the most primitive mineralized tissues of the dermal skeleton, which formed adjacent to the basal lamina [47]. Furthermore, in teleosts and tetrapods, SPARC is involved in maturation of collagen type I and III fibrils and remains one of the major noncollagenous proteins in bone, dentin, and enameloid [39, 51]. They also propose that the association of SPARC with mineralized cartilage in mammals suggests that the machinery involved in the mineralization of the more primitive dermal skeletal (SPARC and fibrillar collagen) was acquired for endoskeletal cartilage mineralization, which eventually evolved to endochondral bone [48].

The creation and diversification of SCPP proteins is very likely to have followed the origin of SPARCL1 by reiterative tandem gene duplication. The SCPPs would then have evolved at the latest before ray-finned (Actinopterygii) and lobe-finned (Sarcopterygii) first diverged, inasmuch as OPN exists in both lineages [52]. The intrinsically disordered nature of the SCPPs may have allowed for the variation seen in their sequences because genes for disordered proteins often exhibit higher evolutionary rates [22]. Presumably this is true because, unlike tightly folded proteins, there are only a few essential residues that must be conserved to ensure folding; in other words, the functional constraints are weak. In addition to having all phase-0 introns, neither exon duplication nor deletions have altered the reading frame. Donoghue et al. [77] posit that the diversity of bone, dentin, enamel, or enameloid tissues in the early vertebrates was due to a lack of SCPP diversity and a corresponding lack of mineralization control. As the SCPPs evolved, the tissues formed became more alike, because of an increased regulation of mineralization [77]. Interestingly, although different lineages have developed functionally equivalent tissues such as teeth in teleosts and tetrapods, they use different sets of SCPPs. For example, the enameloid of teleost teeth is compositionally different from tetrapod enamel and none of the seven fugu SCPP genes are orthologous to tetrapod SCPP genes. This suggests that traits such as teeth were maintained by phenogenetic drift, whereas the SCPP genes for enamel or enameloid arose independently by parallel gene duplication [49].

The above summary of SCPP protein phylogeny is based predominantly on the reports by Kawasaki et al. [47, 48, 50, 51]. Although the relationship between SPARC, SPARCL1, and SCPPs is no longer subject to debate, the exact details and timing of the development of each gene is by no means certain. For example, the analysis of EMP genes by Sire et al. [88, 89] placed the ancestral AMBN/AMEL duplication event at >600 Mya, that is before the appearance of vertebrates. This would mean that the SPARC/SPARCL1 duplication occurred even earlier and further implies that SCPPs had already diverged prior to the development of vertebrate mineralization [88]. This contradicts the origin of mineralization proposed by Kawasaki and colleagues, but accords with the report by Delgado et al. [17]. The presence of enamel/enameloid and dentin-like structures in the earliest mineralized vertebrates (~500 Mya) also suggests that tissue-specific SCPPs had already evolved prior to the advent of any skeletal mineralization [77, 88]. These discrepancies indicate that much work remains to be done in determining the evolutionary origins of bone-related proteins, work that will most likely be dependent on the accumulation of more sequence data and a clearer dating of the second WGD.

12.6 Small Leucine-Rich Proteoglycans

Small leucine-rich proteoglycans (SLRPs) are ECM molecules that contain chondroitin/dermatan sulfate or keratan sulfate glycosaminoglycan chains. Members of the SLRP family include biglycan, decorin, lumican, osteoadherin, osteoglycin, proline arginine-rich and leucine-rich protein, keratocan, chondroadherin, podocan, and epiphycan [44, 66]. Several of the SLRPs have been identified in developing and mature bones and teeth, although their expression, except for osteoadherin, is not limited to mineralized tissues [66, 80, 96]. The SLRPs typically have a negatively charged glycosylated amino-terminal and a central domain that contains leucine-rich repeats (LRR), flanked by cysteine clusters [66]. In vitro and in vivo studies on the role of SLRPs, mostly biglycan and decorin, in mineralized tissue have shown that SLRPs can regulate collagen fibrillogenesis, direct osteoblast/clast cell behavior, and nucleate or inhibit mineralization [10, 67, 80, 93, 96].

SLRPs are a branch of the LRR protein superfamily of which more than 100 have been identified [44, 66]. The SLRPs have been further subdivided into four classes, with class IV, containing chondroadherin, being most distantly related. Phylogenetic analysis [44] comparing human SLRPs with those of the tunicate, *C. intestinalis*, suggests that, like the SCPPs, modern vertebrate SLRPs arose as the result of tandem and large-scale/whole-genome duplications. According to Huxley-Jones et al. [44], class I–III and class IV SLRPs had already diverged before the urochordates. Meanwhile, SLRPs in classes I-III diverged from a common ancestor after the divergence of urochordates had divided [44]. More detailed divergence dates await analysis of SLRPs from more species.

12.7 Directed Evolution of Apatite Binding Peptides

Understanding the details of the interactions between proteins and crystals is inherently difficult. In the case of mineralized tissues, tissue heterogeneity, a lack of protein structural data, the multifunctionality of associated proteins, and the complicated mineral structure of biological hydroxyapatite (HAP) make the problem particularly difficult. To generate more tractable systems, scientists mimic the process of evolution on a rapid time scale, using many biological display platforms, including bacteria [15, 87], viruses [90, 91], yeast [5, 75], mRNA [83, 101], and ribosomes [33, 37] to identify specific peptide and protein ligands for a variety of targets [2, 45, 54, 69, 87, 91, 109]. Sequences identified by these methods are often easier to investigate because they have been selected for a single trait (e.g., binding, catalytic efficiency) in well-defined environments (biological buffers) and can be very short (seven amino acids). Using these methods will help identify functional information associated with protein–protein and protein–crystal interface interactions.

Of these methods, phage display is one of the most popular, because it is fast and readily allows users to link phenotype and genotype [57, 69, 87, 91, 100]. The phage, typically M13 bacteriophage, is a bacterial virus made up of single-stranded DNA encapsulated by multiple coat proteins. The insertion of randomized gene sequences into the phage genome creates a highly diverse, combinatorial library of peptides (up to 10^{11} random sequences) that can be displayed on the surface coat proteins [32, 57, 76, 87, 91, 100]. To isolate the best binding peptides for a given target, the phage library pool goes through several rounds of selection in which nonbinding or weakly binding phage are removed. Recently, phage display has been successfully employed to identify important binding motif information between protein and crystal interfaces [57, 65, 81, 87, 100]. Some of the peptide binding motifs can also modulate crystal nucleation [32, 65].

Phage display has also been used to identify ligands for various synthetic HAP crystal surfaces. Table 12.2 shows the sequences of identified HAP binding peptides [4, 32, 85]. Even though the binding peptide sequences for the apatite crystal differ, they also exhibit characteristics in the major bone- and tooth- associated proteins that suggest that they may be useful as model systems for studying bone-related proteins. Gungormus et al. [32] have identified two disulfide bond constrained 7mer peptides, one of which is a strong binder, HABP1 (CMLPHHWGC) that inhibits mineralization, at the same time increasing the rate of conversion of amorphous calcium phosphate to octacalcium phosphate in mineralization studies in vitro. Circular dichroism studies indicate that like many SCPPs, HABP1 has conformational instability that may be crucial for its activity. Roy et al. [53] have isolated the peptide HA 6–1 (SVSVGMKPSPRP) now considered a "super infectious" sequence [53]. This sequence has greater binding affinity for hydroxyapatite and tooth mineral over calcium carbonate and amorphous calcium phosphate [85]. Sequence analysis of HA 6–1 has identified homology between that sequence and phosphate-binding proteins; this implies that HA 6–1 interacts with phosphate ions of hydroxyapatite (HAP). Recently, single crystal HAP binding peptides have been identified. The dominant 12mer peptide (NPYHPTIPQSVH: termed CLP12) selected against well-defined single HAP crystals. It possessed repeating proline residues at positions having an i and i + 3n relationship (positions 2, 5, and 8) and at periodic hydroxylated residues (positions 3, 6, and 10), somewhat reminiscent of the Pro-X-Y repeats found in amelogenin. When other phage libraries were used, the resulting sequences showed similar features in terms of amino acid/functional group composition. Because of the negatively charged surface of the HAP crystal at pH 7.5, the resulting HAP-binding peptides possessed mainly positively charged residues [34]. When phage display was performed on the single crystal HAP in acidic pH, the HAP surfaces became slightly positively charged and the resulting binding sequences exhibited tripeptide repeats of (–OH)(–OH)(–COOH) (–OH: hydroxylated amino acid residues; –COOH: carboxylated amino acid rcsidues). The best binding sequences showed a sequence similar to that found at the N-terminus of statherin. Interestingly, the (–OH)(–OH)(–COOH) motif is similar to the SXE motifs found in SCPPs and was isolated by phage display, even though it does not bear any phosphorylated serines. Phage display libraries currently do not contain phosphorylated series, but work

Table 12.2. Hydroxyapatite Binding Pept ides

Name	Sequence	Library used	Reference
HABP1	CMLPHHWGC	7mer constrained (pIII)	[32]
HABP2	CNPGFAQAC	12mer peptide (pIII)	[32]
HA 6–1	SVSVGMKPSPRP	12mer peptide (pIII)	[85]
CLP12	NPYHPTIPQSVH	12mer peptide (pIII)	[4]
CLP7	CNYPTLKSC	7mer constrained	[4]
CLP8	VAPASPDS	8mer pVIII	
DPLP8	VPASSEAS	8mer pVIII	
DPLP12	ATDTSDKLSMVK	12mer	

is underway to include such posttranslationally modified amino acids [59].

12.8 Value and Application of Evolutionary Studies

Research into the evolution of mineralizing proteins can provide useful information for biology and medicine. For example, sequence analysis that identifies evolutionarily conserved residues in specific proteins and conserved motifs in protein families has made it possible to isolate sequences that are critical for enamel genes [88, 89]. Another example is the utilization of a motif from DMP1 to create synthetic proteins that allow studies on the effects of motif location on CaP mineralization [94]. More broadly, having recognized the conserved anionic nature of BGP, MGP, and the SCPPs and its importance for interacting with bone mineral, scientists have begun using polyanionic molecules to study and direct CaP mineralization, as well as to design new bone moieties for targeted drug delivery [35, 58, 73, 98]. Evolutionary analysis based on gene and protein sequences also allows better searches for new mineralization proteins.

Finally, by understanding the beginnings of mineralization, components can be identified that are necessary to create biomineralized systems. For example, the distribution of SCPPs suggests that they do not specify the crystal type; rather crystal type is determined by the ionic environment. Another example is the bird SCPP, OC116, which associates with calcium carbonate rather than calcium phosphate to form eggshell. Osteopontin associates with calcium phosphate and calcium carbonate in eggshells and otoconia, and with calcium oxalate in urinary stones [30, 51, 99]. The sequences of proteins that are involved in calcium carbonate mineralization in invertebrates share characteristics with bone/tooth-related proteins. This suggests that toolkits for calcium mineralization are similar throughout the animal kingdom [60]. In other words, evolutionary analysis of mineral-related proteins from vertebrates also has implications for biomineralization in nonvertebrates.

12.9 Conclusion

The origins and evolutionary pathway of vertebrate mineralization remain a subject of debate [77]. However, with each sequenced genome, the picture is becoming clearer. Findings from evolutionary studies can then be integrated with those from other biological disciplines to help understand how mineralized tissues form and to aid in the creation of new molecules for the regulation of mineralized tissue.

Acknowledgment

This work was supported by a National Science Foundation Early Career Development Award (DMR-0747713), start-up funds from the Nanoscience and Nanotechnology Institute at the University of California, Berkeley, and the Laboratory Directed Research and Development Fund from the Lawrence Berkeley National Laboratory.

References

1. Aouacheria A, Cluzel C, Lethias C, Gouy M, Garrone R, Exposito JY (2004) Invertebrate data predict an early emergence of vertebrate fibrillar collagen clades and an anti-incest model. J Biol Chem 279: 47711–47719
2. Arnold FH, Wintrode PL, Miyazaki K, Gershenson A (2001) How enzymes adapt: lessons from directed evolution. Trends Biochem Sci 26:100–106
3. Bailey WJ, Kim J, Wagner GP, Ruddle FH (1997) Phylogenetic reconstruction of vertebrate Hox cluster duplications. Mol Biol Evol 14:843–853
4. Bertozzi CR, Song J, Lee S-W (2006) Hydroxyapatite-binding peptides for bone growth and inhibition. World Patent WO/2006/062776
5. Boder ET, Wittrup KD (1997) Yeast surface display for screening combinatorial polypeptide libraries. Nat Biotechnol 15:553–557
6. Boot-Handford RP, Tuckwell DS (2003) Fibrillar collagen: the key to vertebrate evolution? A tale of molecular incest. Bioessays 25:142–151
7. Boot-Handford RP, Tuckwell DS, Plumb DA, Rock CF, Poulsom R (2003) A novel and highly conserved collagen (pro alpha 1(XXVII)) with a unique expression pattern and unusual molecular characteristics establishes a new clade within the vertebrate fibrillar collagen family. J Biol Chem 278:31067–31077

8. Boskey AL (2008) Mechanism of mineralization of collagen-based connective tissues. In: Sigel A, Sigel H, Sigel RKO (eds) Biomineralization from nature to application. Wiley, West Sussex, pp 457–505
9. Boskey AL, Gadaleta S, Gundberg C, Doty SB, Ducy P, Karsenty G (1998) Fourier transform infrared microspectroscopic analysis of bones of osteocalcin-deficient mice provides insight into the function of osteocalcin. Bone 23:187–196
10. Boskey AL, Spevak L, Doty SB, Rosenberg L (1997) Effects of bone CS-proteoglycans, DS-decorin, and DS-biglycan on hydroxyapatite formation in a gelatin gel. Calcif Tissue Int 61:298–305
11. Cancela ML, Ohresser MCP, Reia JP, Viegas CSB, Williamson MK, Price PA (2001) Matrix Gla protein in *Xenopus laevis*: molecular cloning, tissue distribution, and evolutionary considerations. J Bone Miner Res 16: 1611–1621
12. Chain FJ, Ilieva D, Evans BJ (2008) Duplicate gene evolution and expression in the wake of vertebrate allopolyploidization. BMC Evol Biol 8:43
13. Chenu C, Colucci S, Grano M, Zigrino P, Barattolo R, Zambonin G, Baldini N, Vergnaud P, Delmas PD, Zallone AZ (1994) Osteocalcin induces chemotaxis, secretion of matrix proteins, and calcium-mediated intracellular signaling in human osteoclast-like cells. J Cell Biol 127:1149–1158
14. Cluzel C, Lethias C, Garrone R, Exposito JY (2004) Distinct maturations of N-propeptide domains in fibrillar procollagen molecules involved in the formation of heterotypic fibrils in adult sea urchin collagenous tissues. J Biol Chem 279:9811–9817
15. Daugherty PS, Chen G, Olsen MJ, Iverson BL, Georgiou G (1998) Antibody affinity maturation using bacterial surface display. Protein Eng 11:825–832
16. Dehal P, Boore JL (2005) Two rounds of whole genome duplication in the ancestral vertebrate. Plos Biol 3:1700–1708
17. Delgado S, Casane D, Bonnaud L, Laurin M, Sire JY, Girondot M (2001) Molecular evidence for precambrian origin of amelogenin, the major protein of vertebrate enamel. Mol Biol Evol 18:2146–2153
18. Delmas P, Tracy R, Riggs B, Mann K (1984) Identification of the noncollagenous proteins of bovine bone by two-dimensional gel electrophoresis. Calcif Tissue Int 36:308–316
19. Donoghue PC, Sansom IJ (2002) Origin and early evolution of vertebrate skeletonization. Microsc Res Tech 59:352–372
20. Dowd TL, Rosen JF, Li L, Gundberg CM (2003) The three-dimensional structure of bovine calcium ion-bound osteocalcin using HNMR spectroscopy. Biochemistry 42:7769–7779
21. Ducy P, Desbois C, Boyce B, Pinero G, Story B, Dunstan C, Smith E, Bonadio J, Goldstein S, Gundberg C, Bradley A, Karsenty G (1996) Increased bone formation in osteocalcin-deficient mice. Nature 382:448–452
22. Dunker AK, Brown CJ, Lawson JD, Iakoucheva LM, Obradovic Z (2002) Intrinsic disorder and protein function. Biochemistry 41:6573–6582
23. Exposito J-Y, Larroux C, Cluzel C, Valcourt U, Lethias C, Degnan BM (2008) Demosponge and sea anemone fibrillar collagen diversity reveals the early emergence of A/C clades and the maintenance of the modular structure of type V/XI collagens from sponge to human. J Biol Chem 283:28226–28235
24. Exposito JY, Cluzel C, Garrone R, Lethias C (2002) Evolution of collagens. Anat Rec 268:302–316
25. Exposito JY, van der Rest M, Garrone R (1993) The complete intron/exon structure of Ephydatia mulleri fibrillar collagen gene suggests a mechanism for the evolution of an ancestral gene module. J Mol Evol 37:254–259
26. Fisher LW, Fedarko NS (2003) Six genes expressed in bones and teeth encode the current members of the SIBLING family of proteins. Connect Tissue Res 44: 33–40
27. Fisher LW, Torchia DA, Fohr B, Young MF, Fedarko NS (2001) Flexible structures of SIBLING proteins, bone sialoprotein, and osteopontin. Biochem Biophys Res Commun 280:460–465
28. Force A, Lynch M, Pickett FB, Amores A, Yan Y-l, Postlethwait J (1999) Preservation of duplicate genes by complementary, degenerative mutations. Genetics 151:1531–1545
29. Fraser JD, Price PA (1988) Lung, heart, and kidney express high-levels of messenger-RNA for the vitamin K-dependent matrix Gla-protein – implications for the possible functions of matrix Gla protein and for the tissue distribution of the gamma-carboxylase. J Biol Chem 263:11033–11036
30. Gautron J, Hincke MT, Mann K, Panheleux M, Bain M, McKee MD, Solomon SE, Nys Y (2001) Ovocalyxin-32, a novel chicken eggshell matrix protein. Isolation, amino acid sequencing, cloning, and immunocytochemical localization. J Biol Chem 276:39243–39252
31. Gron P, Hay DI (1976) Inhibition of calcium phosphate precipitation by human salivary secretions. Arch Oral Biol 21:201–205
32. Gungormus M, Fong H, Kim IW, Evans JS, Tamerler C, Sarikaya M (2008) Regulation of in vitro calcium phosphate mineralization by combinatorially selected hydroxyapatite-binding peptides. Biomacromolecules 9:966–973
33. Hanes J, Jermutus L, Weber-Bornhauser S, Bosshard HR, Pluckthun A (1998) Ribosome display efficiently selects and evolves high-affinity antibodies in vitro from immune libraries. Proc Natl Acad Sci U S A 95: 14130–14135
34. Harding IS, Rashid N, Hing KA (2005) Surface charge and the effect of excess calcium ions on the hydroxyapatite surface. Biomaterials 26:6818–6826
35. Hartgerink JD, Beniash E, Stupp SI (2001) Self-assembly and mineralization of peptide-amphiphile nanofibers. Science 294:1684–1688
36. He G, Dahl T, Veis A, George A (2003) Nucleation of apatite crystals in vitro by self-assembled dentin matrix protein 1. Nat Mater 2:552–558
37. He M, Taussig MJ (2007) Eukaryotic ribosome display with in situ DNA recovery. Nat Methods 4:281–288

38. Hoang QQ, Sicheri F, Howard AJ, Yang DSC (2003) Bone recognition mechanism of porcine osteocalcin from crystal structure. Nature 425:977–980
39. Hohenester E, Sasaki T, Giudici C, Farndale RW, BÃchinger HP (2008) Structural basis of sequence-specific collagen recognition by SPARC. Proc Natl Acad Sci U S A 105:18273–18277
40. Holt C, Sawyer L (1988) Primary and predicted secondary structures of the caseins in relation to their biological functions. Protein Eng 2:251–259
41. Hufton AL, Groth D, Vingron M, Lehrach H, Poustka AJ, Panopoulou G (2008) Early vertebrate whole genome duplications were predated by a period of intense genome rearrangement. Genome Res 18: 1582–1591
42. Hunter GK, Hauschka PV, Poole AR, Rosenberg LC, Goldberg HA (1996) Nucleation and inhibition of hydroxyapatite formation by mineralized tissue proteins. Biochem J 317(pt 1):59–64
43. Huq NL, Cross KJ, Ung M, Reynolds EC (2005) A review of protein structure and gene organisation for proteins associated with mineralised tissue and calcium phosphate stabilisation encoded on human chromosome 4. Arch Oral Biol 50:599–609
44. Huxley-Jones J, Robertson DL, Boot-Handford RP (2007) On the origins of the extracellular matrix in vertebrates. Matrix Biol 26:2–11
45. Joo H, Lin ZL, Arnold FH (1999) Laboratory evolution of peroxide-mediated cytochrome P450 hydroxylation. Nature 399:670–673
46. Kasahara M (2007) The 2R hypothesis: an update. Curr Opin Immunol 19:547–552
47. Kawasaki K, Buchanan AV, Weiss KM (2007) Gene duplication and the evolution of vertebrate skeletal mineralization. Cells Tissues Organs 186:7–24
48. Kawasaki K, Suzuki T, Weiss KM (2004) Genetic basis for the evolution of vertebrate mineralized tissue. Proc Natl Acad Sci U S A 101:11356–11361
49. Kawasaki K, Suzuki T, Weiss KM (2005) Phenogenetic drift in evolution: the changing genetic basis of vertebrate teeth. Proc Natl Acad Sci U S A 102:18063–18068
50. Kawasaki K, Weiss KM (2003) Mineralized tissue and vertebrate evolution: the secretory calcium-binding phosphoprotein gene cluster. Proc Natl Acad Sci U S A 100:4060–4065
51. Kawasaki K, Weiss KM (2006) Evolutionary genetics of vertebrate tissue mineralization: the origin secretory calcium-binding and evolution of the phosphoprotein family. J Exp Zoolog B Mol Dev Evol 306B:295–316
52. Kawasaki K, Weiss KM (2008) SCPP gene evolution and the dental mineralization continuum. J Dent Res 87:520–531
53. Kolb G, Boiziau C (2005) Selection by phage display of peptides targeting the HIV-1 TAR element. RNA Biol 2:28–33
54. Kuchner O, Arnold FH (1997) Directed evolution of enzyme catalysts. Trends Biotechnol 15:523–530
55. Laize V, Martel P, Viegas CSB, Price PA, Cancela ML (2005) Evolution of matrix and bone gamma-carboxyglutamic acid proteins in vertebrates. J Biol Chem 280:26659–26668
56. Lee NK, Sowa H, Hinoi E, Ferron M, Ahn JD, Confavreux C, Dacquin R, Mee PJ, McKee MD, Jung DY, Zhang Z, Kim JK, Mauvais-Jarvis F, Ducy P, Karsenty G (2007) Endocrine regulation of energy metabolism by the skeleton. Cell 130:456–469
57. Lee S-W, Mao C, Flynn CE, Belcher AM (2002) Ordering of quantum dots using genetically engineered viruses. Science 296:892–895
58. Li X, Chang J (2008) Preparation of bone-like apatite-collagen nanocomposites by a biomimetic process with phosphorylated collagen. J Biomed Mater Res A 85A:293–300
59. Liu CC, Mack AV, Tsao M-L, Mills JH, Lee HS, Choe H, Farzan M, Schultz PG, Smider VV (2008) Protein evolution with an expanded genetic code. Proc Natl Acad Sci 105:17688–17693
60. Livingston BT, Killian CE, Wilt F, Cameron A, Landrum MJ, Ermolaeva O, Sapojnikov V, Maglott DR, Buchanan AM, Ettensohn CA (2006) A genome-wide analysis of biomineralization-related proteins in the sea urchin *Strongylocentrotus purpuratus*. Dev Biol 300:335–348
61. Lowenstam HA, Weiner S (1989) On biomineralization. Oxford University Press, New York
62. Lundin L-G, Larhammar D, Hallböök F (2003) Numerous groups of chromosomal regional paralogies strongly indicate two genome doublings at the root of the vertebrates. J Struct Funct Genomics 3:53–63
63. Luo GB, Ducy P, McKee MD, Pinero GJ, Loyer E, Behringer RR, Karsenty G (1997) Spontaneous calcification of arteries and cartilage in mice lacking matrix GLA protein. Nature 386:78–81
64. Lynch M, Conery JS (2000) The evolutionary fate and consequences of duplicate genes. Science 290:1151–1155
65. Mao C, Solis DJ, Reiss BD, Kottmann ST, Sweeney RY, Hayhurst A, Georgiou G, Iverson B, Belcher AM (2004) Virus-based toolkit for the directed synthesis of magnetic and semiconducting nanowires. Science 303: 213–217
66. Matsushima N, Ohyanagi T, Tanaka T, Kretsinger RH (2000) Super-motifs and evolution of tandem leucine-rich repeats within the small proteoglycans – biglycan, decorin, lumican, fibromodulin, PRELP, keratocan, osteoadherin, epiphycan, and osteoglycin. Proteins 38:210–225
67. Mochida Y, Duarte WR, Tanzawa H, Paschalis EP, Yamauchi M (2003) Decorin modulates matrix mineralization in vitro. Biochem Biophys Res Commun 305:6–9
68. Morvan-Dubois G, Le Guellec D, Garrone R, Zylberberg L, Bonnaud L (2003) Phylogenetic analysis of vertebrate fibrillar collagen locates the position of zebrafish alpha 3(I) and suggests an evolutionary link between collagen alpha chains and hox clusters. J Mol Evol 57:501–514
69. Mullaney BP, Pallavicini MG (2001) Protein-protein interactions in hematology and phage display. Exp Hematol 29:1136–1146
70. Nakao M, Nishiuchi Y, Nakata M, Kimura T, Sakakibara S (1994) Synthesis of human osteocalcins – gamma-carboxyglutamic acid at position-17 is essential for a calcium-dependent conformational transition. Peptide Res 7:171–174

71. Nakatani Y, Takeda H, Kohara Y, Morishita S (2007) Reconstruction of the vertebrate ancestral genome reveals dynamic genome reorganization in early vertebrates. Genome Res 17:1254–1265
72. Ohno S (1970) Evolution by gene duplication. Springer, New York
73. Olszta MJ, Cheng XG, Jee SS, Kumar R, Kim YY, Kaufman MJ, Douglas EP, Gower LB (2007) Bone structure and formation: a new perspective. Mater Sci Eng R Rep 58:77–116
74. Panopoulou G, Poustka AJ (2005) Timing and mechanism of ancient vertebrate genome duplications – the adventure of a hypothesis. Trends Genet 21:559–567
75. Peterson KR, Clegg CH, Huxley C, Josephson BM, Haugen HS, Furukawa T, Stamatoyannopoulos G (1993) Transgenic mice containing a 248-Kb yeast artificial chromosome carrying the human beta-globin locus display proper developmental control of human globin genes. Proc Natl Acad Sci U S A 90: 7593–7597
76. Petrenko VA, Smith GP, Gong X, Quinn T (1996) A library of organic landscapes on filamentous phage. Protein Eng 9:797–801
77. Donoghue PC, Samson IJ, Downs JP (2006) Early evolution of vertebrate skeletal tissues and cellular interactions, and the canalization of skeletal development. J Exp Zoolog B Mol Dev Evol 306B:278–294
78. Pinto JP, Ohresser MCP, Cancela ML (2001) Cloning of the bone Gla protein gene from the teleost fish *Sparus aurata*. Evidence for overall conservation in gene organization and bone-specific expression from fish to man. Gene 270:77–91
79. Puzas JE (2004) Site-specific mineralized matrix formation by osteoblasts. In: Bronner F, Farach-Carson MC (eds) Bone formation. Springer, London
80. Rehn AP, Cerny R, Sugars RV, Kaukua N, Wendel M (2008) Osteoadherin is upregulated by mature osteoblasts and enhances their in vitro differentiation and mineralization. Calcif Tissue Int 82:454–464
81. Reiss BD, Mao CB, Solis DJ, Ryan KS, Thomson T, Belcher AM (2004) Biological routes to metal alloy ferromagnetic nanostructures. Nano Lett 4:1127–1132
82. Ritter NM, Farachcarson MC, Butler WT (1992) Evidence for the formation of a complex between osteopontin and osteocalcin. J Bone Miner Res 7:877–885
83. Roberts RW (1999) Totally in vitro protein selection using mRNA-protein fusions and ribosome display. Curr Opin Chem Biol 3:268–273
84. Rowe PSN, Kumagai Y, Gutierrez G, Garrett IR, Blacher R, Rosen D, Cundy J, Navvab S, Chen D, Drezner MK, Quarles LD, Mundy GR (2004) MEPE has the properties of an osteoblastic phosphatonin and minhibin. Bone 34:303–319
85. Roy MD, Stanley SK, Amis EJ, Becker ML (2008) Identification of a highly specific hydroxyapatite-binding peptide using phage display. Adv Mater 20:1830
86. Sabatini L, Ota T, Azen E (1993) Nucleotide sequence analysis of the human salivary protein genes HIS1 and HIS2, and evolution of the STATH/HIS gene family. Mol Biol Evol 10:497–511
87. Sarikaya M, Tamerler C, Jen AKY, Schulten K, Baneyx F (2003) Molecular biomimetics: nanotechnology through biology. Nat Mater 2:577–585
88. Sire JY, Davit-Beal T, Delgado S, Gu X (2007) The origin and evolution of enamel mineralization genes. Cells Tissues Organs 186:25–48
89. Sire JY, Delgado S, Fromentin D, Girondot M (2005) Amelogenin: lessons from evolution. Arch Oral Biol 50:205–212
90. Smith GP (1985) Filamentous fusion phage – novel expression vectors that display cloned antigens on the virion surface. Science 228:1315–1317
91. Smith GP, Petrenko VA (1997) Phage display. Chem Rev 97:391–410
92. Smith MCM, Burns N, Sayers JR, Sorrell JA, Caskems SR, Hendrix, RW, Engel J (1998) Bacteriophage collagen. Science 279:1831g
93. Sugars RV, Milan AA, Brown JO, Waddington RJ, Hall RC, Embery G (2003) Molecular interaction of recombinant decorin and biglycan with type I collagen influences crystal growth. Connect Tissue Res 44: 189–195
94. Tsuji T, Onuma K, Yamamoto A, Iijima M, Shiba K (2008) Direct transformation from amorphous to crystalline calcium phosphate facilitated by motif-programmed artificial proteins. Proc Natl Acad Sci U S A 105:16866–16870
95. Wada H, Okuyama M, Satoh N, Zhang SC (2006) Molecular evolution of fibrillar collagen in chordates, with implications for the evolution of vertebrate skeletons and chordate phylogeny. Evol Dev 8:370–377
96. Waddington RJ, Roberts HC, Sugars RV, Schonherr E (2003) Differential roles for small leucine-rich proteoglycans in bone formation. Eur Cell Mater 6:12–21; discussion
97. Walsh JB (1995) How often do duplicated genes evolve new functions? Genetics 139:421–428
98. Wang D, Miller SC, Kopecková P, Kopecek J (2005) Bone-targeting macromolecular therapeutics. Adv Drug Deliv Rev 57:1049–1076
99. Wesson JA, Johnson RJ, Mazzali M, Beshensky AM, Stietz S, Giachelli C, Liaw L, Alpers CE, Couser WG, Kleinman JG, Hughes J (2003) Osteopontin is a critical inhibitor of calcium oxalate crystal formation and retention in renal tubules. J Am Soc Nephrol 14:139–147
100. Whaley SR, English DS, Hu EL, Barbara PF, Belcher AM (2000) Selection of peptides with semiconductor binding specificity for directed nanocrystal assembly. Nature 405:665–668
101. Wilson DS, Keefe AD, Szostak JW (2001) The use of mRNA display to select high-affinity protein-binding peptides. Proc Natl Acad Sci U S A 98:3750–3755
102. Yagami K, Suh JY, Enomoto-Iwamoto M, Koyama E, Abrams WR, Shapiro IM, Pacifici M, Iwamoto M (1999) Matrix GLA protein is a developmental regulator of chondrocyte mineralization and, when constitutively expressed, blocks endochondral and intramembranous ossification in the limb. J Cell Biol 147:1097–1108
103. Yamada Y, Avvedimento VE, Mudryj M, Ohkubo H, Vogeli G, Irani M, Pastan I, Decrombrugghe B (1980)

The collagen gene – evidence for its evolutionary assembly by amplification of a DNA segment containing an exon of 54 bp. Cell 22:887–892
104. Yamakoshi Y, Hu JC-C, Iwata T, Kobayashi K, Fukae M, Simmer JP (2006) Dentin sialophosphoprotein is processed by MMP-2 and MMP-20 in vitro and in vivo. J Biol Chem 281:38235–38243
105. Yokoyama S, Yokoyama R (1989) Molecular evolution of human visual pigment genes. Mol Biol Evol 6: 186–197
106. Yu-Lee LY, Richter-Mann L, Couch CH, Stewart AF, Mackinlay AG, Rosen JM (1986) Evolution of the casein multigene family: conserved sequences in the 5′ flanking and exon regions. Nucleic Acids Res 14: 1883–1902
107. Zhang GJ, Cohn MJ (2006) Hagfish and lancelet fibrillar collagens reveal that type II collagen-based cartilage evolved in stem vertebrates. Proc Natl Acad Sci U S A 103:16829–16833
108. Zhang J (2003) Evolution by gene duplication: an update. Trends Ecol Evol 18:292–298
109. Zhao HM, Giver L, Shao ZX, Affholter JA, Arnold FH (1998) Molecular evolution by staggered extension process (StEP) in vitro recombination. Nat Biotechnol 16:258–261

13. Osteogenesis Imperfecta

Paul Arundel and Nicolas J. Bishop

13.1 Introduction

Osteogenesis imperfecta (OI) is a group of rare heritable disorders characterized by varying degrees of low bone mass and bone fragility. Overall, OI has an estimated prevalence of between 1 in 10,000 and 1 in 20,000 [4, 59]. A Danish study of a geographically defined population found the point prevalence at birth to be 21.8 in 100,000. Mild forms of OI, however, may not be evident at birth and can be easily overlooked in older children.

OI can be a source of considerable morbidity in the early years of life with many affected children suffering recurrent fractures, and the consequent pain and immobilization. However, bone fragility (and sometimes bone pain) persists throughout life and long-term morbidity is a concern, particularly in post-menopausal women and elderly men. Bone mass accretion in childhood and puberty is crucial in determining peak bone mass. This means that the management of the condition through childhood and adolescence is likely to have an impact on long-term morbidity as well as on the outcomes seen in the pediatric clinic. The burden of disease throughout life remains high for many of those who are moderately to severely affected, notwithstanding improvements in the medical and surgical management of OI. There is still no cure, but new therapeutic approaches continue to be investigated. Understanding of the genetics and pathophysiology of the condition continues to expand.

13.2 Nosology and Biology

A widely accepted classification system that distinguishes between four clinical types was originally proposed and modified by Sillence and colleagues [107, 108]. It has undergone further modification, incorporating three further subtypes of OI that have been recognized on both clinical and histological grounds (see Table 13.1) [42, 43, 61, 124].

Simply described, type I OI is mild, type II is lethal, type III is severe with progressive bony deformity, and type IV is intermediate between types I and III. The clinical phenotype within each of these types of OI is, to a degree, variable in terms of other features such as ligamentous laxity, scleral hue, presence of Wormian bones, dentinogenesis imperfecta, and hearing loss.

More recently, types V, VI, and VII have been described. Type V presents with moderate to severe skeletal deformity and is characterized by both clinical findings (hyperplastic callus formation at fracture sites; calcification of the interosseous membranes of the forearm and lower leg; a typical bowing deformity of the forearm with reduction in supination/pronation; and

F. Bronner et al. (eds.), *Bone and Development*, Topics in Bone Biology 6,
DOI 10.1007/978-1-84882-822-3_13,

Table 13.1. Classification of osteogenesis imperfecta

Type	Clinical severity	Typical features	Typical molecular mechanism
I	Mild	Stature normal or slightly short; little or no limb deformity; blue sclera; ligamentous laxity; hearing loss; dentinogenesis imperfecta	Autosomal dominant; haploid insufficiency; nonfunctional *COL1A1* allele; usually due to premature stop codon
II	Perinatal, lethal	Pronounced deformities; multiple fractures at birth; micromelia; broad long bones; beading of the ribs; undermineralized skull; dark sclera	Autosomal dominant; glycine substitution in *COL1A1* or *COL1A2*
III	Severely deforming	Very short stature; severe scoliosis; cystic change at epiphyses; characteristic triangular facies; gray sclera; dentinogenesis imperfecta; dental malocclusion	Autosomal dominant; glycine substitution in *COL1A1* or *COL1A2*
IV	Moderately deforming	Marked heterogeneity; moderate short stature; variable degree of scoliosis; white or gray sclera; dentinogenesis imperfecta	Autosomal dominant; glycine substitution in *COL1A1* or *COL1A2*
V	Moderately deforming	Mild to moderate short stature; mineralized interosseous membrane of forearm; limited supination/pronation; dislocation of radial head; hyperplastic callous; no dentinogenesis imperfecta; "mesh-like" pattern of bone lamellation	Autosomal dominant; no abnormality of type 1 collagen, *COL1A1* or *COL1A2*
VI	Moderately to severely deforming	Moderate short stature; scoliosis; white sclera; no dentinogenesis imperfecta; "fish-scale" pattern of bone lamellation; accumulation of osteoid	No abnormality of type 1 collagen, *COL1A1* or *COL1A2*
VII	Lethal to moderately deforming	Variable phenotype; congenital fractures; rhizomelia; coxa vara; white sclera; no dentinogenesis imperfecta	Autosomal recessive; frameshift or intronic mutation in *CRTAP*; variable CRTAP loss determines clinical phenotype
VIII	Lethal to severely deforming	Severe growth deficiency; extreme skeletal undermineralization; platyspondyly and scoliosis; bulbous metaphyses; long phalanges; white sclera	Autosomal recessive; *LEPRE1* mutation

a tendency to radial head dislocation) and a characteristic mesh-like appearance of lamellae when bone biopsy specimens are viewed under polarized light [42]. Inheritance is autosomal dominant, although the genetic or proteomic defects are unknown. Type VI presents with moderate to severe skeletal deformity and is characterized by a typical histological appearance – excessive osteoid and a "fish scale" appearance of the lamellae. The condition has an autosomal recessive pattern of inheritance and screening of type 1 collagen DNA and protein has proved negative. Subjects do not have dentinogenesis imperfecta (DI) or blue sclera and do not respond as well to bisphosphonate therapy when compared with other types of OI [43]. Type VII OI has been observed in a Native American community in Quebec and has been found to be due to a reduction in the expression of cartilage-associated protein (CRTAP) (see below). It is moderately to severely deforming in type and is characterized by rhizomelia and coxa vara [61, 124].

The majority of individuals with OI (90%) have a mutation of one of the genes that encode type 1 collagen – *COL1A1* or *COL1A2*. Although the genotype–phenotype correlation is still not fully understood, the nature and location of mutations does, to some degree, explain the clinical heterogeneity of the condition [72]. Typically, mild forms of OI are caused by defects of collagen production that are the result of stop, frameshift, or splice site mutations in *COL1A1* or *COL1A2* [113, 129]. These mutations classically result in a *quantitative* defect, as the resulting mRNA is removed by the process of nonsense-mediated decay [16, 17]. More severe forms of OI typically arise from mutations that result in the substitution of an amino acid in either the α1 or α2 chain (coded for by the *COL1A1* or *COL1A2* genes, respectively). These *qualitative* mutations directly affect the structure of the type 1 collagen molecule by interference with helix formation and have an effect on cross-linking. Severely affected individuals usually have a point mutation affecting conserved glycine in either *COL1A1* or *COL1A2*. Normal triple helix formation depends upon every third amino acid in the α1 and α2 helical regions being a glycine residue [51]. Substitution, therefore, causes a delay in the folding of the procollagen triple helix, which results in the posttranslational over-modification of its constituent chains. The presence of these over-modified products is manifest as altered electrophoretic mobility.

Over 800 different mutations in *COL1A1* and *COL1A2* have been identified, but genotype–phenotype correlations have proven difficult to explain fully. The latest data suggest that, commensurate with the complex assembly and interactions of type 1 collagen, both the nature and location of mutations are important in determining the phenotype and draw particular attention to the likely importance of disruptions to collagen–matrix interaction [72]. There is still a surprising degree of phenotypic variation between individuals with substitutions of the same residue. This is probably explained by modifying the genetic and, perhaps, environmental factors. Much of the detail of these is at present poorly understood. A database of mutations of type 1 collagen genes is maintained at http://www.le.ac.uk/genetics/collagen.

Inheritance of most cases of OI is autosomal dominant as a result of the nature of the defects in *COL1A1* and *COL1A2*. Some cases, particularly of lethal and severe forms of OI, do not seem to have a dominant mode of inheritance.

Some recurrences of apparently sporadic mutations in siblings can be explained by germline or somatic mosaicism. Somatic mosaics may be positively identified by sequencing parental DNA.

Over the last few years, mutations in genes other than *COL1A1* and *COL1A2* have been found in individuals with a range of OI phenotypes. *CRTAP* and *LEPRE1* code for CRTAP and prolyl-3-hydroxylase (P3H1), respectively, which together form a complex with cyclophilin B (or peptidylproyl isomerase B) in the rough endoplasmic reticulum [7]. This complex is involved in the posttranslational 3-hydroxylation of a single proline residue in the α1 chain of type 1 collagen. Homozygous mutations of CRTAP have been found in individuals with a variety of OI phenotypes that range from lethal to the less severe classical type VII phenotype [7, 8, 80]. Mutations in *LEPRE1* similarly result in a lethal to severe bone phenotype characterized by significant growth deficiency, skeletal under-mineralization, bulbous metaphyses, thin ribs, a round face, and white sclera [7, 19]. Whether individuals with *CRTAP* and *LEPRE1* mutations can be reliably distinguished from those with classical OI on clinical and radiological grounds alone is currently unclear [7]. Both forms of OI are inherited in an autosomal recessive manner. This probably explains the relatively high empirical risk of "germline mosaicism" in 6% of the cases who had informed genetic counseling in the past. It has been proposed to classify all the cases of OI caused by *CRTAP* and *LEPRE1* mutations as OI types VII and VIII, respectively [19].

13.2.1 Animal Models

A variety of murine models have been utilized to study the pathophysiology of OI [35]. Insertion of the moloney murine leukemia virus into intron 1 of *COL1A1* has resulted in the Mov13 mouse. Heterozygous Mov13 mice correspond to humans with a null allele of *COL1A1* and have a mild OI phenotype [10]. In contrast, the naturally occurring murine *oim* frameshift mutation results in failure of the proα2(I) chain to incorporate into the type 1 collagen heterotrimer, the consequent production of α1 homotrimers. This leads to a severe phenotype that corresponds most closely to the human type III OI clinical phenotype [25]. Brittle (BrtlIV) mice were produced by crossing wild-type mice with mice containing a mutation that results in a glycine substitution in the α1 chain. The phenotype of Brittle mice resembles human OI because it varies from moderate to severe and lethal, corresponding to types III and IV OI, respectively [36]. Other transgenic mouse models, with phenotypes that correspond to severe/lethal OI phenotypes are available [55, 102, 110].

13.2.2 Biomechanics of Brittle Bones

Collagen fibres contribute to the ductility and toughness of bone, whereas the mineral component provides stiffness. Bone fragility arises from abnormal type 1 collagen production in OI, and corresponding mouse models. The changed mechanical properties of the collagen due to the mutation in *oim* mice and the effect of ionizing radiation on bone toughness demonstrate that collagen structure has a major effect on bone quality [20, 28, 29, 74, 78]. The size of this effect is surprising, because, in general, size and distribution of the stiffer component of composite materials is normally more important for determining the mechanical properties. Collagen fibrils, however, play an important role because they affect the size and orientation of mineral crystals [28, 37]. In OI, extrafibrillar crystals tend to be larger and collagen-associated crystals tend to be smaller than in controls [115, 119], yet bone in OI has a higher mineral density than in controls [11]. The complexity of the interactions of collagen with other determinants of bone strength indicates that one cannot regard the material properties of bone in OI as solely due to an abnormal organic matrix [122].

13.3 Clinical Approach

It is crucial for a child with OI to be both accurately diagnosed and assessed by the multidisciplinary team. This provides a guide to management and a baseline to evaluate the changes, and helps to establish a relationship of trust among the team, family, and child.

13.3.1 History

As in all fields of medicine, an accurate and detailed history is a prerequisite for the diagnosis of OI and its complications. The specific aspects of the medical history to which one must attend in cases of suspected OI are listed as follows:

Fractures – number, site, mechanism, degree of trauma, age at first fracture, and timing of most recent fracture.

Dislocations – number, mechanism, and degree of trauma.

Capacity for exercise – distance that a child can walk, or, if mild, whether the child can run and keep up with peers.

Activities of nonambulant children – range of daily activities and amount of assistance required from caregiver.

Back pain or stiffness – timing, relationship to exercise, degree of restriction, night-waking.

Neurological symptoms related to basilar invagination or raised intracranial pressure – headaches (commonly occipital or vertical), most pronounced on waking and worsening with straining; increasing clumsiness; increased difficulty with fine motor tasks; dysphagia; symptoms of cranial nerve palsies (especially VIII, IX, and X); and weakness, paresthesia, or loss of sensation in the extremities [75, 106].

Diet – foods containing calcium and vitamin D, including dairy produce, and details of supplements containing either.

Previous surgery – for example, intramedullary rodding or spinal surgery.

Family history – approximately half of all mildly affected individuals will have a family history.

Features to enquire about in other family members include: short stature in adulthood, fractures, dislocations, teeth that chip or crack, hernias, early-onset osteoporosis, and hearing loss. It is also important to identify any consanguinity or whether the child is from a community with a known increased risk of OI owing to a founder effect.

One area of particular importance is development. Infants with mild forms of OI will often walk well after the age of 12 months; in those more severely affected, the delay can be considerably greater. Attainment of motor milestones appears to be predictive of later walking [30, 33]. Apart from interruptions in the opportunities for normal development, such as those that arise from fractures and hospitalization, the causes of delay in motor development include joint hypermobility, muscle weakness, bone pain, and deformity.

One should actively seek to identify any functional consequences of OI that may have an impact on a child's schooling or socialization. In addition to issues of mobility, one should enquire about the difficulties in fine motor tasks, such as holding a pencil or doing up buttons.

13.3.2 Examination

Deformity of long bones, typically bowing with or without shortening, is common, but varies with the severity of the disease. It is important to examine the lower limb bones for bowing deformities and to monitor progression of any deformities both clinically and radiologically, requesting mechanical axis views wherever appropriate. Severe deformity is, of course, often managed jointly with the orthopedic team.

Deformity of the spine is also common, especially in moderate or severe OI. Compression fractures may be evident as areas of flattening in the otherwise smooth curvature of the flexed spine. An increased anterio-posterior diameter of the chest or shortening of the spine are other indicators of crush fractures. Apposition of the lower ribs and the iliac crest may also occur. Scoliosis or kyphosis may be evident clinically, but changes in vertebral morphology that might predict spinal deformity may only be evident radiologically (Fig. 13.1). Once the degree of curvature in scoliosis reaches 30°, it is unlikely to correct spontaneously and curvature >60° has significant negative effects on pulmonary function [128]. Regular monitoring of the spine in all children with OI is therefore a key role for the responsible physician.

Growth should be monitored closely throughout childhood in all OI patients. It is uncommon for children with even mild OI to be over the 50th percentile for height. Birthweight is commonly normal or in the lower half of the normal range for gestation [120].

Abnormalities of the skull can include widely patent anterior and posterior fontanelles and sutural diastasis in infancy. Hydrocephalus is a recognized complication. Brachycephaly and flattening of the skull are often present and can be extreme in cases of severe OI, particularly if there has been insufficient attention to positioning, e.g., side-lying in early life. Basilar invagination denotes the migration of the upper cervical vertebrae into the depression caused by the elevation of the floor of the posterior cranial fossa (see Fig. 13.2). This is an uncommon, but serious complication seen in moderate to severe OI and may be accompanied by certain characteristic skull shapes [90].

Ligamentous laxity is a common feature of OI. This is manifest clinically as joint hypermobility. A useful tool for quantification of the degree of hypermobility is the Beighton Scale. Severe hypermobility can result in dislocations of, for example, the hip or the radial head.

"Flat footedness" is a common and important problem arising from joint hypermobility, with

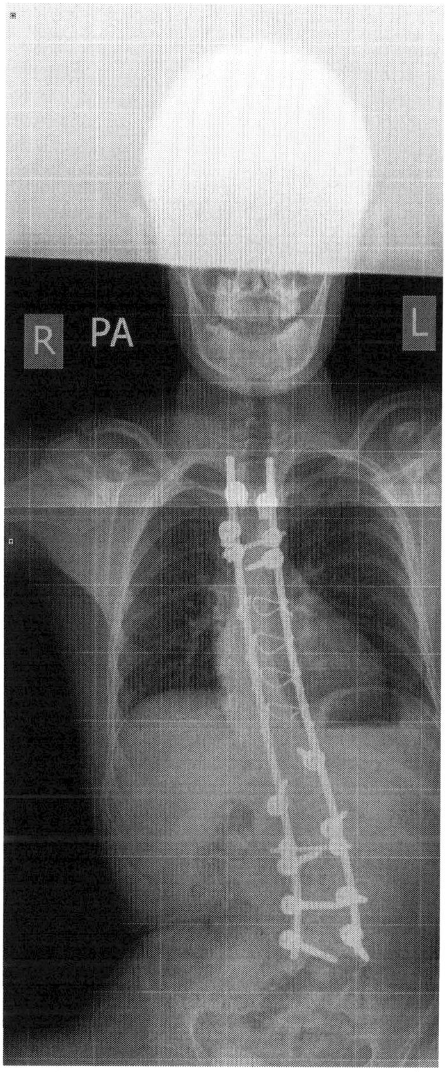

Figure 13.1. Radiograph of the spine showing scoliosis and typical instrumentation.

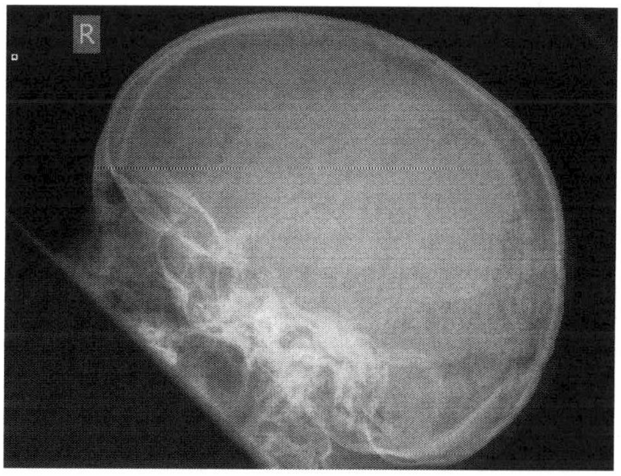

Figure 13.2. Lateral skull radiograph showing basilar invagination.

ankle inversion and "rolling in" of the medial malleoli in severe cases. It can have an impact on mobility directly or indirectly by injuries that have been sustained as a consequence of joint instability. It is usually addressed by ensuring that footwear is supportive, and with the introduction of an insole where necessary. Shortening of the tendo-achilles is seen in severely affected individuals.

Muscle strength is reduced in OI. This can be assessed clinically, but may also be quantified by measuring grip strength with a dynamometer.

Scleral hue is variable in OI. It is important to recognize that blue sclerae are common in infants under 6 months of age, and as such are not pathognomic. Blue sclerae tend to persist in types I and III OI, but tend to lighten with increasing age in type IV. In severely affected and lethal cases of OI, the sclerae often have an unmistakable dark gray or black hue. In adulthood, arcus corneae may be evident.

Skin is stiffer and less elastic than normal [44], but in severe type III OI, may appear translucent.

Constipation is a problem that should be actively looked for and remedied, although treatment can be difficult. It is particularly common and should therefore be anticipated in patients with severe OI in whom reduced mobility, acetabular protrusion, and pelvic deformity may play a role.

13.3.2.1 Dental Manifestations

Dental manifestations of OI include delayed primary dentition, dentinogenesis imperfecta (DI), and malocclusion [49].

Primary dentition may be delayed, with first teeth appearing after 12 months of age in more severely affected infants. In adulthood, unerupted first and second molars occur commonly.

DI is common in OI [85]. Teeth appear translucent owing to abnormal dentin and can either be pink, yellow, or gray in color. The dental phenotype does not run true within families and is not related to the severity of the skeletal phenotype. Although the enamel is normal, teeth chip and crack more easily owing to the relative lack of support from the dentine matrix [39, 66]. Dental treatment should be carried out by an experienced dentist, and generally consists of prevention of dental fracture with appropriate crowns, which also serve a cosmetic purpose in permanent dentition. Malocclusion with a significant overbite is common, especially in type III OI, and may require orthognathic surgery [111].

13.4 Differential Diagnosis

Conditions that can be confused with OI include various rare genetic conditions that share the characteristic of brittle bones. Most, however, can be differentiated by their clinical or biochemical features, and in some cases, the diagnosis can be confirmed by genetic analysis (see Table 13.2). Idiopathic juvenile osteoporosis (IJO) presents typically in the prepubertal age group with metaphyseal fractures, vertebral crush fractures, and neo-osseous osteoporosis [109, 114]. The histomorphometric features of IJO also distinguish it from OI [95]. Familial osteoporosis can usually be identified by family history, but may be difficult to distinguish from OI [21, 104, 116]. Secondary causes of osteoporosis are usually evident from the clinical context.

13.4.1 Nonaccidental Injury

Physicians are commonly asked to exclude the diagnosis of OI in cases of nonaccidental injury (NAI). The diagnosis of NAI is usually clear from the history, examination, and social background of the case or from the radiological evidence when fractures are present. Similarly, the diagnosis of OI will usually be evident to an experienced clinician when presented with the clinical and radiological evidence. However, the distinction between mild OI and NAI can be very difficult, especially because no biochemical or genetic test can reliably identify all cases of OI (see "Testing for Osteogenesis Imperfecta") [9].

Given that unexplained bony injury in an infant or young child is far more common owing to NAI than OI, the likelihood of missing a case of OI is low. However, if missed, the effects for the family and child are profound.

Table 13.2. Skeletal disorders resembling osteogenesis imperfecta

Condition	Severity of bone fragility	Typical features	Pathophysiology
Bruck syndrome	Moderate to severe	Congenital joint contractures; scoliosis	Autosomal recessive; deficiency of telopeptide lysyl hydroxylase; mutation in *PLOD2* in some cases; other cases linked to 17p12
Cole-Carpenter syndrome	Severe	Short stature; osteoporosis; metaphyseal fractures; craniosynostosis; hydrocephalus; ocular proptosis; distinctive facial features	Inheritance unclear; no abnormality of type 1 collagen
Hypophosphatasia	Mild to severe	Low alkaline phosphatase activity; very variable clinical expression; early loss of teeth	Autosomal recessive or dominant.; mutation in *ALPL*
Idiopathic hyperphosphatasia or juvenile Paget disease	Severe	Raised alkaline phosphatase activity; very variable phenotype; thickened skull; widened diaphyses; progressive deformity; scoliosis; deafness	Autosomal recessive; osteoprotegerin deficiency owing to mutation in *TNFRSF11B* in the majority of cases
Panostotic fibrous dysplasia	Severe	Characteristic lesions in all bones	Somatic mutation in *GNAS*
Osteoporosis pseudoglioma syndrome	Moderate	Congenital blindness	Autosomal recessive; mutation in *LRP5*
Idiopathic juvenile osteoporosis	Mild to moderate	Transient osteoporosis (though functional impairment may persist); presentation in prepubertal child; metaphyseal fractures; neo-osseous osteoporosis; no extraskeletal manifestations	Nonhereditary; unknown etiology in majority of cases; minority of cases owing to heterozygous mutation in *LRP5*

13.5 Testing for Osteogenesis Imperfecta

Testing for OI is either by analysis of genomic DNA or RNA, or by biochemical analysis of type 1 procollagen expression in cultured fibroblasts. RNA and collagen analyses require skin fibroblasts obtained by biopsy and careful handling of the sample. DNA analysis has the advantage of requiring only blood or saliva samples.

The collagen produced by cultured fibroblasts is analyzed by isolating isotopically labeled cells and subjecting them to gel electrophoresis. This allows identification of quantitative and qualitative abnormalities, including collagen overmodification. However, even when the test is carried out correctly, up to 20% of abnormalities may be missed [57]. Mutations in either *CRTAP* or *LEPRE1* result in type 1 procollagen with altered electrophoretic mobility. Individuals with these mutations can be identified, but are not easily differentiated from classical OI.

Mutational analysis is done by conformation-sensitive capillary electrophoresis or direct sequencing. The latter is done because highly sensitive and automated direct sequencing is becoming an ever more attractive first-line choice [18, 90]. Direct sequencing may not pick up the rare cases of large deletions or duplications, but multiple-ligation-dependent probe amplification or high-density array analysis, can be employed to cover these eventualities. RNA/cDNA analysis from fibroblasts also detects large deletions or duplications, but is neither sufficiently sensitive or specific to compete with direct sequencing of DNA [57, 90].

When another gene is involved, as in <10% of the cases, *COL1A1* and *COL1A2* analysis may not be helpful. At present, individuals with OI due to other genetic defects that affect posttranslational modification of collagen, such as those with *CRTAP* and *LEPRE1* mutations, cannot be reliably distinguished from those with *COL1A1* or *COL1A2* mutations on clinical, radiological, or biochemical grounds. *CRTAP* and *LEPRE1* mutation analysis will continue to be useful in selected cases, as in consanguineous parentage, or when the siblings are affected and in whom there is a failure to identify *COL1A1* or *COL1A2* mutations.

At present, no test alone is sufficiently sensitive and specific to match the clinical needs. The shortfall can be minimized by employing several tests, but this involves more laboratory time and higher cost [9].

13.6 Biochemistry

Standard biochemical analyses are rarely useful in establishing the diagnosis or severity of OI. Serum calcium and phosphate concentrations are typically normal. Elevated concentrations of serum alkaline phosphatase occur after a fracture, especially with excessive callus formation in type V OI. They have also been observed in patients with type VI OI [43]. The bone formation markers procollagen type 1 N- and C-terminal propeptides have been reported as low in children with mild and nonlethal OI [12, 67], but there is no evidence that they are helpful in establishing diagnosis. Urinary concentrations of the resorption marker type 1 N-terminal telopeptide tend to be higher in more severe cases, but when normalized to urinary creatinine and adjusted for serum creatinine, the difference disappears. The unadjusted difference in telopeptide concentrations may be due to the less well-developed musculature in severe OI [121]. Markers of bone formation and resorption do, however, respond to antiresorptive therapy and may be helpful in monitoring response.

13.7 Imaging

Radiography assesses the gross structural changes in the long bones and spine that may not be evident clinically. Although not specific for OI, Wormian bones are present in around 60% of the cases [120]. Basilar invagination can be identified with a plain lateral skull radiograph.

Dual energy X-ray absorptiometry (DXA) measures the bone area and bone density (BMC) in individuals with OI and is used to calculate areal bone mineral density (aBMD) and monitor the changes over time or in response to intervention. These data also make it possible to evaluate how the BMC of individuals with OI varies with disease severity. Individuals with mild OI commonly have an aBMD that is within the normal range for their age; when adjusted for body size, it tends to be lower than predicted. Bone density assessed by DXA can be normal in cases with thoracic crush fractures (Arundel and Bishop, unpublished).

Quantitative computed tomography can distinguish between the BMD of cortical and trabecular bone. Children with OI have been reported to have reduced bone area in one study [58], but not in another [77].

Magnetic resonance imaging (MRI) and computer tomography (CT) scanning are useful in the investigation of basal skull abnormalities, such as basilar impression and invagination. MRI may also have a role in identifying the upper thoracic vertebral crush fractures that are not well demonstrated by plain X-rays.

13.8 Histomorphometry

Histomorphometric studies of transiliac bone biopsies in children with OI have shown fewer and thinner trabeculae and reduced cortical bone width. Bone remodeling rates are increased, but the amount of new bone formed during remodeling is reduced [96]. Thus the reduced bone surface seems to offset the high rate of bone turnover to result in "normal" bone turnover in the blood. Additionally, the number of trabeculae does not increase with age. This suggests either a failure to form new trabeculae during endochondral ossification or a loss of previously formed trabeculae.

Some centers, including our own, obtain percutaneous transiliac bone biopsies prior to the commencement of bisphosphonate therapy for diagnosis and thus can review the effects of medical intervention. In particular, bone biopsy is diagnostic for OI types V and VI.

13.9 Medical Therapy

Over the years, numerous therapies for OI, including calcitonin, growth hormone, and vitamin D supplementation have been tried, but the introduction of bisphosphonate therapy has constituted the major advance.

13.9.1 Growth Hormone and Calcitonin

Recombinant growth hormone (rGH) therapy has some benefit in terms of increasing bone mass, vertebral size, and linear growth, but does not lead to a reduction in fracture incidence or other outcome parameters [5, 71, 73]. Concerns exist with regard to increasing bone turnover in a condition that already has high bone turnover. Moreover, subjects who have not responded with linear growth to rGH treatment tend to respond with decreased trabecular thickness [73]. Thus, there is no strong reason to utilize rGH therapy because children with OI seem to have essentially sufficient growth hormone secretion [69,70]. Therefore, the rGH therapy does not currently have a role in the standard treatment of OI, although it might, if in combination with bisphosphonates.

The antiresorptive effect of calcitonin is similar to that of bisphosphonates, but its side effects have limited its long-term use. It is now rarely prescribed in OI.

13.9.2 Bisphosphonates

The first reports of bisphosphonate therapy in individuals with OI were published in the late 1980s [31], and were followed by a series of studies that established the substantial benefits of cyclical intravenous bisphosphonates when combined with targeted surgery and a dedicated multidisciplinary approach to increasing mobility. This approach has subsequently been supported by a number of randomized trials with the result that bisphosphonates now constitute the mainstay of OI medical management.

13.9.2.1 Mechanism of Action

Bisphosphonates are pyrophosphate analogs that get incorporated into the bone and inhibit osteoclastic bone resorption. In the case of nitrogen-containing bisphosphonates, the principal mechanism of action is on the mevalonate pathway and the inhibition of protein prenylation.

Subjects treated with intravenous pamidronate have bone with increased cortical thickness, reduced cortical porosity and increased cancellous bone volume, but no increase in the number of trabeculae (see Fig. 13.3) [97]. In other words, there is improvement in the quality of new bone, but not in the mechanical strength of individual bones. Crush fractures of vertebral bodies are a manifestation of reduced bone

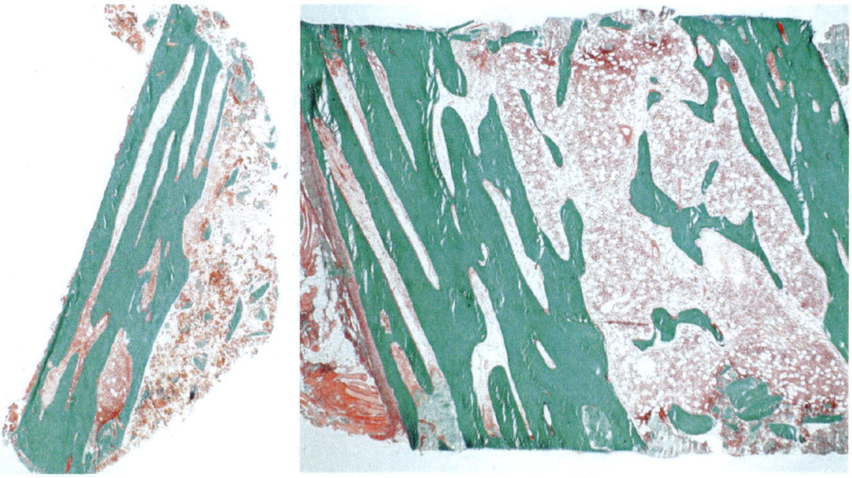

Figure 13.3. Transiliac bone biopsy specimens from the same child; pretreatment (*left*), and following 2 years of pamidronate therapy (*right*) showing increase in cortical bone volume without obvious reduction in cortical porosity. (Courtesy of David Hughes, Royal Hallamshire Hospital, Sheffield, UK).

strength, but can be overcome with bisphosphonate therapy [64].

13.9.2.2 Observational Studies

Cyclical administration of pamidronate in both infants and children leads to improved linear growth and vertebral morphometry, increased metacarpal cortical thickness and greater BMD, as well as to a reduction in the markers of bone resorption [6, 41, 88, 130]. Pamidronate therapy has also led to improvements in function, such as mobility, grip strength, and pain scores [41, 63, 79]. There are few data regarding the effects of treatment on long bone deformity. To achieve therapy benefits, cyclical treatment for 2 to 4 years was required, which was greater in individuals with a milder OI phenotype [92]. These studies have been limited by the lack of robust controls, although they have been compared with prior studies with no therapy [88].

To date, it is unclear whether the functional improvements [92] are due to medical therapy or the result of other interventions such as intensive physiotherapy. Similar uncertainty exists regarding the "quality of life" findings such as reduced pain. The potential effect of nonmedical intervention has been reported in a study of supervised training in children with mild to moderate OI, who showed improved muscle force and a reduction in subjective fatigue [118].

13.9.2.3 Randomized Controlled Trials

There have been relatively few randomized controlled trials (RCT) examining the outcomes of bisphosphonate treatment in OI and the number of subjects is small when compared with those in the observational studies. Available reports have however confirmed the benefits of bisphosphonate therapy in terms of vertebral morphometry, BMD, and fracture risk [40, 56, 65, 99], as well as the relatively swift resolution of vertebral deformity in treated infants [103]. However, RCTs have not shown the same improvements in function and pain reduction as some observational studies [56, 65, 99]. This failure goes against the experience of many clinicians, but it may be difficult to resolve this contradiction with further RCTs, given the other benefits of bisphosphonate therapy.

A number of studies have looked at the effect of other bisphosphonates including neridronate, olpadronate, alendronate, and more recently, zoledronate [2, 14, 68, 82]. Broadly speaking, these have similar, but less well-characterized effects than pamidronate.

13.9.2.4 Discontinuation of Therapy

Therapy has the greatest effects on bone mass during the first 2 years [65, 93]. Prolonged treatment in growing bone leads to dense metaphyseal bands in long bones, which are thought to represent a mixture of calcified cartilage and bone tissue [91] and may contribute to the increase in strength of treated bone [94]. When treatment is discontinued, the density of the newly formed metaphyseal bone returns to "normal" and may therefore become another zone of weakness. Fractures at these points have been described. Therefore, treatment should either be "tailed-off" or continued until completion of growth [23, 91].

The benefits of bisphosphonates appear to be greatest for children with OI who have not completed their growth, but improvements of BMD in adult populations have been reported [24].

13.9.2.5 Complications Associated with Bisphosphonate Therapy

Almost all children will undergo an acute-phase reaction during the first cycle of bisphosphonate treatment, but this does not recur and can be ameliorated with prophylactic anti-pyretics. Treatment will also result in a modest transient fall in serum calcium concentrations, but with a compensatory rise of serum parathyroid hormone (PTH) and 1, 25 dihydroxyvitamin D concentrations in vitamin D-replete individuals.

Concerns exist about the adverse effects of bisphosphonates on the mechanical strength of bones that result from reduced micro-crack repair and alterations in metaphyseal modeling [62]. It is difficult to know how important such potential effects are, because interpretation of fracture rates in studies of bisphosphonate therapy can be difficult because of the variation in fracture incidence in untreated children with OI and because the increased mobility in treated children may lead to fracture.

Delayed healing of osteotomies has been associated in one study [84] with prior pamidronate therapy, but delayed healing of fractures has been attributed to improved mobility rather than pamidronate therapy.

The association of osteonecrosis of the jaw (ONJ) with bisphosphonate therapy, most notably with the potent bisphosphonate zoledronate, and typically in individuals with an underlying malignancy [76] has given rise to concerns, but so far, no bisphosphonate-associated ONJ has been reported for individuals with OI. It would seem prudent, however, to ensure good dental hygiene prior to starting bisphosphonate therapy and to explain the risks to individuals and parents.

Other undesirable effects of bisphosphonate treatment include osteomalacia and osteopetrosis, reported so far only in Paget's disease [3] or following the administration of an extremely high dose [127].

As some bisphosphonates continue to be excreted decades after administration [86], the possibility of late onset side-effects remains. This is of particular concern with regard to the skeletal health of infants of women with OI who have been treated with bisphosphonates for prolonged periods. As yet, there is no evidence that such infants suffer adverse effects [83], but an appropriate balancing of risks and benefits and explanation of those to individuals and families is indicated.

13.9.2.6 Surgical Management

The majority of individuals with OI can be managed conservatively but often improved function or a reduction of deformity can only be achieved with surgery. Any decision to intervene surgically should be taken in consultation with all the relevant members of the multidisciplinary team. The fragility and size of bones in OI can present significant difficulties to the surgeon working with the bone. The outcomes of surgical interventions have improved significantly since the advent of bisphosphonate therapy. In particular, intramedullary rodding is now able to take place at a much younger age than before (from around 18 months), thereby enabling earlier weight-bearing with all the attendant advantages. The quality of the bones after treatment with bisphosphonates is, however, not normal and can itself present challenges to the orthopedic surgeon.

For many with mild disease, the only surgical interventions are those required to manage the effects of fractures. However, for those who are more severely affected, surgery can be a prerequisite to the achievement and maintenance of adequate mobility. Correction of long bone deformity traditionally has been achieved with multiple osteotomies and intramedullary nailing. More recently, distraction osteogenesis has been demonstrated to be effective and safe in achieving the correction of limb-length discrepancy together with deformity [100].

Intramedullary rodding of the lower limbs is used both to stabilize the long bones and to correct deformity. A variety of devices have been used, including expanding or telescopic rods and straight (rush) rods [15, 26, 32, 52, 53, 81, 112]. The former are preferred for use in the femur and the latter, by some, for use in the tibia. Below knee orthoses may be required to prevent bowing and fracture of the bone, especially when they have outgrown the rod. The need for revision of rods due to damage from trauma is always a possibility as are a number of complications including rod migration, loosening of a terminal T piece, infection, and pseudoarthrosis. The likely reoperation rate, the incidence of complications, and the number of joints needing to be opened for their insertion are all factors that influence the choice of a particular rod. Coxa vara warrants mention as a complication of OI that presents particular difficulties to the orthopedic surgeon [1].

Upper limb surgery is uncommon but may be required to improve or preserve hand function, especially in severe forms of OI. Scoliosis is common in OI and, if allowed to progress, can be severe [54]. Once the curvature of the spine reaches 30° then it is unlikely to correct spontaneously and surgical intervention should be considered. If there is any role for nonoperative management (e.g., soft cast bracing), then it is limited to more mild degrees of scoliosis. Surgery is generally intended to prevent progression or reduce pain but may be successful in achieving some correction of deformity. The choice of approach in terms of halo traction, posterior fusion, and instrumentation depends on the severity of the scoliosis and the age of the patient (see Fig. 13.3). Such surgery is difficult; reported results have been variable and thus ought to be undertaken only by those with appropriate experience and support (Fig. 13.3).

Basilar invagination is a slowly progressive but serious complication of OI. It is most commonly, but not exclusively, found in moderate to severe disease and can be complicated by communicating hydrocephalus and brain stem compression [22], sometimes with catastrophic consequences such as tetraplegia or respiratory arrest. Flattening of the occiput may be an indicator of risk for this complication insomuch as it may reflect the degree of weakness of the bony tissue constituting the skull base. In some cases high dose bisphosphonate therapy may reverse early basilar invagination, but the appropriateness of such an approach depends on careful and expert consideration of clinical details alongside the imaging data and be predicated on frequent monitoring.

More commonly a surgical approach is required. Depending on the presentation and radiological findings, surgery involves either a posterior fossa or anterior approach prior to occipitocervical fusion. Even with apparently successful surgery, however, basilar invagination may progress in up to 80% of patients [101]. This has lead to the advocacy of approaches that attempt to stabilize the base of the skull with regard to the thorax.

Protrusion of the acetabulum is another complication that can present a surgical challenge [123]. Successful treatment with multiple osteotomies has been reported [125].

Regarding the general approach to surgery in individuals with OI, it is important that particular care is taken in theatre. In addition to careful handling in order to avoid fractures or hyperextension of hypermobile joints, consideration must be given to abnormalities of the airway, the presence of thoracic deformity, teeth that break easily and the propensity to bruising and bleeding. Drugs that cause muscle fasciculation, such as succinylcholine, should be avoided to prevent fractures. The possibility of cardiovascular or restrictive pulmonary problems must also be considered. Malignant hyperpyrexia in response to inhalational anesthetics is reported as being associated with OI [38]. There is an increased risk of intraoperative hyperthermia but this rarely progresses to malignant hyperthermia [98]. The relationship between OI and malignant hyperpyrexia is not clear and may well be coincidental [13, 89].

13.9.2.7 Transitional Care

As with all chronic childhood conditions, the transition to adult services is crucial in maintaining continuity of care and may define how the individual will relate to adult health care services in the future. A cornerstone of good transitional care is the communication between the pediatric and adult services.

13.10 Management of Severely Affected Infants

Compromised respiratory function at birth owing to a combination of pulmonary hypoplasia and impaired mechanical function of the rib cage as a result of bone disease is frequently seen in severely affected infants. It requires respiratory support on neonatal intensive care, along with prompt therapy to strengthen the skeleton. This needs to be followed by expert physiotherapy and occupational therapy to enable the child to progress safely through motor milestones. An account of the detailed management of these infants is beyond the scope of this chapter.

13.11 Problems in Adulthood

13.11.1 Hearing Impairment

Impaired hearing is common in OI and is, for many, the feature that most interferes with everyday life. Population studies have found hearing loss in up to 59% of individuals with OI [45, 60]. The onset is typically in the second or third decade. In a Finnish national survey, the mean age of onset was 23.9 years (range 12–45 years), with the youngest age being 10 years [45]. The hearing impairment typically proceeds from a conductive loss to a type that is most commonly mixed, but is also sensorineural in a significant number. Sometimes rapid progression of hearing loss can result in anacusis within only a few years of presentation [45]. In spite of some reports, there is no clear association of hearing impairment with mutation types or severity of OI [45, 60, 87, 105, 107]. Expression within families is also variable [45]. In the absence of clear predictors of hearing loss, individuals with OI should receive baseline investigation for hearing impairment at 10 years of age, and have screening audiograms every 3 years thereafter [60]. Hearing aids can ameliorate any loss. In selected cases, stapes surgery may be beneficial, but results are not as good as with otosclerosis, notwithstanding the similarities of the conditions [34, 50].

13.11.2 Cardiovascular and Respiratory

The incidence of congenital heart malformations appears no higher in OI than in the general population [46]. Mitral valve prolapse may or may not be more common in OI than in the general population [46, 126], but is rarely clinically important. Similarly, aortic root dilatation is perhaps more common in OI, but is usually mild [46].

Historically, mortality in adulthood has been related to pulmonary complications arising from chest deformities. It is therefore reasonable to anticipate that the benefits of bisphosphonates in terms of improved vertebral morphology, together with improvements in spinal surgery, will translate into reduced adult morbidity and mortality.

13.11.3 Pregnancy

Women with OI tend to suffer from loss of bone mass during pregnancy and immediately following delivery. This may result in vertebral compression fractures that typically become clinically manifested during or after the second pregnancy. Pregnancy itself is otherwise often uneventful. There is an increased incidence of breech presentation of fetuses with OI, but overall, there appears to be no clear advantage to delivery by Caesarean section [27].

13.12 Future Prospects

Experience with bisphosphonate regimens in OI continues to grow, but other therapies may become available that lead to improved outcomes. Despite the potential synergy between rGH and bisphosphonates, it is still unclear whether there is a role for combined use. Because of its anabolic effect on bone, PTH has promise, but the development of osteosarcoma in young rats treated with PTH has limited its experimental use in children [117].

Osteomesenchymal cell engraftment occurred with some positive effects when bone marrow transplantation was performed in children with severe OI [47, 48], but the clinical benefits seem too limited to justify such serious intervention. Gene-based and stem cell therapies as yet remain at the preclinical stage.

References

1. Aarabi M, Rauch F, Hamdy RC, Fassier F (2006) High prevalence of coxa vara in patients with severe osteogenesis imperfecta. J Pediatr Orthop 26(1): 24–82
2. Adami S, Gatti D, Colapietro F, Fracassi E, Braga V, Rossini M, Tato L (2003) Intravenous neridronate in adults with osteogenesis imperfecta. J Bone Miner Res 18(1):126–310
3. Adamson BB, Gallacher SJ, Byars J, Ralston SH, Boyle IT, Boyce BF (1993) Mineralisation defects with pamidronate therapy for Paget's disease. Lancet 342(8885):1459–6140
4. Andersen PE Jr, Hauge M (1989) Osteogenesis imperfecta: a genetic, radiological, and epidemiological study. Clin Genet 36(4):250–525
5. Antoniazzi F, Bertoldo F, Mottes M, Valli M, Sirpresi S, Zamboni G, Valentini R, Tato L (1996) Growth hormone treatment in osteogenesis imperfecta with quantitative defect of type I collagen synthesis. J Pediatr 129(3):432–943
6. Astrom E, Soderhall S (1998) Beneficial effect of bisphosphonate during five years of treatment of severe osteogenesis imperfecta. Acta Paediatr 87(1):64–86
7. Baldridge D, Schwarze U, Morello R, Lennington J, Bertin TK, Pace JM, Pepin MG, Weis M, Eyre DR, Walsh J, Lambert D, Green A, Robinson H, Michelson M, Houge G, Lindman C, Martin J, Ward J, Lemyre E, Mitchell JJ, Krakow D, Rimoin DL, Cohn DH, Byers PH, Lee B (2008) CRTAP and LEPRE1 mutations in recessive osteogenesis imperfecta. Hum Mutat 29:1435–1442
8. Barnes AM, Chang W, Morello R, Cabral WA, Weis M, Eyre DR, Leikin S, Makareeva E, Kuznetsova N, Uveges TE, Ashok A, Flor AW, Mulvihill JJ, Wilson PL, Sundaram UT, Lee B, Marini JC (2006) Deficiency of cartilage-associated protein in recessive lethal osteogenesis imperfecta. N Engl J Med 355(26): 2757–6274

9. Bishop N, Sprigg A, Dalton A (2007) Unexplained fractures in infancy: looking for fragile bones. Arch Dis Child 92(3):251–625
10. Bonadio J, Saunders TL, Tsai E, Goldstein SA, Morris-Wiman J, Brinkley L, Dolan DF, Altschuler RA, Hawkins JE Jr, Bateman JF et al (1990) Transgenic mouse model of the mild dominant form of osteogenesis imperfecta. Proc Natl Acad Sci U S A 87(18):7145–9714
11. Boyde A, Travers R, Glorieux FH, Jones SJ (1999) The mineralization density of iliac crest bone from children with osteogenesis imperfecta. Calcif Tissue Int 64(3):185–910
12. Brenner RE, Schiller B, Vetter U, Ittner J, Teller WM (1993) Serum concentrations of procollagen I C-terminal propeptide, osteocalcin and insulin-like growth factor-I in patients with non-lethal osteogenesis imperfecta. Acta Paediatr 82(9):764–776
13. Brownell AK (1988) Malignant hyperthermia: relationship to other diseases. Br J Anaesth 60(3):303–830
14. Brumsen C, Hamdy NA, Papapoulos SE (1997) Long-term effects of bisphosphonates on the growing skeleton. Studies of young patients with severe osteoporosis. Medicine (Baltimore) 76(4):266–823
15. Brunelli PC, Novati P (1993) Complications of elongating intramedullary rodding in osteogenesis imperfecta. Am J Med Genet 45(2):275
16. Byers PH (2002) Killing the messenger: new insights into nonsense-mediated mRNA decay. J Clin Invest 109(1):3–6
17. Byers PH (2000) Osteogenesis imperfecta: perspectives and opportunities. Curr Opin Pediatr 12(6): 603–960
18. Byers PH, Krakow D, Nunes ME, Pepin M (2006) Genetic evaluation of suspected osteogenesis imperfecta (OI). Genet Med 8(6):383–838
19. Cabral WA, Chang W, Barnes AM, Weis M, Scott MA, Leikin S, Makareeva E, Kuznetsova NV, Rosenbaum KN, Tifft CJ, Bulas DI, Kozma C, Smith PA, Eyre DR, Marini JC (2007) Prolyl 3-hydroxylase 1 deficiency causes a recessive metabolic bone disorder resembling lethal/severe osteogenesis imperfecta. Nat Genet 39(3):359–635
20. Camacho NP, Hou L, Toledano TR, Ilg WA, Brayton CF, Raggio CL, Root L, Boskey AL (1999) The material basis for reduced mechanical properties in oim mice bones. J Bone Miner Res 14(2):264–722
21. Cardon LR, Garner C, Bennett ST, Mackay IJ, Edwards RM, Cornish J, Hegde M, Murray MA, Reid IR, Cundy T (2000) Evidence for a major gene for bone mineral density in idiopathic osteoporotic families. J Bone Miner Res 15(6):1132–7113
22. Charnas LR, Marini JC (1993) Communicating hydrocephalus, basilar invagination, and other neurologic features in osteogenesis imperfecta. Neurology 43(12): 2603–8260
23. Cheung MS, Glorieux FH (2008) Osteogenesis imperfecta: update on presentation and management. Rev Endocr Metab Disord 9(2):153–610
24. Chevrel G, Schott AM, Fontanges E, Charrin JE, Lina-Granade G, Duboeuf F, Garnero P, Arlot M, Raynal C, Meunier PJ (2006) Effects of oral alendronate on BMD in adult patients with osteogenesis imperfecta: a 3-year randomized placebo-controlled trial. J Bone Miner Res 21(2):300–630
25. Chipman SD, Sweet HO, McBride DJ Jr, Davisson MT, Marks SC Jr, Shuldiner AR, Wenstrup RJ, Rowe DW, Shapiro JR (1993) Defective pro alpha 2(I) collagen synthesis in a recessive mutation in mice: a model of human osteogenesis imperfecta. Proc Natl Acad Sci U S A 90(5):1701–5170
26. Chockalingam S, Bell MJ (2002) Technique of exchange of Sheffield telescopic rod system. J Pediatr Orthop 22(1):117–911
27. Cubert R, Cheng EY, Mack S, Pepin MG, Byers PH (2001) Osteogenesis imperfecta: mode of delivery and neonatal outcome. Obstet Gynecol 97(1):66–96
28. Currey JD (2003) Role of collagen and other organics in the mechanical properties of bone. Osteoporos Int 14(suppl 5):S29–36
29. Currey JD, Foreman J, Laketic I, Mitchell J, Pegg DE, Reilly GC (1997) Effects of ionizing radiation on the mechanical properties of human bone. J Orthop Res 15(1):111–711
30. Daly K, Wisbeach A, Sanpera I Jr, Fixsen JA (1996) The prognosis for walking in osteogenesis imperfecta. J Bone Joint Surg Br 78(3):477–840
31. Devogelaer JP, Malghem J, Maldague B, Nagant de Deuxchaisnes C (1987) Radiological manifestations of bisphosphonate treatment with APD in a child suffering from osteogenesis imperfecta. Skeletal Radiol 16(5):360–336
32. Engelbert RH, Helders PJ, Keessen W, Pruijs HE, Gooskens RH (1995) Intramedullary rodding in type III osteogenesis imperfecta. Effects on neuromotor development in 10 children. Acta Orthop Scand 66(4):361–436
33. Engelbert RH, Uiterwaal CS, Gulmans VA, Pruijs H, Helders PJ (2000) Osteogenesis imperfecta in childhood: prognosis for walking. J Pediatr 137(3):397–402
34. Ferekidis E, Stavroulaki P, Vossinakis I, Yiotakis J, Manolopoulos L, Adamopoulos G (2000) Stapedotomy in osteogenesis imperfecta patients. J Laryngol Otol 114(6):424–842
35. Forlino A, Marini JC (2000) Osteogenesis imperfecta: prospects for molecular therapeutics. Mol Genet Metab 71(1–2):225–322
36. Forlino A, Porter FD, Lee EJ, Westphal H, Marini JC (1999) Use of the Cre/lox recombination system to develop a non-lethal knock-in murine model for osteogenesis imperfecta with an alpha1(I) G349C substitution. Variability in phenotype in BrtlIV mice. J Biol Chem 274(53):37923–33791
37. Fratzl P, Paris O, Klaushofer K, Landis WJ (1996) Bone mineralization in an osteogenesis imperfecta mouse model studied by small-angle x-ray scattering. J Clin Invest 97(2):396–402
38. Furderer S, Stanek A, Karbowski A, Eckardt A (2000) [Intraoperative hyperpyrexia in patients with osteogenesis imperfecta]. Z Orthop Ihre Grenzgeb 138(2): 136–913
39. Gage JP, Francis MJ, Whitaker GE, Smith R (1986) Dentine is biochemically abnormal in osteogenesis imperfecta. Clin Sci (Lond) 70(4):339–436

40. Gatti D, Antoniazzi F, Prizzi R, Braga V, Rossini M, Tato L, Viapiana O, Adami S (2005) Intravenous neridronate in children with osteogenesis imperfecta: a randomized controlled study. J Bone Miner Res 20(5):758–673
41. Glorieux FH, Bishop NJ, Plotkin H, Chabot G, Lanoue G, Travers R (1998) Cyclic administration of pamidronate in children with severe osteogenesis imperfecta. N Engl J Med 339(14):947–592
42. Glorieux FH, Rauch F, Plotkin H, Ward L, Travers R, Roughley P, Lalic L, Glorieux DF, Fassier F, Bishop NJ (2000) Type V osteogenesis imperfecta: a new form of brittle bone disease. J Bone Miner Res 15(9):1650–8165
43. Glorieux FH, Ward LM, Rauch F, Lalic L, Roughley PJ, Travers R (2002) Osteogenesis imperfecta type VI: a form of brittle bone disease with a mineralization defect. J Bone Miner Res 17(1):30–83
44. Hansen B, Jemec GB (2002) The mechanical properties of skin in osteogenesis imperfecta. Arch Dermatol 138(7):909–191
45. Hartikka H, Kuurila K, Korkko J, Kaitila I, Grenman R, Pynnonen S, Hyland JC, Ala-Kokko L (2004) Lack of correlation between the type of COL1A1 or COL1A2 mutation and hearing loss in osteogenesis imperfecta patients. Hum Mutat 24(2):147–514
46. Hortop J, Tsipouras P, Hanley JA, Maron BJ, Shapiro JR (1986) Cardiovascular involvement in osteogenesis imperfecta. Circulation 73(1):54–61
47. Horwitz EM, Prockop DJ, Fitzpatrick LA, Koo WW, Gordon PL, Neel M, Sussman M, Orchard P, Marx JC, Pyeritz RE, Brenner MK (1999) Transplantability and therapeutic effects of bone marrow-derived mesenchymal cells in children with osteogenesis imperfecta. Nat Med 5(3):309–133
48. Horwitz EM, Prockop DJ, Gordon PL, Koo WW, Fitzpatrick LA, Neel MD, McCarville ME, Orchard PJ, Pyeritz RE, Brenner MK (2001) Clinical responses to bone marrow transplantation in children with severe osteogenesis imperfecta. Blood 97(5): 1227–3121
49. Huber MA (2007) Osteogenesis imperfecta. Oral Surg Oral Med Oral Pathol Oral Radiol Endod 103(3):314–230
50. Hultcrantz M, Saaf M (2007) Stapes surgery in osteogenesis imperfecta: a clinical study of 16 patients. Adv Otorhinolaryngol 65:222–522
51. Kadler KE, Holmes DF, Trotter JA, Chapman JA (1996) Collagen fibril formation. Biochem J 316(pt 1):1–11
52. Karbowski A, Schwitalle M, Brenner R, Lehmann H, Pontz B, Worsdorfer O (2000) Experience with Bailey-Dubow rodding in children with osteogenesis imperfecta. Eur J Pediatr Surg 10(2):119–214
53. Karbowski A, Schwitalle M, Eckardt A (1998) [Experiences with different telescope nails in treatment of pediatric osteogenesis imperfecta]. Zentralbl Chir 123(11):1252–6125
54. Karbowski A, Schwitalle M, Eckardt A (1999) [Scoliosis in patients with osteogenesis imperfecta: a federal nation-wide cross-sectional study]. Z Orthop Ihre Grenzgeb 137(3):219–222
55. Khillan JS, Olsen AS, Kontusaari S, Sokolov B, Prockop DJ (1991) Transgenic mice that express a mini-gene version of the human gene for type I procollagen (COL1A1) develop a phenotype resembling a lethal form of osteogenesis imperfecta. J Biol Chem 266(34):23373–92337
56. Kok DH, Sakkers RJ, Janse AJ, Pruijs HE, Verbout AJ, Castelein RM, Engelbert RH (2007) Quality of life in children with osteogenesis imperfecta treated with oral bisphosphonates (Olpadronate): a 2-year randomized placebo-controlled trial. Eur J Pediatr 166(11): 1155–6111
57. Korkko J, Ala-Kokko L, De Paepe A, Nuytinck L, Earley J, Prockop DJ (1998) Analysis of the COL1A1 and COL1A2 genes by PCR amplification and scanning by conformation-sensitive gel electrophoresis identifies only COL1A1 mutations in 15 patients with osteogenesis imperfecta type I: identification of common sequences of null-allele mutations. Am J Hum Genet 62(1):98–110
58. Kovanlikaya A, Loro ML, Hangartner TN, Reynolds RA, Roe TF, Gilsanz V (1996) Osteopenia in children: CT assessment. Radiology 198(3):781–478
59. Kuurila K, Grenman R, Johansson R, Kaitila I (2000) Hearing loss in children with osteogenesis imperfecta. Eur J Pediatr 159(7):515–951
60. Kuurila K, Kaitila I, Johansson R, Grenman R (2002) Hearing loss in Finnish adults with osteogenesis imperfecta: a nationwide survey. Ann Otol Rhinol Laryngol 111(10):939–496
61. Labuda M, Morissette J, Ward LM, Rauch F, Lalic L, Roughley PJ, Glorieux FH (2002) Osteogenesis imperfecta type VII maps to the short arm of chromosome 3. Bone 31(1):19–25
62. Land C, Rauch F, Glorieux FH (2006) Cyclical intravenous pamidronate treatment affects metaphyseal modeling in growing patients with osteogenesis imperfecta. J Bone Miner Res 21(3):374–937
63. Land C, Rauch F, Montpetit K, Ruck-Gibis J, Glorieux FH (2006) Effect of intravenous pamidronate therapy on functional abilities and level of ambulation in children with osteogenesis imperfecta. J Pediatr 148(4): 456–640
64. Land C, Rauch F, Munns CF, Sahebjam S, Glorieux FH (2006) Vertebral morphometry in children and adolescents with osteogenesis imperfecta: effect of intravenous pamidronate treatment. Bone 39(4): 901–690
65. Letocha AD, Cintas HL, Troendle JF, Reynolds JC, Cann CE, Chernoff EJ, Hill SC, Gerber LH, Marini JC (2005) Controlled trial of pamidronate in children with types III and IV osteogenesis imperfecta confirms vertebral gains but not short-term functional improvement. J Bone Miner Res 20(6):977–896
66. Lindau BM, Dietz W, Hoyer I, Lundgren T, Storhaug K, Noren JG (1999) Morphology of dental enamel and dentine-enamel junction in osteogenesis imperfecta. Int J Paediatr Dent 9(1):13–21
67. Lund AM, Hansen M, Kollerup G, Juul A, Teisner B, Skovby F (1998) Collagen-derived markers of bone metabolism in osteogenesis imperfecta. Acta Paediatr 87(11):1131–7113
68. Maasalu K, Haviko T, Martson A (2003) Treatment of children with osteogenesis imperfecta in Estonia. Acta Paediatr 92(4):452–545

69. Marini JC, Bordenick S, Chrousos GP (1995) Endocrine aspects of growth deficiency in OI. Connect Tissue Res 31(4):S55–7S5
70. Marini JC, Bordenick S, Heavner G, Rose S, Hintz R, Rosenfeld R, Chrousos GP (1993) The growth hormone and somatomedin axis in short children with osteogenesis imperfecta. J Clin Endocrinol Metab 76(1):251–625
71. Marini JC, Chrousos GP (1997) Growth hormone treatment of children with types III and IV osteogenesis imperfecta. J Bone Miner Res 12:S527
72. Marini JC, Forlino A, Cabral WA, Barnes AM, San Antonio JD, Milgrom S, Hyland JC, Korkko J, Prockop DJ, De Paepe A, Coucke P, Symoens S, Glorieux FH, Roughley PJ, Lund AM, Kuurila-Svahn K, Hartikka H, Cohn DH, Krakow D, Mottes M, Schwarze U, Chen D, Yang K, Kuslich C, Troendle J, Dalgleish R, Byers PH (2007) Consortium for osteogenesis imperfecta mutations in the helical domain of type I collagen: regions rich in lethal mutations align with collagen binding sites for integrins and proteoglycans. Hum Mutat 28(3): 209–221
73. Marini JC, Hopkins E, Glorieux FH, Chrousos GP, Reynolds JC, Gundberg CM, Reing CM (2003) Positive linear growth and bone responses to growth hormone treatment in children with types III and IV osteogenesis imperfecta: high predictive value of the carboxy-terminal propeptide of type I procollagen. J Bone Miner Res 18(2):237–423
74. McBride DJ Jr, Choe V, Shapiro JR, Brodsky B (1997) Altered collagen structure in mouse tail tendon lacking the alpha 2(I) chain. J Mol Biol 270(2):275–824
75. Menezes AH (2008) Specific entities affecting the craniocervical region: osteogenesis imperfecta and related osteochondrodysplasias: medical and surgical management of basilar impression. Childs Nerv Syst 24(10):1169–7112
76. Migliorati CA, Siegel MA, Elting LS (2006) Bisphosphonate-associated osteonecrosis: a long-term complication of bisphosphonate treatment. Lancet Oncol 7(6):508–154
77. Miller ME, Hangartner TN (1999) Bone density measurements by computed tomography in osteogenesis imperfecta type I. Osteoporos Int 9(5):427–342
78. Misof K, Landis WJ, Klaushofer K, Fratzl P (1997) Collagen from the osteogenesis imperfecta mouse model (oim) shows reduced resistance against tensile stress. J Clin Invest 100(1):40–54
79. Montpetit K, Plotkin H, Rauch F, Bilodeau N, Cloutier S, Rabzel M, Glorieux FH (2003) Rapid increase in grip force after start of pamidronate therapy in children and adolescents with severe osteogenesis imperfecta. Pediatrics 111(5 pt 1):e601–3
80. Morello R, Bertin TK, Chen Y, Hicks J, Tonachini L, Monticone M, Castagnola P, Rauch F, Glorieux FH, Vranka J, Bachinger HP, Pace JM, Schwarze U, Byers PH, Weis M, Fernandes RJ, Eyre DR, Yao Z, Boyce BF, Lee B (2006) CRTAP is required for prolyl 3- hydroxylation and mutations cause recessive osteogenesis imperfecta. Cell 127(2):291–304
81. Mulpuri K, Joseph B (2000) Intramedullary rodding in osteogenesis imperfecta. J Pediatr Orthop 20(2):267–723
82. Munns CF, Rajab MH, Hong J, Briody J, Hogler W, McQuade M, Little DG, Cowell CT (2007) Acute phase response and mineral status following low dose intravenous zoledronic acid in children. Bone 41(3):366–730
83. Munns CF, Rauch F, Ward L, Glorieux FH (2004) Maternal and fetal outcome after long-term pamidronate treatment before conception: a report of two cases. J Bone Miner Res 19(10):1742–5174
84. Munns CF, Rauch F, Zeitlin L, Fassier F, Glorieux FH (2004) Delayed osteotomy but not fracture healing in pediatric osteogenesis imperfecta patients receiving pamidronate. J Bone Miner Res 19(11): 1779–8176
85. O'Connell AC, Marini JC (1999) Evaluation of oral problems in an osteogenesis imperfecta population. Oral Surg Oral Med Oral Pathol Oral Radiol Endod 87(2):189–916
86. Papapoulos SE, Cremers SC (2007) Prolonged bisphosphonate release after treatment in children. N Engl J Med 356(10):1075–6107
87. Paterson CR, Monk EA, McAllion SJ (2001) How common is hearing impairment in osteogenesis imperfecta? J Laryngol Otol 115(4):280–228
88. Plotkin H, Rauch F, Bishop NJ, Montpetit K, Ruck-Gibis J, Travers R, Glorieux FH (2000) Pamidronate treatment of severe osteogenesis imperfecta in children under 3 years of age. J Clin Endocrinol Metab 85(5):1846–5180
89. Porsborg P, Astrup G, Bendixen D, Lund AM, Ording H (1996) Osteogenesis imperfecta and malignant hyperthermia. Is there a relationship? Anaesthesia 51(9): 863–586
90. Primorac D, Rowe DW, Mottes M, Barisic I, Anticevic D, Mirandola S, Gomez Lira M, Kalajzic I, Kusec V, Glorieux FH (2001) Osteogenesis imperfecta at the beginning of bone and joint decade. Croat Med J 42(4):393–415
91. Rauch F, Cornibert S, Cheung M, Glorieux FH (2007) Long-bone changes after pamidronate discontinuation in children and adolescents with osteogenesis imperfecta. Bone 40(4):821–782
92. Rauch F, Munns C, Land C, Glorieux FH (2006) Pamidronate in children and adolescents with osteogenesis imperfecta: effect of treatment discontinuation. J Clin Endocrinol Metab 91(4):1268–7124
93. Rauch F, Travers R, Glorieux FH (2006) Pamidronate in children with osteogenesis imperfecta: histomorphometric effects of long-term therapy. J Clin Endocrinol Metab 91(2):511–651
94. Rauch F, Travers R, Munns C, Glorieux FH (2004) Sclerotic metaphyseal lines in a child treated with pamidronate: histomorphometric analysis. J Bone Miner Res 19(7):1191–3119
95. Rauch F, Travers R, Norman ME, Taylor A, Parfitt AM, Glorieux FH (2002) The bone formation defect in idiopathic juvenile osteoporosis is surface-specific. Bone 31(1):85–98
96. Rauch F, Travers R, Parfitt AM, Glorieux FH (2000) Static and dynamic bone histomorphometry in children with osteogenesis imperfecta. Bone 26(6):581–958
97. Rauch F, Travers R, Plotkin H, Glorieux FH (2002) The effects of intravenous pamidronate on the bone tissue

of children and adolescents with osteogenesis imperfecta. J Clin Invest 110(9):1293–9129
98. Ryan CA, Al-Ghamdi AS, Gayle M, Finer NN (1989) Osteogenesis imperfecta and hyperthermia. Anesth Analg 68(6):811–481
99. Sakkers R, Kok D, Engelbert R, van Dongen A, Jansen M, Pruijs H, Verbout A, Schweitzer D, Uiterwaal C (2004) Skeletal effects and functional outcome with olpadronate in children with osteogenesis imperfecta: a 2-year randomised placebo-controlled study. Lancet 363(9419):1427–3141
100. Saldanha KA, Saleh M, Bell MJ, Fernandes JA (2004) Limb lengthening and correction of deformity in the lower limbs of children with osteogenesis imperfecta. J Bone Joint Surg Br 86(2):259–625
101. Sawin PD, Menezes AH (1997) Basilar invagination in osteogenesis imperfecta and related osteochondrodysplasias: medical and surgical management. J Neurosurg 86(6):950–690
102. Schnieke A, Harbers K, Jaenisch R (1983) Embryonic lethal mutation in mice induced by retrovirus insertion into the alpha 1(I) collagen gene. Nature 304(5924): 315–230
103. Senthilnathan S, Walker E, Bishop NJ (2008) Two doses of pamidronate in infants with osteogenesis imperfecta. Arch Dis Child 93(5):398–400
104. Shapiro JR, Burn VE, Chipman SD, Velis KP, Bansal M (1989) Osteoporosis and familial idiopathic scoliosis: association with an abnormal alpha 2(I) collagen. Connect Tissue Res 21(1–4):117–213; discussion 124
105. Sillence D (1981) Osteogenesis imperfecta: an expanding panorama of variants. Clin Orthop Relat Res 159: 11–25
106. Sillence DO (1994) Craniocervical abnormalities in osteogenesis imperfecta: genetic and molecular correlation. Pediatr Radiol 24(6):427–340
107. Sillence DO (1988) Osteogenesis imperfecta nosology and genetics. Ann N Y Acad Sci 543: 1–15
108. Sillence DO, Senn A, Danks DM (1979) Genetic heterogeneity in osteogenesis imperfecta. J Med Genet 16(2):101–116
109. Smith R (1995) Idiopathic juvenile osteoporosis: experience of twenty-one patients. Br J Rheumatol 34(1):68–77
110. Stacey A, Bateman J, Choi T, Mascara T, Cole W, Jaenisch R (1988) Perinatal lethal osteogenesis imperfecta in transgenic mice bearing an engineered mutant pro-alpha 1(I) collagen gene. Nature 332(6160): 131–613
111. Stenvik A, Larheim TA, Storhaug K (1985) Incisor and jaw relationship in 27 persons with osteogenesis imperfecta. Scand J Dent Res 93(1):56–60
112. Stockley I, Bell MJ, Sharrard WJ (1989) The role of expanding intramedullary rods in osteogenesis imperfecta. J Bone Joint Surg Br 71(3):422–742
113. Stover ML, Primorac D, Liu SC, McKinstry MB, Rowe DW (1993) Defective splicing of mRNA from one COL1A1 allele of type I collagen in nondeforming (type I) osteogenesis imperfecta. J Clin Invest 92(4): 1994–2002
114. Teotia M, Teotia SP, Singh RK (1979) Idiopathic juvenile osteoporosis. Am J Dis Child 133(9):894–900
115. Traub W, Arad T, Vetter U, Weiner S (1994) Ultrastructural studies of bones from patients with osteogenesis imperfecta. Matrix Biol 14(4):337–435
116. Treves R, Harang H, Bertin P, Bonnet C, Arnaud M, Desproges-Gotteron R (1992) Adolescent osteoporosis disclosing familial osteopenia. Clin Rheumatol 11(4): 558–651
117. Vahle JL, Sato M, Long GG, Young JK, Francis PC, Engelhardt JA, Westmore MS, Linda Y, Nold JB (2002) Skeletal changes in rats given daily subcutaneous injections of recombinant human parathyroid hormone (1–34) for 2 years and relevance to human safety. Toxicol Pathol 30(3):312–231
118. Van Brussel M, Takken T, Uiterwaal CS, Pruijs HJ, Van der Net J, Helders PJ, Engelbert RH (2008) Physical training in children with osteogenesis imperfecta. J Pediatr 152(1):111–116; 116.e1
119. Vetter U, Eanes ED, Kopp JB, Termine JD, Robey PG (1991) Changes in apatite crystal size in bones of patients with osteogenesis imperfecta. Calcif Tissue Int 49(4):248–520
120. Vetter U, Pontz B, Zauner E, Brenner RE, Spranger J (1992) Osteogenesis imperfecta: a clinical study of the first ten years of life. Calcif Tissue Int 50(1): 36–41
121. Vieira NE, Goans RE, Weiss GH, Hopkins E, Marini JC, Yergey AL (2000) Calcium kinetics in children with osteogenesis imperfecta type III and IV: pre- and post-growth hormone therapy. Calcif Tissue Int 67(2): 97–100
122. Viguet-Carrin S, Garnero P, Delmas PD (2006) The role of collagen in bone strength. Osteoporos Int 17(3):319–336
123. Violas P, Fassier F, Hamdy R, Duhaime M, Glorieux FH (2002) Acetabular protrusion in osteogenesis imperfecta. J Pediatr Orthop 22(5):622–562
124. Ward LM, Rauch F, Travers R, Chabot G, Azouz EM, Lalic L, Roughley PJ, Glorieux FH (2002) Osteogenesis imperfecta type VII: an autosomal recessive form of brittle bone disease. Bone 31(1):12–81
125. Wenger DR, Abrams RA, Yaru N, Leach J (1988) Obstruction of the colon due to protrusio acetabuli in osteogenesis imperfecta: treatment by pelvic osteotomy. Report of a case. J Bone Joint Surg Am 70(7):1103–7110
126. White NJ, Winearls CG, Smith R (1983) Cardiovascular abnormalities in osteogenesis imperfecta. Am Heart J 106(6):1416–2140
127. Whyte MP, Wenkert D, Clements KL, McAlister WH, Mumm S (2003) Bisphosphonate-induced osteopetrosis. N Engl J Med 349(5):457–643
128. Widmann RF, Bitan FD, Laplaza FJ, Burke SW, DiMaio MF, Schneider R (1999) Spinal deformity, pulmonary compromise, and quality of life in osteogenesis imperfecta. Spine 24(16):1673–8167
129. Willing MC, Deschenes SP, Slayton RL, Roberts EJ (1996) Premature chain termination is a unifying mechanism for COL1A1 null alleles in osteogenesis imperfecta type I cell strains. Am J Hum Genet 59(4):799–809
130. Zeitlin L, Rauch F, Plotkin H, Glorieux FH (2003) Height and weight development during four years of therapy with cyclical intravenous pamidronate in children and adolescents with osteogenesis imperfecta types I, III, and IV. Pediatrics 111(5 pt 1): 1030–6103

14. Fibrodysplasia Ossificans Progressiva: Developmental Implications of a Novel Metamorphogene

Frederick S. Kaplan, Jay C. Groppe, Petra Seemann, Robert J. Pignolo, and Eileen M. Shore

14.1 Introduction

Robust developmental novelty often results from polymorphisms or mutations in the regulatory regions of genes that control major morphogenetic signaling pathways [77]. It is much more unusual for developmental novelty to arise from mutations in the protein-coding region of such genes, because they often lead to embryonic death or catastrophic postnatal phenotypes.

Fibrodysplasia ossificans progressiva (FOP) is the result of a recurrent heterozygous missense mutation in the protein-coding region of the bone morphogenetic (BMP) protein type I receptor, Activin receptor A, type I/Activin-like kinase 2 (ACVR1/ALK2) [91]. This mutation (ACVR1 c.617G > A; R206H) leads to a plethora of pathologic developmental processes, including:

- dysregulated skeletal morphogenesis
- abnormal tissue repair
- skeletal metamorphosis of connective tissues
- oncogenesis (benign skeletal neoplasms)
- degenerative joint disease

In this chapter, by describing the clinical and molecular features of classic FOP in a developmental context, we hope to provide a more comprehensive understanding of the unique phenotype of the FOP mutation.

14.2 Clinical Features of Classic FOP

Two clinical features define classic FOP: congenital malformations of the great toes and progressive heterotopic ossification in characteristic anatomic patterns [13, 49, 52] (Fig. 14.1). Individuals with FOP appear normal at birth, except for malformations of the great toes, which are present in all classically affected individuals. In their first decade, children with FOP develop painful inflammatory soft tissue swellings (or flare-ups) that progressively transform the tissue into an armament-like encasement of heterotopic bone [12, 13]. Ribbons, sheets, and plates of heterotopic bone replace skeletal muscles and other connective tissues by a process of endochondral ossification that leads to the formation of a highly ramified second skeleton and resultant permanent immobility [55, 59, 69, 87]. Minor traumas such as intramuscular immunizations, mandibular blocks for dental work, muscle fatigue, blunt muscle traumas from bumps, bruises, falls, or

F. Bronner et al. (eds.), *Bone and Development*, Topics in Bone Biology 6,
DOI 10.1007/978-1-84882-822-3_14,

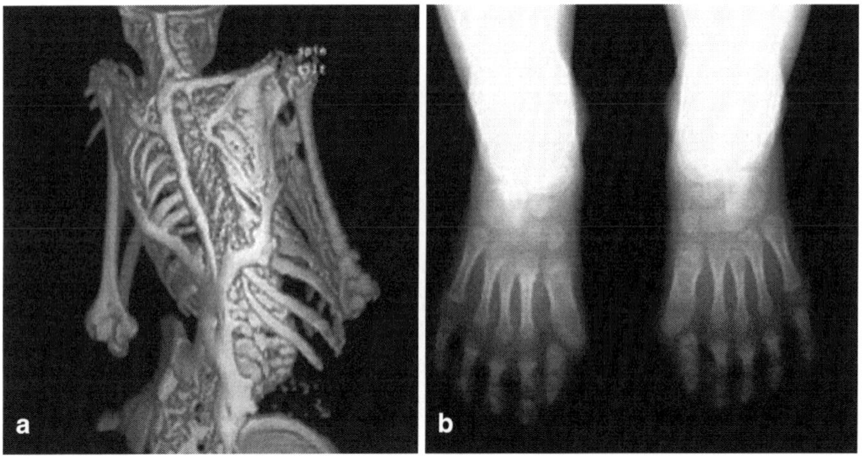

Figure 4.1. Characteristic clinical features of FOP. (**a**) Extensive heterotopic bone formation typical of FOP as seen in a three-dimensional reconstructed computed tomography (CT) scan of the back of a 12-year-old child. (**b**) Anterioposterior radiograph of the feet of a 3-year-old child that shows symmetrical great toe malformations (source: Shore et al. [91]. Copyright held by the authors).

influenza-like illnesses can trigger painful flare-ups that lead to progressive heterotopic ossification. Surgical attempts to remove heterotopic bone commonly lead, instead, to explosive new bone growth [28, 39, 43, 51, 63, 68, 71, 78, 79, 81].

Heterotopic ossification in FOP progresses in characteristic anatomic and temporal patterns that mimic normal embryonic skeletal formation. FOP involvement is seen first in the dorsal, axial, cranial, and proximal regions of the body and later in the ventral, appendicular, caudal, and distal regions [12]. Several skeletal muscles characterized by slow-twitch fibers that are generally resistant to fatigue (including the diaphragm, tongue, and extraoccular muscles) are spared. Cardiac and smooth muscles are also not involved.

Bone formation in FOP is episodic, but disability is cumulative. Most patients are confined to a wheelchair by the third decade of life and require lifelong assistance in performing activities of daily living. Severe weight loss often results from ankylosis of the jaw, and pneumonia or right-sided congestive heart failure complicates rigid fixation of the chest wall. The severe disability of FOP results in low reproductive fitness. The median lifespan is 41 years, with death often resulting from complications of thoracic insufficiency [47, 62].

14.3 Diagnosis and Misdiagnosis of FOP

FOP is a very rare disease and, therefore, is often misdiagnosed [60]. Most clinicians recognize the rapidly developing soft tissue swellings, but fail to associate this with the malformed great toes. When this is not done, FOP is commonly misdiagnosed as progressive juvenile fibromatosis, lymphedema, or soft tissue sarcomas. Children often undergo unnecessary and harmful diagnostic biopsies that exacerbate the progression of the condition [60]. FOP can be diagnosed clinically and by genetic testing (see following section), even before radiographic evidence of heterotopic ossification is seen, if soft tissue lesions are associated with symmetrical malformations of the great toes [57].

In addition to malformations of the great toes, early developmental anomalies are frequently observed in the cervical spine, thumbs, and femoral necks [49, 82]. Proximal medial tibial osteochondromas are a prominent feature of the condition [16]. Early degenerative arthritis is common [13]. Each of these clinical features provides important insights into the biologic activity of the classic FOP mutation that will be discussed in this chapter.

14.4 Epidemiologic, Genetic, and Environmental Factors in FOP

FOP is rare, with a worldwide prevalence of approximately one in two million individuals. There is no ethnic, racial, gender, or geographic predisposition. Most cases arise as a result of a spontaneous new mutation. Fewer than ten multigenerational families have been identified worldwide. Genetic transmission is autosomal dominant and can be inherited from mothers or fathers with complete penetrance [89, 90].

Both genetic and environmental factors affect the phenotype of FOP. In three pairs of monozygotic twins with FOP, congenital malformations of the great toes were found to be identical in each pair [33]. However, postnatal heterotopic ossification varied greatly, depending on life history and environmental exposure; this indicates that genetic factors strongly affect disease phenotype during prenatal development, whereas environmental factors strongly influence postnatal progression of heterotopic ossification [33].

14.5 FOP and the BMP Signaling Pathway

On the basis of the classic FOP phenotype, i.e., great toe malformations and progressive heterotopic endochondral ossification, it has been inferred that the primary molecular pathology in FOP involves skeletal patterning and heterotopic bone formation. Because these two processes are strongly associated, the BMP signaling pathway may be involved in the pathogenesis of the disease [56]. A series of discoveries using in vitro systems has provided compelling evidence that in FOP the BMP signaling pathway is profoundly dysregulated.

The findings include, but are not limited to:

- increased expression of BMP4 [25, 72, 80, 86]
- failure to upregulate multiple BMP antagonists [1]
- failure to regulate BMP concentration in the extracellular space [85]
- an increase in the concentration of BMP type I receptors at the cell surface [85]
- failure to appropriately internalize and degrade BMP type I receptors [45, 46, 85]
- ligand-independent BMP signaling through the SMAD pathway [5, 21]
- ligand-dependent BMP signaling through both the SMAD and the p38 MAPK pathways [5, 21]

14.6 The FOP Gene

Genome-wide linkage analysis of five small, two-generation families led to assigning the FOP gene to chromosome 2q23–24. Because this region includes the gene encoding Activin receptor A type I/activin-like kinase 2 (ACVR1/ALK2) [91] and because dysregulated BMP signaling had been shown to be the basis for the pathogenesis of FOP, ACVR1/ALK2 has become a prime candidate. It is one of seven activin-like kinases (ALKs) in humans [48]. These serine–threonine transmembrane receptors help specify cell fate during embryonic development and postnatal life in a wide variety of tissues [18, 31, 32, 83, 94].

An identical heterozygous missense mutation (c.617G > A;R206H) was identified in the glycine serine (GS) activation domain of ACVR1/ALK2 in all classically affected FOP patients worldwide [91]. This single nucleotide mutation transforms a morphogen receptor gene into a metamorphogene and provides a permissive genetic background for all developmental and postnatal phenotypic features of classic FOP. The mutant protein activates ACVR1/ALK2 signaling in the absence of ligand and permits robust signaling in the presence of ligand [88]. Identification of the mutant transmembrane receptor, which remarkably contains only a single substituted amino acid residue, has provided the basis for elucidating the molecular pathophysiology of dysregulated BMP signaling and the resultant skeletal metamorphosis in FOP [53].

Although ACVR1/ALK2 has been recognized as a BMP receptor, investigations of its function in embryonic development and in cell differentiation have been limited [103]. The fact that ACVR1/ALK2 is expressed in many tissues, including skeletal muscle and chondrocytes, provides support for ascribing to it the phenotypic effects in FOP. Constitutive activation of ACVR1/ALK2 induces alkaline phosphatase activity in C2C12 skeletal muscle satellite cells, upregulates BMP4, downregulates BMP antagonists, expands cartilage elements, induces ectopic chondrogenesis and stimulates joint fusions, findings similar to those seen in FOP [2, 91, 103]. Constitutively active ACVR1/ALK2 expression in embryonic chick limb buds induces expansion of the chondrogenic anlage and leads to joint fusions; this suggests that promiscuous ACVR1/ALK2 signaling alters cell fate and induces undifferentiated mesenchyme to form cartilage and bone [88, 103]. Enhanced ACVR1/ALK2 activation in FOP is also supported by findings that have shown increased pathway-specific SMAD phosphorylation and expression of BMP transcriptional targets in FOP cells [24, 88]. This was further strengthened by rescuing in zebra fish embryos the ACVR1/ALK2 loss of function phenotype with a mutant FOP ACVR1 [88].

Connective tissue progenitor (CTP) cells (SHED cells; stem cells obtained from discarded human exfoliated deciduous teeth of FOP patients and controls) transmitted BMP signals through both the SMAD and p38 mitogen-activated protein kinase (MAPK) pathways and responded to BMP4 treatment by inducing BMP responsive genes [5]. FOP cells showed ligand-independent BMP signaling, as well as ligand-dependent hyperresponsiveness to BMP stimulation. Further, FOP cells showed more rapid differentiation to an osteogenic phenotype than did control cells [5]. These findings strongly support the concept that both ligand-independent and ligand-dependent dysregulation of BMP signaling occur in FOP cells.

The seminal role of inflammation in triggering heterotopic ossification in BMP-permissive environments was brought out in one study, where the activity of circulating monocytes and tissue macrophages was inhibited pharmacologically and genetically [42]. As a result, inflammation-induced heterotopic ossification was substantially abrogated. In a subsequent study, local inflammation was sufficient to stimulate heterotopic ossification in a BMP4-permissive transgenic mouse model [67]. Finally, the conditional activation of inflammatory pathways in a constitutively active ALK2 mouse model led to the activation of heterotopic ossification at sites of inflammation [101].

14.7 Atypical FOP Phenotypes Caused by Novel Mutations in the FOP Gene

Recently, patients with FOP-like heterotopic ossification and/or toe malformations were identified with clinical features unusual for FOP. The atypical FOP patients form two classes: FOP-plus (classic defining features of FOP plus one or more atypical features) and FOP-variants (major variations in one or both of the two classic defining features of FOP). All patients examined had heterozygous ACVR1 missense mutations in conserved amino acids. While the recurrent c.617G > A; R206H mutation was found in all cases of classic FOP and in most cases of FOP-plus, novel ACVR1 mutations occurred in the FOP variants and in two cases of FOP-plus [58].

14.8 Protein Homology Mapping of the FOP Gene

Protein homology modeling of the mutant ACVR1/ALK2 receptor in FOP predicts changes in both ligand-independent and ligand-dependent BMP signaling in FOP cells [29, 91]. The classic FOP mutation (ACVR1 c.617G > A;R206H) replaces an arginine residue with a histidine residue at amino acid 206 in the glycine-serine (GS) domain of ACVR1/ALK2; it leads to loss of autoinhibition of the receptor.

The GS domain of all TGF-β/BMP type I receptors is a critical site for the activation of pathway-specific SMAD signaling proteins by constitutively active TGF-β/BMP type II receptors. FKBP12 binds and stabilizes the inactive conformation of all TGF-β/BMP type I receptors, including ACVR1/ALK2. When bound to the GS domain, FKBP12 prevents leaky activation of type I receptors in the absence of ligand [10, 36, 37, 95]. Importantly,

FKBP12 also serves as a docking protein for SMAD/SMURF complexes that mediate ubiquitination, internalization, and degradation of ACVR1/ALK2 [19, 97]. Consequently, FKBP12 regulates the concentration of ACVR1/ALK2 and its BMP type I receptor oligomerization partners (ALK3 and/or ALK6) at the cell membrane.

Protein modeling of the FOP mutation predicts that FKBP12 binding and/or activity is impaired. This in turn enhances ligand-independent and ligand-dependent BMP signaling, with both changes affecting BMP signal dysregulation as demonstrated in FOP cells [29, 88] (Fig. 14.2). As a result, the interaction of FKBP12 with the GS

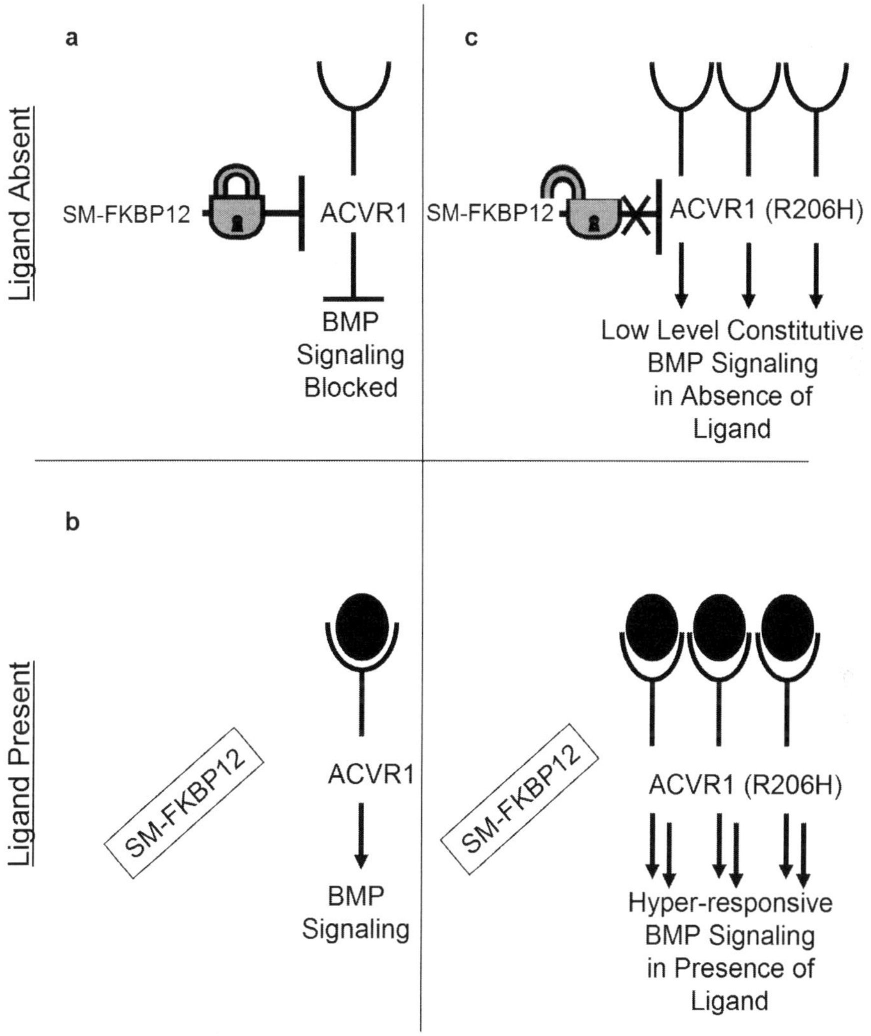

Figure 14.2. Hypothetical schema of bone morphogenetic protein (BMP) signaling in fibrodysplasia ossificans progressiva (FOP) cells. In control cells (**a**), in the absence of ligand, the Smad/Smurf-FKBP12 (SM-FKBP12) complex binds activin receptor IA (ACVR1; a BMP type I receptor) and prevents its promiscuous phosphorylation by the constitutively active type II BMP receptor (not shown). SM-FKBP12 also promotes ubiquitin associated degradation of ACVR1 in the absence of ligand, thus maintaining low steady-state levels of ACVR1 at the cell membrane. Following ligand binding in control cells (**b**), SM-FKBP12 dissociates from ACVR1, thus allowing the constitutively active BMP type II receptor (not shown) to phosphorylate ACVR1, promoting Smad 1, 5, and 8 phosphorylation and downstream BMP signaling. In FOP cells, SM-FKBP12 does not bind to the mutant receptor [ACVR1 (R206H)]. The failure to bind impairs BMP signaling (**c**). Additionally, since the SM-FKBP12 complex does not seem able to properly target the mutant ACVR1 (R206H) receptor for ubiquitin-associated degradation, ACVR1 may be expected to accumulate at the cell surface. Thus, in the presence of ligand (**d**), hyper-responsive BMP signaling may occur. Arrows, signaling promoted; blunt-end lines, signaling inhibited; lock, SM-FKBP12 binding to ACVR1; X, SM-FKBP12 binding to ACVR1 impaired; open cups, extracellular ligand-binding domain of ACVR1; filled-in circles, BMP ligand; filled-in circles inside open cups, BMP ligand binding to ACVR1 (modified from Kaplan et al. [52], Copyright 2008, with permission from Elsevier).

domain is likely to be altered and lead to promiscuous ACVR1/ALK2 activity [88]. Moreover, loss of autoinhibition of ACVR1/ALK2 is likely to change not only the intensity, but also the timing and duration of BMP signaling, thus creating new repertoires of BMP activity.

To better understand the molecular constraints and functional implications of the FOP mutation, wild-type and mutant ACVR1 activities were modeled [29]. Because homology between the cytoplasmic domains of all activin-like kinases is extensive, it was possible to develop reliable structure-based homology models of wild-type and mutant ACVR1 receptor kinases. In the wild-type ACVR1 model and in the template crystal structures (TβRI), the conserved arginine at codon 206 appears to form a salt bridge with an invariant aspartate residue at codon 269 [29]. Although lysine, a conservative substitution in BMPRIA and BMPRIB, can be readily accommodated, histidine at residue 206 (as occurs in FOP) would participate in a salt bridge with aspartate (residue 269) only if the intracellular pH were lowered and extensive structural rearrangement were to occur [29]. Protein modeling predicts that substitution with histidine, and only histidine, creates a pH-sensitive switch within the activation domain of the receptor that leads to ligand-independent activation of ACVR1 in FOP, as well as to conditional hyperactivity of the receptor at low intracellular pH [29] (Fig. 14.3).

pH-sensitive switches have been postulated for numerous proteins regulated by conformational changes. On protonation or deprotonation, these switches can produce small but important shifts. Consisting of only pairs or small clusters of residues, these switches induce major rearrangements in the tertiary or quaternary structure of proteins resulting from the amplification of the small displacements by secondary structure elements (α-helices, β-strands) that act as hinges and levers [29].

Histidine is a common element of pH-sensitive molecular switches, because the pKa of its imidazole group (approximately 6.0) allows the side chain to protonate and deprotonate within the physiological pH range. As the pH decreases from approximately 7.4 to the lower end of the physiologic range, the histidine side chain becomes partially ionized, going from an uncharged to a positively charged state. Histidine is unique in this respect, because the four other side chain groups (two other basic and two acidic) that participate in ion pairs remain fully charged over the entire range of physiological pH [29].

A fundamental aspect of the mutant switch is that it is responsive only in the R206H mutant context, i.e., when the pH-sensitive residue histidine replaces arginine. Because the mutation results in loss of regulation, only histidine would seem to have an activating effect at this site, with the clinical features of FOP the result of this substitution. Substitution at any of the 17 nonbasic residues at codon 206 has no observable effect, rendering such changes silent or lethal. However, because the residues on both sides of the salt bridge have been maintained through evolution, this structural element, by endowing the receptor with added stability, must play an important functional role [29].

The most crucial test of this role is to determine whether the ligand-independent activity of the ACVR1 R206H mutant kinase is sufficiently increased when the histidine side chain is partially ionized. Preliminary data strongly support this hypothesis [29] (Fig. 14.3).

If the concept of an aberrant switch is confirmed, a therapeutic approach might alter pH sensitivity of the histidine side chain. Conceivably, flare-ups of FOP result from trauma-associated hypoxia that lowers intracellular pH and turns on the switch. If so, modulation of the intracellular pH might suppress flare-ups of FOP or diminish heterotopic ossification [29]. Interestingly, generation of a hypoxic environment triggered by BMP2 in muscle in a murine model has been shown to be a critical step in the formation of heterotopic bone [73]. Thus, development of therapeutic approaches that eliminate hypoxic stress may block heterotopic bone formation.

The canonical ACVR1 (R206H) mutation in classic FOP, protein structure homology modeling of the novel missense mutations found in patients who have atypical FOP, including FOP-plus and FOP variants, predicts that each of the amino acid substitutions in these novel mutations leads to a loss of autoinhibition of the receptor through one of two mechanisms: by affecting binding of FKBP12 to the receptor or by affecting conformation of the kinase domain

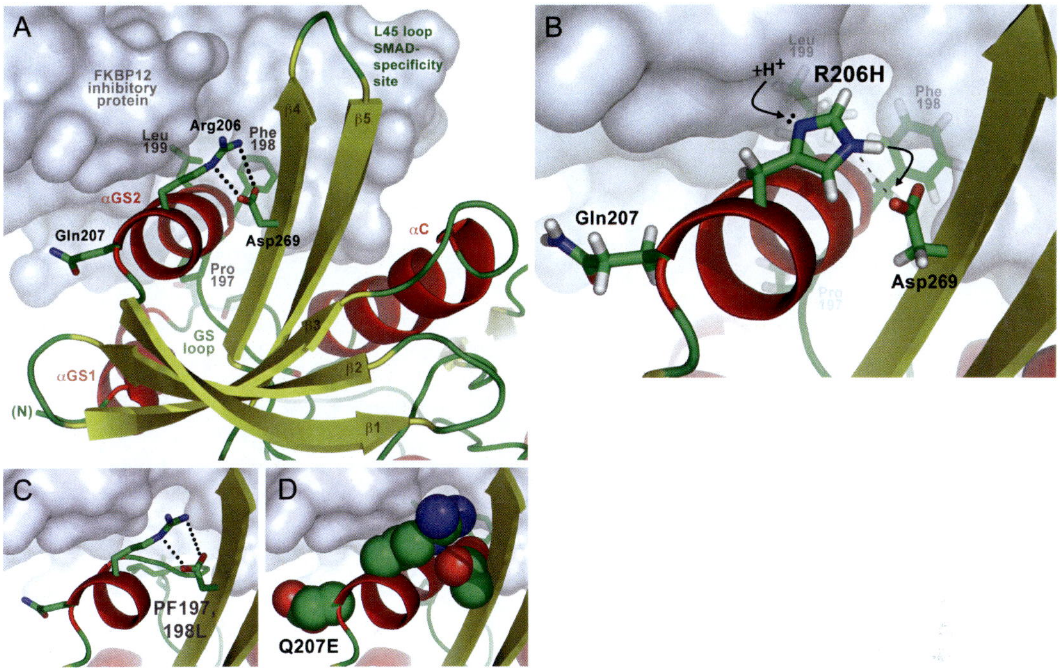

Figure 14.3. Structure-based homology models of wildtype and mutant ACVR1/ALK2 receptor kinases. (**a**) Overview of the N-lobe of the wildtype kinase, comprised of a five-stranded β-sheet scaffold, the conserved αC helix impinging on the catalytic site, and the juxtamembrane, helix-loop-helix GS (glycine, serine-rich) subdomain. The latter element regulates the activity of the enzyme by switching from an inhibitory to a substrate-binding (SMAD) mode, a transition requiring dissociation of an inhibitory protein (*grey surface*) and phosphorylation of the hydroxyl side chains of serine and threonine residues of the GS loop (*behind, in fog*) by a constitutively active type II BMP receptor kinase. In addition to the phosphorylated loop of the GS subdomain, another highly flexible loop extending from the β-sheet scaffold (L45 loop) participates in recruitment of the SMAD substrate and imparts specificity to the interaction. Arginine 206, a conserved basic residue and the site of substitution with histidine in the classic FOP mutation, forms an ion pair (*dotted lines*) with an acidic residue (aspartate 269) invariant amongst the seven type I receptor kinases of the TGF-β superfamily. Substitution of the adjacent residue (Gln207) with aspartate constitutively activates type I kinases in transgenic model organisms. At the opposite end of the αGS2 helix, two bulky hydrophobic residues (Phe198, Leu199) bind the inhibitory protein (FKBP12) within a hydrophobic pocket. The larger C-lobe of the kinases is mainly α-helical and primarily serves as a structural scaffold (*not shown*). (**b**) Close-up view of the αGS2 helix-FKBP12 interface with the R206H mutant linked to the classic form of FOP. Hydrogen atoms were added (*silver*) to emphasize the geometry of the imidazole ring of the histidine side chain relative to the carboxylate of the invariant aspartate, inasmuch as angular orientation is not conducive for ion pair formation. Moreover, under standard physiological conditions, the imidazole ring is neutral, requiring proton binding to become charged. At the lower range of physiological pH, however, the positively charged ring is thought to align the shared hydrogen atom of the ion pair with a carbonyl oxygen of the aspartate, rotating αGS2 in a lever-like fashion that results in displacement of the two hydrophobic side chains at the opposite end of the helix required for FKBP12 binding and inhibition. (**c**) Close-up view of the αGS2 helix-FKBP12 interface with the PF197, 198L mutant linked to a variant form of FOP. In the homology model, αGS2 is reduced to a single turn by substitution of proline 197 and phenylalanine 198, which precede and form the N-terminus of the helix with a leucine residue. As a result, the entire binding interface is lost, essentially abolishing interaction with the inhibitory protein. (**d**) Close-up view of the αGS2 helix-FKBP12 interface with the Q207E mutant linked to an atypical form of FOP. Side chain atoms are represented as space-filling spheres to depict the tolerance with the FKBP12 surface. An acidic residue introduced adjacent to arginine 206, acting in cis, would likely compete for ion pair formation with the invariant aspartate lying in trans. Transient formation of the non-native ion pair is thought to diminish binding of the FKBP12 inhibitory protein through steric conflict. Based on homology modeling, the three mutations highlighted here may diminish or abolish FKBP12 binding. Other mutations linked to variant or atypical forms of FOP lie adjacent to either the GS regulatory region or the active site of the kinase and thus should be able to alter the geometry of the active site, disrupting key regulatory interactions required to maintain the kinase in an autoinhibited state.

of the receptor [58] (Fig,14.3). Studies by X-ray crystallography of the receptors, now under way, are likely to shed information at the atomic level on the pathologic mechanisms of action of the various forms of FOP.

The missense mutation that causes FOP opens a "trap-door" in BMP signaling. That "trap-door" bypasses feedback mechanisms that regulate and constrain a critical morphogenetic signaling pathway.

Table 14.1. Pathologic processes of the FOP metamorphogene

ACVR1/ALK2 c.617G>A; R206H					
Pathologic process	**Dysregulated morphogenesis**		**Oncogenesis**	**Metamorphosis**	**Degeneration**
Phenotype	Orthotopic fusion of facet joints (cervical spine) & costovertebral joints	Digital malformations	Osteochondromas	Heterotopic ossification	Degenerative arthritis
Temporal expression:	Mid-embryonic	Late-embryonic	Early Post-natal	First decade Post natal	Second decade Post-natal
Spatial expression	Vertebral anlagen	Limb bud mesenchyme	Growth plate & perichondrium	Muscles tendon ligament, and aponeurosis	Articular cartilage
Trigger	Endogenous ligands?	Endogenous ligands?	Physical stress?	Inflammation; hypoxia; pH	Physical stress?
Responding cell	Skeletal anlagen cell?	Mesenchymal precursor cells; chondrocytes	Growth plate chondrocytes and perichondrial cells	Connective tissue progenitor cells?	Articular chondrocytes or pre-chondrocytes

FOP is particularly instructive because it is caused by a single nucleotide mutation in the protein-coding region of a BMP type I receptor that vastly alters not only body plan, but tissue response to injury. It is rare and perhaps unique that a single nucleotide mutation so vastly alters the identity of tissues and organ systems as a result of an inflammatory trigger and permits metamorphosis into other tissues and organs. Genetic diseases do not usually create new functional tissue or organs, but in FOP soft connective tissues undergo a profound metamorphosis into mature heterotopic bone. Metamorphosis thus joins the ranks of wound healing, regeneration, oncogenesis, and aging as a key biological process that is unmasked by a single point mutation [53].

We will now review the four processes, morphogenesis, metamorphosis, oncogenesis, and degeneration that are dysregulated by the FOP metamorphogene and describe how these features emerge from dysregulation of the BMP signaling pathway and interacting pathways (Table 14.1).

14.9 FOP and Morphogenesis

Congenital features of genetic disorders often provide clues to the underlying etiology and developmental pathways of those diseases. Similarly, as pointed out earlier, dysregulation of highly conserved signaling pathways provides insight into the role of those pathways in the morphogenesis of normal tissues and organs. In a seminal experiment, Brunet and colleagues showed that enhanced BMP activity during embryogenesis prevents the formation of all diarthrodial joints [7]. Malformations of the great toes are characteristic of FOP, but malformations of other diarthrodial joints are also common in FOP. These include the temporomandibular joints (TMJs), costovertebral joints (CVJ), hips, and cervical facet joints [49, 58].

In addition to the shortened, monophalangeal great toe, sometimes associated with a hallux valgus, seen in all FOP patients, approximately 50% also have shortened thumbs and clinodactyly of the little fingers [13, 49]. There is overlap of FOP-associated limb malformations with brachydactyly type A2 and C (BDA2, MIM #112600; BDC, MIM #113100), two conditions that are also associated with mutations in the BMP signaling pathway. BDA2 is characterized by a shortened index finger and variable clinodactyly of the little finger. In some patients, the feet are affected to variable degrees [20]. In some patients, the feet display a short, broad, and laterally deviated first toe [66]. BDC is a more severe brachydactyly involving the middle phalanges of the index, middle, and little finger, as well as shortening of the first metacarpal. BDA2 and BDC seem to represent related phenotypes of a common underlying molecular defect; this is consistent with the fact that both diseases are linked to the same signaling cascade, i.e., GDF5 and its receptor BMPR1B [65, 66, 76, 84]. Mice that lack BMPR1B and limb-specific BMPR1A develop nearly no skeletal anlagen [74, 98, 100]. Unfortunately, no data are available for knock-out of ACVR1 in the limb, because knock-out of ACVR1 is lethal in mice before limbs develop; no conditional studies have been performed in limbs to date [70]. Since ACVR1 is expressed in the limb mesenchyme, ACVR1 most likely acts together with BMPRIA or BMPR1B during limb development [99]. Conceivably, dominant negative mutations of BMPR1B or mutations of GDF5 that cause loss of function shift the balance toward increased ACVR1 signaling. A similar condition might apply for activating mutations of ACVR1. This would explain the overlapping features of limb malformations in FOP and BDA2 and BDC.

Malformations of the cervical spine are seen in nearly all classically affected FOP patients [82]. Neck stiffness and decreased range of motion are noted early in life in most children with FOP, even before occurrence of heterotopic ossification. Characteristic anomalies of the cervical spine include large posterior elements, tall, narrow vertebral bodies, and variable fusions of the facet joints between C2 and C7. Most notably, these characteristic anomalies of the cervical spine are strikingly similar to those seen in mice with homozygous deletions of the gene encoding Noggin, a BMP antagonist, even though Noggin mutations do not cause FOP [82, 96].

14.10 FOP and Metamorphosis

Much attention has been devoted to the establishment of pattern and form during embryogenesis [4, 6, 15, 17, 30, 61, 64]. However, little attention has been devoted to the dramatic and pathologic transformation of a normal tissue or organ system after morphogenesis has taken place [53].

FOP exemplifies the pathological and promiscuous transformation of one normal tissue or organ into another, called metamorphosis, a pathological process in which the normal structure and function of one tissue or organ is replaced by that of another tissue or organ [53]. This differs from the transformation of one mature cell into another [11].

The pathologic stages of skeletal metamorphosis in FOP have been well described [26, 27, 53, 59, 75]. Skeletal metamorphosis in FOP begins with a destructive stage in which a soft tissue injury triggers an inflammatory mononuclear cell infiltrate, proceeds to muscle cell injury and death, and is replaced with a highly angiogenic fibroproliferative lesion that matures through an endochondral process and culminates in the formation of new heterotopic bone. As the process of metamorphosis spreads to contiguous and adjacent sites, the new skeletal elements ramify to form a disabling second skeleton of heterotopic bone.

Metamorphosis is at the far end of a spectrum of cellular and tissue responses to injury that include repair and regeneration, adaptive biological processes that involve inflammatory stimuli. In mammals, the regenerative response is blunted, and most tissues respond to injury with a repair process that involves the formation of scar tissue. Bone, however, is one of the few tissues that responds to injury with complete regeneration [53].

It has been known for a century that embryogenesis of the skeleton and its regeneration following injury are closely related. As indicated earlier, inflammatory signals are not needed for skeletal formation, but are needed for skeletal regeneration and heterotopic ossification [42, 67, 101]. Moreover, BMP2 activity is required to initiate skeletal regeneration following fractures [101]. BMP stimulation of the prostaglandin pathway, through the action of cyclooxygenase 2, is known to be essential for fracture healing, thus linking the BMP signaling pathway with the skeletal regeneration-inflammatory pathway, but this is true only postnatally, not during embryonic morphogenesis. Thus, the same signaling pathway that exhibits robustness and refractoriness to stochastic changes during morphogenesis has evolved to be exquisitely sensitive to environmental signals postnatally [8, 53].

The fact that BMP4 is chemotactic to monocytes further implicates an association between inflammation of the BMP pathway and postnatal skeletal regeneration [53]. When recombinant BMPs are implanted subcutaneously, they stimulate heterotopic ossification with an inflammatory response that is nearly identical to that in FOP lesions [27]. During disease flare-ups (Kaplan et al., unpublished), endogenous prostanoids derived from local tissues are elevated in the serum of FOP patients. While BMP signaling is necessary for skeletal formation, regeneration in addition requires an inflammatory response [54]. An inflammatory response may also have a permissive function for skeletal metamorphosis [54]. Inflammatory stimuli also trigger heterotopic ossification in a BMP permissive environment [67].

In FOP and BMP-induced skeletal metamorphosis, mature connective tissue cells do not transdifferentiate into bone cells. Rather, they are replaced with normal functioning bone tissue via a complex pathologic process [41]. Stem cells and progenitor cells must therefore lie at the very heart of metamorphosis [53].

Hematopoietic cells have been implicated in the skeletal metamorphosis of FOP, and their replacement has been postulated as a possible cure [50]. However, the definitive contribution of hematopoietic cells to the pathogenesis of skeletal metamorphosis has, until recently, remained obscure. Examination of a patient with FOP who coincidentally developed intercurrent aplastic anemia demonstrated that bone marrow transplantation does not cure FOP, most likely because the hematopoietic cell population is not the target, or at least not the dominant target, of the intrinsic dysregulation of the BMP signaling pathway in FOP. However, following transplantation of bone marrow from a normal donor, immunosuppression of the immune system appeared to ameliorate activation of skeletal metamorphosis in a genetically susceptible host. Moreover, even a normal functioning immune system seems sufficient to trigger an FOP flare-up in a genetically susceptible host [50].

The question of which cells contribute to the fibroproliferative and chondrogenic mesenchymal anlagen in skeletal metamorphosis is fascinating, important, and unresolved. Two independent approaches have shown that such cells are not of hematopoietic origin, but arise from a different pool of CTP cells that have a vascular origin, at least in part [34, 67]. To definitively determine the origin of these cells will require detailed lineage-tracing experiments in transgenic mice with stable lineage markers. This will be facilitated by developing a knock-in mouse that replicates the FOP mutation and is sensitive to dysregulated BMP signaling [9].

Taken together, skeletal metamorphosis appears to be a stem-cell or progenitor-cell disorder triggered by inflammatory stimuli on a background of dysregulated BMP signaling [53, 67]. One normal tissue is replaced with another, but first nearly all vestiges of the original tissue, except its soft tissue scaffolding, neurovascular infrastructure, and progenitor cell repository are destroyed and then replaced (Fig. 14.4).

14.11 FOP and Oncogenesis

The clinical and pathological features of skeletal metamorphosis are often mistaken for oncogenesis, especially in the early stages [60]. According to a recent worldwide survey nearly 90% of FOP patients were initially misdiagnosed, most commonly with soft tissue sarcoma or aggressive juvenile fibromatosis. Moreover, 50% of the misdiagnosed patients experienced permanent and lifelong harm as a result of diagnostic and therapeutic errors [60].

Malignant degeneration has not been reported in FOP lesions or as a consequence of skeletal metamorphosis in FOP, but benign osteochondral neoplasms are actually common and are poorly recognized features of the condition [16]. Among the least explored functions of the FOP metamorphogene (ACVR1 c.617G > A; R206H) is its ability to stimulate benign osteochondral neoplasms or osteochondromas. Osteochondromas are associated with dysregulated BMP signaling and have been considered an atypical feature of FOP, but may be under-diagnosed because of their often asymptomatic nature. According to a recent study [16], 90% of FOP patients had osteochondromas of the proximal tibia and nearly 100% had one or more asymptomatic osteochondromas at other sites. Benign osteochondral neoplasms are therefore a common feature of FOP in addition to skeletal malformations and skeletal metamorphosis.

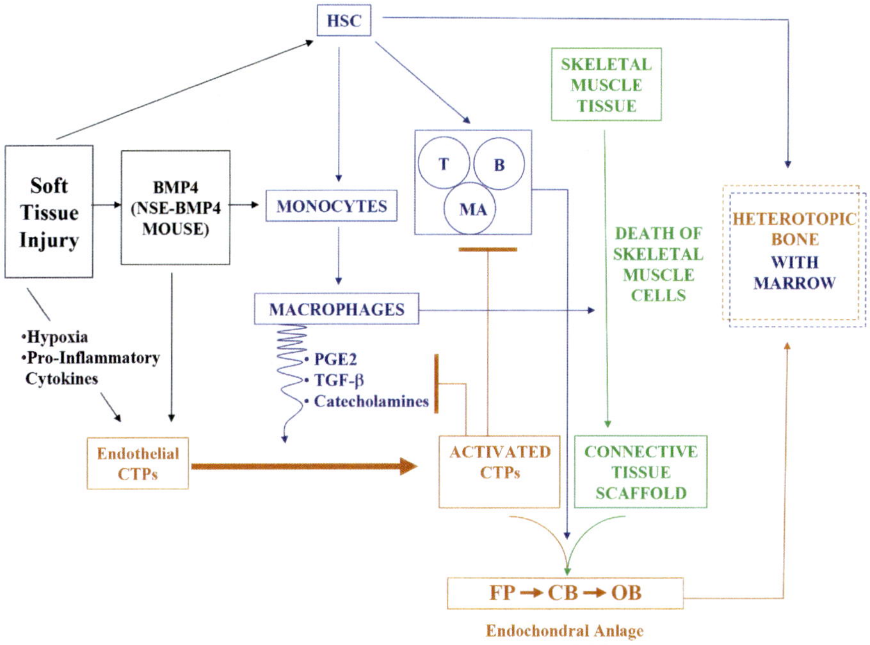

Figure 14.4. Working model of BMP-associated heterotopic ossification. Injury to skeletal muscle and connective tissues leads to monocyte invasion, macrophage inactivation, tissue hypoxia, and upregulation of inflammatory cytokines and osteogenic factors, including BMPs that recruit endothelial cells to form the heterotopic anlagen. Wound hypoxia and inflammatory cytokine contribute to the angiogenic response in wound healing. Hypoxia-related pH changes may further sensitize *FOP* cells to ambient levels of BMPs which further mobilize endothelial progenitor cells. The inflammatory reaction to muscle injury, the secretion of BMPs, and the cross-talk between cells of the innate and adaptive immune system stimulate the induction and propagation of an ectopic skeletal element. *CTPs* connective tissue progenitor cells; *HSC* hematopoietic stem cells; *T* T-cells; *B* B-cells; *MA* mast cells; *FP* fibroproliferative cells; *CB* chondroblasts; *OB* osteoblasts; PGE_2 prostaglandin E2; *TGFβ* transforming growth factor-beta; *blue lines*, hematopoietic-derived pathways; *brown lines*, CTP-derived pathways; *blunt-end lines* signify inhibitory pathways; *arrows* signify stimulatory pathways (modified from Lounev et al.[67]).

FOP is one of a small number of hereditary disorders with osteochondromas. The most common disorder is multiple hereditary exostosis (MHE; OMIM#13700), an autosomal dominant condition characterized by numerous osteochondromas that occur predominantly at the metaphyses and less commonly at the diaphyses of long bones. Deformities of the hands, forearms, and legs occur frequently secondary to MHE lesions. Patients with MHE also exhibit defective modeling of the metaphyses of long bones, leading to shortening [16].

MHE is caused by mutations in the EXT1 or EXT2 genes, which encode tumor suppressors and glycosylstransferases involved in the biosynthesis of heparan sulfate, an essential component of heparan sulfate proteoglycans. Cell surface heparan sulfate proteoglycans bind to and modulate the activity of a vast array of growth factors and cell surface receptors (including BMPs) that direct cellular proliferation, differentiation, adhesion, and intracellular signaling [16, 40].

Cell surface heparan sulfate proteoglycans play a significant role in the local distribution of secreted morphogens (such as Ihh and BMPs) to receptive cells by establishing morphogen gradients and linking exostosis formation in MHE to the Indian hedgehog (Ihh)/parathyroid hormone-related peptide (PTHrP) pathway. EXT1 deficiency in mice leads to defective heparan sulfate proteoglycan synthesis, defective Ihh transport, and increased levels of intracellular Ihh in perichondrial cells. The abnormal modulation of the tightly regulated Ihh/PTHrP negative feedback loop may constitute a molecular model of osteochondroma formation in patients with MHE [16].

In FOP, the molecular mechanism of osteochondroma formation differs from that of MHE,

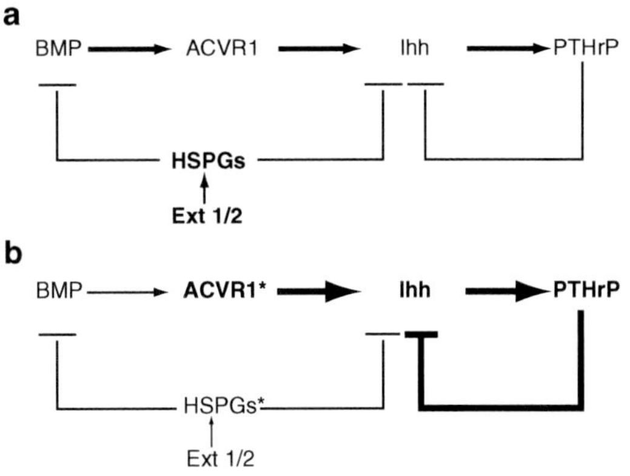

Figure 14.5. Working schema of the molecular pathogenesis of osteochondroma formation in multiple hereditary exostosis (MHE) and fibrodysplasia ossificans progressive (FOP). (**a**) Normal regulation of the BMP/Ihh/PTHrP pathway. Arrows signify stimulation and lines ending in bars signify inhibition. (**b**) For MHE, abnormal EXT1/2 (EXT1/2*) leads to deficient synthesis of heparan sulfate proteoglycans (HSPGs*), resulting in increased Ihh and BMP activity via diminished inhibition (*unbolded lines and bars*). For FOP, constitutively active ACVR1 (ACVR1*) is postulated to cause hyperstimulation of Ihh (*left bolded arrow*) and, subsequently, of PTHrP (*right bolded arrow*). In both MHE and chicken models that have FOP-like features, hyperactive Ihh results in abnormal regulation of chondrocyte differentiation and osteochondromal formation (adapted from Deirmengian et al. [16]).

even though it involves the same feedback loops as in the growth plate and perichondrium. In FOP, the dysregulated activation of ACVR1/ALK2 seems to increase Ihh secretion in perichondrial cells [16] (Fig. 14.5).

Studies of the developing chick limb have shown that Ihh expression is activated by robustly expressed ACVR1 in the limb perichondrium and periosteum [103]. Transfection of constitutively active ACVR1 results in dramatic upregulation of Ihh at the perichondrium and a delay in the temporal and anatomic pattern of chondrocyte differentiation [103], as also true in FOP. These findings make it likely that the BMP signaling pathway contributes significantly to the Ihh/PTHrP feedback loop.

It is thus reasonable to suggest the osteochondroma formation in both FOP and MHE is mediated by disruption of the BMP/Ihh/PTHrP negative feedback loop at the perichondrium. In FOP, this feedback loop is dysregulated directly through the increased activity of mutated ACVR1, whereas in MHE, the feedback loop is affected indirectly through reduction in heparan sulfated proteoglycans, leading to a functional increase in BMP and Ihh morphogens that regulate BMP/Ihh/PTHrP signaling [16] (Fig. 14.5). Additional studies are needed to determine the timing of gene expression during development and postnatal life.

14.12 FOP and Degenerative Joint Disease

The expression of the FOP metamorphogene in articular cartilage cells plays a role in the fate of the diarthrodial joint. Individuals with FOP develop degenerative joint disease early in life, some by the end of the first decade [13].

Toe malformations are ubiquitous in patients with FOP, but some children with FOP are born with normally appearing interphalangeal joints of the great toe that rapidly fuse, not with heterotopic bone, but as a result of a rapid loss of articular cartilage and intraarticular ankylosis early in life [13].

Most patients with FOP develop early degenerative joint disease at weightbearing and non-weightbearing joints in the elbows, wrists, fingers, hips, knees, and feet. The temporomandibular joints (TMJs) and the CVJ are also affected with early degenerative changes. Interestingly, FOP patients with less severe heterotopic ossification often develop degenerative changes early in life. This may be because the later, overwhelming extraarticular ankylosis has not yet masked the degenerative changes. Alternatively, stress shielding across an extraarticular ankylosis may provide protection for articular chondrocytes when decreased lifespan or altered cell fate is genetically programmed [55].

Intersecting morphogenetic pathways such as those involved in Wnt, Hedgehog, Fibroblast growth factor, and Notch signaling play important roles in the formation and maturation of diarthrodial joints [23, 35, 93]. How does mutant ACVR1 expression affect those interacting pathways in the embryonic development of the joints? These and other questions on the role of the FOP metamorphogene will provide important insight on the role of the BMP pathway and interacting pathways in degenerative joint diseases. Knock-in animal models of the FOP metamorphogene may be a means to study these questions [9].

14.13 Prevention and Treatment of Skeletal Metamorphosis in FOP

Definitive treatments and cures for FOP are not yet available, but the discovery of the FOP gene and insights into its mechanism of action suggest four plausible approaches to the treatment and/or prevention of FOP [48, 52]:

1. blocking the overactive ACVR1/ALK2-mediated BMP signaling pathway, by means of monoclonal antibodies, by signal transduction inhibitors, inhibitory RNA, or secreted antagonists
2. blocking the inflammatory triggers
3. blocking the responding CTP cells
4. altering inductive and/or conducive microenvironments that promote heterotopic ossification.

These points have been discussed [48, 52]. In this chapter, we will highlight only one approach, that of blocking the ACVR1/ALK2 signaling pathway.

(a) Signal transduction inhibitor (STI) strategy

Small molecule STIs are invaluable for investigating signal transduction pathways and can be developed into therapeutic agents with the potential of modifying the natural history of the disease [14, 22, 44, 48, 52, 101, 102]. Residues close to the ATP-binding site of ACVR1/ALK2 may provide selectivity even between closely related receptor serine threonine kinases such as ALK3 (BMPRIA) and ALK6 (BMPRIB) [101].

Dorsomorphin has been identified as a small molecule inhibitor of type I BMP receptors ALK2, ALK3, and ALK6, blocking BMP-mediated SMAD 1, 5, 8 phosphorylation, target gene transcription, and osteogenic differentiation [102].But because of Dorsomorphin's toxicity, newer analogs such as DM 3189 are being explored [101]. Dorsomorphin and its derivatives inhibit SMAD activation, but do not appreciably affect the ability of BMPs to activate p38 MAP kinases [3, 102].

(b) Monoclonal Antibody Strategy

FOP cells express higher levels of some BMP cell surface receptors with a resulting decrease in receptor internalization and degradation [85]. FOP cells also exhibit a ligand-dependent increase in signaling [88]. FOP cells may therefore respond to ligand stimulation.

The BMP type I receptor ALK3 may be a signaling partner of ALK2 in the heterotetrametric signaling complex involved in FOP pathogenesis. The development of effective antibodies and therapeutic blocking antibodies would be helpful in assessing the specific role of mutant ALK2 in heterotopic ossification. Preliminary findings indicate that blocking ligand-dependent signaling may modulate disease-causing BMP signaling in FOP.

(c) Small Inhibitory RNA (siRNA) Strategy

FOP is the result of a missense mutation in one of the two alleles of ACVR1/ALK2. Inhibiting messenger RNA from the mutant allele without perturbing messenger RNA from the normal allele seems plausible and might become an effective therapy.

14.14 Conclusions

FOP is a rare genetic disorder that provides insight into the cellular and genetic regulation of skeletal and extraskeletal bone formation. The single nucleotide missense mutation that causes classic FOP induces a metamorphogene that dysregulates the highly conserved BMP signaling pathway involved in normal tissue development and repair. This metamorphogene regulates chondroosseous differentiation which, in turn, affects morphogenesis, metamorphosis, oncogenesis, and tissue maintenance and repair. The FOP metamorphogene and its encoded receptor are not only therapeutic targets, but the mechanism of their action helps understand developmental and repair processes subject to regulation by ACVR1 signaling. Comprehensive understanding of these processes has important implications for developmental and regenerative medicine [38].

Acknowledgments

Work by the authors discussed in this chapter was supported in part by the International Fibrodysplasia Ossificans Progressiva Association, the Center for Research in FOP and Related Disorders, the Ian Cali Endowment for FOP Research, the Whitney Weldon Endowment for FOP Research, the Isaac & Rose Nassau Professorship of Orthopaedic Molecular Medicine, by grants from the Rita Allen Foundation and the US National Institutes of Health (NIH R01-AR41916).

References

1. Ahn J, Serrano de la Peña L, Shore EM, Kaplan FS (2003) Paresis of a bone morphogenetic protein-antagonist response in a genetic disorder of heterotopic skeletogenesis. J Bone Joint Surg 85-A:667–674
2. Akiyama S, Katagiri T, Namiki M, Yamaji N, Yamamoto N, Miyama K, Shibuya H, Ueno N, Wozney JM, Suda T (1997) Constitutively active BMP type I receptors transduce BMP2 signals without the ligand in C2C12 myoblasts. Exp Cell Res 235:362–369
3. Anderson GJ, Darshan D (2008) Small-molecule dissection of BMP signaling. Nature Chem Biol 4: 15–16
4. Barkai N, Shilo B-Z (2007) Variability and robustness in bimolecular systems. Mol Cell 28:755–760
5. Billings PC, Fiori JL, Bentwood JL, O'Connell MP, Jiao X, Nussbaum B, Caron RJ, Shore EM, Kaplan FS (2008) Dysregulated BMP signaling and enhanced osteogenic differentiation of connective tissue progenitor cells from patients with fibrodysplasia ossificans progressiva. J Bone Miner Res 23:305–313
6. Birnbaum KD, Alvarado AS (2008) Slicing across kingdoms: regeneration in plants and animals. Cell 132: 697–710
7. Brunet LJ, McMahon JA, McMahon AP, Harland RM (1998) Noggin, cartilage morphogenesis, and joint formation in the mammalian skeleton. Science 280: 1455–1457
8. Carlson BM (2005) Some principles of regeneration in mammalian systems. Anat Rec B New Anat 287B:4–13
9. Chakkalakal SA, Zhang D, Raabe T, Richa J, Hankenson K, Kaplan FS, Shore EM (2008) ACVR1 knock-in mouse model for fibrodysplasia ossificans progressiva. J Bone Miner Res 23(suppl 1)
10. Chen Y-G, Liu F, Massague J (1997) Mechanism of TGF-β receptor inhibition by FKBP12. EMBO J 16:3866–3876
11. Cobaleda C, Jochum W, Busslinger M (2007) Conversion of mature B cells into T cells by dedifferentiation to uncommitted progenitors. Nature 449:473–477
12. Cohen RB, Hahn GV, Tabas J, Peeper J, Levitz CL, Sando A, Sando N, Zasloff M, Kaplan FS (1993) The natural history of heterotopic ossification in patients who have fibrodysplasia ossificans progressiva. J Bone Joint Surg 75-A:215–219
13. Connor JM, Evans DA (1982) Fibrodysplasia ossificans progressiva. The clinical features and natural history of 34 patients. J Bone Joint Surg 64(1):76–83
14. Cuny GD, Yui PB, Laha JK, Xing X, Liu J-F, Lai CS, Deng DY, Sachidanandan C, Bloch KD, Peterson RT (2008). Structure-activity relationship study of bone morphogenetic protein (BMP) signaling inhibitors. Bioorg Med Chem Lett 18(15):8366–8377
15. Davis SR, Meltzer PS (2007) Modeling synovial sarcoma: timing is everything. Cancer Cell 11:305–307
16. Deirmengian GK, Hebela NM, O'Connell M, Glaser DL, Shore EM, Kaplan FS, Deirmengian GK (2008) Proximal tibial osteochondromas in patients with fibrodysplasia ossificans progressiva. J Bone Joint Surg Am 90:366–374
17. De Robertis EM (2008) Evo-Devo: variations on ancestral themes. Cell 132:185–195
18. Derynck R, Akhurst RJ (2007) Differentiation plasticity regulated by the TGF-β family proteins in development and disease. Nature Cell Biol 9:1000–1004
19. Ebisawa T, Fukuchi M, Murakami G, Chiba T, Tanaka K, Imamura T, Miyazono K (2001) Smurf 1 interacts with transforming growth factor-β type I receptor through Smad7 and induces receptor degradation. J Biol Chem 276:12477–12480
20. Everman DB, Bartels CF, Yang Y, Yanamandra N, Goodman FR, Mendoza-Londono JR, Savarirayan R, White SM, Graham JM Jr, Gale RP, Svarch E, Newman WG, Kleckers AR, Francomano CA, Govindaiah V, Singh L, Morrison S, Thomas JT, Warman ML (2002) The mutational spectrum of brachydactyly type C. Am J Med Genet 112(3):291–296
21. Fiori JL, Billings PC, Serrano de la Peña L, Kaplan FS, Shore EM (2006) Dysregulation of the BMP-p38 MAPK signaling pathway in cells from patients with fibrodysplasia ossificans progressiva (FOP). J Bone Miner Res 21:902–909
22. Fishman MC, Porter JA (2005) A new grammar for drug discovery. Nature 437:491–493
23. Fuentealba LC, Eivers E, Ikeda A, Hurtado C, Kuroda H, Pera EM, De Robertis EM (2007) Integrating patterning signals: Wnt/GSK3 regulates the duration of the BMP/SMAD1 signal. Cell 131:980–993
24. Fukada T, Kohda M, Kanomata K, Nojima J, Kamizono J, Oda H, Nakayama K, Ohtake A, Miyazono K, Jimi E, Owan I, Okazaki Y, Katagiri T (2007) A constitutively activated BMP receptor, ALK2, induces heterotopic ossification in patients with fibrodysplasia ossificans progressiva. J Bone Miner Res 22(suppl 1):S10
25. Gannon FH, Kaplan FS, Olmsted E, Finkel G, Zasloff MA, Shore EM (1997) Bone morphogenetic

protein 2/4 in early fibromatous lesions of fibrodysplasia ossificans progressiva. Hum Pathol 28:339–343
26. Gannon FH, Valentine BA, Shore EM, Zasloff MA, Kaplan FS (1998) Acute lymphocytic infiltration in an extremely early lesion of fibrodysplasia ossificans progressiva. Clin Orthop Rel Res 346:19–25
27. Glaser DL, Economides AN, Wang L, Liu X, Kimble RD, Fandl JP, Wilson JM, Stahl N, Kaplan FS, Shore EM (2003) In vivo somatic cell gene transfer of an engineered noggin mutein prevents BMP4-induced heterotopic ossification. J Bone Joint Surg 85-A:2332–2342
28. Glaser DL, Rocke DM, Kaplan FS (1998) Catastrophic falls in patients who have fibrodysplasia ossificans progressiva. Clin Orthop Rel Res 346:110–116
29. Groppe JC, Shore EM, Kaplan FS (2007) Functional modeling of the ACVR1 (R206H) mutation in FOP. Clin Orthop Rel Res 462:87–92
30. Haldar M, Hancock JD, Coffin CM, Lessnick SL, Capecchi MR (2007) A conditional mouse model of synovial sarcoma: insights into a myogenic origin. Cancer Cell 11:375–388
31. Harradine KA, Akhurst RJ (2006) Mutations of TGF-β signaling molecules in human disease. Ann Med 38:403–414
32. Hartung A, Sieber C, Knaus P (2006) Yin and Yang in BMP signaling: impact on the pathology of diseases and potential for tissue regeneration. Signal Transduct 6:314–328
33. Hebela N, Shore EM, Kaplan FS (2005) Three pairs of monozygotic twins with fibrodysplasia ossificans progressiva: the role of environment in the progression of heterotopic ossification. Clin Rev Bone Miner Metab 3:205–208
34. Hegyi L, Gannon FH, Glaser DL, Shore EM, Kaplan FS, Shanahan CM (2003) Stromal cells of fibrodysplasia ossificans progressiva lesions express smooth muscle lineage markers and the osteogenic transcription factor Runx2/Cbfa-1: clues to a vascular origin of heterotopic ossification. J Pathol 201:141–148
35. Herpin A, Cunningham C (2007) Cross-talk between the bone morphogenetic protein pathway and other major signaling pathways results in tightly regulated cell-specific outcomes. FEBS J 274:2977–2985
36. Huse M, Chen Y-G, Massague J, Kuriyan J (1999) Crystal structure of the cytosplasmic domain of the type I TGF-β receptor in complex with FKBP12. Cell 96:425–436
37. Huse M, Muir TW, Xu L, Chen YG, Kuriyan J, Massagué J (2001) The TGF-β receptor activation process: an inhibitor-to-substrate binding switch. Mol Cell 8: 671–682
38. Ingber DE, Levin M (2007) What lies at the interface of regenerative medicine and developmental biology? Development 134:2541–2547
39. Janoff HB, Zasloff MA, Kaplan FS (1996) Submandibular swelling in patients with fibrodysplasia ossificans progressiva. Otolaryngol Head Neck Surg 114:599–604
40. Jiao X, Billings PC, O'Connell MP, Kaplan FS, Shore EM, Glaser DL (2007) Heparan sulfate proteoglycans (HSPGs) modulate BMP2 osteogenic bioactivity in C2C12 cells. J Biol Chem 282(2):1080–1086
41. Kan L, Hu M, Gomes WA, Kessler JA (2004) Transgenic mice overexpressing BMP4 develop a fibrodysplasia ossificans progressiva (FOP)-like phenotype. Am J Pathol 165:1107–1115
42. Kan L, Liu Y, McGuire TL, Berger DMP, Atwatramani RB, Dymecki SM, Kessler JA (2009) Dysregulation of local stem/progenitor cells as a common cellular mechanism for heterotopic ossification. Stem Cells, 27: 150–156
43. Kaplan FS (2005) Fibrodysplasia ossificans progressiva: an historical perspective. Clin Rev Bone Miner Metab 3:179–181
44. Kaplan FS (2006) The key to the closet is the key to the kingdom: a common lesson of rare diseases. Orphan Dis Update 24(3):1–9
45. Kaplan FS, Fiori JL, Ahn J, Billings PC, Shore EM (2005) Dysregulation of BMP4 receptor trafficking and signaling in fibrodysplasia ossificans progressiva. Clin Rev Bone Miner Metab 3:217–223
46. Kaplan FS, Fiori J, Serrano de la Peña L, Ahn J, Billings PC, Shore EM (2006) Dysregulation of the BMP4 signaling pathway in fibrodysplasia ossificans progressiva. Ann N Y Acad Sci 1068:54–65
47. Kaplan FS, Glaser DL (2005) Thoracic insufficiency syndrome in patients with fibrodysplasia ossificans progressiva. Clin Rev Bone Miner Metab 3:213–216
48. Kaplan FS, Glaser DL, Pignolo RJ, Shore EM (2004) A new era of fibrodysplasia ossificans progressiva (FOP): a druggable target for the second skeleton. Exp Opin Biol Ther 7:705–712
49. Kaplan FS, Glaser DL, Shore EM, Deirmengian GK, Gupta R, Delai P, Morhart P, Smith R, Le Merrer M, Rogers JG, Connor JM, Kitterman JA (2005) The phenotype of fibrodysplasia ossificans progressiva. Clin Rev Bone Miner Metab 3:183–188
50. Kaplan FS, Glaser DL, Shore EM, Pignolo RJ, Xu M, Zhang Y, Senitzer D, Forman SJ, Emerson SG (2007) Hematopoietic stem-cell contribution to ectopic skeletogenesis. J Bone Joint Surg Am 89:347–357
51. Kaplan FS, Hahn GV, Zasloff MA (2004) Heterotopic ossification. J Am Acad Orthop Surg 12:116–125
52. Kaplan FS, LeMerrer M, Glaser DL, Pignolo RJ, Goldsby RE, Kitterman JA, Groppe J, Shore EM (2008) Fibrodysplasia ossificans progressiva. Best Pract Res Clin Rheumatol 22:191–205
53. Kaplan FS, Shore EM (2007) Morphogen receptor genes and metamorphogenes: skeleton keys to metamorphosis. Ann N Y Acad Sci 1116:113–133
54. Kaplan FS, Shore EM, Gupta R, Billings PC, Glaser DL, Pignolo RJ, Graf D, Kamoun M (2005) Immunological features of fibrodysplasia ossificans progressiva and the dysregulated BMP4 Pathway. Clin Rev Bone Miner Metab 3:189–193
55. Kaplan FS, Strear CM, Zasloff MA (1994) Radiographic and scintigraphic features of modeling and remodeling in the heterotopic skeleton of patients who have fibrodysplasia ossificans progressiva. Clin Orthop Rel Res 304:238–247
56. Kaplan FS, Tabas JA, Zasloff MA (1990) Fibrodysplasia ossificans progressiva: a clue from the fly? Calcif Tiss Int 47:117–125

57. Kaplan FS, Xu M, Glaser DL Collins F, Connor M, Kitterman J, Sillence D, Zackai E, Ravitsky V, Zasloff M, Ganguly A, Shore EM (2008) Early diagnosis of fibrodysplasia ossificans progressiva. Pediatrics 121: e1295–e1300
58. Kaplan FS, Xu M, Seemann P, Connor M, Glaser DL, Carroll, L, Delai P, Fastnacht-Urban E, Forman SJ, Gillessen-Kaesbach G, Hoover-Fong J, Köster B, Pauli RM, Reardon W, Zaidi S-A, Zasloff M, Morhart R, Mundlos S, Groppe J, Shore EM (2008) Classic and atypical FOP phenotypes caused by mutations in the BMP type I receptor ACVR1. Hum Mutat 30:379–390
59. Kaplan FS, Zasloff MA (1993) The histopathology of fibrodysplasia ossificans progressiva: an endochondral process. J Bone Joint Surg 75-A:220–230
60. Kitterman JA, Kantanie S, Rocke DM, Kaplan FS (2005) Iatrogenic harm caused by diagnostic errors in fibrodysplasia ossificans progressiva. Pediatrics 116: 654–661
61. Koentges G (2008) Evolution of anatomy and gene control. Nature 451:658–663
62. Kussmaul WG, Esmail AN, Sagar Y, Ross J, Gregory S, Kaplan FS (1998) Pulmonary and cardiac function in advanced fibrodysplasia ossificans progressiva. Clin Orthop Rel Res 346:104–109
63. Lanchoney TF, Cohen RB, Rocke DM, Zasloff MA, Kaplan FS (1995) Permanent heterotopic ossification at the injection site after diphtheria-tetanus-pertussis immunizations in children who have fibrodysplasia ossificans progressiva. J Pediatr 126:762–764
64. Lander AD (2007) Morpheus unbound: reimagining the morphogen gradient. Cell 128:245–256
65. Lehmann K, Seemann P, Boergermann J, Morin G, Reif S, Knaus P, Mundlos S (2006) A novel R486Q mutation in BMPR1B resulting in either a brachydactyly type C/symphalangism-like phenotype or brachydactyly type A2. Eur J Hum Genet 14(12):1248–54
66. Lehmann K, Seemann P, Stricker S, Sammar M, Meyer B, Süring K, Majewski F, Tinschert S, Grzeschik K-H, Müller D, Knaus, P, Nürnberg P, Mundlos S (2003) Mutations in bone morphogenetic protein receptor 1B cause brachydactyly type A2. Proc Natl Acad Sci U S A 100(21):12277–82
67. Lounev VY, Ramachandran R, Wosczyna MN, Yamamoto M, Maidment ADA, Shore EM, Glaser EM, Goldhamer DJ, Kaplan FS (2008) Identification of progenitor cells that contribute to heterotopic skeletogenesis. J Bone Joint Surgery Am 91:652–663
68. Luchetti W, Cohen RB, Hahn GV, Rocke DM, Helpin M, Zasloff M, Kaplan FS (1995) Severe restriction in jaw movement after routine injection of local anesthetic in patients who have fibrodysplasia ossificans progressiva. Oral Surg Oral Med Oral Pathol Oral Radiol Endod 81:21–25
69. Mahboubi S, Glaser DL, Shore EM, Kaplan FS (2001) Fibrodysplasia ossificans progressiva. Pediatr Radiol 31:307–314
70. Mishina Y, Crombie R, Bradley A, Behringer RR (1999) Multiple roles for activin-like kinase-2 signaling during mouse embryogenesis. Dev Biol 213(2):314–26
71. Moriatis JM, Gannon FH, Shore EM, Bilker W, Zasloff MA, Kaplan FS (1997) Limb swelling in patients who have fibrodysplasia ossificans progressiva. Clin Orthop Rel Res 336:247–253
72. Olmsted EA, Kaplan FS, Shore EM (2003) Bone morphogenetic protein 4 regulation in fibrodysplasia ossificans progressiva. Clin Orthop Rel Res 408: 331–343
73. Olmsted-Davis E, Gannon FH, Ozen M, Ittmann MM, Gugala Z, Hipp JA, Moran KM, Fouletier-Dilling CM, Schumara-Martin S, Lindsey RW, Heggeness MH, Brenner MK, Davis AR (2007) Hypoxic adipocytes pattern early heterotopic bone formation. Am J Pathol 170:620–632
74. Ovchinnikov DA, Selever J, Ying W, Chen Y-T, Mishina Y, Martin JF, Behringer RR (2006) BMP receptor type IA in limb bud mesenchyme regulates distal outgrowth and patterning. Dev Biol 295(1):10–3–15
75. Pignolo RJ, Suda RK, Kaplan FS (2005) The fibrodysplasia ossificans progressiva lesion. Clin Rev Bone Miner Metab 3:195–200
76. Plöger F, Seemann P, Schmidt-von Kegler M, Lehmann K, Seidel J, Kjaer KW, Pohl J, Mundlos S (2008) Brachydactyly type A2 associated with a defect in proGDF5 BMP processing. Hum Mol Genet 17(9):1222–1233
77. Prud'homme B, Gompel N, Carroll SB (2007) Emerging principles of regulatory evolution. Proc Natl Acad Sci U S A 104(suppl 1):8605–8612
78. Rocke DM, Zasloff M, Peeper J, Cohen RB, Kaplan FS (1994) Age and joint-specific risk of initial heterotopic ossification in patients who have fibrodysplasia ossificans progressiva. Clin Orthop Rel Res 301:243–248
79. Rosenstirn JA (1918) A contribution to the study of myositis ossificans progressiva. Ann Surg 68:468–520; 591–637
80. Roush W (1996) Protein builds second skeleton. Science 273:1170
81. Scarlett RF, Rocke DM, Kantanie S, Patel JB, Shore EM, Kaplan FS (2004). Influenza-like viral illnesses and flare-ups of fibrodysplasia ossificans progressiva (FOP) Clin Orthop Rel Res 423:275–279
82. Schaffer AA, Kaplan FS, Tracy MR, O'Brien ML, Dormans JP, Shore EM, Harland RM, Kusumi K (2005) Developmental anomalies of the cervical spine in patients with fibrodysplasia ossificans progressiva are distinctly different from those in patients with Klippel-Feil syndrome. Spine 30:1379–1385
83. Schmierer B, Hill CS (2007) TGF-β-SMAD signal transduction: molecular specificity and functional flexibility. Nat Rev Mol Cell Bio 8:970–982
84. Seemann P, Schwappacher R, Kjaer KW, Krakow D, Lehmann K, Dawson K, Stricker S, Pohl J, Plöger F, Staub E, Nickel J, Sebald W, Knaus P, Mundlos S (2005) Activating and deactivating mutations in the receptor interaction site of GDF5 cause symphalangism or brachydactyly type A2. J Clin Invest 115(9):2373–81
85. Serrano de la Peña L, Billings PC, Fiori JL, Ahn J, Shore EM, Kaplan FS (2005) Fibrodysplasia ossificans progressiva (FOP), a disorder of ectopic osteogenesis, misregulates cell surface expression and trafficking of BMPRIA. J Bone Miner Res 20:1168–1176

86. Shafritz AB, Shore EM, Gannon FH, Zasloff MA, Taub R, Muenke M, Kaplan FS (1996) Over-expression of an osteogenic morphogen in fibrodysplasia ossificans progressiva. N Engl J Med 335:555–561
87. Shah PB, Zasloff MA, Drummond D, Kaplan FS (1994) Spinal deformity in patients who have fibrodysplasia ossificans progressiva. J Bone Joint Surg 76-A:1442–1450
88. Shen Q, Xu M, Little SC, Kaplan FS, Mullins MC, Shore EM (2007) Activation of BMP signaling by the FOP ACVR1 R206H mutation. J Bone Miner Res 22(suppl 1):S43
89. Shore EM, Feldman GJ, Xu M, Kaplan FS (2005) The genetics of fibrodysplasia ossificans progressiva. Clin Rev Bone Miner Metab 3:201–204
90. Shore EM, Kaplan FS (2008) Insights from a rare genetic disorder of extra-skeletal bone formation, fibrodysplasia ossificans progressiva (FOP). Bone 43:427–433
91. Shore EM, Xu M, Feldman GJ, Fenstermacher DA, Cho T-J, Choi IH, Connor JM, Delai P, Glaser DL, Le Merrer M, Morhart R, Rogers JG, Smith R, Triffitt JT, Urtizberea JA, Zasloff M, Brown MA, Kaplan FS (2006) A recurrent mutation in the BMP type I receptor ACVR1 causes inherited and sporadic fibrodysplasia ossificans progressiva. Nat Genet 38:525–527
92. Stoick-Cooper CL, Moon RT, Weidinger G (2007) Advances in signaling in vertebrate regeneration as a prelude to regenerative medicine. Genes Dev 21: 1292–1315
93. Verheyen EM (2007) Opposing effects of Wnt and MAPK on BMP/SMAD signal duration. Dev Cell 13:755–756
94. Wagner TU (2007) Bone morphogenetic protein signaling in stem cells – one signal many consequences. FEBS J 274:2968–2976
95. Wang T, Li B-Y, Danielson PD, Shah PC, Rockwell S, Lechleider RJ, Martin J, Manganaro T, Donahoe PK (1996) The immunophilin FKBP12 functions as a common inhibitor of the TGF-β family type I receptors. Cell 86:435–444
96. Xu MQ, Feldman G, LeMerrer M, Shugart YY, Glaser DL, Urtizberea JA, Fardeau M, Connor JM, Triffitt J, Smith R, Shore EM, Kaplan FS (2000) Linkage exclusion and mutational analysis of the noggin gene in patients with fibrodysplasia ossificans progressiva (FOP). Clin Genet 58:291–298
97. Yamaguchi T, Kurisaki A, Yamakawa N, Minakuchi K, Sugino H (2006) FKBP12 functions as an adaptor of the Smad7-Smurf1 complex on activin type I receptor. J Mol Endocrinol 36:569–579
98. Yi SE, Daluiski A, Pederson R, Rosen V, Lyons KM (2000) The type I BMP receptor BMPR1B is required for chondrogenesis in the mouse limb. Development 127(3):621–30
99. Yoon BS, Lyons KM (2004) Multiple functions of BMPs in chondrogenesis. J Cell Biochem 93(1):93–103
100. Yoon BS, Ovchinnikov DA, Yoshii I, Mishina Y, Behringer RR, Lyons KM (2005) BMPR1A and BMPR1B have overlapping functions and are essential for chondrogenesis in vivo. Proc Natl Acad Sci U S A 102(14):5062–7
101. Yu PB, Deng DY, Lai CS, Hong CC, Cuny GD, Bouxsein ML, Hong DW, McManus PM, Katagiri T, Sachidanandan C, Kamiya N, Fukuda T, Mishina Y, Peterson RT, Bloch KD (2008) BMP type I receptor inhibition prevents ectopic ossification in mouse model of fibrodysplasia ossificans progressiva (FOP). Nat Med 14(12):1363–1364
102. Yu PB, Hong CC, Sachidanandan C, Babitt JL, Deng DY, Hoyng SA, Lin HY, Block KD, Peterson RT (2008) Dorsomorphin inhibits BMP signals required for embryogenesis and iron metabolism. Nat Chem Biol 4:33–41
103. Zhang D, Schwarz EM, Rosier RN, Zuscik MJ, Puzas JE, O'Keefe RJ (2003) ALK2 functions as a BMP type I receptor and induces Indian Hedgehog in chondrocytes during skeletal development. J Bone Miner Res 18:1593–1604

15. Bone-Mineral Homeostasis and Associated Pathologies

Meinrad Peterlik

15.1 Introduction

Bone-mineral homeostasis (*homoióstasis* = equilibrium in Greek) is the result of the interplay of two intertwined endocrine circuits formed by the feedback-regulated actions of 1,25-dihydroxyvitamin D_3 (1,25-$(OH)_2D_3$) and parathyroid hormone (PTH). Partially divergent effects of two hormones on calcium and phosphate fluxes in the classical target organs (intestine, kidney, and bone) have to be carefully orchestrated at any time during the life of a vertebrate organism to meet the ever-changing demands of bone growth and functions. This can only be achieved if the input into the system from the outside will allow it to adjust itself to different functional levels, i.e., to promote longitudinal growth during development, to build up an adequate peak bone mass through appositional bone growth until 20–30 years of age, to meet the specific challenge for bone-mineral homeostasis during pregnancy, and finally to maintain structural and functional integrity as long as possible in the face of continuous involutional bone loss throughout adulthood.

15.2 Physiological Aspects

The principles of systemic bone-mineral homeostasis are illustrated in Fig. 15.1. The key to short-term regulation of bone-mineral metabolism is the expression of the extracellular calcium-sensing receptor (CaR) on the plasma membrane of parathyroid gland "chief" cells [120]. The CaR

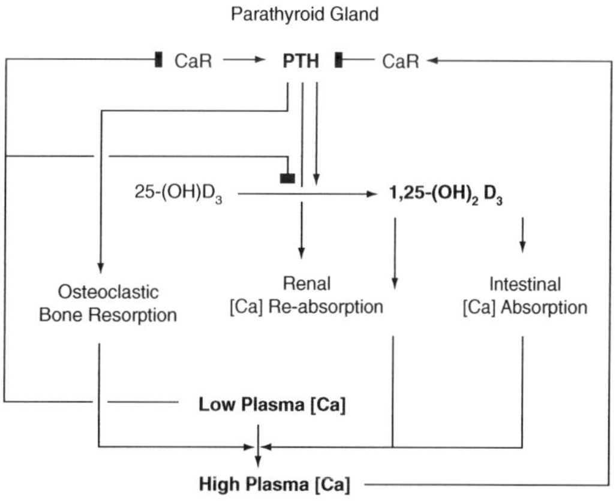

Figure 15.1. Control of systemic bone-mineral homeostasis by PTH and 1,25-$(OH)_2D_3$.

F. Bronner et al. (eds.), *Bone and Development*, Topics in Bone Biology 6,
DOI 10.1007/978-1-84882-822-3_15,

is a 7-membrane spanning G protein-coupled receptor, which "senses" and transduces signals from variations in plasma Ca^{2+} to intracellular pathways that regulate the synthesis of PTH, among other cellular functions. Parathyroid gland cells can thus rapidly respond to minute alterations of plasma Ca^{2+} by appropriate changes in PTH secretion. PTH in turn will control the rate of Ca reabsorption in the kidney so that plasma Ca^{2+} can be maintained within physiological range.

During fetal development, bone-mineral homeostasis is maintained through the actions of PTH on fetal bone and kidney and of the parathyroid hormone-related peptide (PTHrP) on placental mineral-ion transport [63]. Both hormones signal through the same G protein-coupled receptor, the PTH/PTHrP receptor. PTHrP also plays a key role in the regulation of endochondral bone development. PTHrP is produced by perichondrial cells and chondrocytes, and in a feedback loop with Indian hedge hog, regulates the pace of chondrocytes, differentiation at sites at which perichondrial cells first differentiate into osteoblasts [66]. Block of PTHrP intracellular signaling at the level of the nucleus causes severe skeletal growth retardation by impairment of endochondral bone formation [87]. Notably, the CaR also has a key role in embryonic development of the skeleton as recently shown in the elegant study of Chang et al. [21]. Selective deletion of the *CaR* on chondrocytes in mice between embryonic day 16–18 caused delayed development of the growth plate.

At term, blood cord levels of PTHrP exceed those of PTH by far. However, the presence of both hormones is required to maintain fetal blood calcium at higher than maternal levels and thereby provide sufficient calcium for the normal development and mineralization of bone during gestation [63]. The CaR may play a dual role in regulating blood calcium in the fetus. In the parathyroid gland, the CaR may be responsible for the suppression of PTH release in response to elevated fetal blood calcium. Since the CaR is expressed in placental tissue, it may play a role in promoting calcium transfer across the placenta.

Vitamin D seems to have no major impact on fetal bone and mineral metabolism. Utilizing a *VDR* knockout mouse model, Kovacs et al. [64] found that VDR is not required by fetal mice to regulate placental calcium transfer, circulating mineral levels, and skeletal mineralization. This indicates that the VDR-mediated effects of 1,25-$(OH)_2D_3$ on bone and mineral metabolism are redundant and that Ca^{2+} can subsume the role of vitamin D [30]. In other words, as long as Ca^{2+} homeostasis in the fetus is maintained by unimpaired signaling from PTH/PTHrP, maternal vitamin D deficiency has no negative effect on bone development and mineralization.

This is certainly not the case during postnatal development and throughout adult life. At that time, long-term regulation of bone-mineral metabolism needs strong input from the vitamin D endocrine system. Whether synthesized in the epidermis or absorbed from the diet, vitamin D_3 is converted in the liver to 25-hydroxyvitamin D_3 (25-$(OH)D_3$). Serum levels of this vitamin D compound are considered a reliable indicator for the vitamin D status of an individual. Whether 25-$(OH)D_3$ is further hydroxylated in the kidney to either 24,25-dihydroxyvitamin D_3 (24,25-$(OH)_2D_3$) or to 1,25-$(OH)_2D_3$ depends on the requirements for long-term bone-mineral homeostasis: With mineral metabolism at equilibrium, activity of the *CYP24A1*-encoded enzyme, 25-$(OH)D_3$–24-hydroxylase, is high; therefore, 24,25-$(OH)_2D_3$ is the predominant circulating vitamin D metabolite. However, when the organism is in need of calcium and phosphate, the *CYP27B1*-encoded 25-(OH)D-1α-hydroxylase in renal proximal tubular cells is upregulated by PTH, as well as by low serum [Ca^{2+}] and phosphate. 1,25-$(OH)_2D_3$ then stimulates calcium and phosphate uptake across the intestinal mucosa and the renal tubular epithelium. In addition, 1,25-$(OH)_2D_3$, in concert with elevated PTH, promotes osteoclast differentiation and activation, causing calcium and phosphate mobilization from bone. Together, this will restore systemic bone-mineral homeostasis to normal levels (Fig. 15.1).

Altogether, outside input is necessary to allow the 1,25-$(OH)_2D_3$/PTH endocrine system to function at varying steady-state levels of efficiency. To achieve this requires adequate supply of (a) Ca^{2+} and inorganic phosphate for mineralization of newly formed bone and (b) vitamin D_3 so that the circulating levels of 25-$(OH)D_3$ are adequate to produce sufficient quantities of

$1,25\text{-}(OH)_2D_3$ not only in the kidney but also at many extrarenal sites, as detailed below.

15.3 Pathophysiological Aspects

15.3.1 Dysfunction of Short-Term Regulation of Mineral Metabolism

PTH plays a unique role in short-term regulation of calcium homeostasis. This explains why ablation of parathyroid gland tissue, a frequent accident during thyroid surgery, causes acute hypocalcemia. The precipitous fall of plasma Ca^{2+} that occurs within minutes following parathyroidectomy lowers the threshold for neuromuscular excitation–contraction coupling with the well-known symptoms of tetanic spasms of skeletal muscles. Ca^{2+} infusion will resolve the acute situation. However, long-term maintenance of normal plasma $[Ca^{2+}]$ requires the administration of $1,25\text{-}(OH)_2D_3$ or of one of its hypercalcemic analogs, such as $1\alpha\text{-}(OH)D_3$, to avoid adverse effects on bone health.

15.3.2 Long-Term Dysfunction of Bone-Mineral Homeostasis

A compromised vitamin D status and an inadequate supply of mineral ions are risk factors not only for bone diseases such as rickets, osteomalacia, or osteoporosis, but also for malignant, chronic inflammatory, autoimmune, metabolic, and cardiovascular diseases [97]. Why vitamin D and calcium deficits are pathogenic for so many chronic diseases remains an enigma, particularly because even under these conditions, systemic homeostatic mechanisms maintain the plasma Ca^{2+} and $1,25\text{-}(OH)_2D_3$ levels within the normal range [47, 90, 91]. Studies from our laboratory on the expression of the 25-hydroxyvitamin D-1α-hydroxylase (25-(OH)D-1α-hydroxylase) in human colon carcinoma cells has suggested that tumor progression can be inhibited by autocrine/paracrine effects of endogenously synthesized $1,25\text{-}(OH)_2D_3$, and that this antitumor defense mechanism is impaired at low-plasma levels of 25-(OH)D [26, 60]. This notion can now be extended to a general concept of a local control by $1,25\text{-}(OH)_2D_3$ of cell functions in health and disease, because a widespread expression of the 25-(OH)D-1α-hydroxylase is found in nonrenal tissues and cellular systems [139]. Moreover, the pioneering work of Brown and colleagues on the expression, function, and tissue distribution of the extracellular calcium-sensing receptor (CaR) has added to the understanding of the role played by extracellular Ca^{2+} as first messenger for many cellular responses under normal and pathological conditions [120].

15.3.2.1 Definition of the Vitamin D Status

As mentioned earlier, the serum level of 25-(OH)D[1] is considered a reliable indicator of the vitamin D status of a person. Outright vitamin D deficiency or depletion inevitably causes rickets or osteomalacia and is indicated by 25-(OH)D concentrations below 10 nM. The term vitamin D insufficiency or inadequacy is used to describe a condition in which vitamin D supply is suboptimal and where 25-(OH)D levels are inversely related to the incidence of many chronic diseases [97]. Importantly, low-serum 25-(OH)D has been shown to be a reliable predictor of all-cause mortality [33]. Conservative calculations of the set point between vitamin D insufficiency and optimal vitamin D supply suggested a value of 30 nM 25-(OH)D [23], but there is increasing evidence that for optimal health outcomes, serum 25-(OH)D should be maintained between 60 and 100 nM [11, 28, 44, 51].

Vitamin D insufficiency is frequently observed in individuals with limited sun exposure, as in the chronically ill, immobilized, or housebound elderly people. Yet, a compromised vitamin D status is also common in the free-living normal population at any age. In a large multicenter study on the calcium and vitamin D status of more than 1,000 healthy Austrian men and women, 19–79 years of age, 26% had 25-(OH)D levels below 30 nM [67]. Similar reports from the USA, Great Britain, and Finland [27, 54, 70] lend support to the inference that vitamin D insufficiency is widespread in adults of the Western world.

[1]The term 25-(OH)D is used to denote the sum of $25\text{-}(OH)D_3$ and $25\text{-}(OH)D_2$, the latter from dietary sources.

15.3.2.2 Calcium Insufficiency

The levels of daily calcium intake as a preventative against osteoporosis vary according to age, sex, and hormonal status [41]. A minimum of 1,000 mg calcium per day is required for healthy adults until age 60, whereas higher values apply to people of advanced age, to pregnant or nursing women, or after menopause. Evidence is accumulating that calcium malnutrition is not only encountered in the elderly [6] but is also widespread in the young. A recent survey on the calcium, vitamin D, and bone status of a healthy adult population in Austria [67] found that 87% of the study participants did not meet the current recommendations on calcium intake. Comparable results have been reported by, among others, Ma et al. [78] who had analyzed data from a national survey in the USA.

15.3.2.3 Prevalence of Combined Vitamin D and Calcium Insufficiency

As already mentioned, in a population-based cross-sectional study on the calcium and vitamin D status of healthy adults of both sexes [67, 68], in over 80% of the cohort daily calcium consumption was below recommended levels, and 26% had to be considered vitamin D-insufficient. When the calcium intake was calculated according to 25-(OH)D serum levels, 23% of the entire cohort were found to exhibit combined vitamin D and calcium insufficiency [97]. Such individuals have a high risk for osteoporosis but also for many cancers, because calcium and vitamin D status act largely together in the pathogenesis of these diseases [97, 98].

15.3.2.4 Inorganic Phosphate Insufficiency

Because inorganic phosphate is readily available in the diet, and its absorption from the stomach is by passive nonsaturable diffusion, cases of long-term phosphate insufficiency are relatively rare. Nevertheless, it has been estimated that about 2% of hospital patients have mild or severe hypophosphatemia (i.e., serum phosphate concentration <1.0 mg/100 mL) and show symptoms of skeletal disorders (osteomalacia and osteoporosis), disturbances of renal electrolyte metabolism and dysfunction of the nervous, respiratory, and cardiovascular system [80].

15.3.2.5 Relevance of Adequate 25-(OH)D Levels for Organ-Specific Control of Cell Functions

Conversion of 25-(OH)D_3 to 1,25-$(OH)_2D_3$ is catalyzed by the *CYP27B1*-encoded enzyme 25-(OH)D-1α-hydoxylase and occurs primarily in the kidney (Fig. 15.2). However, many extrarenal cells also biosynthesize 1,25-$(OH)_2D_3$. Examples are normal and neoplastic epithelial cells of the skin [103], gastrointestinal tract [60, 107, 113], and reproductive organs [7, 39, 114]. Other sites of 1,25-$(OH)_2D_3$ biosynthesis include osteoblasts and osteoclasts [4, 125], as well as cells of the vascular [138], central nervous [36], and immune systems [50, 117] (Fig. 15.2).

Renal CYP27B1 activity is tightly regulated by serum Ca^{2+} and PTH, as well as by feedback inhibition from 1,25-$(OH)_2D_3$ (Fig. 15.2). Therefore, circulating 1,25-$(OH)_2D_3$ can be maintained in the normal range, 75–200 pM, even when serum levels of 25-(OH)D are relatively low [47]. Extrarenal synthesis of 1,25-$(OH)_2D_3$ is, however, regulated differently. Expression of *CYP27B1* at extrarenal sites can be modulated independently of circulating PTH, Ca^{2+} [58], or 1,25-$(OH)_2D_3$ [1, 72]. In other words, 25-(OH)D-1α-hydroxylase activity depends largely on ambient 25-(OH)D levels (Fig. 15.2). This may explain why the incidence of vitamin D insufficiency-related chronic diseases is correlated primarily with low-serum 25-(OH)D and only to a lesser extent with low 1,25-$(OH)_2D_3$: This is true for osteoporosis [22], cancer [104], particularly of the colorectum [37], breast [8], and prostate gland [124], and for cardiovascular disease [33]. Indeed, when serum levels of 25-(OH)D are low, CYP27B1 activity in extrarenal cellular systems may not be high enough to achieve steady-state tissue concentrations of 1,25-$(OH)_2D_3$ necessary to regulate cellular growth, differentiation, and function. Therefore, vitamin D insufficiency plays an important pathogenic role in many common chronic diseases [97].

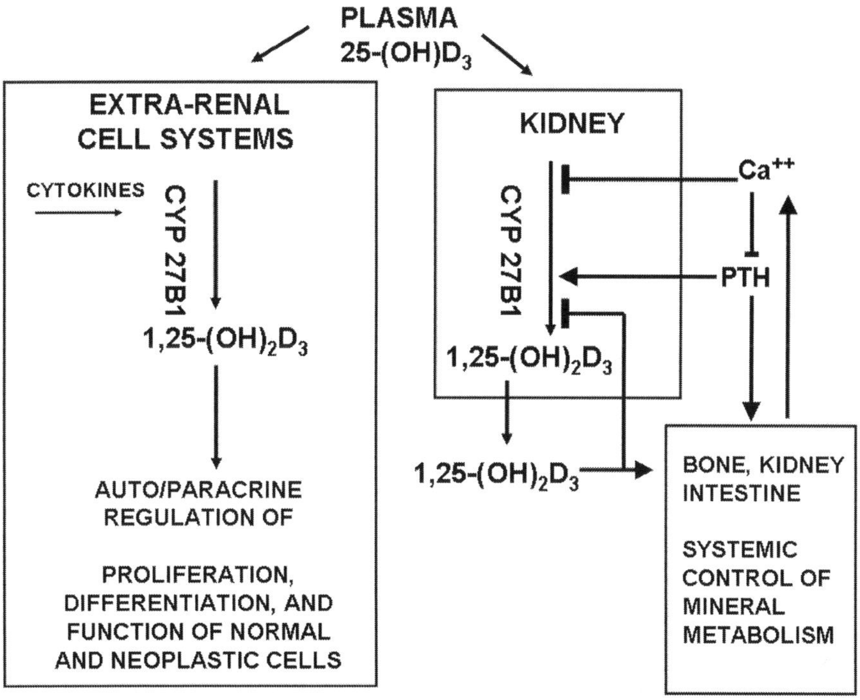

Figure 15.2. Systemic (*right*) vs. autocrine/paracrine (*left*) actions of 1,25-$(OH)_2D_3$.

15.3.2.6 Relevance of Adequate Calcium Intake for Extracellular Ca^{2+} Homeostasis and Control of Cellular Functions

An inadequate calcium intake not only has negative effects on bone health but also increases the risk of certain types of cancer, hypertension, metabolic and cardiovascular diseases, autoimmune disorders, and neuromuscular dysfunctions [97]. It was difficult to understand what were the signals from calcium status and how they were transduced to organs and cell systems distant from the intestinal lumen, until Brown and colleagues [16] cloned an extracellular calcium-sensing receptor (CaR) from the bovine parathyroid gland. Other cells that express this receptor include human osteoblasts [115], renal [16], gastric [48], and large intestinal epithelial cells [60], mammary gland [24], ovarian [84], prostate gland [112], pancreatic duct [106], and islet cells [118], as well as monocytes, macrophages, and dendritic cells [135]. Furthermore, in many regions of the brain, neuronal and glial cells express the CaR [137]. The CaR transduces minute changes in extracellular fluid Ca^{2+} concentrations to stimulatory and inhibitory G proteins of many intracellular signaling pathways. Consequently, when extracellular Ca^{2+} drops, as when there is inadequate dietary supply, not only will the parathyroid gland release more PTH but cellular homeostasis and functions in many other tissues and biological systems will be also affected. CaR-mediated changes affect proliferation, differentiation, apoptosis, hormone secretion, and inflammatory responses and thus contribute to the pathogenesis of chronic diseases (see later).

15.4 Pathogenesis of Vitamin D and Calcium Insufficiency-Related Diseases

15.4.1 Bone Diseases

15.4.1.1 Rickets and Osteomalacia

The prevention of rickets and osteomalacia by vitamin D has been attributed to the stimulation by 1,25-$(OH)_2D_3$ of transcellular calcium and

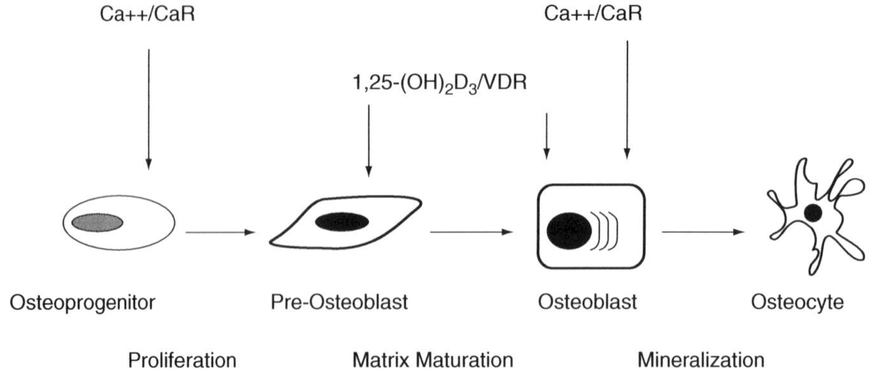

Figure 15.3. Differential effects of 1,25-$(OH)_2D_3$ and Ca^{2+} on osteoblast proliferation and maturation.

phosphate absorption. However, mineralization of the organic matrix depends primarily on growth factor-stimulated osteoprogenitor cells and their further maturation into differentiated osteoblasts. This process is tightly controlled by VDR-mediated effects of 1,25-$(OH)_2D_3$ on temporal expression of genes that encode the noncollagenous matrix proteins necessary for initiation of the mineralization process [94] (cf. Fig. 15.3). Osteoblasts, because of their CYP27B1 activity [4, 125], are an important source of 1,25-$(OH)_2D_3$ In vitamin D deficiency, however, it is the lack of endogenously produced 1, 25-$(OH)_2D_3$ that severely compromises osteoblast differentiation and mineralization of the organic matrix.

It is also important to recall that rickets is not only due to a lack of vitamin D, but also due to calcium deficiency [99]. Otherwise, the disease would not be prevalent in tropical countries with ample sunlight but insufficient calcium intake from cereal-based diets [5, 123]. Hereditary hypophosphatemias provide another example of rickets being caused by a disturbance of mineral metabolism rather than by impaired VDR action. Persistence of hypertrophic chondrocytes at the epiphyseal growth plate is observed in both X-linked and autosomal-dominant hypophosphatemic rickets. Utilizing two mouse models of disturbed mineral metabolism, Sabbagh et al. [111] provided convincing evidence that hypophosphatemia leads to rickets by impairing caspase-mediated apoptosis of hypertrophic chondrocytes.

15.4.1.2 Osteoporosis

Vitamin D insufficiency and calcium malnutrition are important risk factors of involutional osteoporosis in both males and females [108]. This is illustrated by, among others, a recent report from Looker and Mussolino [77] that hip fractures in older adults were associated with low serum levels of 25-(OH)D and calcium. The need for both vitamin D_3 and calcium to prevent and treat osteoporosis [14] is because the formation of mineralized bone depends on signaling from Ca^{2+}/CaR and 1,25$(OH)_2D_3$/VDR [34, 96]. As illustrated in Fig. 15.3, activation of the CaR by an increase in extracellular Ca^{2+} first stimulates preosteoblasts to proliferate [134] and produce collagen. Then, signaling from 1,25$(OH)_2D_3$/VDR promotes osteoblast differentiation through phases of matrix maturation and mineralization [94]. At this stage, signaling from the CaR seems to be particularly important for orderly bone formation by regulating crystal growth and preventing excessive mineralization [34].

Low 25-(OH)D is detrimental to bone health, not only because it impairs osteoblast differentiation, but because it also leads to secondary hyperparathyroidism. Particularly in the elderly, serum 25-(OH)D levels are inversely correlated with PTH secretion [67]. One explanation for this phenomenon could be that in vitamin D insufficiency, CYP27B1-mediated production of 1,25$(OH)_2D_3$ in parathyroid gland cells may be too low to effectively suppress PTH secretion and subsequent action on osteoclasts [109].

15.4.2 Cancer

Vitamin D insufficiency and poor calcium nutrition are risk factors for various types of malignancy. For example, in ecological studies, using solar UV-B exposure as an index of vitamin D_3 photoproduction in the skin, Grant [45] showed a highly significant inverse relationship between UV-B and mortality in 15 types of cancer. Pilz et al. [104] found that low serum 25-(OH)D levels predict fatal cancer in general. Many observational studies have reported a strong association between a low vitamin D status and cancer incidence or mortality from colon, rectal, breast, prostate, and ovarian cancer [42]. There is firm evidence that colorectal [25, 133] and breast cancers [74, 83, 116] are associated also with poor calcium nutrition. In addition, low calcium intake may contribute to the development of gastric [136], endometrial [119], renal [53], and ovarian cancers [62], and multiple myeloma [52].

The study of Lappe et al. [71] on the effect of calcium and vitamin D on cumulative risk of cancer of the breast, lung, colon, uterus, lymphoid, and myeloid system provides an impressive example of the efficacy of combined calcium and vitamin D supplementation in cancer prevention in general. In particular, in a study on the effect of vitamin D and calcium supplementation on recurrence of colorectal adenomas, Grau et al. [46] found that calcium supplementation was effective in patients only if their 25-(OH)D values were normal. Conversely, high-25-(OH)D levels were associated with a reduced risk of adenoma recurrence only among subjects on calcium supplements. Cho et al. [25] concluded from an analysis of pooled primary data from ten cohort studies, in which more than half a million individuals were followed up for 6–16 years, that optimal risk reduction for colorectal cancer necessitates high intakes of both vitamin D and calcium. In premenopausal women, Bérubé et al. [9] found that there were highly significant negative associations between total intakes of vitamin D and calcium with mammographic breast density, which is a positive indicator of breast cancer risk. It is noteworthy that higher intake of one nutrient was related to lower breast density only in the presence of higher intake of the other nutrient. This strongly suggests that only high intake of vitamin D and calcium combined is an effective regimen for prevention of breast cancer.

1,25-$(OH)_2D_3$ exerts antiproliferative effects on cancer cells by modulating the transcriptional activity of key genes involved in cell cycle control [29]. 1,25-$(OH)_2D_3$ may also suppress tumor growth and progression indirectly by facilitating immunocytotoxic killing of tumor cells. 1,25-$(OH)_2D_3$ reduces levels of immunosuppressive $CD34^+$ lymphocytes, which normally limit the cytotoxic activity of infiltrating tumor-specific $CD8^+$ T lymphocytes [129]. The nearly ubiquitous expression of *CYP27B1* and the importance of intrinsic 1,25-$(OH)_2D_3$ production to control cell proliferation may explain why vitamin D insufficiency increases the risk of malignancies in many organs and biological systems.

The CaR is an essential part of an intricate network of calcium signaling pathways that control normal and cancer cell growth [19, 110, 120]. Depending on cell-specific coupling to appropriate G proteins, activation of the CaR by elevated extracellular Ca^{2+} reduces the rate of cellular proliferation as in human colon carcinoma [20, 59] or ovarian surface epithelial cells [10]. However, it may also stimulate cell growth as in Leydig cancer cells [122] and protect from apoptosis, as in prostate cancer cells [75].

Three modes of interaction between 1,25-$(OH)_2D_3$ and calcium in modulating cell growth have been identified in the colon mucosa: (a) antiproliferative signaling pathways from the VDR and CaR converge on the same downstream elements in the canonical *Wnt* pathway. 1,25$(OH)_2D_3$ and Ca^{2+} inhibit cell division and induce differentiation by suppressing the T cell proliferation factor (TCF)-4/β-catenin activity and subsequent upregulation of *E-cadherin* [20, 95] (Fig. 15.4). (b) High-luminal calcium not only inhibits cellular growth by activating the CaR, but at the same time suppresses the vitamin D catabolizing enzyme 25-(OH)D-24-hydroxylase (CYP24) (Fig. 15.1); this very likely leads to higher steady-state local concentrations of 1,25$(OH)_2D_3$ [58, 92]. (c) 1,25$(OH)_2D_3$ may upregulate expression of the CaR [17] and thus augment CaR-mediated antiproliferative responses to high extracellular $[Ca^{2+}]$.

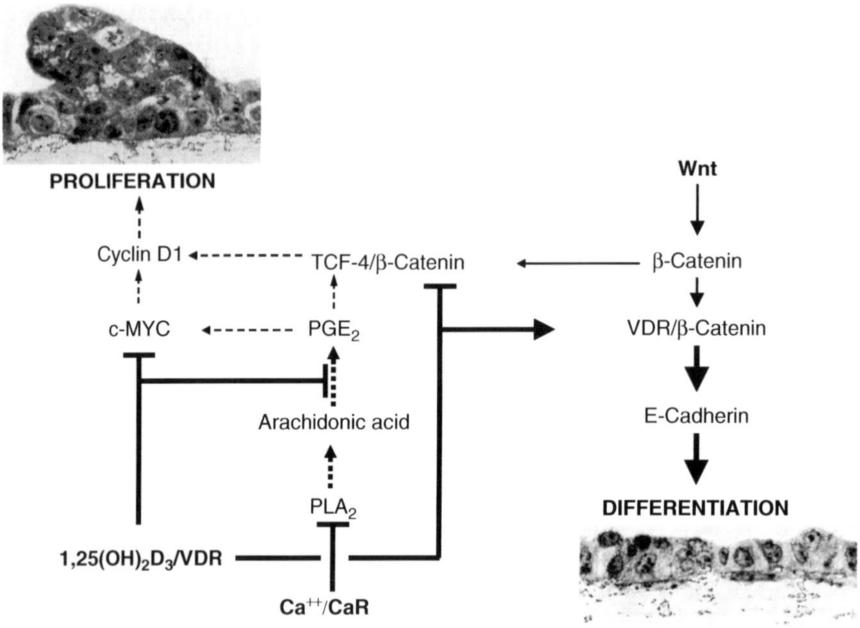

Figure 15.4. Cooperative signaling from 1,25-$(OH)_2D_3$/VDR and Ca^{2+}/CaR inhibits proliferation and promotes differentiation of human colon cancer cells.

15.4.3 Diabetes Mellitus Type I

A compromised vitamin D status increases the risk for autoimmune diseases, such as inflammatory bowel disease [40], rheumatoid arthritis [85], systemic lupus erythematodes [61], multiple sclerosis [89], and type I diabetes mellitus [55]. This effect can be attributed to the reduced capability of immunoregulatory cells to produce 1,25-$(OH)_2D_3$, with the result that the immunomodulatory and antiinflammatory actions of the hormone are severely compromised [49]. A link between inadequate calcium supply and a specific infectious or chronic inflammatory disease in humans has not yet been established, even though calcium homeostasis may be a prerequisite for normal function of the immune system. Support for this assumption comes from experimental animal studies that provide evidence for an essential role of calcium in the suppression of autoimmune responses [18, 81].

The importance of vitamin D_3 supplementation for the prevention of diabetes mellitus type I in humans is highlighted by the study of Hypponen et al. [55] who showed that regular intake of daily doses of 2,000 IU vitamin D_3 during the first year of life, as recommended for the prophylaxis of rickets, is associated with an 88% risk reduction of autoimmune diabetes mellitus in later life.

15.4.4 Hypertension

Diastolic as well as systolic blood pressure in adult males is inversely related to bone-mineral content and density at various skeletal sites [86]. Considering bone-mineral density as a surrogate marker for exposure to calcium and vitamin D, this suggests that both vitamin D and calcium play a role in the regulation of blood pressure. This concept has been substantiated by many observational, interventional, and experimental studies [82], but the exact mechanisms of the antihypertensive action of calcium and vitamin D are not yet known.

1,25-$(OH)_2D_3$ is a potent inhibitor of renin expression in rat juxtaglomerular cells [73] and may therefore play a role in the regulation of blood pressure. However, three large prospective cohort studies found that high vitamin D intake is not associated with a lowered risk of incident hypertension [38]. Also, two earlier observational studies had reported that systolic blood pressure in normotensive middle-aged men was not related to 25-(OH)D levels [65, 76]. Conceivably, normal blood pressure can be maintained at suboptimal 25-(OH)D levels if enough 1,25-$(OH)_2D_3$ is produced in renal tubular cells to suppress renin synthesis by a paracrine effect on juxtaglomerular cells. This may no longer be the case in advancing age, when renal *CYP27B1* is no longer under stringent control from the Ca^{2+}/PTH axis [3]. In this situation, the amount of available 25-$(OH)D_3$ will ultimately determine the amount of 1,25-$(OH)_2D_3$ that is produced in the kidney and thus the extent of its antihypertensive effect. This inference agrees with a recent report [57] that the age-related increase in systolic blood pressure in white Americans having 25-(OH)D serum concentrations above 80 nM was 20% lower than in those with 25-(OH)D levels below 50 nM.

Evidence from a very large number of observational studies and randomized clinical trials indicates that low dietary calcium constitutes a significant risk factor for primary hypertension. Conversely, dietary calcium lowers diastolic blood pressure in healthy adults. In patients with mild to moderate hypertension, dietary calcium has an even greater effect on systolic blood pressure [82]. Calcium appears to be particularly effective in reducing the age-related increase in blood pressure [57]. Dobnig et al. [32] conducted a randomized, double-blind, multicenter study on the effect of daily high-dose calcium supplements in healthy, elderly adults and observed a substantial reduction of systolic and diastolic blood pressure after 1 year of treatment in individuals who were in the upper third of prestudy blood pressure values. No further improvement was seen by calcium plus vitamin D supplementation.

Whether changes in dietary calcium affect blood pressure via the action of the CaR on endothelial and smooth vascular cells of human arteries [88] are not known. Alternatively, activation of the renal CaR, leading to enhanced prostaglandin E_2 synthesis and natriuresis with subsequent reduction in plasma volume, may account for the blood pressure-lowering effect of elevated extracellular calcium [126].

15.4.5 Cardiovascular Disease

Vitamin D and calcium insufficiencies have been correlated not only with cardiovascular risk factors, such as obesity, hypertension, metabolic syndrome, and diabetes mellitus type 2 [79], but also with incident cardiovascular symptoms, including angina, coronary insufficiency, myocardial infarction, transient ischemic attack, and stroke [43, 127], and with greater mortality from chronic cardiovascular disease [15, 33, 105].

Cardiomyocytes as well as vascular endothelial and smooth muscle cells express the VDR and are endowed with a functional CaR, but the mechanisms by which vitamin D and calcium insufficiencies can cause heart failure are poorly understood. In a rat model of cardiac hypertrophy, the cardioprotective effect of 1,25-$(OH)_2D_3$ was associated with VDR-mediated suppression of several genes that were upregulated in the course of the hypertrophic process [132]. Activation of the CaR on rat neonatal ventricular cardiomyocytes had a biphasic effect on DNA, suggesting that the receptor could play a role in maintaining cellular homeostasis [121].

Vascular endothelial cells convert 25-$(OH)D_3$ to 1,25-$(OH)_2D_3$ [138], which most likely acts in a paracrine fashion on VDR-bearing vascular smooth muscle cells. Vitamin D may therefore play a regulatory role in vascular functions [93]. This view is strongly supported by the identification of 176 genes in human coronary artery smooth muscle cells that are sensitive to 1,25-$(OH)_2D_3$, including those involved in regulating smooth muscle cell growth, thrombogenicity, fibrinolysis, and endothelial regeneration [130].

Human smooth muscle and endothelial cells in large and small arteries express the CaR, but its function in the cardiovascular system has not been defined. Molostvov et al. [88] suggested that arterial calcification, a major cause of premature cardiovascular mortality, may be the result of CaR activation. Thus, one cannot exclude that calcium supplementation may cause adverse vascular events that compromise, at least in part, its beneficial action on cardiovascular risk [13].

15.4.6 Chronic Kidney Disease

Chronic kidney failure is associated with severe complications from breakdown of systemic regulation of bone and mineral metabolism. The syndrome of renal osteodystrophy is mainly caused by decreasing renal production of 1,25-$(OH)_2D_3$ and subsequent development of secondary hyperparathyroidism. In addition, lack of 1,25-$(OH)_2D_3$ is responsible for the high incidence of peripheral vascular disease, coronary artery disease, left ventricular hypertrophy, and high mortality in patients with end-stage renal failure [2]. This may be the reason that for a long time no attention was paid to the possibility that these patients may also have low 25-(OH)D serum levels. Only recently, LaClair et al. [69] reported a prevalence of vitamin D insufficiency, i.e., serum 25-(OH)D below 10 ng/mL, in more than 70% of patients who had moderate to severe chronic kidney disease and were not yet on dialysis. In another study, Elder and Mackun observed low levels of serum 25-(OH)D in patients with chronic kidney disease, particularly in women, patients with diabetes mellitus, and patients on peritoneal dialysis [35]. These findings clearly suggest that patients with end-stage renal disease will suffer not only from the consequences of severe systemic 1,25-$(OH)_2D_3$ deficiency, i.e., renal osteodystrophy, but are also at high risk for diseases that are caused by insufficient production of 1,25-$(OH)_2D_3$ at the extrarenal sites [56]. This could explain why young patients on hemodialysis have a 500-fold higher risk for cardiovascular diseases than age-matched healthy individuals [131].

15.4.7 Neuromuscular Dysfunction

In elderly people with relatively low serum 25-(OH)D, supplementation with either vitamin D or calcium had a significant beneficial effect on postural sway, reaction time, and balance [31, 100], as well as on musculoskeletal functions [100, 102] and physical performance [128]. Optimal improvement of neuromuscular functions was achieved when vitamin D and calcium supplementation was combined, as indicated by the highest decrease in the number of falls [12, 101]. As is known, falls account for about one-half of osteoporotic fractures in the elderly.

The mechanisms by which vitamin D and calcium modulate neuromuscular functions are far from being understood. 25-(OH)D-1α-hydroxylase is expressed in neurons and glial cells of many structures of the central nervous system [36]. The CaR is also widely distributed in the central nervous system [137]. This makes it very likely that nervous functions are modulated by extracellular Ca^{2+} and the autocrine/paracrine actions of 1,25-$(OH)_2D_3$. Whether vitamin D and calcium could have direct effects on muscular functions is not clear, because skeletal muscle cells do not express the CaR or the 25-(OH)D-1α-hydroxylase. They express, however, the VDR and may therefore be sensitive to fluctuations of plasma 1,25-$(OH)_2D_3$ within the normal range, rather than to changes in 25-(OH)D serum levels. Even in the absence of the CaR, extracellular Ca^{2+} may modulate skeletal muscle functions through L-type Ca^{2+} channels or other Ca^{2+} entry mechanisms.

15.5 Conclusion

Studies on expression of the *CYP27B1*-encoded 25-(OH)-D-1α-hydroxylase at extrarenal sites and on cell-specific function of the CaR have led to a general understanding of how locally produced 1,25-$(OH)_2D_3$ and extracellular Ca^{2+} jointly act as key regulators of cellular proliferation, differentiation, and function in many organs and cell systems. Under conditions of vitamin D and calcium insufficiency, cooperative signaling from 1,25-$(OH)_2D_3$-activated VDR and from Ca^{2+}/CaR is necessarily impaired, leading to alterations of cellular growth and function in bone and many extraskeletal sites. This explains why perturbation of bone-mineral homeostasis is associated not only with osteoporosis and osteomalacia, but also with many other chronic diseases, such as colorectal and breast cancer, insulin-dependent diabetes mellitus, hypertension, cardiovascular disease, and neuromuscular dysfunction.

References

1. Anderson PH, O'Loughlin PD, May BK, Morris HA (2005) Modulation of CYP27B1 and CYP24 mRNA expression in bone is independent of circulating $1,25(OH)_2D_3$ levels. Bone 36:654–662
2. Andress DL (2006) Vitamin D in chronic kidney disease: a systemic role for selective vitamin D receptor activation. Kidney Int 69:33–43
3. Armbrecht HJ, Hodam TL, Boltz MA, Kumar VB (1999) Capacity of a low calcium diet to induce the renal vitamin D 1alpha-hydroxylase is decreased in adult rats. Biochem Biophys Res Commun 255:731–734
4. Atkins GJ, Anderson PH, Findlay DM, Welldon KJ, Vincent C, Zannettino AC et al (2007) Metabolism of vitamin D_3 in human osteoblasts: evidence for autocrine and paracrine activities of 1alpha,25-dihydroxyvitamin D_3. Bone 40:1517–1528
5. Balasubramanian K, Rajeswari J, Gulab, Govil YC, Agarwal AK, Kumar A et al (2003) Varying role of vitamin D deficiency in the etiology of rickets in young children vs. adolescents in northern India. J Trop Pediatr 49:201–206
6. Barrett-Connor E (1989) The RDA for calcium in the elderly: too little, too late. Calcif Tissue Int 44:303–307
7. Becker S, Cordes T, Diesing D, Diedrich K, Friedrich M (2007) Expression of 25-hydroxyvitamin D_3-1alpha-hydroxylase in human endometrial tissue. J Steroid Biochem Mol Biol 103:771–775
8. Bertone-Johnson ER, Chen WY, Holick MF, Hollis BW, Colditz GA, Willett WC et al (2005) Plasma 25-hydroxyvitamin D and 1,25-dihydroxyvitamin D and risk of breast cancer. Cancer Epidemiol Biomarkers Prev 14:1991–1997
9. Berube S, Diorio C, Masse B, Hebert-Croteau N, Byrne C, Cote G et al (2005) Vitamin D and calcium intakes from food or supplements and mammographic breast density. Cancer Epidemiol Biomarkers Prev 14:1653–1659
10. Bilderback TR, Lee F, Auersperg N, Rodland KD (2002) Phosphatidylinositol 3-kinase-dependent, MEK- independent proliferation in response to CaR activation. Am J Physiol Cell Physiol 283:C282–C288
11. Bischoff-Ferrari HA, Giovannucci E, Willett WC, Dietrich T, Dawson-Hughes B (2006) Estimation of optimal serum concentrations of 25-hydroxyvitamin D for multiple health outcomes. Am J Clin Nutr 84:18–28
12. Bischoff HA, Stahelin HB, Dick W, Akos R, Knecht M, Salis C et al (2003) Effects of vitamin D and calcium supplementation on falls: a randomized controlled trial. J Bone Miner Res 18:343–351
13. Bolland MJ, Barber PA, Doughty RN, Mason B, Horne A, Ames R et al (2008) Vascular events in healthy older women receiving calcium supplementation: randomised controlled trial. BMJ 336:262–266
14. Boonen S, Lips P, Bouillon R, Bischoff-Ferrari HA, Vanderschueren D, Haentjens P (2007) Need for additional calcium to reduce the risk of hip fracture with vitamin D supplementation: evidence from a comparative metaanalysis of randomized controlled trials. J Clin Endocrinol Metab 92:1415–1423
15. Bostick RM, Kushi LH, Wu Y, Meyer KA, Sellers TA, Folsom AR (1999) Relation of calcium, vitamin D, and dairy food intake to ischemic heart disease mortality among postmenopausal women. Am J Epidemiol 149: 151–161
16. Brown EM, Gamba G, Riccardi D, Lombardi M, Butters R, Kifor O et al (1993) Cloning and characterization of an extracellular Ca(2+)-sensing receptor from bovine parathyroid. Nature 366:575–580
17. Canaff L, Hendy GN (2002) Human calcium-sensing receptor gene. Vitamin D response elements in promoters P1 and P2 confer transcriptional responsiveness to 1,25-dihydroxyvitamin D. J Biol Chem 277:30337–30350
18. Cantorna MT, Humpal-Winter J, DeLuca HF (1999) Dietary calcium is a major factor in 1,25-dihydroxycholecalciferol suppression of experimental autoimmune encephalomyelitis in mice. J Nutr 129:1966–1971
19. Capiod T, Shuba Y, Skryma R, Prevarskaya N (2007) Calcium signalling and cancer cell growth. Subcell Biochem 45:405–427
20. Chakrabarty S, Wang H, Canaff L, Hendy GN, Appelman H, Varani J (2005) Calcium sensing receptor in human colon carcinoma: interaction with Ca(2+) and 1,25-dihydroxyvitamin D_3. Cancer Res 65:493–498
21. Chang W, Tu C, Chen TH, Bikle D, Shoback D (2008) The extracellular calcium-sensing receptor (CaSR) is a critical modulator of skeletal development. Sci Signal 1:ra1
22. Chapuy MC, Arlot ME, Duboeuf F, Brun J, Crouzet B, Arnaud S et al (1992) Vitamin D_3 and calcium to prevent hip fractures in the elderly women. N Engl J Med 327:1637–1642
23. Chapuy MC, Preziosi P, Maamer M, Arnaud S, Galan P, Hercberg S et al (1997) Prevalence of vitamin D insufficiency in an adult normal population. Osteoporos Int 7:439–443
24. Cheng I, Klingensmith ME, Chattopadhyay N, Kifor O, Butters RR, Soybel DI et al (1998) Identification and localization of the extracellular calcium-sensing receptor in human breast. J Clin Endocrinol Metab 83:703–707
25. Cho E, Smith-Warner SA, Spiegelman D, Beeson WL, van den Brandt PA, Colditz GA et al (2004) Dairy foods, calcium, and colorectal cancer: a pooled analysis of 10 cohort studies. J Natl Cancer Inst 96:1015–1022
26. Cross HS, Bareis P, Hofer H, Bischof MG, Bajna E, Kriwanek S et al (2001) 25-Hydroxyvitamin D_3-1alpha-hydroxylase and vitamin D receptor gene expression in human colonic mucosa is elevated during early cancerogenesis. Steroids 66:287–292
27. Dawson-Hughes B, Harris SS, Dallal GE (1997) Plasma calcidiol, season, and serum parathyroid hormone concentrations in healthy elderly men and women. Am J Clin Nutr 65:67–71
28. Dawson-Hughes B, Heaney RP, Holick MF, Lips P, Meunier PJ, Vieth R (2005) Estimates of optimal vitamin D status. Osteoporos Int 16:713–716
29. Deeb KK, Trump DL, Johnson CS (2007) Vitamin D signalling pathways in cancer: potential for anticancer therapeutics. Nat Rev Cancer 7:684–700

30. Demay MB, Sabbagh Y, Carpenter TO (2007) Calcium and vitamin D: what is known about the effects on growing bone. Pediatrics 119(suppl 2):S141–S144
31. Dhesi JK, Jackson SH, Bearne LM, Moniz C, Hurley MV, Swift CG et al (2004) Vitamin D supplementation improves neuromuscular function in older people who fall. Age Ageing 33:589–595
32. Dobnig H, Pfeifer M, Begerow B, Suppan K (2005) Calcium, not vitamin D decreases blood pressure effectively in elderly subjects with low vitamin D levels; a randomized, double-blind, multi-center study. In: Abstracts of the Annual Meeting of the American Endocrine Society, San Diego
33. Dobnig H, Pilz S, Scharnagl H, Renner W, Seelhorst U, Wellnitz B et al (2008) Independent association of low serum 25-hydroxyvitamin D and 1,25-dihydroxyvitamin D levels with all-cause and cardiovascular mortality. Arch Intern Med 168:1340–1349
34. Dvorak MM, Siddiqua A, Ward DT, Carter DH, Dallas SL, Nemeth EF et al (2004) Physiological changes in extracellular calcium concentration directly control osteoblast function in the absence of calciotropic hormones. Proc Natl Acad Sci U S A 101:5140–5145
35. Elder GJ, Mackun K (2006) 25-Hydroxyvitamin D deficiency and diabetes predict reduced BMD in patients with chronic kidney disease. J Bone Miner Res 21:1778–1784
36. Eyles DW, Smith S, Kinobe R, Hewison M, McGrath JJ (2005) Distribution of the vitamin D receptor and 1 alpha-hydroxylase in human brain. J Chem Neuroanat 29:21–30
37. Feskanich D, Ma J, Fuchs CS, Kirkner GJ, Hankinson SE, Hollis BW et al (2004) Plasma vitamin D metabolites and risk of colorectal cancer in women. Cancer Epidemiol Biomarkers Prev 13:1502–1508
38. Forman JP, Bischoff-Ferrari HA, Willett WC, Stampfer MJ, Curhan GC (2005) Vitamin D intake and risk of incident hypertension: results from three large prospective cohort studies. Hypertension 46:676–682
39. Friedrich M, Rafi L, Mitschele T, Tilgen W, Schmidt W, Reichrath J (2003) Analysis of the vitamin D system in cervical carcinomas, breast cancer and ovarian cancer. Recent Results Cancer Res 164:239–246
40. Froicu M, Weaver V, Wynn TA, McDowell MA, Welsh JE, Cantorna MT (2003) A crucial role for the vitamin D_3 receptor in experimental inflammatory bowel diseases. Mol Endocrinol 17:2386–2392
41. Gagel RF (1993) Mineral and vitamin D RDA for infants children and adults. In: Favus MJ (ed) Primer on the metabolic bone diseases and disorders of mineral metabolism, 2nd edn. Raven Press, New York, pp 413
42. Garland CF, Garland FC, Gorham ED, Lipkin M, Newmark H, Mohr SB et al (2006) The role of vitamin D in cancer prevention. Am J Public Health 96:252–261
43. Giovannucci E, Liu Y, Hollis BW, Rimm EB (2008) 25-hydroxyvitamin D and risk of myocardial infarction in men: a prospective study. Arch Intern Med 168:1174–1180
44. Gorham ED, Garland CF, Garland FC, Grant WB, Mohr SB, Lipkin M et al (2005) Vitamin D and prevention of colorectal cancer. J Steroid Biochem Mol Biol 97: 179–194
45. Grant WB (2006) The likely role of vitamin D from solar ultraviolet-B irradiance in increasing cancer survival. Anticancer Res 26:2605–2614
46. Grau MV, Baron JA, Sandler RS, Haile RW, Beach ML, Church TR et al (2003) Vitamin D, calcium supplementation, and colorectal adenomas: results of a randomized trial. J Natl Cancer Inst 95:1765–1771
47. Hansen KE, Jones AN, Lindstrom MJ, Davis LA, Engelke JA, Shafer MM (2008) Vitamin D insufficiency: disease or no disease? J Bone Miner Res 23:1052–1060
48. Hebert SC, Cheng S, Geibel J (2004) Functions and roles of the extracellular Ca^{2+}-sensing receptor in the gastrointestinal tract. Cell Calcium 35:239–247
49. Hewison M, Burke F, Evans KN, Lammas DA, Sansom DM, Liu P et al (2007) Extra-renal 25-hydroxyvitamin D_3-1alpha-hydroxylase in human health and disease. J Steroid Biochem Mol Biol 103:316–321
50. Hewison M, Freeman L, Hughes SV, Evans KN, Bland R, Eliopoulos AG et al (2003) Differential regulation of vitamin D receptor and its ligand in human monocyte-derived dendritic cells. J Immunol 170:5382–5390
51. Hintzpeter B, Mensink GB, Thierfelder W, Muller MJ, Scheidt-Nave C (2008) Vitamin D status and health correlates among German adults. Eur J Clin Nutr 62:1079–1089
52. Hosgood HD III, Baris D, Zahm SH, Zheng T, Cross AJ (2007) Diet and risk of multiple myeloma in Connecticut women. Cancer Causes Control 18:1065–1076
53. Hu J, Mao Y, White K (2003) Diet and vitamin or mineral supplements and risk of renal cell carcinoma in Canada. Cancer Causes Control 14:705–714
54. Hypponen E, Power C (2007) Hypovitaminosis D in British adults at age 45 y: nationwide cohort study of dietary and life style predictors. Am J Clin Nutr 85:860–868
55. Hypponen E, Laara E, Reunanen A, Jarvelin MR, Virtanen SM (2001) Intake of vitamin D and risk of type 1 diabetes: a birth-cohort study. Lancet 358: 1500–1503
56. Jones G (2007) Expanding role for vitamin D in chronic kidney disease: importance of blood 25-OH-D levels and extra-renal 1alpha-hydroxylase in the classical and nonclassical actions of 1alpha,25-dihydroxyvitamin D_3. Semin Dial 20:316–324
57. Judd SE, Nanes MS, Ziegler TR, Wilson PW, Tangpricha V (2008) Optimal vitamin D status attenuates the age-associated increase in systolic blood pressure in white Americans: results from the third National Health and Nutrition Examination Survey. Am J Clin Nutr 87: 136–141
58. Kállay E, Bises G, Bajna E, Bieglmayer C, Gerdenitsch W, Steffan I et al (2005) Colon-specific regulation of vitamin D hydroxylases – a possible approach for tumor prevention. Carcinogenesis 26:1581–1589
59. Kállay E, Bonner E, Wrba F, Thakker RV, Peterlik M, Cross HS (2003) Molecular and functional characterization of the extracellular calcium-sensing receptor in human colon cancer cells. Oncol Res 13:551–559

60. Kállay E, Kifor O, Chattopadhyay N, Brown EM, Bischof MG, Peterlik M et al (1997) Calcium-dependent c-myc proto-oncogene expression and proliferation of Caco-2 cells: a role for a luminal extracellular calcium-sensing receptor. Biochem Biophys Res Commun 232: 80–83
61. Kamen DL, Cooper GS, Bouali H, Shaftman SR, Hollis BW, Gilkeson GS (2006) Vitamin D deficiency in systemic lupus erythematosus. Autoimmun Rev 5:114–117
62. Koralek DO, Bertone-Johnson ER, Leitzmann MF, Sturgeon SR, Lacey JV Jr, Schairer C et al (2006) Relationship between calcium, lactose, vitamin D, and dairy products and ovarian cancer. Nutr Cancer 56: 22–30
63. Kovacs CS (2008) Fetal calcium metabolism. In: Rosen CJ (ed) Primer on the metabolic bone diseases and disorders of mineral metabolism, 7th edn. American Society for Bone and Mineral Research, Washington, DC, pp 108–113
64. Kovacs CS, Woodland ML, Fudge NJ, Friel JK (2005) The vitamin D receptor is not required for fetal mineral homeostasis or for the regulation of placental calcium transfer in mice. Am J Physiol Endocrinol Metab 289:E133–E144
65. Kristal-Boneh E, Froom P, Harari G, Ribak J (1997) Association of calcitriol and blood pressure in normotensive men. Hypertension 30:1289–1294
66. Kronenberg HM (2006) PTHrP and skeletal development. Ann N Y Acad Sci 1068:1–13
67. Kudlacek S, Schneider B, Peterlik M, Leb G, Klaushofer K, Weber K et al (2003) Assessment of vitamin D and calcium status in healthy adult Austrians. Eur J Clin Invest 33:323–331
68. Kudlacek S, Schneider B, Peterlik M, Leb G, Klaushofer K, Weber K et al (2003) Normative data of bone mineral density in an unselected adult Austrian population. Eur J Clin Invest 33:332–339
69. LaClair RE, Hellman RN, Karp SL, Kraus M, Ofner S, Li Q et al (2005) Prevalence of calcidiol deficiency in CKD: a cross-sectional study across latitudes in the United States. Am J Kidney Dis 45:1026–1033
70. Lamberg-Allardt CJ, Outila TA, Karkkainen MU, Rita HJ, Valsta LM (2001) Vitamin D deficiency and bone health in healthy adults in Finland: could this be a concern in other parts of Europe? J Bone Miner Res 16:2066–2073
71. Lappe JM, Travers-Gustafson D, Davies KM, Recker RR, Heaney RP (2007) Vitamin D and calcium supplementation reduces cancer risk: results of a randomized trial. Am J Clin Nutr 85:1586–1591
72. Lechner D, Kállay E, Cross HS (2007) 1Alpha,25-dihydroxyvitamin D3 downregulates CYP27B1 and induces CYP24A1 in colon cells. Mol Cell Endocrinol 263:55–64
73. Li YC, Kong J, Wei M, Chen ZF, Liu SQ, Cao LP (2002) 1,25-Dihydroxyvitamin D_3 is a negative endocrine regulator of the renin-angiotensin system. J Clin Invest 110:229–238
74. Lin J, Manson JE, Lee IM, Cook NR, Buring JE, Zhang SM (2007) Intakes of calcium and vitamin D and breast cancer risk in women. Arch Intern Med 167:1050–1059
75. Lin KI, Chattopadhyay N, Bai M, Alvarez R, Dang CV, Baraban JM et al (1998) Elevated extracellular calcium can prevent apoptosis via the calcium-sensing receptor. Biochem Biophys Res Commun 249:325–331
76. Lind L, Hanni A, Lithell H, Hvarfner A, Sorensen OH, Ljunghall S (1995) Vitamin D is related to blood pressure and other cardiovascular risk factors in middle-aged men. Am J Hypertens 8:894–901
77. Looker AC, Mussolino ME (2008) Serum 25-hydroxyvitamin d and hip fracture risk in older U.S. White adults. J Bone Miner Res 23:143–150
78. Ma J, Johns RA, Stafford RS (2007) Americans are not meeting current calcium recommendations. Am J Clin Nutr 85:1361–1366
79. Martins D, Wolf M, Pan D, Zadshir A, Tareen N, Thadhani R et al (2007) Prevalence of cardiovascular risk factors and the serum levels of 25-hydroxyvitamin D in the United States: data from the third national health and nutrition examination survey. Arch Intern Med 167:1159–1165
80. Massry SG (1978) The cinical syndrome of phosphate depletion. In: Massry SG, Ritz E, Rapado A (eds). Homeostasis of phosphate and other minerals. Plenum Press, New York, pp 301–307
81. Mathieu C, Van Etten E, Gysemans C, Decallonne B, Kato S, Laureys J et al (2001) In vitro and in vivo analysis of the immune system of vitamin D receptor knockout mice. J Bone Miner Res 16:2057–2065
82. McCarron DA, Reusser ME (1999) Finding consensus in the dietary calcium-blood pressure debate. J Am Coll Nutr 18:398S–405S
83. McCullough ML, Rodriguez C, Diver WR, Feigelson HS, Stevens VL, Thun MJ et al (2005) Dairy, calcium, and vitamin D intake and postmenopausal breast cancer risk in the Cancer Prevention Study II Nutrition Cohort. Cancer Epidemiol Biomarkers Prev 14: 2898–2904
84. McNeil L, Hobson S, Nipper V, Rodland KD (1998) Functional calcium-sensing receptor expression in ovarian surface epithelial cells. Am J Obstet Gynecol 178:305–313
85. Merlino L, Curtis J, Mikuls TR, Cerhan JR, Criswell LA, Saag KG (2004) Vitamin D intake is inversely associated with rheumatoid arthritis. Results from the Iowa Women's Health Study. Arthr Rheumat 50:72–77
86. Metz JA, Morris CD, Roberts LA, McClung MR, McCarron DA (1999) Blood pressure and calcium intake are related to bone density in adult males. Br J Nutr 81:383–388
87. Miao D, Su H, He B, Gao J, Xia Q, Zhu M et al (2008) Severe growth retardation and early lethality in mice lacking the nuclear localization sequence and C-terminus of PTH-related protein. Proc Natl Acad Sci U S A 105:20309–20314
88. Molostvov G, James S, Fletcher S, Bennett J, Lehnert H, Bland R et al (2007) Extracellular calcium-sensing receptor is functionally expressed in human artery. Am J Physiol Renal Physiol 293:F946–F955

89. Munger KL, Levin LI, Hollis BW, Howard NS, Ascherio A (2006) Serum 25-hydroxyvitamin D levels and risk of multiple sclerosis. JAMA 296:2832–2838
90. Need AG, Nordin BE (2008) Misconceptions – vitamin D insufficiency causes malabsorption of calcium. Bone 42:1021–1024
91. Need AG, O'Loughlin PD, Morris HA, Coates PS, Horowitz M, Nordin BE (2008) Vitamin D metabolites and calcium absorption in severe vitamin D deficiency. J Bone Miner Res 23:1859–1863
92. Nittke T, Selig S, Kállay E, Cross HS (2008) Nutritional calcium modulates colonic expression of vitamin D receptor and pregnane X receptor target genes. Mol Nutr Food Res 52:45–51
93. Norman PE, Powell JT (2005) Vitamin D, shedding light on the development of disease in peripheral arteries. Arterioscler Thromb Vasc Biol 25:39–46
94. Owen TA, Aronow MS, Barone LM, Bettencourt B, Stein GS, Lian JB (1991) Pleiotropic effects of vitamin D on osteoblast gene expression are related to the proliferative and differentiated state of the bone cell phenotype: dependency upon basal levels of gene expression, duration of exposure, and bone matrix competency in normal rat osteoblast cultures. Endocrinology 128: 1496–1504
95. Palmer HG, Gonzalez-Sancho JM, Espada J, Berciano MT, Puig I, Baulida J et al (2001) Vitamin D_3 promotes the differentiation of colon carcinoma cells by the induction of E-cadherin and the inhibition of beta-catenin signaling. J Cell Biol 154:369–387
96. Panda DK, Miao D, Bolivar I, Li J, Huo R, Hendy GN et al (2004) Inactivation of the 25-hydroxyvitamin D 1alpha-hydroxylase and vitamin D receptor demonstrates independent and interdependent effects of calcium and vitamin D on skeletal and mineral homeostasis. J Biol Chem 279:16754–16766
97. Peterlik M, Cross HS (2005) Vitamin D and calcium deficits predispose for multiple chronic diseases. Eur J Clin Invest 35:290–304
98. Peterlik M, Grant WB, Cross HS (2009) Calcium, vitamin D, and cancer. Anticancer Res. 29:3687-3698
99. Pettifor JM (2004) Nutritional rickets: deficiency of vitamin D, calcium, or both? Am J Clin Nutr 80: 1725S–1729S
100. Pfeifer M, Begerow B, Minne HW, Abrams C, Nachtigall D, Hansen C (2000) Effects of a short-term vitamin D and calcium supplementation on body sway and secondary hyperparathyroidism in elderly women. J Bone Miner Res 15:1113–1118
101. Pfeifer M, Begerow B, Minne HW, Schlotthauer T, Pospeschill M, Scholz M et al (2001) Vitamin D status, trunk muscle strength, body sway, falls, and fractures among 237 postmenopausal women with osteoporosis. Exp Clin Endocrinol Diabetes 109:87–92
102. Pfeifer M, Begerow B, Minne HW, Suppan K, Fahrleitner-Pammer A, Dobnig H (2009) Effects of a long-term vitamin D and calcium supplementation on falls and parameters of muscle function in community-dwelling older individuals. Osteoporos Int 20: 315–322
103. Pillai S, Bikle DD, Elias PM (1988) 1,25-Dihydroxyvitamin D production and receptor binding in human keratinocytes varies with differentiation. J Biol Chem 263: 5390–5395
104. Pilz S, Dobnig H, Winklhofer-Roob B, Riedmuller G, Fischer JE, Seelhorst U et al (2008) Low serum levels of 25-hydroxyvitamin D predict fatal cancer in patients referred to coronary angiography. Cancer Epidemiol Biomarkers Prev 17:1228–1233
105. Pilz S, Marz W, Wellnitz B, Seelhorst U, Fahrleitner-Pammer A, Dimai HP et al (2008) Association of vitamin D deficiency with heart failure and sudden cardiac death in a large cross-sectional study of patients referred for coronary angiography. J Clin Endocrinol Metab 93:3927–3935
106. Racz GZ, Kittel A, Riccardi D, Case RM, Elliott AC, Varga G (2002) Extracellular calcium sensing receptor in human pancreatic cells. Gut 51:705–711
107. Radermacher J, Diesel B, Seifert M, Tilgen W, Reichrath J, Fischer U et al (2006) Expression analysis of CYP27B1 in tumor biopsies and cell cultures. Anticancer Res 26:2683–2686
108. Riggs BL, Khosla S, Melton LJ III (1998) A unitary model for involutional osteoporosis: estrogen deficiency causes both type I and type II osteoporosis in postmenopausal women and contributes to bone loss in aging men. J Bone Miner Res 13:763–773
109. Ritter CS, Armbrecht HJ, Slatopolsky E, Brown AJ (2006) 25-Hydroxyvitamin D_3 suppresses PTH synthesis and secretion by bovine parathyroid cells. Kidney Int 70:654–659
110. Rodland KD (2004) The role of the calcium-sensing receptor in cancer. Cell Calcium 35:291–295
111. Sabbagh Y, Carpenter TO, Demay MB (2005) Hypophosphatemia leads to rickets by impairing caspase-mediated apoptosis of hypertrophic chondrocytes. Proc Natl Acad Sci U S A 102:9637–9642
112. Sanders JL, Chattopadhyay N, Kifor O, Yamaguchi T, Brown EM (2001) Ca(2+)-sensing receptor expression and PTHrP secretion in PC-3 human prostate cancer cells. Am J Physiol Endocrinol Metab 281: E1267–E1274
113. Schwartz GG, Eads D, Rao A, Cramer SD, Willingham MC, Chen TC et al (2004) Pancreatic cancer cells express 25-hydroxyvitamin D-1 alpha-hydroxylase and their proliferation is inhibited by the prohormone 25-hydroxyvitamin D_3. Carcinogenesis 25:1015–1026
114. Schwartz GG, Whitlatch LW, Chen TC, Lokeshwar BL, Holick MF (1998) Human prostate cells synthesize 1,25-dihydroxyvitamin D_3 from 25-hydroxyvitamin D_3. Cancer Epidemiol Biomarkers Prev 7:391–395
115. Shalhoub V, Grisanti M, Padagas J, Scully S, Rattan A, Qi M et al (2003) In vitro studies with the calcimimetic, cinacalcet HCl, on normal human adult osteoblastic and osteoclastic cells. Crit Rev Eukaryot Gene Expr 13:89–106
116. Shin MH, Holmes MD, Hankinson SE, Wu K, Colditz GA, Willett WC (2002) Intake of dairy products, calcium, and vitamin D and risk of breast cancer. J Natl Cancer Inst 94:1301–1311

117. Sigmundsdottir H, Pan J, Debes GF, Alt C, Habtezion A, Soler D et al (2007) DCs metabolize sunlight-induced vitamin D3 to 'program' T cell attraction to the epidermal chemokine CCL27. Nat Immunol 8:285–293
118. Squires PE, Harris TE, Persaud SJ, Curtis SB, Buchan AM, Jones PM (2000) The extracellular calcium-sensing receptor on human beta-cells negatively modulates insulin secretion. Diabetes 49:409–417
119. Terry P, Vainio H, Wolk A, Weiderpass E (2002) Dietary factors in relation to endometrial cancer: a nationwide case-control study in Sweden. Nutr Cancer 42:25–32
120. Tfelt-Hansen J, Brown EM (2005) The calcium-sensing receptor in normal physiology and pathophysiology: a review. Crit Rev Clin Lab Sci 42:35–70
121. Tfelt-Hansen J, Hansen JL, Smajilovic S, Terwilliger EF, Haunso S, Sheikh SP (2006) Calcium receptor is functionally expressed in rat neonatal ventricular cardiomyocytes. Am J Physiol Heart Circ Physiol 290: H1165–H1171
122. Tfelt-Hansen J, Yano S, John Macleod R, Smajilovic S, Chattopadhyay N, Brown EM (2005) High calcium activates the EGF receptor potentially through the calcium-sensing receptor in Leydig cancer cells. Growth Factors 23:117–123
123. Thacher TD, Fischer PR, Pettifor JM, Lawson JO, Isichei CO, Reading JC et al (1999) A comparison of calcium, vitamin D, or both for nutritional rickets in Nigerian children. N Engl J Med 341:563–568
124. Tuohimaa P, Tenkanen L, Ahonen M, Lumme S, Jellum E, Hallmans G et al (2004) Both high and low levels of blood vitamin D are associated with a higher prostate cancer risk: a longitudinal, nested case-control study in the Nordic countries. Int J Cancer 108:104–108
125. van Driel M, Koedam M, Buurman CJ, Hewison M, Chiba H, Uitterlinden AG et al (2006) Evidence for auto/paracrine actions of vitamin D in bone: 1alpha-hydroxylase expression and activity in human bone cells. FASEB J 20:2417–2419
126. Wang D, An SJ, Wang WH, McGiff JC, Ferreri NR (2001) CaR-mediated COX-2 expression in primary cultured mTAL cells. Am J Physiol Renal Physiol 281: F658–F664
127. Wang TJ, Pencina MJ, Booth SL, Jacques PF, Ingelsson E, Lanier K et al (2008) Vitamin D deficiency and risk of cardiovascular disease. Circulation 117:503–511
128. Wicherts IS, van Schoor NM, Boeke AJ, Visser M, Deeg DJ, Smit J et al (2007) Vitamin D status predicts physical performance and its decline in older persons. J Clin Endocrinol Metab 92:2058–2065
129. Wiers K, Wright MA, Vellody K, Young MR (1998) Failure of tumor-reactive lymph node cells to kill tumor in the presence of immune-suppressive CD34+ cells can be overcome with vitamin D3 treatment to diminish CD34+ cell levels. Clin Exp Metastasis 16:275–282
130. Wu-Wong JR, Nakane M, Ma J, Ruan X, Kroeger PE (2006) Effects of Vitamin D analogs on gene expression profiling in human coronary artery smooth muscle cells. Atherosclerosis 186:20–28
131. Wu-Wong JR, Tian J, Nakane M, Ma J, Fey TA, Kroeger P et al (2006) Cardiovascular disease in chronic kidney failure: the role of VDR activators. Curr Opin Investig Drugs 7:206–213
132. Wu J, Garami M, Cheng T, Gardner DG (1996) 1,25$(OH)_2$-vitamin D_3, and retinoic acid antagonize endothelin-stimulated hypertrophy of neonatal rat cardiac myocytes. J Clin Invest 97:1577–1588
133. Wu K, Willett WC, Fuchs CS, Colditz GA, Giovannucci EL (2002) Calcium intake and risk of colon cancer in women and men. J Natl Cancer Inst 94:437–446
134. Yamaguchi T, Chattopadhyay N, Kifor O, Butters RR Jr, Sugimoto T, Brown EM (1998) Mouse osteoblastic cell line (MC3T3-E1) expresses extracellular calcium (Ca2+o)-sensing receptor and its agonists stimulate chemotaxis and proliferation of MC3T3-E1 cells. J Bone Miner Res 13:1530–1538
135. Yamaguchi T, Olozak I, Chattopadhyay N, Butters RR, Kifor O, Scadden DT et al (1998) Expression of extra cellular calcium (Ca2+o)-sensing receptor in human peripheral blood monocytes. Biochem Biophys Res Commun 246:501–506
136. Yang CY, Cheng MF, Tsai SS, Hsieh YL (1998) Calcium, magnesium, and nitrate in drinking water and gastric cancer mortality. Jpn J Cancer Res 89:124–130
137. Yano S, Brown EM, Chattopadhyay N (2004) Calcium-sensing receptor in the brain. Cell Calcium 35:257–264
138. Zehnder D, Bland R, Chana RS, Wheeler DC, Howie AJ, Williams MC et al (2002) Synthesis of 1,25-dihydroxyvitamin D_3 by human endothelial cells is regulated by inflammatory cytokines: a novel autocrine determinant of vascular cell adhesion. J Am Soc Nephrol 13:621–629
139. Zehnder D, Bland R, Williams MC, McNinch RW, Howie AJ, Stewart PM et al (2001) Extrarenal expression of 25-hydroxyvitamin D_3-1 alpha-hydroxylase. J Clin Endocrinol Metab 86:888–894

16. Interrelationship Between Bone and Other Tissues: Brain–Bone Axis and Bone-Adipo Axis

Shu Takeda

16.1 Introduction

It has been widely assumed that bone metabolism is controlled mostly by the local environment and does not affect the metabolism of other tissues. In other words, bone was thought to constitute an independent domain from the rest of the body. However, the discovery of neuronal control of bone mass by leptin has shed light on a novel pathway that controls bone metabolism [32]. Furthermore, the recent discovery that osteocalcin modified by OST-PTP regulates glucose metabolism opened a new domain linked to skeletal biology [39]. These unexpected relationships are an outgrowth from the wealth of genetically modified mouse models. Most of these pathways are still far from being fully explored, but the identification of a network between bone and other organs has attracted much attention from basic and clinical scientists.

16.2 Leptin and Bone

Leptin, a 16-kDa peptide hormone, is synthesized by adipocytes and affects appetite and energy metabolism by binding to the leptin receptor that is located in the hypothalamus [1, 2]. *ob/ob* mice that lack functional leptin and *db/db* mice that lack a functional leptin receptor are obese and sterile. Notwithstanding their hypogonadism – the most common cause of osteoporosis – *ob/ob* mice and *db/db* mice have a high bone mass [15]. Importantly, *ob/ob* mice fed on a low fat diet have high bone mass at 1 month of age, when their weight is still normal. Therefore, high bone mass is due to the absence of leptin and not the result of the obesity of the *ob/ob* and db/db mice. Mouse models of lipodystrophy, such as A-ZIP transgenic mice expressing a dominant-negative protein inhibiting B-ZIP adipocyte transcription factors or $Ppar\gamma^{hyp/hyp}$ mice carrying a hypomorphic mutation at the PPARγ2 locus [10, 18] also display a high bone mass phenotype. It is therefore apparent that low serum leptin levels induce an increase in bone mass regardless of body weight. Moreover, a leptin transgene can correct the high bone mass of these lipodystrophic mice. Consequently, a leptin signaling defect is both necessary and sufficient to develop high bone mass [18] (Fig. 16.1).

F. Bronner et al. (eds.), *Bone and Development*, Topics in Bone Biology 6,
DOI 10.1007/978-1-84882-822-3_16,

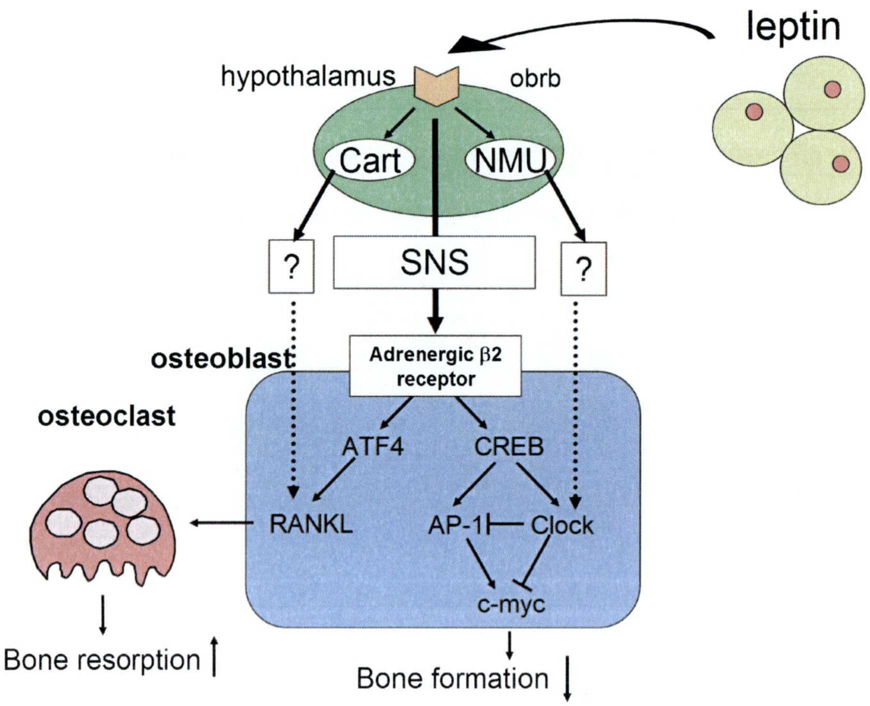

Figure 16.1. Regulation of bone remodeling by neuropeptides.

16.3 Regulation of Bone Remodeling by Leptin

Histomorphometric analyses have revealed a nearly twofold increase in trabecular bone volume in *ob/ob* (or db/db) mice when compared with wild-type (WT) littermates [15]. This phenotype is observed in both sexes, in growing and remodeling animals, and in long bones as well as in vertebrae. The high bone mass phenotype of leptin signaling-deficient mice is due to a massive increase in bone turnover, with both bone formation and bone resorption rates increasing, and with formation exceeding resorption. Leptin's action on appetite and reproduction depends on its binding to a specific receptor located on hypothalamic neurons [1, 2]. Detailed analysis reveals that leptin receptor-deficient osteoblasts proliferate and differentiate normally. In contrast, an intracerebroventricular (ICV) infusion of leptin to *ob/ob* mice or wild-type mice decreases bone mass, even with a minimal dose that does not affect body weight [15].

These findings show:

First, that leptin regulates bone formation in mice through the central nervous system. This is important because of the controversy regarding the peripheral and central mode of leptin action on bone remodeling. Several reports have indicated that leptin stimulates osteoblastic proliferation and differentiation in vitro, and that peripheral injection of supra-physiological amounts of leptin to WT animals is correlated with a gain in bone mass [12, 44]. Unfortunately, the leptin doses in these experiments were pharmacological. However, transgenic mice that overexpress leptin in osteoblasts or have an osteoblast-specific deletion of the leptin receptor exhibit no overt bone abnormalities. This demonstrates that the physiological role of peripheral leptin on bone remodeling is limited or absent [18, 56].

Second, the inhibitory action of leptin on bone formation is one of its most important functions; the fact that similar amounts of leptin were needed to affect body weight and bone mass suggests that leptin's anorexigenic and antiosteogenic functions are equally important in vivo [18].

16.4 Leptin and Bone Remodeling in Human Subjects

Follow-up studies have revealed that leptin has a regulatory role in bone remodeling not just in mice but also in sheep and rats [25, 50]. Furthermore, a human patient with a mutation in the leptin gene also displayed a high bone mass phenotype, and patients with congenital generalized lipodystrophy, whose serum leptin levels are extremely low due to the absence of adipocytes, exhibit accelerated bone maturation [18]. Clinical epidemiologic studies have also confirmed that the negative association between serum leptin level and bone mass in human patients is independent of fat mass and other covariates [45, 51]. Other cross-sectional studies, however, have failed to show a negative association between serum leptin levels and bone mass or BMD [23, 45, 62]. These discrepancies may be related to differences in race, gender, age, or body mass index. Indeed, in a few recent studies in men, the leptin level was inversely correlated to BMD, an association that became apparent only after adjustment of BMD for body weight [46, 54].

16.5 Leptin, the Sympathetic Nervous System, and Bone Remodeling

There are two regions in the hypothalamus, the arcuate (ARC) and ventromedial hypothalamic (VMH) nuclei, which are rich in leptin receptors [60]. Destruction of ARC by monosodium glutamate in WT mice induces obesity, but not high bone mass [58]. In contrast, destruction of VMH by gold thioglucose in WT mice recapitulates the bone phenotype of *ob/ob* mice: high bone mass due to an increase in bone formation. Moreover, in *ob/ob* mice whose VMH neurons have been lesioned, leptin ICV infusion decreases body weight, but does not affect bone formation parameters or bone mass. Conversely, leptin ICV fails to decrease body weight, but decreases bone mass and bone formation in *ob/ob* mice whose ARC neurons have been lesioned [58]. In accordance with these findings, l/l mice, a model of gain of function in leptin signaling harboring a Y985L substitution in the leptin receptor, have low bone mass, but their appetite and energy expenditure are normal. The actions of leptin on appetite and bone formation can therefore be clearly dissociated.

The nature of the downstream mediator between the VMH nucleus and osteoblasts has been studied with a parabiotic model. Two *ob/ob* mice were surgically fusioned, with one ICV-infused with leptin [58]. The infused mouse exhibited the expected decrease in bone mass, yet the bone mass of the contralateral mouse was never affected. Although this result does not completely rule out the possibility that the mediators of leptin action on bones are humoral in nature, it is more consistent with a neurally mediated signal. One of the many abnormalities displayed by *ob/ob* mice is low sympathetic activity [8]. This suggests that the sympathetic nervous system (SNS) mediates the regulation of bone mass by leptin. Consistent with an influence of the SNS on bone remodeling, many osteoblasts reside next to sympathetic neurons in bone marrow and specifically express the beta 2-adrenergic receptor (adrb2) [58]. Indeed, mice treated with isoproterenol, a beta agonist, display a massive decrease in bone mass, and mice whose SNS signaling is blocked either genetically (Adr$\beta 2^{-/-}$ mice or dopamine beta hydroxylase$^{-/-}$ mice) or pharmacologically (WT mice treated with β-blocker) all exhibit a high bone mass phenotype [17,58]. Importantly, the bone phenotype observed in these mice cannot be rescued by leptin ICV infusion; this demonstrates that the SNS, via Adrβ2, mediates leptin regulation of bone mass (Fig. 16.1). Adr$\beta 2^{-/-}$ mice have normal body and fat pads and have none of the endocrine abnormalities of *ob/ob* and db/db mice. Therefore, the bone abnormality is caused by the SNS signaling defect and is not secondary to other abnormalities. Thus, SNS is a major, if not the only, pathway responsible for leptin's inhibition of bone formation.

Leptin and SNS also regulate osteoclastic resorption [17] (Fig. 16.1). In addition to increased bone formation, adrb$2^{-/-}$ mice show a significant decrease in the number of tartrate-resistant acid phosphatase (TRAP)-positive multinucleated osteoclasts, a result of a defect in osteoclast differentiation. Although Adrb2 is also expressed by osteoclasts, any attempt to demonstrate a direct effect of the SNS on osteoclasts or osteoclast precursors has failed. Rather, SNS and Adrb2 activation activate protein kinase A. This in turn phosphorylates ATF4, an essential transcription factor for osteoblastic differentiation and function that induces *Rankl* (receptor activator of NFkappaB ligand) expression [17]. The bone resorption phenotype cannot be corrected by leptin ICV infusion; this indicates that leptin signaling also uses the SNS to regulate bone resorption through its action on osteoblasts. Because osteoclasts exist in *adrb2*$^{-/-}$ mice, SNS signaling cannot be essential for osteoclast differentiation; nevertheless, SNS is important for bone remodeling (see below).

16.6 SNS and Bone Remodeling: Clinical Implications

In mice, ovariectomy-induced [58], unloading-induced [35, 40], or depression-induced [65] bone loss are ameliorated by concomitant treatment with β-blockers. As for leptin's regulation of bone remodeling, clinical observations indicate that the influence of SNS on bone mass is also true for humans. For instance, patients with reflex sympathetic dystrophy, a disease characterized by localized high sympathetic activity, develop a severe and localized osteoporosis that can be treated with β-blockers [37]. Interestingly, traumatic brain injury (TBI) enhances healing of a fracture in the appendicular skeleton. Recently, it was shown that the norepinephrine content of bone is decreased in TBI via cannabinoid receptor 1 signaling, and the TBI-induced stimulation of osteogenesis is restrained by a β agonist [59].

Many epidemiological studies have also confirmed the effect of β-blockers on fracture. Reports conflict on whether β-blockers prevent or have no effect on osteoporotic fractures, but a recent meta-analysis of eight studies has demonstrated that β-blockers protect against any fractures (pooled relative risk = 0.86), especially against hip fractures (28% relative fracture risk reduction) [64].

Discrepancies may be due to the amount of β-blocker used: a low dose of propranolol that did not affect cardiovascular functions was sufficient to increase bone formation and to prevent bone loss. As the dose was increased, its beneficial effect was progressively decreased [7]. The specificity of the β-blocker may also be relevant. Mouse osteoblasts do not normally express the adrenergic receptor 1 (adrβ1), and adrβ1$^{-/-}$ mice do not show a bone phenotype; adrβ1$^{-/-}$; adrβ2$^{-/-}$ double mutant mice display a low bone mass phenotype [48]. This suggests that the adrβ1 receptor counteracts the effect of adrβ2 on bone remodeling via an osteoblast-independent mechanism.

Considering the widespread use of β-blockers in clinical medicine, β-blockers may be useful to treat osteoporosis. However, most studies addressing the relation of β-blockers to osteoporotic fracture have been observational; long-term prospective randomized trials that take into account the specificity and dosage of the β-blocker(s) are needed.

16.7 Regulation of Bone Remodeling by Neuropeptides Affecting Appetite: Cocaine- and Amphetamine-Regulated Transcript (Cart) and MC4R

The phenotypic discrepancy observed between *ob/ob* mice (increase in bone resorption) and ovariectomized-*adrb2* mice (decrease in bone resorption) suggests that in addition to the SNS, there must be other molecules that control bone resorption whose expression is regulated by leptin. Cart is a neuropeptide precursor protein involved in the regulation of food intake and energy expenditure. It is broadly expressed in the central nervous system, including the hypothalamus and peripheral organs such as the pancreas and adrenal glands [20]. Because cart expression is virtually undetectable in hypothalamic neurons of *ob/ob* mice, it may be positively regulated by leptin and could therefore act as its mediator [14, 36]. Cart$^{-/-}$ mice do not present changes in body weight or reproduction [4], but have low bone mass. Osteoblast numbers and bone formation rates are normal, but the number of osteoclasts and the area of bone resorption are nearly doubled in *Cart*$^{-/-}$ bones [17]. In agreement with the absence of cart expression in bone cells, the *Cart*$^{-/-}$ phenotype is not bone cell autonomous, as *Cart*$^{-/-}$ bone marrow macrophages differentiate normally into osteoclasts and *Cart*$^{-/-}$ bone marrow stromal cells can normally support osteoclastogenesis in co-culture experiments [17]. Further analysis has revealed that *Cart*$^{-/-}$ bones exhibit an increase in *Rankl* expression; this indicates that CART does not affect bone resorption by acting directly on osteoclasts, but by modulating *Rankl* expression in osteoblasts [17] (Fig. 16.1). Considering that *Cart* expression is not detectable in *ob/ob* mice, the increase in bone resorption in *ob/ob* mice can be attributed to a negative influence of CART on bone resorption. It has been shown that *Cart* polymorphism affects bone mass in postmenopausal women; CART therefore also regulates bone remodeling in humans [24]. Identification of a CART receptor will make it possible to analyze the mechanism of how CART acts on bone resorption.

16.8 The Melanocortin 4 Receptor

Melanocortins, which are produced by the processing of propiomelanocortin, regulate food intake and energy expenditure through the melanocortin 3 (MC3) and melanocortin 4 (MC4) receptors [11]. MC4R is implicated in the regulation of appetite by leptin, and mutations in *Mc4r* are the most common single genetic mutations that cause human obesity [11]. Interestingly, patients with mutations in *Mc4r* and *Mc4r*$^{-/-}$ mice display high bone mass, but normal bone formation parameters. This high bone mass is caused by a decrease in osteoclast number and function [17]. Moreover, Mc4r inactivation leads to a nearly twofold increase in hypothalamic *Cart* expression [17]. Likewise, serum CART levels are significantly increased in patients heterozygous for mutations inactivating Mc4R [3]. Furthermore, the fact that decreasing *Cart* expression genetically in *Mc4r*$^{-/-}$ mice rescues their bone phenotype clearly demonstrates that *Cart* overexpression is the cause of the high bone mass [3]. Accordingly, Rankl expression is normalized in *Cart/Mc4r* compound homozygote mutant mice. Because *Cart* polymorphism affects bone mass in human patients [24], regulation of bone resorption by CART and MC4R seems to be conserved in humans as well.

16.9 Neuromedin U

Neuromedin U (NMU) is a neuropeptide produced in the gastrointestinal tract, spinal cord, and brain structures [9]. NMU inhibits food intake by a leptin-independent mechanism, as demonstrated by the fact that NMU ICV decreased body weight in WT and *ob/ob* mice [27]. Accordingly, *Nmu*$^{-/-}$ mice are hyperphagic and obese and also have a high bone mass with an increase in bone formation that is similar to that in *ob/ob* mice [55].

This phenotype is not cell-autonomous, because *Nmu*$^{-/-}$ osteoblasts are indistinguishable from WT osteoblasts. Because treatment of WT osteoblasts with NMU does not affect proliferation or differentiation, NMU must have a central role in the regulation of bone formation [55]. Indeed, ICV infusion of NMU in NMU$^{-/-}$ mice and WT mice decreases bone formation and bone volume in both [55].

Importantly, ICV infusion of NMU in *ob/ob* mice decreases bone volume in WT mice, but ICV infusion of leptin in NMU$^{-/-}$ mice increases bone mass; hence NMU is a mediator of leptin's action on bone formation [55]. Furthermore, treatment of NMU$^{-/-}$ mice with the β-agonist isoproterenol does not decrease their bone mass. Therefore, NMU mediates the regulation of bone formation by leptin and SNS; NMU in the hypothalamus affects only the leptin-dependent negative regulator of osteoblast proliferation, namely the molecular clock [22] (Fig. 16.1). The mechanism that links NMU in the hypothalamus and the clock in bone is not known. One way to address this question is by parabiosis. Human genomic polymorphism in the *Nmu* coding region alters body weight [26] and may affect bone mass. Mice deficient for the NMU receptor are not obese (NMUR2) [66]. If this pathway also exists in humans, NMU antagonists might become candidates to treat bone-loss disorders without inducing an increase in body weight.

16.10 Npy

Neuropeptide Y (NPY) is expressed in the central and peripheral nervous system and has various functions, including regulation of food intake. So far, five receptors (Y1, 2, 4, 5, and 6) have been identified as NPY receptors [42]. In addition, the Y signaling system has many ligands, including NPY, peptide YY (PYY), and pancreatic polypeptide (PP) [42]. An increase in NPY expression in the hypothalamus leads to increased food intake and obesity in mice on a high sucrose diet [30]. In knockout mice, Y1 and Y5 are important for appetite regulation [42]. In contrast, $Y2^{-/-}$ or hypothalamic-specific $Y2^{-/-}$ mice develop a high bone mass with an increase in bone formation. Thus, Y2 signaling acts on bone formation via the central nervous system [6]. However, $NPY^{-/-}$ mice show normal bone mass. Therefore, it is not clear which ligand(s) is (are) involved [19].

$Y1^{-/-}$ mice have high bone mass because bone formation is increased, as are osteoclast surfaces [5]. However, hypothalamus-specific $Y1^{-/-}$ mice show normal bone mass; this suggests that Y1 receptor signaling affects bone remodeling peripherally. Accordingly, treatment of WT mouse calvarial osteoblasts with NPY markedly reduces cell numbers, but this is abolished in $Y1^{-/-}$ cultures. Therefore, Y1 seems to regulate bone mass by acting directly on bone cells. Interestingly, germline deletion of Y2 significantly reduces the expression of Y1 in osteoblasts. This explains the high bone mass in Y2-deficient mice [43]. Though $Y4^{-/-}$ mice have normal bone, Y2/Y4 double mutant mice display a higher bone mass than $Y2^{-/-}$ mice, owing to an increase in the bone formation rate. Because serum leptin levels in Y2/Y4 double mutant mice are lower than in Y2 single mutant mice, leptin signaling may indirectly act on bone remodeling in Y2/Y4 double mutant mice [52]. To date, there is no evidence of Y receptor signaling interacting with SNS to remodel bone.

16.11 Regulation of Glucose Metabolism by Bone Cells

An endocrine organ needs feedback from its target to regulate its hormone output. Regulation of bone remodeling by adipokines like leptin implies that bone regulates fat metabolism via adipocytes function [39] (Fig. 16.2).

The gene Esp encodes a tyrosine phosphatase, OST-PTP, which is expressed in osteoblasts and testes. $Esp^{-/-}$ mice show no remarkable bone phenotype [13], but $Esp^{-/-}$ mice die perinatally due to hypoglycemia [39]. Detailed analyses have failed to detect Esp expression in β cells of the pancreas, adipocytes, muscle, liver, or brain; only osteoblasts and testes express this enzyme. The glucose level of $Esp^{-/-}$ mice was only a third of that in controls. The pancreatic islet cells had increased from 60 to 300% over that in controls so that the serum insulin level at birth was twice that of the controls and glucose tolerance was raised. $Esp^{-/-}$ mice also had double the normal level of adiponectin, a hormone that regulates adipocyte insulin sensitivity. This may explain the increase in insulin sensitivity. On the other hand, leptin and resistin expression are unchanged in the mutants who are lean, whose energy expenditure is increased, and whose serum triglyceride and free fatty acid levels are lowered, with food intake normal. In the experiment, WT mice, on a high fat diet or when their satiety center (the VMH nucleus) was inhibited by gold thioglucose, became obese and developed hyperglycemia, glucose intolerance, and insulin resistance. In contrast, $Esp^{-/-}$ mice so treated remained lean and did not develop

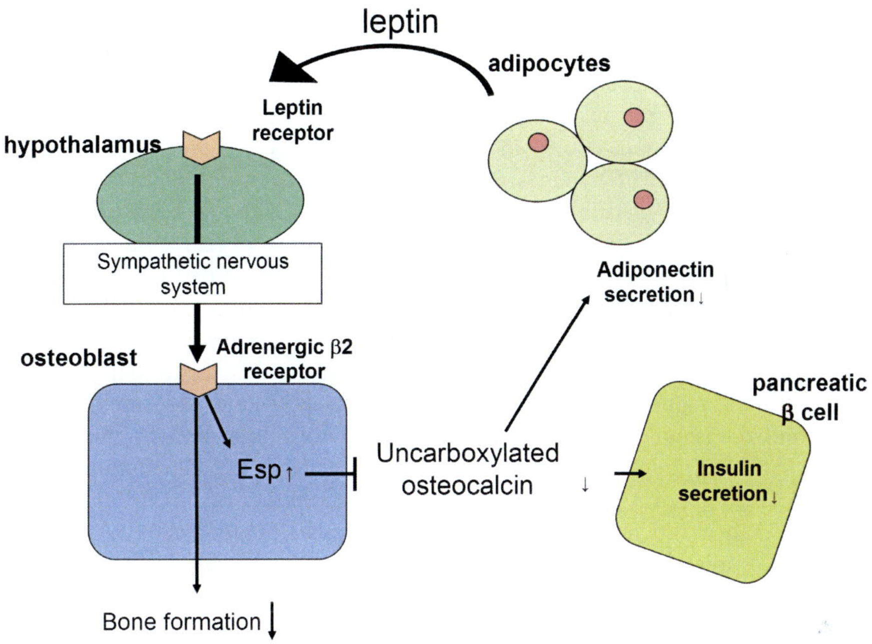

Figure 16.2. Regulation of glucose metabolism by osteoblast.

glucose intolerance or insulin resistance. Thus, $Esp^{-/-}$ mice clearly display an increase in insulin secretion and sensitivity.

Conversely, mice overexpressing Esp (Esp transgenic mice) only in osteoblasts showed poor insulin secretion because of reduced β cell proliferation and small islets. They also showed lower adiponectin expression in fat. As a result, Esp transgenic mice developed glucose intolerance, insulin resistance, and hyperglycemia. These results demonstrate that Esp in osteoblasts regulates insulin sensitivity through adiponectin expression in fat; this finding indicates links between bone, pancreas, and fat [38] (Fig. 16.2).

There are two possible ways by which the pancreas can be regulated by fat and/or bone. One is a neuronal network from osteoblast to pancreatic islets or fat, as in the regulation of pancreatic islet proliferation by the liver [29]. The other is hormonal regulation with the hormone secreted from osteoblasts acting on pancreatic islets or fat. This has been shown to be the case when pancreatic islets were co-cultured with osteoblasts and insulin secretion was upregulated by 40% [39]. Yet, glucagon expression was unchanged; the effect was therefore specific to insulin. Also, when adipocytes were co-cultured with osteoblasts, adiponectin expression was induced. Moreover, the supernatant of cultured osteoblasts, but not of fibroblasts, had the same effect on pancreatic islets and adipocytes. These findings clearly demonstrate the existence of an osteoblastic hormone that acts on islet cells and adipocytes. In agreement with the in vivo observations, osteoblasts from $Esp^{-/-}$ mice enhanced insulin secretion more than WT osteoblasts. One may therefore conclude that osteoblasts secrete a hormone that regulates glucose metabolism and that its activity is regulated by Esp.

Osteocalcin (Ocn) is the seventh most abundant protein in the human body and the most abundant noncollagenous protein in bone tissue. It has only 49 amino acids, a −9 charge, and the sequence of amino acids is highly conserved from swordfish to humans [41]. Ocn not only accumulates in bone as a matrix protein but is also secreted into the general circulation. $Ocn^{-/-}$ mice develop a mild bone abnormality [16] and are hyperglycemic, hypoinsulinemic, glucose intolerant, insulin resistant, and obese. The mice develop a disturbance in glucose metabolism before becoming obese. Glucose intolerance therefore is not secondary to obesity. Furthermore, in $Ocn^{-/-}$ mice, insulin content, beta cell proliferation in the pancreas, and serum adiponectin concentration all were decreased. The absence of Ocn expression in pancreas or fat suggests that Ocn is a candidate for the regulation of pancreas and fat.

Indeed, when co-cultured with islet cells or adipocytes, $Ocn^{-/-}$ osteoblasts failed to induce insulin and adiponectin expression. Furthermore, addition of recombinant osteocalcin to the culture medium significantly increased insulin secretion from islet cells and adiponectin expression from adipocytes. Most importantly, injection of recombinant Ocn ameliorated the glucose intolerance and improved insulin secretion in $Ocn^{-/-}$ mice. Serum adiponectin was reduced not only in $Ocn^{-/-}$ mice but also in $Ocn^{+/-}$/Adiponectin$^{+/-}$ heterozygous mice. Yet, it was unchanged in either of the single heterozygous mice; this demonstrates a genetic interaction of Ocn with adiponectin. Ocn therefore is both necessary and sufficient for osteoblastic regulation of insulin secretion and adiponectin expression. Ocn is modified post-translationally by a vitamin K dependent carboxylation of two of its glutamic acid residues on the pre-osteocalcin molecule secreted by osteoblasts [41]. This carboxylation enhances the binding affinity of osteocalcin to bone mineral (hydroxyapatite). However, loss or gain of function experiments in mice have failed to indicate a physiological role for Ocn in the mineralization of the extracellular matrix. Patients with vitamin K deficiency have less carboxylated Ocn and are at increased risk for vertebral fracture, independent of bone mineral density. Ocn must therefore play a role in the maintenance of bone quality [63]. Interestingly, carboxylated osteocalcin does not affect adiponectin or insulin expression in adipocytes or islets, whereas uncarboxylated osteocalcin does. Some results suggest, however, that carboxylated osteocalcin acts like uncarboxylated osteocalcin, but less so. The phenotype of $Ocn^{-/-}$ mice is a mirror image of that of $Esp^{-/-}$ mice. OST-PTP may therefore use Ocn to regulate glucose metabolism.

Several lines of evidence support this hypothesis. The removal of one allele of Ocn in $Esp^{-/-}$ mice completely rescued their metabolic abnormalities, i.e., hypoglycemia, increased insulin sensitivity and secretion, and islet proliferation. Moreover, although the total amount of osteocalcin is the same in $Esp^{-/-}$ and WT mice, the serum concentration of uncarboxylated "metabolically active" osteocalcin was elevated in $Esp^{-/-}$ mice. How OST-PTP regulates carboxylation is not known. In conclusion, OST-PTP affects osteocalcin carboxylation. Uncarboxylated osteoblasts secrete osteocalcin that in turn regulates glucose metabolism (Fig. 16.2). However, given the lack of an Esp homolog in humans, it is unclear whether carboxylase also affects glucose metabolism in humans.

16.12 Osteocalcin as a Potential Therapeutic for Diabetes

The serum concentration of uncarboxylated "metabolically active" Ocn is approximately 7 ng/mL in WT mice. A detailed dose–response analysis of the effect of uncarboxylated Ocn on insulin secretion and insulin sensitivity revealed that the addition of Ocn to a culture medium, at concentrations from 0.03 to 0.3 ng/mL, significantly increased insulin expression in islets, whereas higher concentrations of Ocn inhibited insulin secretion [21]. To induce adiponectin expression in adipocytes requires Ocn concentrations higher than 1 ng/mL. Ocn infusion to WT mice at rates between 0.3 and 3 ng/h significantly increases serum insulin and decreases serum glucose, whereas Ocn infusions of 3–30 ng/h induce adiponectin expression and raise insulin sensitivity. The difference in Ocn concentration needed to regulate insulin vs. that needed to regulate adiponectin indicates that Ocn acts differently on islets and adipocytes. This may be due to differences in receptor sensitivity to uncarboxylated Ocn. Because Ocn lowers the serum glucose level at an infusion rate as low as 0.3 ng/h, Ocn may become useful for the treatment of diabetes.

16.13 Leptin Regulates Glucose Metabolism Through Osteoblasts via the SNS

Because *ob/ob* mice display hyperinsulinemia at 2 weeks of age, when their body weight and insulin sensitivity are still normal, leptin seems to inhibit insulin secretion either by directly acting on the pancreas or indirectly through the central nervous system via unidentified mechanisms [33]. Addition of recombinant leptin to cultured islets decreases insulin secretion modestly. In contrast, in mice deficient in the neuron-specific leptin receptor (LepR), the serum insulin concentration is doubled. This clearly demonstrates that the leptin-dependent regulatory pathway of insulin secretion involves the central nervous system [28].

Because leptin modulates osteoblast proliferation through the SNS and osteocalcin regulates insulin secretion, whereas stimulation of the SNS inhibits insulin secretion [47], leptin may regulate insulin secretion through the SNS via osteoblasts. This inference derives support from the above-mentioned studies with $LepR^{-/-}$ mice [28], but a definitive resolution requires analysis of glucose metabolism in osteoblast-specific $Adrb2^{-/-}$ mice; these mice are hypoglycemic because their serum insulin level is raised. Moreover, whereas propranolol treatment increased serum insulin level in WT mice (see above), this did not alter the serum insulin in osteoblast-specific $Adrb2^{-/-}$ mice. Moreover, leptin ICV treatment decreased glucose-stimulated insulin secretion in WT mice, but not in osteoblast-specific $Adrb2^{-/-}$ mice. Osteoblast-specific $Adrb2^{+/-}$/ob/+ compound heterozygous mice exhibit hyperinsulinemia and hypoglycemia, while single heterozygous mice had a normal glucose metabolism. It is therefore quite likely that the major leptin-dependent regulatory pathway of insulin secretion involves the SNS and adrb2 of osteoblasts.

Interestingly, sympathomimetic treatment of osteoblasts induced Esp expression without affecting Ocn or caroboxylase expression. In addition, total Ocn serum concentration was similar in WT, *ob/ob,* and osteoblast-specific $Adrb2^{-/-}$ mice, but uncarboxylated "metabolically active" Ocn was significantly increased in *ob/ob* and osteoblast-specific $Adrb2^{-/-}$ mice. This indicates that leptin and SNS regulate Esp expression. Esp in turn carboxylates Ocn to enable it to regulate glucose metabolism. When one allele of the Esp gene is deleted, serum insulin levels in *ob/ob* mice go up further, presumably because of an increase in "metabolically active" Ocn. If both alleles of Ocn are deleted, *ob/ob* mice again become hyperinsulinemic. These results demonstrate the fundamental role that osteocalcin plays in the leptin/SNS-dependent regulation of insulin secretion (Fig. 16.2).

16.14 Clinical Implications of the Skeletal Regulation of Glucose Metabolism

In human subjects, the Ocn level predicts how far fasting plasma glucose (FPG) will rise. Neither the bone formation marker, P1NP, nor the bone resorption marker, NTX, is affected [49]. Ocn, but not bone alkaline phosphatase, is negatively correlated with FPG and HbA1c in both men and postmenopausal women with diabetes. It is positively correlated with serum adiponectin level in postmenopausal diabetic women, even after adjustment for age, duration of diabetes, and body mass index [31]. Furthermore, in nondiabetic subjects, Ocn is negatively correlated with FPG [34]. Thus, regulation of glucose metabolism by osteocalcin is conserved in humans and mice.

In contrast, the role of vitamin K in glucose metabolism is elusive. Theoretically, vitamin K, which stimulates γ-carboxylation of Ocn, would diminish Ocn's metabolic activity. However, people with low vitamin K intake show low serum insulin levels and administration of menaquinone for 1 week increased insulin secretion. It is apparent, therefore, that vitamin K improves insulin secretion [58]. The specific function of carboxylation in the metabolic activity of Ocn is not known.

16.15 Conclusions

Some important questions remain to be addressed. For bone homeostasis to occur, a feedback signal from bone to the hypothalamus is necessary [57]. What is the nature of this signal? The sensing mechanism by which osteoblasts regulate insulin secretion is also not known. More fundamentally, why did the skeleton acquire the ability to affect other organs? The glucose metabolism of human patients with primary hyperparathyroidism is impaired, but their serum Ocn levels are higher, an apparent contradiction [61]. Mouse studies have led to a new research area that links skeletal, neuronal, and metabolic biology. Analysis of these signals, a new field of integrative biology, may bring light to the relationship between the skeleton and the other organs it modulates. From the clinical viewpoint, neuronal pathways that regulate bone remodeling and endocrine pathways originating from the skeleton that regulate glucose and fat metabolism have become attractive targets for the development of therapies for osteoporosis, diabetes, and obesity.

References

1. Ahima RS, Flier JS (2000) Leptin. Annu Rev Physiol 62: 413–437
2. Ahima RS, Osei SY (2004) Leptin signaling. Physiol Behav 81:223–241
3. Ahn JD, Dubern B, Lubrano-Berthelier C, Clement K, Karsenty G (2006) Cart overexpression is the only identifiable cause of high bone mass in melanocortin 4 receptor deficiency. Endocrinology 147:3196–3202
4. Asnicar MA, Smith DP, Yang DD, Heiman ML, Fox N, Chen YF et al (2001) Absence of cocaine- and amphetamine-regulated transcript results in obesity in mice fed a high caloric diet. Endocrinology 142:4394–4400
5. Baldock PA, Allison SJ, Lundberg P, Lee NJ, Slack K, Lin EJ et al (2007) Novel role of Y1 receptors in the coordinated regulation of bone and energy homeostasis. J Biol Chem 282:19092–19102
6. Baldock PA, Sainsbury A, Couzens M, Enriquez RF, Thomas GP, Gardiner EM et al (2002) Hypothalamic Y2 receptors regulate bone formation. J Clin Invest 109:915–921
7. Bonnet N, Laroche N, Vico L, Dolleans E, Benhamou CL, Courteix D (2006) Dose effects of propranolol on cancellous and cortical bone in ovariectomized adult rats. J Pharmacol Exp Ther 318:1118–1127
8. Bray GA, York DA (1998) The MONA LISA hypothesis in the time of leptin. Recent Prog Horm Res 53:95–117
9. Brighton PJ, Szekeres PG, Willars GB (2004) Neuromedin U and its receptors: structure, function, and physiological roles. Pharmacol Rev 56:231–248
10. Cock TA, Back J, Elefteriou F, Karsenty G, Kastner P, Chan S et al (2004) Enhanced bone formation in lipodystrophic PPARgamma(hyp/hyp) mice relocates haematopoiesis to the spleen. EMBO Rep 5:1007–1012
11. Cone RD (2006) Studies on the physiological functions of the melanocortin system. Endocr Rev 27: 736–749
12. Cornish J, Callon KE, Bava U, Lin C, Naot D, Hill BL et al (2002) Leptin directly regulates bone cell function in vitro and reduces bone fragility in vivo. J Endocrinol 175:405–415
13. Dacquin R, Mee PJ, Kawaguchi J, Olmsted-Davis EA, Gallagher JA, Nichols J et al (2004) Knock-in of nuclear localised beta-galactosidase reveals that the tyrosine phosphatase Ptprv is specifically expressed in cells of the bone collar. Dev Dyn 229:826–834
14. Douglass J, McKinzie AA, Couceyro P (1995) PCR differential display identifies a rat brain mRNA that is transcriptionally regulated by cocaine and amphetamine. J Neurosci 15:2471–2481
15. Ducy P, Amling M, Takeda S, Priemel M, Schilling AF, Beil FT et al (2000) Leptin inhibits bone formation through a hypothalamic relay: a central control of bone mass. Cell 100:197–207
16. Ducy P, Desbois C, Boyce B, Pinero G, Story B, Dunstan C et al (1996) Increased bone formation in osteocalcin-deficient mice. Nature 382:448–452
17. Elefteriou F, Ahn JD, Takeda S, Starbuck M, Yang X, Liu X et al (2005) Leptin regulation of bone resorption by the sympathetic nervous system and CART. Nature 434:514–520
18. Elefteriou F, Takeda S, Ebihara K, Magre J, Patano N, Kim CA et al (2004) Serum leptin level is a regulator of bone mass. Proc Natl Acad Sci U S A 101:3258–3263
19. Elefteriou F, Takeda S, Liu X, Armstrong D, Karsenty G (2003) Monosodium glutamate-sensitive hypothalamic neurons contribute to the control of bone mass. Endocrinology 144:3842–3847
20. Elias CF, Lee C, Kelly J, Aschkenasi C, Ahima RS, Couceyro PR et al (1998) Leptin activates hypothalamic CART neurons projecting to the spinal cord. Neuron 21:1375–1385
21. Ferron M, Hinoi E, Karsenty G, Ducy P (2008) Osteocalcin differentially regulates beta cell and adipocyte gene expression and affects the development of metabolic diseases in wild-type mice. Proc Natl Acad Sci U S A 105:5266–5270
22. Fu L, Patel MS, Bradley A, Wagner EF, Karsenty G (2005) The molecular clock mediates leptin-regulated bone formation. Cell 122:803–815
23. Goulding A, Taylor RW (1998) Plasma leptin values in relation to bone mass and density and to dynamic biochemical markers of bone resorption and formation in postmenopausal women. Calcif Tissue Int 63:456–458

24. Guerardel A, Tanko LB, Boutin P, Christiansen C, Froguel P (2006) Obesity susceptibility CART gene polymorphism contributes to bone remodeling in postmenopausal women. Osteoporos Int 17:156–157
25. Guidobono F, Pagani F, Sibilia V, Netti C, Lattuada N, Rapetti D et al (2006) Different skeletal regional response to continuous brain infusion of leptin in the rat. Peptides 27:1426–1433
26. Hainerova I, Torekov SS, Ek J, Finkova M, Borch-Johnsen K, Jorgensen T et al (2006) Association between neuromedin U gene variants and overweight and obesity. J Clin Endocrinol Metab 91:5057–5063
27. Hanada R, Nakazato M, Murakami N, Sakihara S, Yoshimatsu H, Toshinai K et al (2001) A role for neuromedin U in stress response. Biochem Biophys Res Commun 289:225–228
28. Hinoi E, Gao N, Jung DY, Yadav V, Yoshizawa T, Myers MG Jr et al (2008) The sympathetic tone mediates leptin's inhibition of insulin secretion by modulating osteocalcin bioactivity. J Cell Biol 183: 1235–1242
29. Imai J, Katagiri H, Yamada T, Ishigaki Y, Suzuki T, Kudo H et al (2008) Regulation of pancreatic beta cell mass by neuronal signals from the liver. Science 322:1250–1254
30. Kaga T, Inui A, Okita M, Asakawa A, Ueno N, Kasuga M et al (2001) Modest overexpression of neuropeptide Y in the brain leads to obesity after high-sucrose feeding. Diabetes 50:1206–1210
31. Kanazawa I, Yamaguchi T, Yamamoto M, Yamauchi M, Kurioka S, Yano S et al (2009) Serum osteocalcin level is associated with glucose metabolism and atherosclerosis parameters in type 2 diabetes mellitus. J Clin Endocrinol Metab 94:45–49
32. Karsenty G (2006) Convergence between bone and energy homeostases: leptin regulation of bone mass. Cell Metab 4:341–348
33. Kieffer TJ, Habener JF (2000) The adipoinsular axis: effects of leptin on pancreatic beta-cells. Am J Physiol Endocrinol Metab 278:E1–E14
34. Kindblom JM, Ohlsson C, Ljunggren O, Karlsson MK, Tivesten A, Smith U et al (2009) Plasma osteocalcin is inversely related to fat mass and plasma glucose in elderly swedish men. J Bone Miner Res 24(5):785–791
35. Kondo H, Nifuji A, Takeda S, Ezura Y, Rittling SR, Denhardt DT et al (2005) Unloading induces osteoblastic cell suppression and osteoclastic cell activation to lead to bone loss via sympathetic nervous system. J Biol Chem 280:30192–30200
36. Kristensen P, Judge ME, Thim L, Ribel U, Christjansen KN, Wulff BS et al (1998) Hypothalamic CART is a new anorectic peptide regulated by leptin. Nature 393:72–76
37. Kurvers HA (1998) Reflex sympathetic dystrophy: facts and hypotheses. Vasc Med 3:207–214
38. Lee NK, Karsenty G (2008) Reciprocal regulation of bone and energy metabolism. Trends Endocrinol Metab 19:161–166
39. Lee NK, Sowa H, Hinoi E, Ferron M, Ahn JD, Confavreux C et al (2007) Endocrine regulation of energy metabolism by the skeleton. Cell 130:456–469
40. Levasseur R, Sabatier JP, Potrel-Burgot C, Lecoq B, Creveuil C, Marcelli C (2003) Sympathetic nervous system as transmitter of mechanical loading in bone. Joint Bone Spine 70:515–519
41. Lian JB, Gundberg CM (1988) Osteocalcin. Biochemical considerations and clinical applications. Clin Orthop Relat Res (226):267–291
42. Lin S, Boey D, Herzog H (2004) NPY and Y receptors: lessons from transgenic and knockout models. Neuropeptides 38:189–200
43. Lundberg P, Allison SJ, Lee NJ, Baldock PA, Brouard N, Rost S et al (2007) Greater bone formation of Y2 knockout mice is associated with increased osteoprogenitor numbers and altered Y1 receptor expression. J Biol Chem 282:19082–19091
44. Martin A, de Vittoris R, David V, Moraes R, Begeot M, Lafage-Proust MH et al (2005) Leptin modulates both resorption and formation while preventing disuse-induced bone loss in tail-suspended female rats. Endocrinology 146:3652–3659
45. Martini G, Valenti R, Giovani S, Franci B, Campagna S, Nuti R (2001) Influence of insulin-like growth factor-1 and leptin on bone mass in healthy postmenopausal women. Bone 28:113–117
46. Morberg CM, Tetens I, Black E, Toubro S, Soerensen TI, Pedersen O et al (2003) Leptin and bone mineral density: a cross-sectional study in obese and nonobese men. J Clin Endocrinol Metab 88:5795–5800
47. Nonogaki K (2000) New insights into sympathetic regulation of glucose and fat metabolism. Diabetologia 43:533–549
48. Pierroz DD, Bouxsein ML, Rizzoli R, Ferrari SL (2006) Combined treatment with a [beta]-blocker and intermittent PTH improves bone mass and microarchitecture in ovariectomized mice. Bone 39:260–267
49. Pittas AG, Harris SS, Eliades M, Stark P, Dawson-Hughes B (2009) Association between serum osteocalcin and markers of metabolic phenotype. J Clin Endocrinol Metab 94:827–832
50. Pogoda P, Egermann M, Schnell JC, Priemel M, Schilling AF, Alini M et al (2006) Leptin inhibits bone formation not only in rodents, but also in sheep. J Bone Miner Res 21:1591–1599
51. Ruhl CE, Everhart JE (2002) Relationship of serum leptin concentration with bone mineral density in the United States population. J Bone Miner Res 17:1896–1903
52. Sainsbury A, Baldock PA, Schwarzer C, Ueno N, Enriquez RF, Couzens M et al (2003) Synergistic effects of Y2 and Y4 receptors on adiposity and bone mass revealed in double knockout mice. Mol Cell Biol 23:5225–5233
53. Sakamoto N, Nishiike T, Iguchi H, Sakamoto K (2000) Possible effects of one week vitamin K (menaquinone-4) tablets intake on glucose tolerance in healthy young male volunteers with different descarboxy prothrombin levels. Clin Nutr 19:259–263
54. Sato M, Takeda N, Sarui H, Takami R, Takami K, Hayashi M et al (2001) Association between serum leptin concentrations and bone mineral density, and

biochemical markers of bone turnover in adult men. J Clin Endocrinol Metab 86:5273–5276
55. Sato S, Hanada R, Kimura A, Abe T, Matsumoto T, Iwasaki M et al (2007) Central control of bone remodeling by neuromedin U. Nat Med 13:1234–1240
56. Shi Y, Yadav VK, Suda N, Liu XS, Guo XE, Myers MG Jr et al (2008) Dissociation of the neuronal regulation of bone mass and energy metabolism by leptin in vivo. Proc Natl Acad Sci U S A 105:20529–20533
57. Takeda S (2008) Central control of bone remodelling. J Neuroendocrinol 20:802–807
58. Takeda S, Elefteriou F, Levasseur R, Liu X, Zhao L, Parker KL et al (2002) Leptin regulates bone formation via the sympathetic nervous system. Cell 111:305–317
59. Tam J, Trembovler V, Di Marzo V, Petrosino S, Leo G, Alexandrovich A et al (2008) The cannabinoid CB1 receptor regulates bone formation by modulating adrenergic signaling. FASEB J 22:285–294
60. Tartaglia LA (1997) The leptin receptor. J Biol Chem 272:6093–6096
61. Taylor WH, Khaleeli AA (2001) Coincident diabetes mellitus and primary hyperparathyroidism. Diabetes Metab Res Rev 17:175–180
62. Thomas T, Burguera B, Melton LJ III, Atkinson EJ, O'Fallon WM, Riggs BL et al (2001) Role of serum leptin, insulin, and estrogen levels as potential mediators of the relationship between fat mass and bone mineral density in men versus women. Bone 29:114–120
63. Tsugawa N, Shiraki M, Suhara Y, Kamao M, Tanaka K, Okano T (2006) Vitamin K status of healthy Japanese women: age-related vitamin K requirement for gamma-carboxylation of osteocalcin. Am J Clin Nutr 83:380–386
64. Wiens M, Etminan M, Gill SS, Takkouche B (2006) Effects of antihypertensive drug treatments on fracture outcomes: a meta-analysis of observational studies. J Intern Med 260:350–362
65. Yirmiya R, Goshen I, Bajayo A, Kreisel T, Feldman S, Tam J et al (2006) Depression induces bone loss through stimulation of the sympathetic nervous system. Proc Natl Acad Sci U S A 103:16876–16881
66. Zeng H, Gragerov A, Hohmann JG, Pavlova MN, Schimpf BA, Xu H et al (2006) Neuromedin U receptor 2-deficient mice display differential responses in sensory perception, stress, and feeding. Mol Cell Biol 26:9352–9363

17. Mechanobiology of Bone Development and Computational Simulations

Gongfa Chen, Michael Schuetz, and Mark Pearcy

Bone is important because it provides the skeleton structural integrity and enables movement and locomotion. Its development and morphology follow its function. It adapts to changes of mechanical loading and has the ability to repair itself after damage or fracture. The processes of bone development, bone adaptation, and bone regeneration in fracture healing are regulated, in part, by mechanical stimuli that result when the bone is loaded.

"Mechanobiology is the study of how mechanical or physical conditions regulate biologic processes" [13]. It studies how bones, as a load-bearing tissue, are produced, maintained, and regenerated through the active response of cells to the biophysical stimuli in their environment. The mechanobiology of bone growth, adaption, and regeneration is still in an early stage of development and application. Understanding bone mechanobiology can be helpful for the clinical treatment of all conditions that affect bone formation, from congenital deformities to bone fracture.

Both experimental and theoretical methods are employed in mechanobiological investigations. Experimental models can explore the relation between the biological processes and the global mechanical stimuli, like forces and displacements, which are defined at the organ level. Theoretical models, particularly with computational simulations, establish the relationship between the global mechanical factors to the local distribution of strains defined at the tissue level. In this way, the mechanobiological models for bone growth, adaption, and regeneration can be further defined at the tissue level.

This chapter will briefly review the recent development of the mechanobiology of bone growth, adaption, and regeneration.

17.1 Form and Function of Bone

The idea that "form follows function" is a widely accepted concept in modern biology, originated by the German anatomist Julius Wolff [98]. This section will illustrate how bone shape and structure are related to function.

17.1.1 Bone Function

Bone, and hence the skeleton, provides structural support for the body and serves as the body's mineral reservoir. It also provides anchorage for the muscles enabling motion and protects internal organs. The human skeleton has more than 200 bones, which are generally classified into four types according to shape: long, short, flat, or irregular. Bone size and shape match the structural demands placed on bones.

F. Bronner et al. (eds.), *Bone and Development*, Topics in Bone Biology 6,
DOI 10.1007/978-1-84882-822-3_17,

The femur is the largest bone of the human body. It must be strong as it withstands significant mechanical forces during walking, running, jumping, etc. Because it supports compression, bending, and torsion, its shaft is formed like a hollow cylinder, an optimal design for maximum strength with minimum material. For efficiency of movement, the femur must be light, but must have sufficient strength to provide motion and support. Natural selection will favor a bone with minimum mass and maximum bending resistance. The femur must be sufficiently stiff to resist the bending moments without too much distortion, but must also be compliant enough not to fail in a brittle manner in response to impact loads.

The vertebrae of the spinal column are another example of how each bone is formed to match a purpose. The vertebral bodies are cylindrical and consist of a thin external layer of compact (or cortical) bone with a honeycomb-like internal structure known as cancellous (or trabecular) bone. This gives them strength (particularly in compression and torsion) with a minimum of material. The spine is made up of vertebrae with compliant, cartilaginous inter-vertebral discs between the vertebrae that impart flexibility to the spine.

17.1.2 Bone Form

To match the structural demands placed on them, bones optimize their shape at the gross morphological level.

The femur, an example of a long bone (Fig. 17.1), consists of a tubular shaft called the diaphysis; at each end is an epiphysis, which forms a joint with another bone. The diaphysis, comprising the compact bone, is solid and strong. The epiphyses are composed largely of cancellous bone, which is enclosed in a cortical layer. With this optimal structure, the femur can support the compressive forces at the joints that occur in many directions through the epiphyses and the axial compression forces, bending, and torsional moments experienced by the diaphysis.

The shaft of the femur, in the form of a hollow tube with minimal mass, can effectively resist axial compression forces, bending, and torsional moments. In long bones, the direction of loading is variable; a roughly circular section is the best solution to resist bending in all directions (Fig. 17.1c). From the perspective of structural engineering, a hollow section can provide the largest bending resistance for a certain amount of material. For a hollow circular section, the area moment of inertia (I) is equal to $\pi(R^4 - r^4)/4 = (A^2/\pi + 2r^2A)/4$, where R is the external radius, r is the internal radius, and A the area of the hollow section (Fig. 17.1d). Obviously, if the area A is kept the same, i.e., with the same bone mass, the area moment of inertia I is large for a large internal radius r [68]. The area of bone is given by $A = \pi(R - r)(R + r)$; rearrangement yields $(R - r) = A/[\pi(R + r)]$. If A is constant, it follows that if the internal radius is large, the wall of the bone will be thin. With A constant, a large internal radius increases not only the bending resistance (indicated by I), but also the strength of the bone. The largest stress (σ) due to a bending moment (M) is on the external perimeter and is given by $\sigma = \frac{M}{I}R = \frac{4M}{A \cdot R[1+(r/R)^2]}$ With A constant, an increase of r will cause r/R and R to increase, causing the largest stress to decrease.

Size and dimensions of the femoral shaft are necessarily governed by this optimization process [27]. Through mechanical adaptation, a living bone modifies its mass and structure in response to mechanical demand, in an attempt to support mechanical loads with the bone mass efficiently distributed. Too much bone mass leads to uneconomic energy consumption during movement, while too little risks the chance of fracture.

For aging people, both internal and external radii of tubular bones increase, leading to a decrease in wall thickness. Because the area moment of inertia increases as the radii increase, bone mass is effectively optimized [18]. An infinitely large radius with a vanishing thin wall, however, is not a good solution, inasmuch as bones also need to resist other types of loads, such as the impact from perpendicular directions.

Further consideration of the shape of the femur leads to the ends of the femoral shaft, the epiphyses, which are expanded to form the joints. The shape of the epiphyses is affected by the transmission of loads across the joint from one

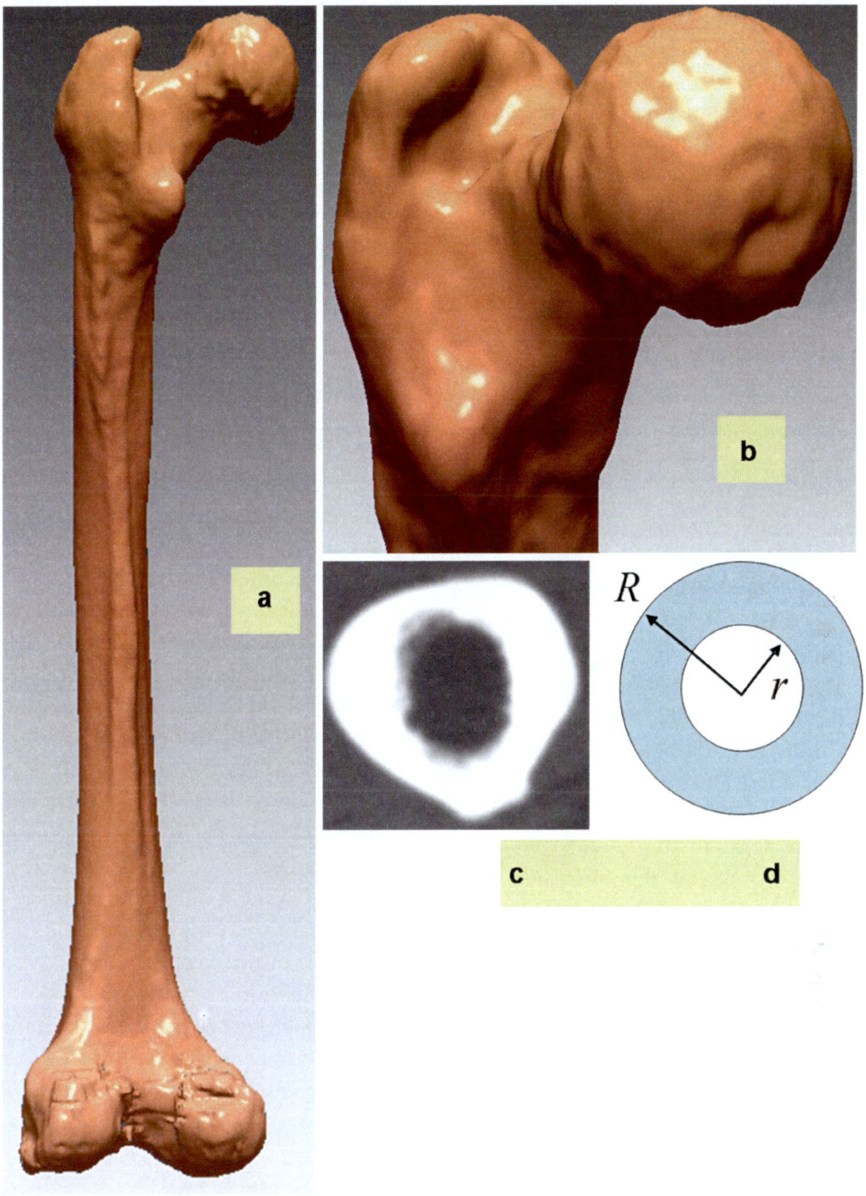

Figure 17.1. A human femur. (**a**) Femur model built from CT scan images; (**b**) proximal head; (**c**) cross-section of diaphysis; (**d**) hollow circular section. Courtesy of Dr. Beat Schmutz, Queensland University of Technology, Australia.

bone to the next. A major feature of the joint is that the ends of the bones are capped with articular cartilage that provides an extremely efficient weight-bearing surface in conjunction with synovial fluid. The cartilage provides a large compliant surface that enables multidirectional loads to be transferred from one bone to the next, thereby reducing the stresses on the subchondral bone. The generally thin layer of subchondral bone underneath the cartilage encases cancellous bone through which the multidirectional loads are transmitted to the dense cortex of the diaphysis as bending, torsion, and compression.

17.1.3 Bone Architecture

At the microscopic level, bone optimizes the architecture of bone tissue. As explained above, the trabecular cascades of the proximal femur, for example (Fig. 17.1b), readily lead the forces and moments to the cortical shell of the diaphysis.

The material properties of bone are greatly affected by its porosity [26, 80]. Most bone tissues have either very low or very high porosity, with few tissues having intermediate porosity. High porosity is characteristic of trabecular bone and low porosity of compact bone. The shafts of long bones and the bone forming a shell around vertebral bodies are compact bone, with porosity around 5–10% [84]. Trabecular bone is porous bone, typically making up the ends of long bones (epiphyses) and constituting the inside of the vertebral bodies. Its porosity ranges from 75 to 95% [80]. The material properties of trabecular and compact bones are listed in Table 17.1.

Bone is anisotropic as it optimizes its architecture by aligning trabeculae with the direction of loading. In the femoral head, Wolff observed that the trabecular trajectories roughly aligned with the direction of the largest principal stress [98]. Trabeculae tend to align with principal stresses in many bones as demonstrated [53]. Material anisotropy, induced by trabecular orientation, makes bone stiffer and stronger in the direction of trabecular alignment. By increasing its load-bearing capacity without increasing mass, trabecular bone significantly improves its structural efficiency.

17.1.4 Structural Optimization in Nature

Because mass in bone is minimized without compromising strength or stiffness, bone tissue is an optimum structure. Mattheck and Reuss demonstrated this by analyzing a tiger claw [58]. Structural engineers have adopted this concept to achieve optimum structural designs by equalizing stresses as much as possible. The result is the Evolutionary Structural Optimization method, which has been successfully applied in structural engineering [101]. Its premise is that additional material should be used only in regions of high stress.

17.2 Mechanobiological Regulation and Simulations of Bone Growth

All bones begin as mesenchymal condensations. By the eighth week after fertilization, the pattern and basic geometry of the skeleton are formed in cartilage and connective tissue membranes; ossification follows. Bone is formed by intramembranous and endochondral ossification.

In intramembranous ossification, some mesenchymal cells are transformed into osteoblasts and replace sheet-like connective tissue membranes by laying down bone. Certain flat bones of the skull and some of the irregular bones are formed in this manner. Endochondral ossification refers to the replacement of hyaline cartilage with bony tissue. This process is composed of a finely balanced cycle of cartilage growth, matrix formation, and calcification of cartilage. Most of the bones of the skeleton are formed in this manner.

This section will discuss the growth and mechanobiological regulation of bones, particularly long bones.

17.2.1 Growth and Ossification of Long Bones [73]

Long bones grow longitudinally by endochondral ossification at the growth plates and in diameter by apposition of bone at the periosteum.

Table 17.1. Material properties of femur (data from [8])

	Density (kg.m^{-3})	Young's modulus (GPa)	Breaking strength (MPa)	Ultimate strain
Compact bone	1,990	20	133	0.03
Trabecular bone	140–1,000	0.044–1.531	0.56–22.9	0.50

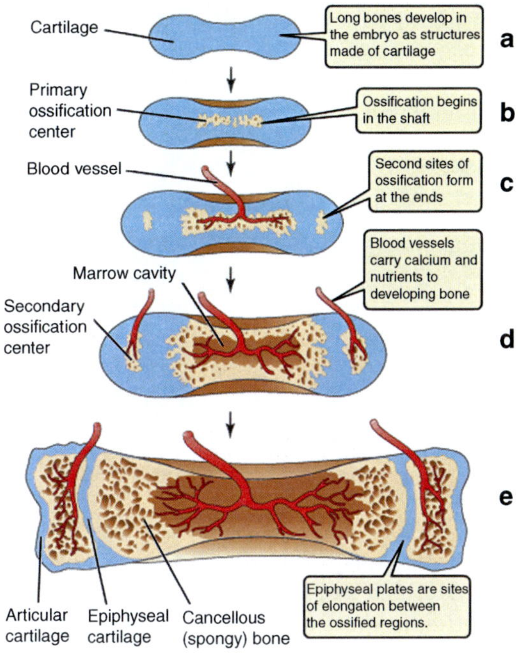

Figure 17.2. Growth and ossification of long bones (Reprinted with permission from Purves et al. [73]).

At the beginning, mesenchymal cells condense and differentiate into the chondrocytes that secrete a matrix and then produce cartilaginous models, or precursors, of the future bones (Fig. 17.2a). These cartilage models are surrounded by the perichondrium and grow by interstitial and appositional growth. During the third month after gestation, a vascular system develops that invades the perichondrium and changes it into periosteum. The ossification starts with a collar of bone that is laid by osteoblasts on the periosteum at the mid-shaft of the bone. At the same time, the cartilage in the center of the diaphysis starts to be denatured and the osteoblasts, together with capillaries, invade this disintegrating cartilage and replace it with cancellous bone, forming a primary ossification center (Fig. 17.2b). Ossification frontiers move from the center toward the bone ends. The embryonic long bones increase their radial dimension by apposition at the periosteum, and the cancellous bone in the center of the diaphysis gradually becomes resorbed to form a marrow cavity (Fig. 17.2c).

The secondary ossification centers emerge in the epiphyses (Fig. 17.2d). This generally occurs after birth. Here, ossification totally replaces the hyaline cartilage except in two regions (Fig. 17.2e). One region is at the articular end of the bone, which remains articular cartilage. The other region is the growth plate, with cartilage remaining between the epiphysis and diaphysis.

Bones grow in length at the growth plate by endochondral ossification. The cartilage on the epiphyseal side continues to grow by mitosis; on the diaphyseal side the cartilage matures, is calcified, and replaced by bone. This process, responsible for increasing the length of the bone, continues throughout childhood and the adolescent years until an individual stops growing. The epiphyseal plate completely ossifies after cartilage growth ceases.

As the skeleton grows in length, the bones must also increase in diameter to support the increasing body weight. The increase in diameter is achieved by intramembranous ossification. Osteoblasts in the periosteum deposit bone around the external bone surface while, simultaneously, osteoclasts in the endosteum resorb bone from the internal surface around the medullary cavity. This process continues even when bones stop growing longitudinally. From that position, the size of the intramedullary cavity increases with age.

17.2.2 Influences of Mechanical Factors on Bone Growth and Development

Mechanical loading influences the process of endochondral growth and ossification. Muscle fibers develop by the eighth week after gestation and the newly formed muscle begins making involuntary contractions. The stresses caused by muscular contractions on skeletal tissue begin to play an essential role in modulating cartilage growth and ossification rates. Muscle paralysis in chick embryos has been found to slow bone growth [42]. Diminished bone growth correlates with reduced muscular activity.

After birth, further growth of bones continues to be strongly influenced by externally applied mechanical forces. The growth of the skeleton is described by the Hueter–Volkmann law, which states, as a result of clinical observations and animal experiments, that growth is hindered by increased compressive stresses and accelerated by reduced loading [9, 87].

In clinical experience, progression of angular deformities of the proximal tibia and progression of the spine in scoliosis are thought to result from unbalanced forces that interact with the load-growth response for bone [34, 88]. Gooding and Neuhauser [39] and McCall et al. [59] reported "tall vertebrae" in patients with paralysis, in accordance with the observation that unloading of the spine leads to increased longitudinal growth [90].

These clinical observations have been verified by animal experiments. Stokes et al. [88] showed that asymmetric loading of rat tail vertebral segments resulted in differential growth on the compression side, when compared with the tension side. Mente et al. [60] further demonstrated that a vertebral wedge deformity created by asymmetrical loading can be corrected by reversal of the load asymmetry.

There is also evidence that the morphologic organization of bone is affected by the accumulated effects of its strain history. Skedros et al. [83] studied the relationships between developmental morphologic variations and the functional strain distribution of the deer calcaneus. Their findings showed that cross-sectional shape changed with age from a quasi-circular to a quasi-elliptical shape, in accordance with the direction of primary bending. Tanck et al. [89] investigated adaptation of trabecular density and architecture in pigs at different ages and found that density adapts to a rapidly increasing load in the early phase of growth, but that improved structural efficiency is the result of adaptation of trabecular architecture later in development.

17.2.3 Computational Simulations of Bone Growth and Development

17.2.3.1 Endochondral Growth and Ossification

The processes of endochondral growth and ossification are regulated by biological factors such as hormones and influenced by mechanical stresses. Carter and associates [16, 86, 99, 100] hypothesized that the normal sequence of cell proliferation followed by maturation and subsequent denaturation and ossification of cartilage is promoted in regions of high shear stress and inhibited in regions of intermittent hydrostatic stress. The stimulus for ossification was expressed as an osteogenic index. Their hypothesis has been investigated using finite-element models of the femur and sternum. In the femur model, the daily loading history was represented by three separate loading conditions. The development period was divided into five successive stages. The model was initially specified to consist of cartilage and portions of the model were changed to represent the bone regions that had formed.

The osteogenic index was defined as: $O = (\bar{\sigma}_s + k\bar{\sigma}_h)$; $\bar{\sigma}_s$ = octahedral shear (distortional) stress; $\bar{\sigma}_h$ = hydrostatic stress; k = empirical constant. The octahedral stress, $\bar{\sigma}_s$, and hydrostatic stress $\bar{\sigma}_h$ are defined by the principal stresses, σ_1, σ_2, and σ_3, as:

$$\bar{\sigma}_s = \frac{1}{3}\sqrt{(\sigma_1 - \sigma_2)^2 + (\sigma_2 - \sigma_3)^2 + (\sigma_3 - \sigma_1)^2},$$

$$\bar{\sigma}_h = \frac{1}{3}(\sigma_1 + \sigma_2 + \sigma_3). \quad (17.1)$$

A maturation parameter that is linearly related to the osteogenic index [100] is utilized to keep track at different stages of cartilage growth, maturation, and hypertrophy of each element. The element becomes ossified at a critical level of maturation, with ossification starting from the midshaft perichondrium and moving toward the bone ends. Simulations of cartilage maturation and the predicted ossification patterns were found consistent with normal long bone development [100].

Lerner et al. [56] investigated the distribution of mechanical stresses within the growth plate of a rabbit distal femur and verified that the patterns derived from modeling correlated with the experimental patterns of bone growth in five age groups of rabbits and four different loading conditions. Their simulations supported the hypothesis that high compressive stresses relate to lower bone growth rates. A linear relationship between longitudinal growth rate and the rate of cartilage maturation has been proposed, at least for one cartilage region [86].

Ribble et al. [76] used finite element models of the developing proximal femur to demonstrate an inverse relationship between the relative magnitude of the shear stress in the growth plate and the developing neck-shaft angle. In normal development, the relatively high shear stresses in the growth plate indicated a decrease in neck-shaft angle. However, loading conditions representing spasticity, that generated lower shear stresses in the growth plate, were associated with a valgus deformity.

17.2.3.2 Appositional Growth

To study the cross-sectional development and growth of long bones, van der Meulen et al. [94] created computer models of the growth of long bone diaphyses. They related bone surface growth rates to the mechanical stimulus in the skeleton and took into account the two drivers of growth and modeling, biological and mechanical. The total bone apposition rate was modeled as the sum of the biological growth rate and the rate due to mechanobiological factors. Bone apposition and resorption were activated when the change in stimulus reached a trigger level.

17.3 Mechanobiological Regulation of Bone Remodeling and Bone Remodeling Simulations

Mechanical regulation of bone is not only part of bone growth and development, but is the mechanism that changes the internal architecture of bone and its geometry so as to allow bone to adapt to its environment. The process, called bone remodeling (Fig. 17.3), is essential for repair of microscopic damage and to prevent fatigue failure. Thus, it ensures the mechanical and biological integrity of bone.

17.3.1 Remodeling

Remodeling involves resorption of older bone and formation of new bone, accomplished by osteoclasts and osteoblasts, respectively. Frost [32] postulated that osteoclasts and osteoblasts work together in teams of basic multicellular units (BMUs). The remodeling process consists of three principal phases: activation, resorption, and formation (ARF). Activation occurs when a chemical

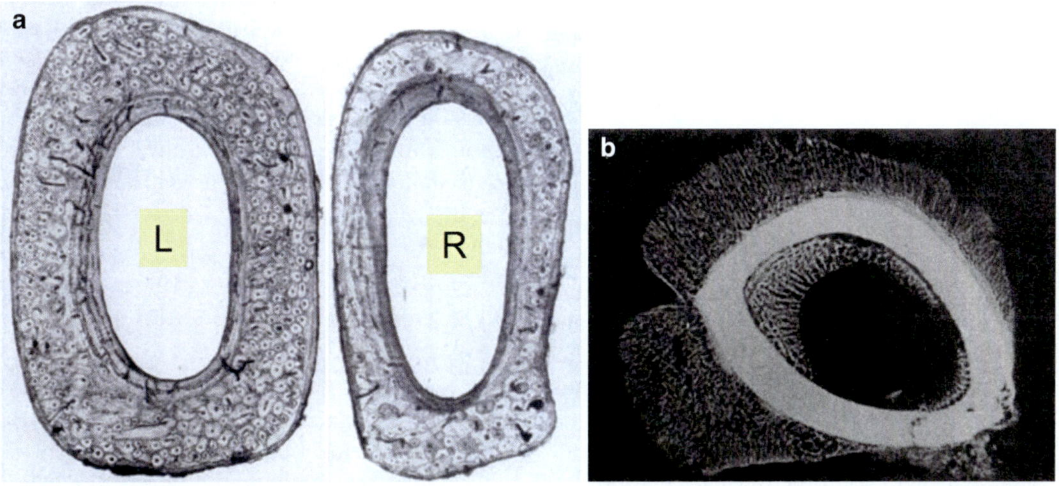

Figure 17.3. Bone resorption and formation. (**a**) Bone resorption. Decrease in cortical area and thickness in a dog model. (L) A metacarpal from the control and (R) a metacarpal after 40 weeks of immobilization (Reprinted with permission and copyright © of the British Editorial Society of Bone and Joint Surgery [93]). (**b**) Bone formation. A section of the mid-shaft of an ulna that was loaded for 36 cycles a day for 24 days (From Rubin and Lanyon [78]. Copyright 1984 by the Journal of Bone and Joint Surgery. Reproduced with permission of the Journal of Bone and Joint Surgery via Copyright Clearance Center).

or mechanical signal causes the local mesenchymal cells to begin producing osteoclasts and osteoblasts [32]. The factor that initiates this process is unknown. When osteoclasts arrive at the surface of bone, they start to resorb it, forming Howship's lacunae in cancellous bone and cutting cones in cortical bone. After the osteoclasts have left their sites of action, osteoblasts derived from mesenchymal cells replace the resorbed tissue with new bone, with typically no change in the bone mass.

Remodeling can result in bone loss if functional loading is reduced (Fig. 17.3a), or in bone gain when functional strains are exceeded (Fig. 17.3b). Functional loading is reduced during prolonged periods of bed rest [55] and as a result of long-term space flights [21, 61]. Bone loss also occurs when fractured bones are stabilized by fixation devices, the plates and screws of which share the load and reduce the strain experienced by the underlying bone [93]. Increased functional loading can occur when physical exercise is increased. Rubin et al. [79] have shown that application of high-frequency, low-magnitude cyclical bone strain can evoke bone formation in animal models of osteoporosis.

17.3.2 Mechanobiological Theories of Bone Remodeling

The capacity of bone tissue to adapt to changing mechanical demands is well documented, but the mechanism by which the cells respond to the mechanical stimuli is not understood.

Mechanical loading strains the bone matrix. The strain must then be sensed by bone cells and translated into a cellular signal that ensures remodeling [54]. Micro-deformation of bone cells and tissue is most likely the result of the mechanotransductive role of strain [12]. Rubin and Lanyon [78] developed in vivo experiments to measure strain in bones exposed to controlled loading conditions. Their findings made it possible to establish a relationship between mechanical loading parameters (i.e., strain magnitude, rate, frequency) and functional adaptation [92]. However, the degree of strain produced by physiological loading is only 0.2–0.3% [78], a much lower value than the deformations needed to obtain a cellular response [11, 62]. Hence, You et al. [102] proposed that bone tissue incorporates a lever system that transduces the small strains of the matrix into a larger signal that bone cells can sense.

Bone is a connective tissue with a porous extracellular matrix that contains living cells with interstitial fluid. Deformation of the bone matrix as in response to mechanical loading induces flow of the interstitial fluid, which may induce shear stresses as the fluid flows over the cells. Several studies of mechanotransduction mechanisms have identified the fluid-induced shear stress as a signal to which bone cells respond [29, 48, 75].

Using simplified models, Piekarski and Munro [69] demonstrated transient pressure gradients in bone tissue induced by mechanical loading and suggested this to be the mechanism that drives load-induced fluid flow within bone. This in turn may enhance the convective transport of nutrients and signaling molecules [28, 49, 50].

Oxygen tension acts as a key regulator of osteoclastic bone resorption, with hypoxia stimulating bone resorption by inducing the formation of large osteoclasts [2, 51, 91]. Diminished locomotory loading induces osteocyte hypoxia, followed by osteoclast formation [28, 41, 63, 95].

When mechanical forces are applied to bone, fluid flow through the lacuno-canalicular system will also induce streaming potentials, i.e., strain-generated potentials [5, 35, 70]. These electrical signals may constitute the physical signals that induce mechanical adaptation. It is as yet uncertain, however, whether streaming potentials are physiologically significant [71]. In one study, the application of a current that either doubled or cancelled the convective current had no effect on the calcium response of bone cells to fluid flow [45].

17.3.3 Computational Simulations of Bone Remodeling

Cowin and Hegedus [25] proposed a general theory of cortical bone remodeling, which was followed by several theoretical models [6, 24, 44]. Many models assume a "remodeling equilibrium," i.e., the bone mass is in equilibrium, undergoing neither net deposition nor resorption. When mechanical stimuli change, the remodeling equilibrium is violated and the error signal drives the remodeling process.

Remodeling can be described by using the apparent density of bone as characteristic of the internal morphology. The rate of change of the apparent density of the bone at a particular location, $d\rho/dt$, can be specified by

$$\frac{d\rho}{dt} = B((S/\rho) - k), \qquad 17.2$$

where B is a constant that characterizes the remodeling speed; $S = S(x,y,z)$ is the mechanical stimulus, and $k = k(x,y,z)$ is the reference value. The mechanical stimulus may be expressed as strain [24], stress [6], or strain energy [44, 97]. Frost [33] introduced minimum effective strain (MES), which is about 0.0008–0.002. Strains below the MES apparently do not evoke bone remodeling. Huiskes et al. [44] and Beaupre et al. [6] called strains below the MES the lazy or dead zone. During remodeling, the Young modulus (E) of a bone is related to its apparent density, ρ, via $E = C\rho^r$, where C is a constant; r is 2–3 for cancellous bone [15, 77] and 5–10 for cortical bone [80].

Numerical analysis can be undertaken using the finite element method (FEM). FEM is a mathematical method by which a set of differential equations can be converted approximately into a set of algebraic equations and solved numerically. The name comes from the process in which a body or structure is divided into very small (or finite) elements to which known properties can be assigned. The elements are connected by nodes through which displacements are transmitted from applied boundary conditions. In this manner, an unknown function in an element is represented by a series of known functions with many unknown variables on the element nodes that are calculated from the boundary conditions. FEM has been commonly applied to solve a broad spectrum of engineering problems. Iterative FEM models have been developed to simulate the process of bone remodeling over time [7, 47, 97]. In this process, the properties of elements are assigned new values at each iteration. The values depend on the particular definition applied to the element and the stresses and strains developed in it. Figure 17.4 illustrates the computational simulation of the remodeling process of the proximal femoral head.

The models of bone remodeling mentioned above are phenomenological in nature, i.e., they describe the stimulus and the response, without taking the biological basis into account [23]. The other type of models are mechanistic, based on the load-induced interstitial fluid flow and the enhanced nutrient transport [43, 64, 85, 96]. At

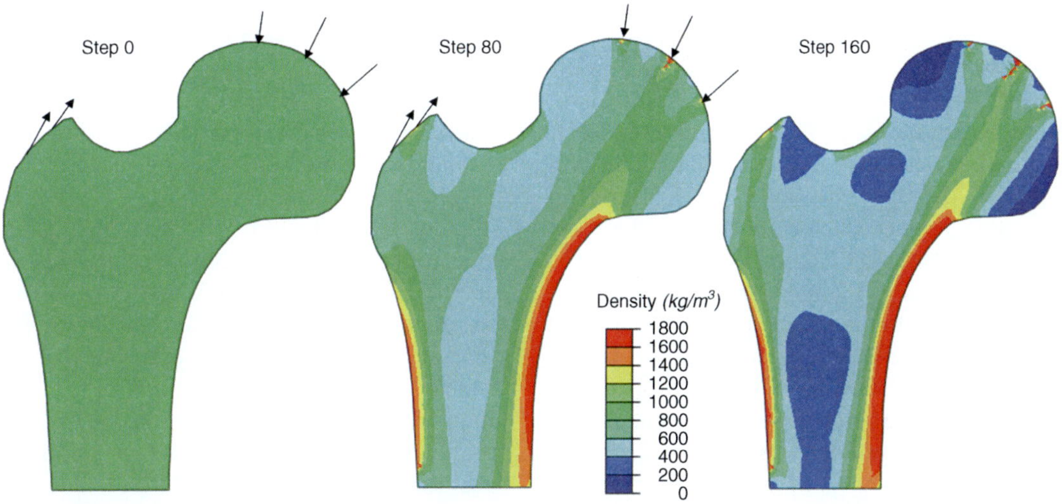

Figure 17.4. Computational simulation of the remodeling process of proximal femur head. Starting from a uniform distribution of bone density at the beginning, the bone responds to simulated physiological loading over time, producing denser bone at sites of larger mechanical stimulus (i.e., strain energy density).

present, the relation between the shear stress induced by interstitial fluid flow and bone remodeling has not been established, and the models are less well developed [22].

17.4 Mechanobiological Regulation and Simulations of Bone Fracture Healing

Following fracture, bone starts a repair process that restores its function and its original anatomical configuration. The healing type and the outcomes of the healing process are modulated by the mechanics at the fracture site. This section reviews the mechanobiological models of bone fracture healing and the computational simulations.

17.4.1 Healing Stages

Bone is formed either by intramembranous ossification or endochondral ossification. Fracture healing has been classified into direct (or primary) fracture healing and indirect (or secondary) fracture healing [17]. In intramembranous ossification, bone segments are rigidly stabilized and mesenchymal precursor cells differentiate directly into bone-forming osteoblasts. This is called direct fracture healing. On the other hand, in a biomechanically flexible environment, bone formation occurs indirectly and fracture healing involves callus formation and a combination of intramembranous and endochondral ossification. Most fractures, even if treated with surgical fixation devices, experience some degree of motion. Indirect fracture healing is the most common and direct fracture healing is rare [30].

Histologically, indirect healing consists of four stages: (1) inflammation, (2) soft callus, (3) hard callus, and (4) remodeling [10].

The inflammation stage starts when a bone fractures and the blood vessels in the bone, periosteum, and surrounding tissues are disrupted. Within approximately 48 h after the fracture incident, a hematoma forms at the fracture site.

The soft callus forms a few days after fracture; the hematoma is replaced by granulation tissue consisting of inflammatory cells, fibroblasts, collagen, osteoblasts, and osteoclasts. Osteoclasts start to remove dead bone and capillaries invade the hematoma. Fibroblasts start to produce cartilaginous tissue and collagen fibers, i.e., the soft callus that links the broken bone fragments together.

Hard callus: As healing progresses, the soft callus converts to woven bone via endochondral ossification. Membranous bone formation occurs between the fracture fragments.

In the remodeling stage, the woven bone is converted into lamellar bone and unwanted bone is removed as the stiffness of the cortex recovers. Both the medullary cavity and the bone geometry are restored during this stage.

17.4.2 Influence of Mechanics on Bone Fracture Healing

Not all fractures heal normally, with delayed union or nonunion resulting. Delayed union refers to a union that is the result of intramedullary callus formation and direct healing. Because the normal external callus has not formed and remodeling ceases before complete union occurs, delayed unions take much longer. Nonunion occurs when neither the endosteal nor the periosteal callus is formed, or both are overcome by bone resorption [57].

The bone fracture healing process is modulated or influenced by many biological and mechanical factors. Nonunion may result from adverse mechanical or biological environments at the fracture site. Poor vascularity and inadequate stability are the major factors that lead to a nonunion. Nonunions may be classified as hypertrophic or atrophic [65].

Radiologically, hypertrophic nonunion shows some callus formation with a visible fracture gap. It is commonly accepted that in hypertrophic nonunion, the fracture site has the needed blood supply and healing response, but without adequate stability. Radiograms of atrophic nonunion typically show little callus formation around a fibrous tissue-filled fracture gap that is considered to be poorly vascularized, although some investigators dispute this [74]. This situation is indicative of a poor environment for bone-forming cells and therefore is likely to lead to poor healing.

Mechanical milieus regulate not only whether a fracture will heal but also the mechanism through which bone union will take place. The main factors that determine the mechanics at the fracture site are stability of the fixation device, the fracture geometry and reduction, and loading at the bone ends. Chao and associates [3, 17], using a rigid configuration and direct contact healing with new periosteal bone formation under axially dynamized stable fixation, have shown that bone can heal by callus-free gap healing. As demonstrated by Goodship et al. [40], if the fixation is too flexible, it can cause excessive inter-fragmentary movement, which may induce a hypertrophic nonunion, whereas more rigid fixation may hinder bone formation and result in atrophic nonunion. Claes et al. [19] investigated the influences of inter-fragmentary movement and gap size on fracture healing and found that a large gap between the bone ends generally leads to nonunions.

17.4.3 Mechanobiological Models of Bone Fracture Healing

The goal of fracture treatment is for the injured limb to regain function quickly, reliably, and safely. Surgical fracture fixation achieves this goal by providing sufficient stability and strength to allow immediate joint mobilization. Understanding the mechanobiology of bone healing is essential for the optimal selection of surgical fracture fixation devices.

For over half a century, researchers have attempted to define rules for the mechanical regulation of tissue changes in fracture healing. Most of these specify ranges of local stress and strain within the fracture callus that control the formation of soft fibrous tissue, cartilage, and bone. In most mechanobiological models, the mechanical stimuli are characterized by the stress and strain invariants. Two stress invariants (distortional stress, $\bar{\sigma}_s$, and hydrostatic stress, $\bar{\sigma}_h$) are defined in (17.1). The corresponding strain invariants are distortional strain and volumetric strain, which are defined by the principal strains.

Pauwels [66] proposed that hydrostatic compression stimulates cartilage formation and that the distortional stress, which induces cell and extracellular matrix elongation, stimulates the development of collagen fibers. Pauwels, however, did not identify the mechanical stimulus for bony tissue formation.

A tissue that ruptures at a certain strain level cannot be formed under strains that exceed that level. Perren and Cordey [67] therefore proposed that tissue differentiation was controlled by the tolerance of various tissues to the inter-fragmentary strain, defined as the inter-fragmentary movement divided by the fracture gap. Because tissues differ in their tolerance to rupture, healing is thought to take place progressively as tissue differentiates from granulation to fibrous to cartilaginous and finally to bony tissue. The limitations of this theory include modeling the fracture as a one-dimensional entity and ignoring the three-dimensional complexity of the callus.

Carter and associates [13, 14] based their mechano-regulation model on the hypothesis that fibro-cartilage forms in regions of tensile strain with a compressive hydrostatic stress, that cartilage develops in regions of compressive hydrostatic stress and low octahedral shear strain, that fibrous tissue forms in regions of tensile strain, and that direct bone formation occurs in regions of low tensile strain and hydrostatic stress. Figure 17.5a shows a graphical conceptualization of these differentiation rules. The prerequisite of appropriate blood supply for bone formation is mentioned, but not included in the model [13].

Claes and Heigele [20] were the first to quantify mechanobiological rules and to distinguish endochondral and intramembranous ossification. In their approach, intramembranous ossification takes place in the regions where distortional strain is less than 5% and hydrostatic pressure below 0.15 MPa, whereas endochondral bone formation occurs in regions with compressive hydrostatic pressures greater than 0.15 MPa and strains smaller than 15%. All other conditions lead to connective or fibrous tissue (see Fig. 17.5b). The requirement for an adequate blood supply has been included in the further development of this model [82].

Prendergast et al. [72] proposed a biophysical scheme where tissue differentiation is regulated by distortional strain and relative fluid velocity. Fibrous tissue forms under high values of distortional strain and relative fluid velocity,

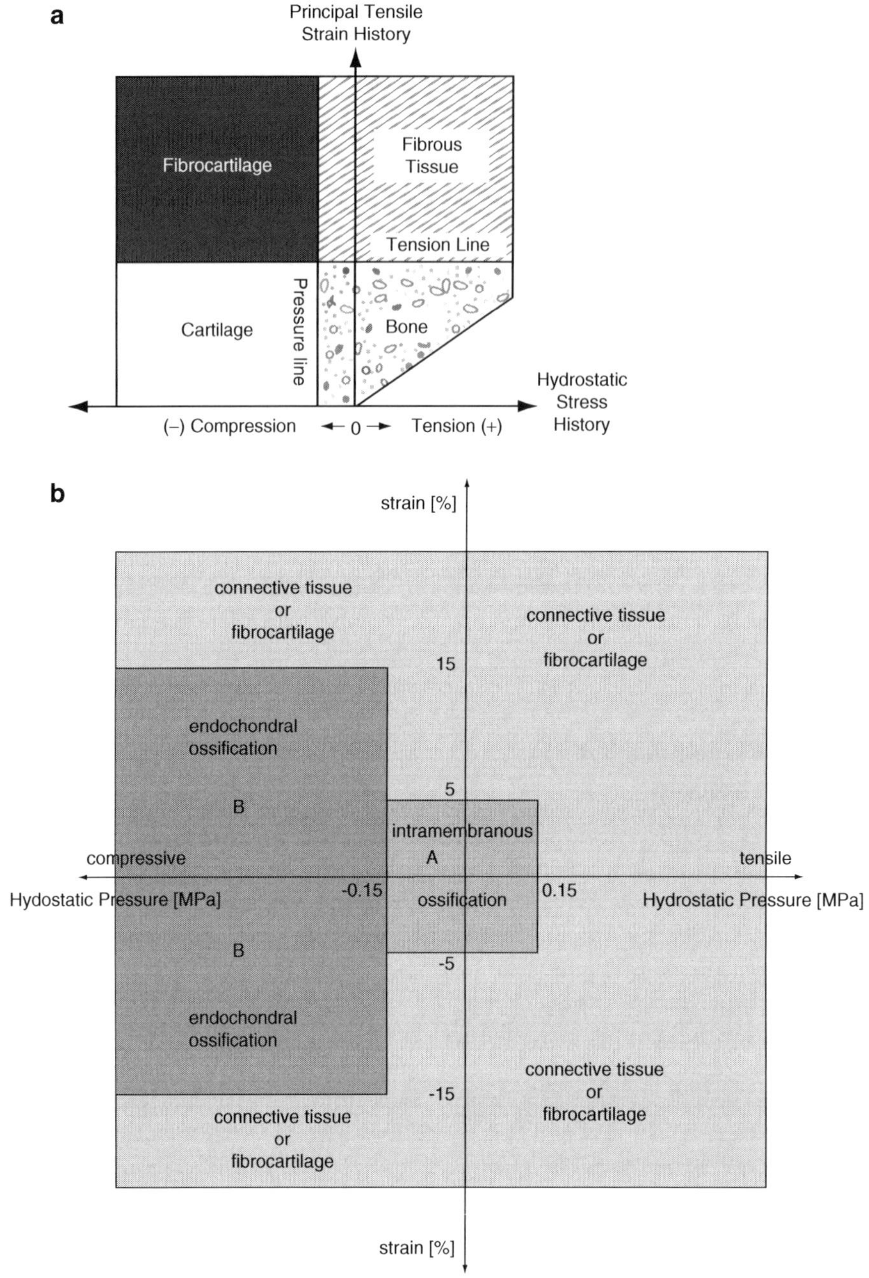

Figure 17.5. Mechanobiological models of bone healing. (**a**) Healing criteria based on principal tensile strain and hydrostatic pressure (Reprinted with permission from ref [13]). (**b**) Healing criteria based on distortional strain and hydrostatic pressure (Reprinted from Claes and Heigele [20], Copyright 1999, with permission from Elsevier).

whereas intermediate values of distortional strain and fluid velocity stimulate growth of cartilaginous tissue. Bone formation only takes place if the values of both are sufficiently low. In the later development of this model [52], cell proliferation and migration determine turnover of tissues and material components. However, the rates of change of material components are arbitrarily decided by a numerical scheme, rather than derived from experimental studies.

The sets of tissue differentiation rules reviewed above generally do not specifically address the biological aspects of the healing process. More recently, several studies have sought to establish mechano-regulation algorithms based on cellular responses [4, 37, 38, 52].

17.4.4 Computational Simulations of Bone Fracture Healing

Carter et al. appear to have been the first to have used FEM to develop a tissue differentiation algorithm and to explore its predictions for bone fracture healing [13, 14]. They examined the relationship between an "osteogenic index" in the callus and the pattern of endochondral bone formation in a two-dimensional FE model. Gardner et al. [36] developed a two-dimensional FE model for a clinical case of fracture healing, based on the direct measurement of interfragmentary movement at four temporal points during healing. Material properties of the callus were assigned for an iterative analysis.

Based on their experimental tests [19] and finite element models [20], Claes and associates developed a healing algorithm [81] using a fuzzy logic method [1]. This model has been tested in several different situations. Figure 17.6 illustrates the simulations of the healing process of one animal model reported by Claes et al. [19]

Isaksson et al. [46] compared several mechanobiological models for bone fracture healing and showed that all yield similar results. It therefore seems that mechanical stimuli can be characterized by distortional strain alone [4, 38].

At present, most available models have been tested on simple problems and with limited applications. Fracture geometries have often been oversimplified and material properties and forces were selected empirically. As yet, no model has been validated and applied to a broad range of examples. Therefore, simulating optimal conditions has remained a remarkable challenge (cf. Epari et al. [31] on fracture healing).

17.5 Summary

Mechanobiology merges mechanics with the science of molecular biology. The premise of mechanobiology is to describe the way cells sense and respond to mechanical forces. Skeletal mechanobiology is complementary to skeletal biomechanics that studies the effects of forces on biological tissues in relation to biological and medical problems. Because bone tissue can grow and adapt, the geometry and material properties of bone structure are constantly modified. To understand and predict bone remodeling and regeneration, the two disciplines have to be integrated.

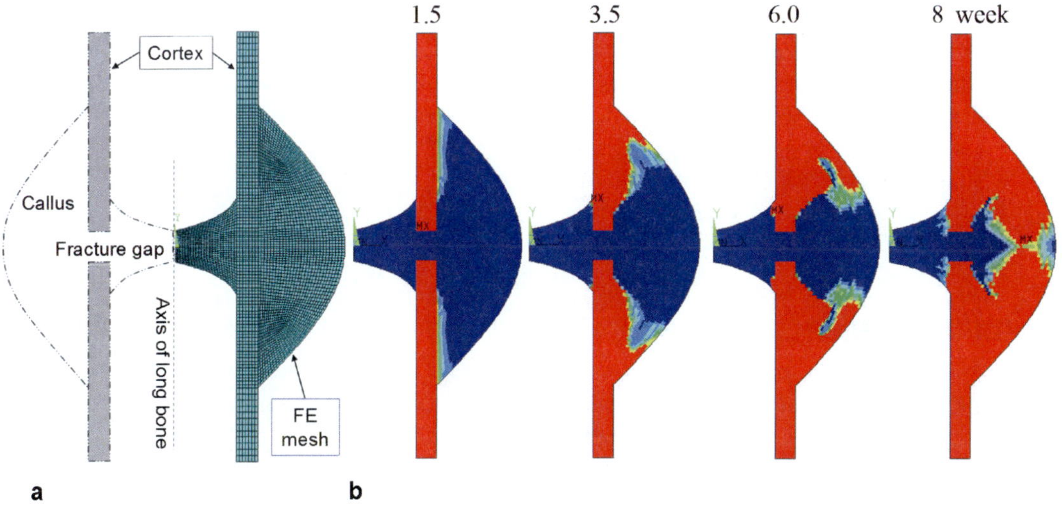

Figure 17.6. Computational simulation of the healing process of a long bone fracture. (**a**) Fracture healing FEM model. (**b**) Simulation of callus growth after operation (Courtesy of Dr. Ulrich Simon and Prof. Lutz Claes, University of Ulm).

Models to describe bone growth, remodeling, and regeneration may be classified as phenomenological or mechanistic. Phenomenological models develop the relationships between mechanical loading and adaptation and formation of bone tissue directly, without taking into account biological mechanisms. Mechanistic models include cell activities that give rise to the processes involved in bone maintenance, turnover, and regeneration. Because mechanistic models attempt to link mechanical and biological causes and effects, they are complex and as yet not well developed.

Most models of bone remodeling and healing reviewed above are phenomenological; examples are Carter's bone remodeling algorithm [13–16] and Claes' bone healing algorithm [81, 82]. Because these models avoid the complexity of biological analyses, they can offer insights into manipulation of the bone response and development of surgical implants. However, because these models were developed by comparing computational and experimental findings, the loading parameters, boundary conditions, and material properties which were empirically chosen have led to inconsistencies between the various algorithms.

Mechanistic models have the promise of linking cell activities and growth factors to mechanical causes, but present the challenge to define the relationship between cause and effect accurately. For example, it is not clear how bone fluid flow causes bone remodeling. At present, many parameters involved in mechanistic models are empirically selected. However, with the increasing publication of relevant findings, models may become available that accurately simulate the processes involved in bone healing, growth, and remodeling. If so, effective clinical interventions may become possible.

Acknowledgments

We thank these of our colleagues for their kind help: Dr. Beat Schmutz (Queensland University of Technology, Australia) for the femur images in Fig. 17.1; Prof. Lutz Claes and Dr. Ulrich Simon (University of Ulm, Germany) for permission to use Fig. 17.6; and Dr. Maria J. Gomez-Benito (University of Zaragoza, Spain) and Dr. Guoxin Ni (Fujian Medical University, China) for their comments on the manuscript.

References

1. Ament C, Hofer EP (2000) A fuzzy logic model of fracture healing. J Biomech 33(8):961–968
2. Arnett TR, Gibbons DC, Utting JC, Orriss IR, Hoebertz A, Rosendaal M, Meghji S (2003) Hypoxia is a major stimulator of osteoclast formation and bone resorption. J Cell Physiol 196(1):2–8
3. Aro HT, Chao EY (1993) Bone-healing patterns affected by loading, fracture fragment stability, fracture type, and fracture site compression. Clin Orthop Relat Res (293):8–17
4. Bailón-Plaza A, van der Meulen MCH (2003) Beneficial effects of moderate, early loading and adverse effects of delayed or excessive loading on bone healing. J Biomech 36(8):1069–1077
5. Bassett CAL, Becker RO (1962) Generation of electric potentials by bone in response to mechanical stress. Science 137(3535):1063–1064
6. Beaupre GS, Orr TE, Carter DR (1990) Approach for time-dependent bone modeling and remodeling-theoretical development. J Orthop Res 8(5):651–661
7. Beaupre GS, Orr TE, Carter DR (1990) Approach for time-dependent bone modeling and remodeling-application. A preliminary remodeling simulation. J Orthop Res 8(5):662–670
8. Black J, Hastings GW (1998) Handbook of biomaterial properties. Chapman and Hall, London
9. Braun JT, Hines JL, Akyuz E, Vallera C, Ogilvie JW (2006) Relative versus absolute modulation of growth in the fusionless treatment of experimental scoliosis. Spine 31(16):1776–1782
10. Brighton CT (1984) The biology of fracture repair. Instr Course Lect 33(2):60–82
11. Burr DB, Milgrom C, Fyhrie D, Forwood M, Nyska M, Finestone A, Hoshaw S, Saiag E, Simkin A (1996) In vivo measurement of human tibial strains during vigorous activity. Bone 18(5):405–410
12 Burr BD, Schaffler MB, Yang KH, Lukoschek M, Sivaneri N, Blaha JD, Radin EL (1989) Skeletal change in response to alterted strain environments: is woven bone a response to elevated strains? Bone 10(13): 223–233
13. Carter DR, Beaupre GS, Giori NJ, Helms JA (1998) Mechanobiology of skeletal regeneration. Clin Orthop Relat Res 355:S41–S55
14. Carter DR, Blenman PR, Beaupre GS (1988) Correlations between mechanical stress history and tissue differentiation in initial fracture healing. J Orthop Res 6(5):736–748
15. Carter DR, Hayes WC (1977) The compressive behavior of bone as a two-phase porous structure. J Bone Joint Surg Am 59(7):954–962

16. Carter DR, Wong M (1988) The role of mechanical loading histories in the development of diarthrodial joints. J Orthop Res 6(6):804–816
17. Chao EY, Aro HT, Lewallen DG, Kelly PJ (1989) The effect of rigidity on fracture healing in external fixation. Clin Orthop Relat Res 241:24–35
18. Chigira M (1996) Mechanical optimization of bone. Med Hypotheses 46(4):327–330
19. Claes L, Augat P, Suger G, Wilke H-J (1997) Influence of size and stability of the osteotomy gap on the success of fracture healing. J Orthop Res 15(4):577–584
20. Claes LE, Heigele CA (1999) Magnitudes of local stress and strain along bony surfaces predict the course and type of fracture healing. J Biomech 32(3): 255–266
21. Collet P, Uebelhart D, Vico L, Moro L, Hartmann D, Roth M, Alexandre C (1997) Effects of 1- and 6-month spaceflight on bone mass and biochemistry in two humans. Bone 20(6):547–551
22. Cowin SC (2002) Mechanosensation and fluid transport in living bone. J Musculoskelet Neuronal Interact 2(3):256–260
23. Cowin SC (2004) Tissue growth and remodeling. Annu Rev Biomed Eng 6(1):77–107
24. Cowin SC, Hart RT, Balser JR, Kohn DH (1985) Functional adaptation in long bones: establishing in vivo values for surface remodeling rate coefficients. J Biomech 18(9):665–671
25. Cowin SC, Hegedus DH, Bone remodelling I (1976) Small strain adaptive elasticity. J Elast 6(3):313–326
26. Currey JD (1988) The effect of porosity and mineral content on the Young's modulus of elasticity of compact bone. J Biomech 21(2):131–139
27. Currey JD (2002) Bones: structure and mechanics, 2nd edn. Princeton University Press, Woodstock
28. Dodd JS, Raleigh JA, Gross TS (1999) Osteocyte hypoxia: a novel mechanotransduction pathway. Am J Physiol Cell Physiol 277(3):C598–C602
29. Donahue TLH, Haut TR, Yellowley CE, Donahue HJ, Jacobs CR (2003) Mechanosensitivity of bone cells to oscillating fluid flow induced shear stress may be modulated by chemotransport. J Biomech 36(9):1363–1371
30. Einhorn TA (1998) The cell and molecular biology of fracture healing. Clin Orthop Relat Res 355(suppl): 7–21
31. Epari DR, Kassi J-P, Schell H, Duda GN (2007) Timely fracture-healing requires optimization of axial fixation stability. J Bone Joint Surg Am 89(7):1575–1585
32. Frost HM (1969) Tetracycline-based histological analysis of bone remodeling. Calcif Tissue Int 3(1): 211–237
33. Frost HM (1983) Determinant of bone architecture: the minimum effective strain. Clin Orthop Relat Res 175:286–292
34. Frost HM (1997) Biomechanical control of knee alignment: some insights from a new paradigm. Clin Orthop Relat Res 335(1):335
35. Fukada E, Yasuda I (1957) On the piezoelectric effect of bone. J Phys Soc Jpn 12(10):1158–1162
36. Gardner TN, Stoll T, Marks L, Mishra S, Knothe Tate M (2000) The influence of mechanical stimulus on the pattern of tissue differentiation in a long bone fracture – an FEM study. J Biomech 33(4):415–425
37. Geris L, Gerisch A, Sloten JV, Weiner R, Oosterwyck HV (2008) Angiogenesis in bone fracture healing: a bioregulatory model. J Theor Biol 251(1): 137–158
38. Gomez-Benito MJ, Garcia-Aznar JM, Kuiper JH, Doblare M (2005) Influence of fracture gap size on the pattern of long bone healing: a computational study. J Theor Biol 235(1):105–119
39. Gooding CA, Neuhauser EB (1965) Growth and development of the vertebral body in the presence and absence of normal stress. Am J Roentgenol Radium Ther Nucl Med 93:388–394
40. Goodship AE, Watkins PE, Rigby HS, Kenwright J (1993) The role of fixator frame stiffness in the control of fracture healing. An experimental study. J Biomech 26(9):1027–1035
41. Gross TS, King KA, Rabaia NA, Pathare P, Srinivasan S (2005) Upregulation of osteopontin by osteocytes deprived of mechanical loading or oxygen. J Bone Miner Res 20(2):250–256
42. Hall BK, Herring SW (1990) Paralysis and growth of the musculoskeletal system in the embryonic chick. J Morphol 206(1):45–56
43. Hazelwood SJ, Martin RB, Rashid MM, Rodrigo JJ (2001) A mechanistic model for internal bone remodeling exhibits different dynamic responses in disuse and overload. J Biomech 34(3):299–308
44. Huiskes R, Weinans H, Grootenboer HJ, Dalstra M, Fudala B, Slooff TJ (1987) Adaptive bone-remodeling theory applied to prosthetic-design analysis. J Biomech 20(11–12):1135–1150
45. Hung CT, Allen FD, Pollack SR, Brighton CT (1996) What is the role of the convective current density in the real-time calcium response of cultured bone cells to fluid flow? J Biomech 29(11):1403–1409
46. Isaksson H, Wilson W, van Donkelaar CC, Huiskes R, Ito K (2006) Comparison of biophysical stimuli for mechano-regulation of tissue differentiation during fracture healing. J Biomech 39(8):1507–1516
47. Jacobs CR, Levenston ME, Beaupre GS, Simo JC, Carter DR (1995) Numerical instabilities in bone remodeling simulations: the advantages of a node-based finite element approach. J Biomech 28(4):449–459
48. Jacobs CR, Yellowley CE, Davis BR, Zhou Z, Cimbala JM, Donahue HJ (1998) Differential effect of steady versus oscillating flow on bone cells. J Biomech 31(11):969–976
49. Knothe Tate ML, Niederer P, Knothe U (1998) In vivo tracer transport through the lacunocanalicular system of rat bone in an environment devoid of mechanical loading. Bone 22(2):107–117
50. Knothe Tate ML, Steck R, Forwood MR, Niederer P (2000) In vivo demonstration of load-induced fluid flow in the rat tibia and its potential implications for processes associated with functional adaptation. J Exp Biol 203(18):2737–2745
51. Koller MR, Bender JG, Miller WM, Papoutsakis ET (1992) Reduced oxygen tension increases hematopoiesis in long-term culture of human stem and progenitor

cells from cord blood and bone marrow. Exp Hematol 20(2):264–270
52. Lacroix D, Prendergast PJ (2002) A mechano-regulation model for tissue differentiation during fracture healing: analysis of gap size and loading. J Biomech 35(9):1163–1171
53. Lanyon LE (1974) Experimental support for the trajectorial theory of bone structure. J Bone Joint Surg Br 56-B(1):160–166
54. Lanyon LE (1993) Osteocytes, strain detection, bone modeling and remodeling. Calcif Tissue Int 53(suppl 1): S102–S107
55. Leblanc AD, Schneider VS, Evans HJ, Engelbretson DA, Krebs JM (1990) Bone mineral loss and recovery after 17 weeks of bed rest. J Bone Miner Res 5(8):843–850
56. Lerner AL, Kuhn JL, Hollister SJ (1998) Are regional variations in bone growth related to mechanical stress and strain parameters? J Biomech 31(4):327–335
57. Marsh D (1998) Concepts of fracture union, delayed union, and nonunion. Clin Orthop Relat Res 355(suppl): S22–S30
58. Mattheck C (1998) Design in nature: learning from trees. Springer, Berlin
59. McCall IW, Galvin E, O'Brien JP, Park WM (1981) Alterations in vertebral growth following prolonged plaster immobilisation. Acta Orthop 52(3):327–330
60. Mente PL, Aronsson DD, Stokes IAF, Iatridis JC (1999) Mechanical modulation of growth for the correction of vertebral wedge deformities. J Orthop Res 17(4): 518–524
61. Morey ER, Baylink DJ (1978) Inhibition of bone formation during space flight. Science 201(4361):1138–1141
62. Murray D, Rushton N (1990) The effect of strain on bone cell prostaglandin E2 release: a new experimental method. Calcif Tissue Int 47(1):35–39
63. Muzylak M, Price J, Horton M (2006) Hypoxia induces giant osteoclast formation and extensive bone resorption in the cat. Calcif Tissue Int 79(5):301–309
64. Nyman JS, Yeh OC, Hazelwood SJ, Martin RB (2004) A theoretical analysis of long-term bisphosphonate effects on trabecular bone volume and microdamage. Bone 35(1):296–305
65. Panagiotis M (2005) Classification of non-union. Injury 36(4 suppl 1):S30–S37
66. Pauwels F (1980) A new theory concerning the influence of mechanical stimuli on the differentiation of the supporting tissues. In: Pauwels F (ed) Biomechanics of the locomotor apparatus: contributions on the functional anatomy of the locomotor apparatus. Springer, Berlin, pp 375–405
67. Perren SM, Cordey J (1980) The concept of interfragmentary strain. In: Uhthoff HK, Stahl E (eds) Current concepts of internal fixation of fractures. Springer, Berlin, pp 63–77
68. Petit MA, Beck TJ, Kontulainen SA (2005) Examining the developing bone: what do we measure and how do we do it? J Musculoskelet Neuronal Interact 5(3):213–224
69. Piekarski K, Munro M (1977) Transport mechanism operating between blood supply and osteocytes in long bones. Nature 269(5623):80–82
70. Pienkowski D, Pollack SR (1983) The origin of stress-generated potentials in fluid-saturated bone. J Orthop Res 1(1):30–41
71. Pollack SR (2001) Streaming potentials in bone. In: Cowin SC (ed) Bone mechanics handbook. CRC, Boca Raton 24.21–24.22.
72. Prendergast PJ, Huiskes R, Soballe K (1997) Biophysical stimuli on cells during tissue differentiation at implant interfaces. J Biomech 30(6):539–548
73. Purves WK, Sadava D, Orians GH, Heller HC (2004) Life: the science of biology, 7th edn. Sinauer Associates, Sunderland
74. Reed AAC, Joyner CJ, Brownlow HC, Simpson AHRW (2002) Human atrophic fracture non-unions are not avascular. J Orthop Res 20(3):593–599
75. Reich KM, Gay CV, Frangos JA (1990) Fluid shear stress as a mediator of osteoblast cyclic adenosine monophosphate production. J Cell Physiol 143(1):100–104
76. Ribble TG, Santare MH, Miller F (2001) Stresses in the growth plate of the developing proximal femur J Appl Biomech 17(2):129–141
77. Rice JC, Cowin SC, Bowman JA (1988) On the dependence of the elasticity and strength of cancellous bone on apparent density. J Biomech 21(2):155–168
78. Rubin CT, Lanyon LE (1984) Regulation of bone formation by applied dynamic loads. J Bone Joint Surg Am 66(3):397–402
79. Rubin C, Turner AS, Bain S, Mallinckrodt C, McLeod K (2001) Low mechanical signals strengthen long bones. Nature 412(6847):603–604
80. Schaffler MB, Burr DB (1988) Stiffness of compact bone: effects of porosity and density. J Biomech 21(1): 13–16
81. Shefelbine SJ, Augat P, Claes L, Simon U (2005) Trabecular bone fracture healing simulation with finite element analysis and fuzzy logic. J Biomech 38(12):2440–2450
82. Simon U, Augat P, Utz M, Claes L (2003) Simulation of tissue development and vascularisation in the callus healing process. Trans Orthop Res Soc 28:O299
83. Skedros JG, Hunt KJ, Bloebaum RD (2004) Relationships of loading history and structural and material characteristics of bone: development of the mule deer calcaneus. J Morphol 259(3):281–307
84. Smit TH, Huyghe JM, Cowin SC (2002) Estimation of the poroelastic parameters of cortical bone. J Biomech 35(6):829–835
85. Steck R, Niederer P, Knothe Tate ML (2003) A finite element analysis for the prediction of load-induced fluid flow and mechanochemical transduction in bone. J Theor Biol 220(2):249–259
86. Stevens SS, Beaupré GS, Carter DR (1999) Computer model of endochondral growth and ossification in long bones: biological and mechanobiological influences. J Orthop Res 17(5):646–653
87. Stokes IAF (2002) Mechanical effects on skeletal growth. J Musculoskelet Neuronal Interact 2(3):277–280
88. Stokes IAF, Spence H, Aronsson DD, Kilmer N (1996) Mechanical modulation of vertebral body growth: implications for scoliosis progression. Spine 21(10): 1162–1167

89. Tanck E, Homminga J, van Lenthe GH, Huiskes R (2001) Increase in bone volume fraction precedes architectural adaptation in growing bone. Bone 28(6): 650–654
90. Taylor JR (1975) Growth of human intervertebral discs and vertebral bodies. J Anat 120(1):49–68
91. Tuncay OC, Ho D, Barker MK (1994) Oxygen tension regulates osteoblast function. Am J Orthod Dentofacial Orthop 105(5):457–463
92. Turner CH (1998) Three rules for bone adaptation to mechanical stimuli. Bone 23(5):399–407
93. Uhthoff HK, Jaworski ZF (1978) Bone loss in response to long-term immobilisation. J Bone Joint Surg Br 60-B(3):420–429
94. van der Meulen MCH, Beaupré GS, Carter DR (1993) Mechanobiologic influences in long bone cross-sectional growth. Bone 14(4):635–642
95. van der Meulen MCH, Globus RK (2005) Progress in understanding disuse osteopenia. Curr Opin Orthop 16(5):325–330
96. Wang L, Fritton SP, Weinbaum S, Cowin SC (2003) On bone adaptation due to venous stasis. J Biomech 36(10): 1439–1451
97. Weinans H, Huiskes R, Grootenboer HJ (1992) The behavior of adaptive bone-remodeling simulation models. J Biomech 25(12):1425–1441
98. Wolff J (1892) The law of bone remodelling, translation of: Das Gesetz der Transformation der Knochen. Springer, New York
99. Wong M, Carter DR (1988) Mechanical stress and morphogenetic endochondral ossification of the sternum. J Bone Joint Surg Am 70(7):992–1000
100. Wong M, Carter DR (1990) A theoretical model of endochondral ossification and bone architectural construction in long bone ontogeny. Anat Embryol 181(6):523–532
101. Xie YM, Steven GP (1997) Evolutionary structural optimization. Springer, London
102. You L, Cowin SC, Schaffler MB, Weinbaum S (2001) A model for strain amplification in the actin cytoskeleton of osteocytes due to fluid drag on pericellular matrix. J Biomech 34(11):1375–1386

Subject Index